S0-AXK-033

ENDOCRINOLOGY

S. A. Binkley

Temple University

HarperCollins*CollegePublishers*

Editor in Chief: Glyn Davies
Acquisitions Editor: Susan McLaughlin
Development Editor: Marla Johnson
Acquisitions Editor: Susan McLaughlin
Design Manager: Teresa J. Delgado
Cover Designer: Kay Petronio

Endocrinology

Copyright ©1995 by HarperCollins College Publishers

All rights reserved. Printed in the United States of America. No part of this book may be used or reproduced in any manner whatsoever without written permission, except in the case of brief quotations embodied in critical articles and reviews. For information address HarperCollins College Publishers, 10 East 53rd Street, New York, NY 10022

Library of Congress Cataloging-in-Publication Data

Binkley, Sue Ann, 1944-
    Endocrinology / S.A. Binkley
    p. cm.
    Includes bibliographical references and index.
    ISBN 0-06-500018-8
    1. Endocrinology. I. Title.
    [DNLM: 1. Endocrinology. WK 100 B313e]
QB187.B573 1993
616.4--dc20
DNLM/DLC
for Library of Congress
                                                                    92-49643
                                                                      CIP

94 95 96 97 9 8 7 6 5 4 3 2 1

Dedicated to

H. Randolph Tatem, III., M.D.

Shelley Binkley, M.D.

Rich Zelter

Basalt and Carbondale emergency crews

Pitkin County Sheriff's Department

Aspen Valley Hospital

Contents in Brief

Contents in Detail

Preface

The purpose of this book is to provide a broad classical introduction to the subject of endocrinology. **Endocrinology** is the study of glands and hormones, and this book focuses on those in vertebrate organisms. Hormones are natural chemicals produced by biological organisms which are used as **chemical messengers** to convey information from one place in the body to another.

There are two major ways by which higher organisms control, integrate, and organize the functions of their bodies. The first is by the nervous system which provides quick transmission of signals from one place to another along nerve processes. The second is by the endocrine system which is organized for less rapid transmission of messages. The means by which the hormones are regulated and the mechanisms by which they act offer amplification—a small signal is converted to a large effect.

But, the subject of endocrinology is not just historical. Endocrinology is a live and active field of research. Ideas are constantly being refined and refuted and replaced by new directions. The words "may" and "possibly" could be added to almost every sentence in this book because every aspect of the subject is open to question and reexamination. Everything has not yet been discovered nor has every issue been resolved. Technological advances open new doors of inquiry and application. There is still room in the house of endocrinology for new generations of endocrinologists.

In writing a new book on an established subject, one hopes to contribute something special. In this regard, I have made a particular effort to include the daily cycles of the hormones and other rhythmic aspects of endocrinology which have, especially in the past two decades, brought a fresh perspective to our understanding of hormone function.

USING THE BOOK

The book is divided into sections based on anatomy and embryology. The sections are subdivided into chapters on the basis of glands and their hormones.

The book begins with introductory material. Next, the reader will find discussion of the amine and peptide hormone which are made first, by neuroendocrine glands located in the head (hypothalamus, pituitary, pineal), and second, by glands that are in or near the gastrointestinal tract (thyroid, thymus, parathyroid, pancreas, and gut). Following the peptide and amine hormones are the pituitary governed glands that secrete steroids (adrenal, ovary, testis). Other endocrine subjects that remain are briefly discussed in conclusion.

History, anatomy, histology, embryology, hormone chemical structures, hormone biosynthesis, hormone metabolism, functions, comparative endocrinology, rhythms, regulation, and principal diseases are general subtopics of the chapters.

Signposts and aids to help the student in finding his or her way through the maze of the subject of endocrinology have been provided: chapter and section openers, headings, key words in bold type, figures (anatomical sketches, biochemical pathways, and regulation schemes), tables of data, end-of-chapter references, glossary of terms and abbreviations, annotated bibliography, and index.

Some hormones are principal "characters" in more than one chapter which is indicated by cross referencing on chapter-opening pages. An overview of the subject can be obtained by looking first at the section and chapter-opening pages.

The field of endocrinology has been subdivided into a diversity of subspecialities. One introductory volume cannot pretend to adequately serve all these areas at the same time. In this book, an attempt has been made to include information from each of the subspecialities to provide a broad background for a student. Neuroendocrinology is the subject of Section II, molecular endocrinology is most discussed in Chapter 2, comparative endocrinology includes especially the melanotropins, Chapter 7, and the pineal, Chapter 8, and clinical endocrinology is represented in chapter subsections on the diseases.

ACKNOWLEDGMENTS

I am grateful to my teachers—Jack W. Hudson, Roy V. Talmage, Michael Menaker, and David C. Klein. Over the years, I learned from the authors of the textbooks that I used in teaching my endocrinology courses and I enjoyed their works—J. T. Bagnara, William Ganong, Mac E. Hadley, Earl Frieden, Francis S. Greenspan, Harry Lipner, and C. Donnell Turner. The imaginative

General Overall Organization of *Endocrinology*

Section	Location of glands	Embryological origin	Main types of hormones	Main functions
I Introduction				
II Hypothalamus Pituitary Pineal	head	ectoderm	amine and peptides	regulation, water balance, growth, and skin color
III Thyroid Thymus Parathyroid Pancreas Gastrointestinal Tract	neck and abdomen	ectoderm, endoderm	amines and peptides	metabolism, minerals, and digestion
IV Adrenals Gonads	abdomen and scrotum	ectoderm mesoderm	amines steroids	sugar, salt and water balance, stress, and reproduction
V Other topics				

questions of my students—biology graduate and undergraduate students, the "medicians" (pre-health professional students), and exercise physiology students—provided a sustaining spark for this project. In particular I appreciate the support of Bruce Umminger and Elvira Doman of the National Science Foundation.

For their help during the preparation of this book, I thank Mildred Brammer (Ithaca College), Charles Bridgman (National Library of Medicine), Mary Anne Brock (Gerontology Research Center of the National Institute of Aging), P. Michael Conn (past editor of *Endocrinology*), Melissa Dolchin (Temple University), August Epple (Thomas Jefferson University), Emily Feinberg (Temple University), Gregory Florant (Temple University), Bruce Goldman (University of Connecticut), Michael Franklin, Nicholas Fry (Temple University), Robert Hilfer (Temple University), Colin Hill (Temple University), Ed and Ann Lingenfelter, John J. Lepri (University of North Carolina), Jennie Loi (Temple University), Al Meier (Louisiana State University), Vincent Menna, Sandra D. Michael (State University of New York), Chris Mills (Computer Forum), Ann Monkiewitz (Computer Forum), Karen Mosher, John Natalini (Quincy College), Louise Odor (University of South Carolina), Mary Jane Potter (Temple University), Shepherd Roberts (Temple University), Colin Scanes (Rutgers), Michael K. Skinner, Stephan Steinlechner (Philipps Universitat Marburg), Steve Takats (Temple University), Roy V. Talmage (University of North Carolina Medical School), Gloria S. Tannenbaum (McGill, Montreal Children's Hospital), Laurie Tompkins (Temple University), Lillian Wainwright (Mount St. Vincent College), Stan Wainwright (Dalhousie University), Donna Wechmann (Temple University), Richard Weisenberg (Temple University), Marcia Welsh (University of South Carolina), Beatrix H. White (Maryland Psychiatric Research Center), Farah Vikoran, Jerry Vriend (University of Manitoba), Larry Yager (Temple

University), and Stover Wiggins.

I thank libraries and librarians for their special help: Christine Balonis (Doylestown Hospital Library), Deborah Beaumont (Temple University), Laura Lane (Temple University), Catherine Mayer (Temple University), and Rena Radovich (Doylestown Hospital Library).

Reviewers were William A. deGraw (University of Nebraska, Omaha), Richard Fehn (California State University, San Bernardino), James P. Holland (Indiana University), Harry W. Jarrett, III (University of Tennessee, Memphis), James Lott (University of North Texas), K. Jean Lucas, M.D., L. Scott Quackenbush (Florida International University), Lavern R. Whisenton (Millersville University of Pennsylvania). Their useful suggestions are greatly appreciated.

I also thank my editors and staff at HarperCollins*CollegePublishers*—Kevin Bradley, Donna Campion, Vicki Cohen, Glyn Davies, Teresa J. Delgado, Juliana Nocker, Amy Spinthourakis, Suzanne Van Cleve. I am grateful to Sandy Schnetzka, Susan Bogle, and Angela Gladfelter at York Production Services. Finally, I am especially grateful for the work of my Acquisitions Editor, Susan McLaughlin; Developmental Editor, Marla Johnson; and my Copy Editor, Maureen Iannuzzi.

Further suggestions are welcome.

S. A. BINKLEY
Biology Department
Temple University
Philadelphia, PA 19122

ABOUT THE COVER

Dr. Frank Lynn Meshberger looked at a photograph of Michelangelo's 1508–1512 fresco which is painted on the ceiling of the Sistine Chapel. He compared the fresco details to Netter's illustrations of the nervous system and concluded that the image that surrounded God and the angels remarkably resembled the shape of the human brain. He saw the billowing red drapery as the cranium and the brain itself was shaped by God and the angels. A dangling angel's leg was in the location of the pituitary gland. Meshberger writes:

[In the neuroanatomical diagram] the pituitary gland is seen lying in the pituitary fossa; the fact that the pituitary is bilobed can be seen grossly....[In the fresco] the pituitary stalk and gland are depicted by the leg and foot of the angel that extends below the base of the picture. Note that the feet of both God and Adam have five toes; however, the angel's leg that represents the pituitary stalk and gland has a bifid foot.

Dr. Meshberger's article, "An interpretation of Michelangelo's *Creation of Adam*," was published in the *Journal of the American Medical Association* (volume 264, pages 1837–1841, 1990). In the article, he shows side-by-side comparisons of the fresco with cartoons of the neuroanatomy and identifies the cranium, brain, pituitary gland, sulci and gyri, pons, optic chiasm, vertebral artery, and spinal cord. Would Michelangelo have done such a thing? Man is supposed to be created in God's image—or is it a bit of heretical wit that Michelangelo may have painted God in the image of the human brain? Would Michelangelo have used the anatomy of the human brain as a symbol? Would it have taken almost five hundred years for someone to notice? Is Eve's knee in the location of the pineal gland? Michelangelo did have the carnal knowledge to paint the anatomy which he had obtained by dissections. He had "flay[ed] dead bodies in order to discover the secrets of anatomy" and he believed that God bestowed intellect on mankind. The photograph is reproduced with permission from *The Sistine Chapel*, Alfred A. Knopf, Inc., ©1991 by Nippon Television Network Corp.

ABOUT THE AUTHOR

S. A. Binkley, Ph.D., was born in Ohio, attended Goodrich High School in Fond du Lac, Wisconsin, and graduated from Broomfield High School in Colorado in 1962. Dr. Binkley graduated Summa cum Laude and Phi Beta Kappa from the University of Colorado in Boulder in 1966 and did graduate work with Jack Hudson and Roy Talmage in the physiology of pack rats and the endocrinology of calcium metabolism at Rice University in Houston. Dr. Binkley's doctorate in 1971 included work on the endocrine function of the pineal gland in the circadian rhythms of house sparrows with Michael Menaker at the University of Texas in Austin in 1971. During a postdoctoral fellowship with David C. Klein at the National Institutes of Health in Washington, D.C., in 1972, the author studied the endocrinology of pineal enzyme rhythms in rats. In 1973 the author began teaching endocrinology to undergraduate pre-health professional students and biology undergraduate and graduate students at Temple University in Philadelphia. At Temple, Dr. Binkley continued to pursue research interests in the endocrine aspects of circadian rhythms (e.g. the perching activity of house sparrows) and the pineal gland (e.g. the regulation of chicken pineal enzymes by light and dark). The work was supported by grants from the National Science Foundation, the National Institutes of Health, and Temple University. Professor Binkley is the author of other books about endocrinology and circadian rhythms: *The Pineal: Endocrine and Nonendocrine Function* ©1988 and *The Clockwork Sparrow* ©1990 (Prentice Hall, Englewood Cliffs, New Jersey).

SECTION I

INTRODUCTION

Endocrinology is a subject of "communication." The body uses the endocrine system of glands to send hormone messages. The effects of the endocrine system are visible and dramatic—hormones regulate body size and color and differences between males and females. This section describes the general ways in which a gland responds to a signal by secreting its particular hormone. The hormone is carried by the blood to a target organ where the hormone then interacts with receptors and exerts its action. The sequences of endocrine events achieve amplification so that a miniscule amount of hormone can have an enormous consequence.

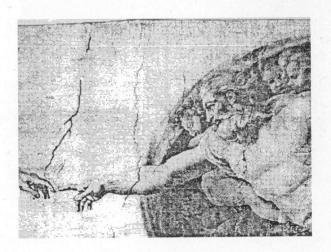

CHAPTER 1

General Concepts and Methods

The first chapter introduces general terminology and key concepts, such as secretion, receptors, and targets which will be referred to throughout the book. It describes the hormones and other chemical messengers that are the subject of endocrinology, the chemistry of these hormones, the anatomy of the endocrine system, and the methods used in endocrinology. It covers the ways in which physiology affects the regulation of the endocrine system and offers an early history of the field.

ENDOCRINOLOGY AND HORMONES

Evolution has produced two fine systems that work together to perform the communicating function in multicellular organisms. The first system is the nervous system. The second system, and the one that is the topic of this book, is the endocrine system, and it is thought of as acting more slowly. The term, **endocrinology**, is defined by Webster's as "the science or study of the endocrine glands and the internal secretions of the body."[1] The word "endocrine" is derived from the Greek (*endo-*, within; *krinein*, to separate). Biologists think of the nervous system as a wiring system in which signals flash from cell to cell with great speed. Appreciation of the interaction of the nervous and endocrine systems has led to a view of the two systems as functioning together to use chemical messengers as signals.

These pedantics aren't much help to the student. The student must still discover what are the endocrine glands and what may be meant by internal secretions. Strict endocrinologists reserve the designation "endocrine glands" for the ductless glands that secrete their products into the bloodstream. Traditionally the classical endocrine glands are the pituitary, the thyroid, the parathyroids, the adrenals, the gonads, and the pancreas. These organs are discrete "glands" with clear boundaries which are readily visible to the naked eye in the internal anatomy of most vertebrates (the vertebrates are the mammals, birds, reptiles, amphibians, and fish). Some cells of other tissues (thymus, pineal, hypothalamus) secrete chemical messengers so that they may be considered to be endocrine. Also, there are cells whose chemical messengers travel in fluids other than blood (e.g., cerebrospinal fluid).

CHEMICAL MESSENGERS

Classical hormones come from the classical endocrine glands. Blakiston's Medical Dictionary defines a **hormone** as "a specific chemical product of an organ or of certain cells of an organ, transported by the blood or other body fluids, and having a specific regulatory effect upon cells remote from its origin."[2] (Figure 1.1). The hormones are all molecules. The word "hormone" comes from a Greek word, *hormaein*, meaning to excite or to arouse.

Scientists may regard hormones more globally by their function as chemical messengers. A **chemical messenger** is a molecule that carries information, that is a signal from one location in the organism's body to another location in the body. Usually chemical messengers are viewed as traveling through fluids. Sometimes chemical messengers that are not classical hormones are called "hormones," but this practice is frowned on by classically oriented endocrinologists.

Ganong[3] divides communication by chemical messengers into four subtypes: (i) endocrine communication using the circulating body fluids, (ii) neural communication via synapses, (iii) paracrine communication when the messengers do not enter the blood stream but act on other cells, and (iv) autocrine communication when the messengers act on the cells from which they were secreted. It is possible for a chemical compound to have autocrine, paracrine, and endocrine effects. For example, testosterone's concentration in cells of the testis affects the rate of testosterone synthesis (autocrine effect), diffusion to other testis cells affects spermatogenesis (paracrine effect), and testosterone circulating through the body affects physiology and behavior (endocrine effect).

KINDS OF CHEMICAL MESSENGERS

All hormones are chemical messengers. However, some scientists might not view all chemical messengers as hormones. The classical hormones which are secreted into the bloodstream by the ductless glands form a subset of chemical messengers. Some names of specific hormones are thyroid hormone, estrogen, and prolactin.

The nervous system also uses chemicals for communication, that is, molecules, in its function. A neuron (nerve cell) communicates with another neuron by secreting a chemical across a synapse, or cleft. A synapse is a space between two neurons. The chemicals that are liberated at nerve endings that cross the synapses are called **neurotransmitters** or neurohumors. They travel from one cell to the next without using the bloodstream. Communication of two cells across a synaptic cleft is only one of the ways that nerve cells work. Examples of some neurotransmitters are acetylcholine and norepinephrine.

Additionally, chemicals, such as ions and small molecules, can pass between adjacent cells

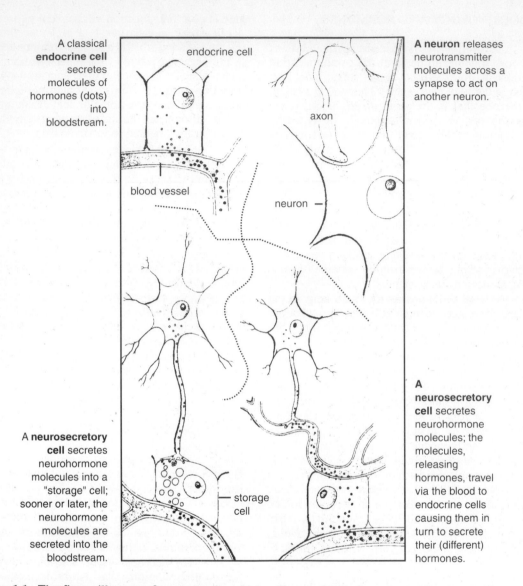

A classical **endocrine cell** secretes molecules of hormones (dots) into bloodstream.

endocrine cell

A neuron releases neurotransmitter molecules across a synapse to act on another neuron.

axon

blood vessel

neuron —

A **neurosecretory cell** secretes neurohormone molecules into a "storage" cell; sooner or later, the neurohormone molecules are secreted into the bloodstream.

storage cell

A neurosecretory cell secretes neurohormone molecules; the molecules, releasing hormones, travel via the blood to endocrine cells causing them in turn to secrete their (different) hormones.

Figure 1.1 The figure illustrates four means by which cells use chemical messengers to communicate. The classical endocrine cell, a neuron, and two arrangements for neurosecretion are shown. With permission, after Guillemin, R.; Burgus, R. The hormones of the hypothalamus. Scientific American 227: 24-33; 1972; p. 30.

where cell membranes contact with **gap junctions**.[4] Neural signals are also transmitted directly from cell to cell, without chemical messengers, by gap junctions.[5] This passage is not considered to be endocrine.

Some molecules are secreted by specialized nerve cells into the bloodstream. The nerve cells that do this are called **neurosecretory cells**. The hormones that are secreted into the blood from neurosecretory cells are called **neurohormones**.

All cells make molecules (e.g., carbon dioxide, urea, histamine, wound hormones, and embryonic inductive substances), and some of these molecules end up in the blood stream. Since the molecules may influence other cells, they can be considered to be chemical messengers. A term has been coined to denote these molecules which are made by all or most cells, **parahormones.** The term "parahormones" has also been used by some endocrinologists to denote the products of glands or chemical messengers that are not established as endocrine glands.

Plants have chemical messengers too. Since they don't have a circulating bloodstream, the plant messenger molecules cannot meet the classic definition of hormones. The word **phytohormones,** or the phrase "plant hormones," has been used to denote chemical messengers in plants. Some examples of phytohormones are auxins and gibberellins.

A particularly interesting group of chemical messengers differs from all the previously described chemical messengers that carry information within an organism—they are chemical messengers between organisms. The molecules in this group are called **pheromones.** These messengers are transmitted through the external environment. They control interactions between individuals. They are species specific. Pheromones include the sex attractants of insects and the chemical signs found in mouse urine.

NEUROENDOCRINOLOGY

The word "neuroendocrinology" has been used to refer to the endocrinology of those glands in which neurosecretion plays a large role or in which the hormones are also putative neurotransmitters. So neuroendocrinology usually includes the endocrinology of the brain, pituitary gland, adrenal medulla, and pineal gland.

The relationships between a hormone, a neurotransmitter, and a neurohormone can be confusing. To reiterate, the classic hormones are secreted by endocrine cells into the bloodstream. Neurotransmitters cross a synapse between two cells. Neurohormones are secreted into the blood by neurosecretory cells (neurons, nerve cells). A region where neurohormones are released and/or stored is called a **neurohemal organ.** In vertebrates, the median eminence of the hypothalamus and the posterior pituitary gland are the only neurohemal organs. There are other neurohemal organs in nonmammalian species: the caudal urophysis of fish, the sinus gland of crustaceans, and the corpus allatum and corpus cardiacum of insects.

ANATOMY

The endocrine glands are readily located, visible organs in the head, torso, and scrotum. The pineal gland lies in the anatomical center of the brain in humans. Descartes thought that this premier location meant the pineal gland was the location of the soul. In birds, some mammals, and lower vertebrates, however, the pineal is located more toward the top of the brain and may even lie just beneath the skull. The pituitary gland is below the brain in all vertebrate species. The thyroid gland is found in the necks of humans and the parathyroids are on the thyroid; but in other species the thyroid is in the chest and the parathyroids are separate. In humans, the thymus is found in the upper chest, and it is large early in development. The pancreas nests among, or overlays, the loops of the intestines. The adrenal glands are located close to the kidneys. Ovaries and testes are collectively called the gonads; the ovaries are in the abdomen; the testes may be either in the abdomen or in the scrotum.

The variations and similarities of a gland and its hormones among species constitute the gland's comparative anatomy. The nerve supply to or from the gland is called the **innervation.** The arteries and veins and capillary beds make up the **vascularization** of the gland.

CELLS AND ORGANELLES

The cells of the endocrine glands have organelles which are used in the synthesis and the secretion of hormones (Figure 1.2). The **nucleus** of each cell contains chromosomes made up of molecules of nucleic acid (DNA), which are used as the blueprint to make hormones and enzymes. In the **cytoplasm** outside the nucleus are organelles (Golgi apparatus, endoplasmic reticulum, mitochondria, phagolysosomes) that are important to the synthesis of hormones.

The **Golgi apparatus** (or body) is near the nucleus.[6] It consists of six or so membrane-bound stacked sacs called "cisternae." The Golgi apparatus processes proteins (e.g., by modifying sugars of glycoproteins).

The **endoplasmic reticulum** (e.r.) is a series of tubules. The membrane walls of the tubules can be either rough (granular, with ribosomes) or smooth (agranular). The structural types of the hormones that are synthesized by an en-

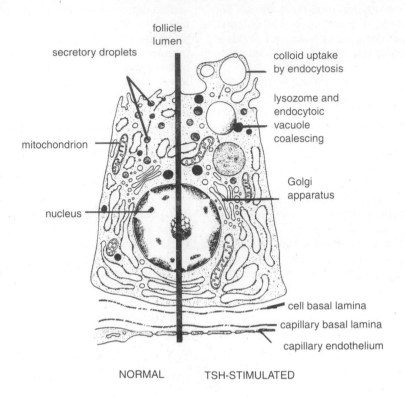

follicle lumen

secretory droplets

colloid uptake by endocytosis

lysozome and endocytoic vacuole coalescing

mitochondrion

Golgi apparatus

nucleus

cell basal lamina

capillary basal lamina

capillary endothelium

NORMAL   TSH-STIMULATED

Figure 1.2 The sketch shows an example of an endocrine cell, the thyroid follicle cell. The left side represents an unstimulated thyroid cell; the right side represents a thyroid cell stimulated by thyroid-stimulating hormone from the pituitary gland. The cell has the usual parts—a nucleus and mitochondria. Cell parts particularly relevant to its endocrine function are the Golgi apparatus, the secretory droplets, cell basal lamina, capillary basal lamina, and capillary endothelium. Anatomical specializations associated with the cell's function in the thyroid gland include the production and uptake of the colloid which occupies thyroid follicle lumens. Modified, with permission, after Fawcett, D.W.; Long; J.A.; Jones, A.L. The ultrastructure of endocrine glands. Rec. Prog. Horm. Res. 25: 315; 1969.

docrine cell are related to the detailed anatomical appearance of the endoplasmic reticulum. Polypeptides are synthesized at the ribosomes. Steroids are synthesized at smooth endoplasmic reticulum.

Mitochondria are organelles responsible for oxidative phosphorylation. In mitochondria, energy is stored in the molecule of ATP (adenosine triphosphate). The mitochondria are the site of some steps in the synthesis of steroids.

Lysosomes are organelles containing digestive enzymes. They function as the cell's digestive system. In the thyroid gland, phagolysozomes are involved in the process of releasing the thyroid hormones from their storage form in thyroglobulin.

The cytoplasm contains other organelles (lipid droplets, vesicles, and vesicles containing secretory granules) that are important to hormone synthesis, storage, and secretion. The cytoplasm also has centrioles, microtubules, and microfilaments that form a dynamic skeleton for the cell and are used in cell division and in movement. **Microtubules** form tracks for the movement of secretory granules to the cell membrane. In turn, the cytoskeleton is affected by hormones.

The **cell membrane**, also called the plasma membrane, is particularly important for hormones because they need to pass through the cell membrane to get out of the cell and into the circulation to deliver their messages. The membranes are made up of proteins, cholesterol, and phospholipids which have a head and two tails. Because the phospholipids have soluble (polar, hydrophilic) phosphate heads and insoluble (nonpolar, hydrophobic) tails, the heads contact the aqueous external fluids and cytoplasm, and the heads sandwich the tails between them. Proteins are embedded like nuggets in the membrane on the inner or outer surface or all the way through the membranes. The proteins give structure to the membrane, they labor as pumps actively transporting ions through the membrane, they form ion channels, they work as enzymes, or they act as receptors. Membrane is recycled.

SECRETION

Endocrine cells secrete their hormones into the extracellular space and then the hormones enter the bloodstream. Walls of capillaries of most endocrine glands (and the kidney and intestine) have tiny pores (20–100 nm diameter, fenestrations) which may facilitate movement of large molecules. In the brain and muscle, in contrast, the fenestrations are absent. The absence of fenestrated capillaries in brain and muscle contribute to the "blood-brain barrier"[7] which protects the brain from outside chemical influences.

Peptide hormones are secreted in the manner of proteins and amines, similar to the secretion processes used by cells that secrete proteins or enzymes and by nerve cells that secrete biogenic amine neurohumors. The proteins (or their precursors called prehormones or prohormones) are synthesized at the endoplasmic reticulum, which is an organelle in the cytoplasm of a cell (Figure 1.3). The proteins pass through another organelle, the Golgi apparatus, where they are packaged into secretory granules in vesicles. The hormones may

be stored and further processed in the vesicles, or the hormones may be secreted from the cells immediately. Secretion involves travel of the dense core vesicles through the cytoplasm of the cell to the cell membrane (Figure 1.4). There, the vesicle releases its contents (granules, the hormones) into the extracellular space by a process called "exocytosis."

The secretion of amine hormones is similar to that of protein hormones. For example, in the adrenal medulla, tyrosine is converted to dopamine in the cytoplasm. The dopamine is concentrated into secretory granules where enzymes convert it to epinephrine and norepinephrine. The hormones are secreted by exocytosis. Membrane is conserved by recycling.

Steroid hormones, in contrast, are synthesized from precursor cholesterol (in lipid droplets). Synthesis is a shuttling affair that takes place in the cytoplasm, smooth endoplasmic reticulum, and mitochondria of steroidal cells. Transit to the bloodstream is simple because the lipid-soluble steroids pass readily through the cell membrane. Thus, the rate of steroid secretion is usually a function of the rate of steroid synthesis. Proteinaceous molecules in the blood stream act as carriers for molecules of steroid hormones.

CHEMISTRY

Most hormones fall into one of a few categories of chemicals: polypeptides, glycoproteins, steroids, and amines (Table 1.1). A great many hormones are proteins. Proteins are assembled from small molecules called **amino acids**. Amino acid residues are bonded together by peptide bonds to make proteins. The hormones made from amino acids are **peptides**, **polypeptides**, or **proteins**. Some hormones contain amino acids and sugars and are classified as **glycoproteins**. Following the convention of Ganong, peptides have 2–10 amino acid residues, polypeptides have 10–99 amino acid residues, and proteins have more than 100 amino acid residues. In practice this fine distinction is not always adhered to, and any compound with two or more amino acids may be referred to as a peptide.

Hormones that are structurally similar to the amino acids are called the **amine hormones**. Iodinated amine hormones from the thyroid also have iodine in their structures.

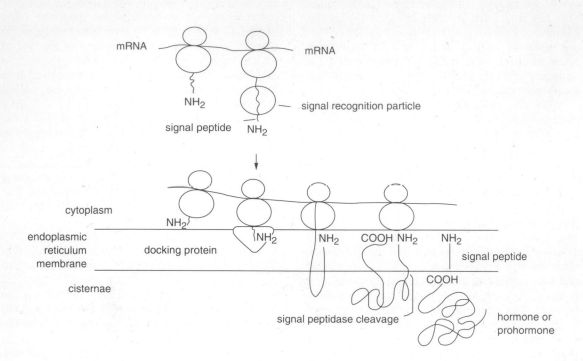

mRNA

mRNA

signal recognition particle

NH_2

signal peptide NH_2

cytoplasm

endoplasmic
reticulum
membrane

cisternae

NH_2

docking protein NH_2 NH_2 COOH NH_2 NH_2

signal peptide

COOH

signal peptidase cleavage

hormone or
prohormone

Figure 1.3 Assembly of peptides begins with their formation at the ribosomes. The ribosomes may be free or, as here, attached to the outside of rough endoplasmic reticulum membranes. The ribosomes read the genetic message carried by a molecule of messenger RNA. The ribosomes "translate" the message into precursors of the protein that is to be secreted. The secretory protein products pass into the cisternal space of the reticulum. From there, the secretory protein products move to the Golgi apparatus. Redrawn and modified, with permission, after Griffen, J.E.; Ojeda, S.R. Textbook of Endocrine Physiology, Second Edition. New York: Oxford University Press; 1992; p. 25.

Hormones made by the testes and ovaries and adrenal glands are **steroids.** Steroids have a distinctive structure with four connected rings and side chains.

A group of chemical messengers is derived from fatty acids; they are collectively called the **prostaglandins.**

It seems at first that there is an overwhelming plethora of hormones. But learning the hormones can be simplified by grouping them into families by structural similarities (Table 1.2).

AMOUNTS

Hormones usually perform their actions in very low concentrations (Table 1.3). This concept,

that hormones act in miniscule amounts, is illustrated by looking at typical hormone concentrations, which fall between 10^{-7} and 10^{-12} Molar. The amount of hormone in the blood may be referred to as the concentration in the blood or the blood level.

The units commonly seen in endocrinology are milligrams (10^{-3} grams), micrograms (10^{-6} grams), nanograms (10^{-9} grams), and picograms (10^{-12} grams). It helps to remember the order of these units if you can recall that the last three are in alphabetical order (micro, nano, pico). The abbreviation mg stands for milligram, ng for nanogram, and pg for picogram. Endocrinologists make use of an even more miniscule amount: the letter "f" ab-

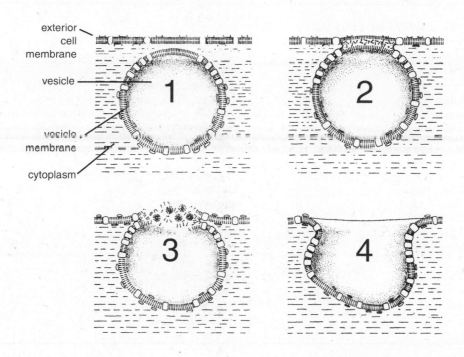

exterior
cell
membrane

vesicle

vesicle
membrane

cytoplasm

Figure 1.4 A molecular model of a secretory event is shown. (1) A mature secretory vesicle. (2) The membranes touch and "fuse." (3) The secretory vesicle discharges its contents. (4) The remaining vesicle membrane fuses with the cell membrane. Redrawn and modified, with permission, after Satir, B. The final steps in secretion. Scientific American 233: 1975; page 37.

breviates the prefix femto- for 10^{-15}, so an fg is a thousandth of a picogram. Thus, decreasing size is indicated in the sequence: milli > micro > nano > pico > femto.

Hormone concentrations have sometimes been given in titers (titres). This term derives from titration methods of hormone assay where the hormone is measured by its interaction with some other substance and given in equivalents based on that substance. The units for titers are usually grams of hormone per cubic centimeter of fluid.

The **half-life** of a hormone is the length of time that it takes half of the hormone to disappear from the blood stream. What makes this concept complicated, is that half-life is affected by everything that affects the level of a hormone in the bloodstream: storage, stability in the blood, selec-

tive concentration by the target, inactivation, and excretion. Stability of hormones, how long they last in the blood, may be influenced by the presence or absence of a carrier molecule in the blood for the hormone. Inactivation of a hormone, which refers to its biological activity, is usually accomplished by enzymes in the liver, kidney, and/or blood. Excretion of hormones is commonly done by the liver and/or kidneys.

CYCLIC NUCLEOTIDES AND GENES

Some compounds are chemically related to the small molecules, or bases, that form DNA (deoxyribonucleic acid) and RNA (ribonucleic acid). The molecules that function as intracellular second messengers are called the cyclic nucleotides.

Table 1.1 Hormones Classified by Biochemical Category

PEPTIDES, POLYPEPTIDES, AND PROTEINS
adrenocorticotropic hormone
angiotensin
calcitonin
cholecystokinin
erythropoietin
gastrin
glucagon
growth hormone
insulin
somatomedins
melanotropin
nerve growth factor
oxytocin
parathormone
prolactin
relaxin
secretin
somatostatin
vasopressin

GLYCOPROTEINS
follicle-stimulating hormone
human chorionic gonadotropin
luteinizing hormone
thyroid-stimulating hormone

STEROIDS
aldosterone
cortisol
estradiol
progesterone
testosterone

AMINES
epinephrine
melatonin
norepinephrine
dopamine
thyroxine
triiodothyronine

Cyclic AMP (cyclic adenosine monophosphate) is one of the cyclic nucleotides.

Genetics are important to endocrinology because genes are responsible for the structures of protein hormones, enzymes that synthesize hormones, and hormone receptors. Genes, the precisely arranged sequences of deoxyribonucleic acid in the nucleus, control the hormones that are produced because they provide the genetic code for the synthesis of the hormones that are made up of amino acids (peptide, polypeptide, and protein hormones). They provide the genetic code for the synthesis of the enzymes that in turn synthesize the other hormones (steroids, amines, prostaglandins, etc.) that are not themselves proteins. Genes also code for the receptor proteins that are on or in the target cells; the expression of the "receptor genes" is regulated by the amount of hormone.

MOLECULAR BIOLOGY

Molecular biology comprises the biochemistry and genetics of the nucleic acids, DNA and RNA. The genetic material, DNA, contains the blueprints for the peptide hormones and for the enzymes involved in the formation of the hormones that aren't peptides (Figure 1.5). The technical advances of molecular biology have enormous potential for endocrine applications. Techniques can be used to synthesize peptide hormones in large quantities. Peptide hormones were previously extracted in miniscule amounts from animals or people. Molecular biology can also be used to further explain how hormones act. The techniques provide means of detecting genetic bases of diseases, and make possible genetic repairs of abnormalities in the synthesis or hormones or their associated substances (receptors, synthesizing enzymes, etc.).

Many of the hormones discussed in this book are peptides or polypeptides. The amino acid sequences of their protein precursors are specified by the sequence of bases in deoxyribonucleic acid (DNA), the genetic material. Those hormones that are small molecules are synthesized from nutrients by the activity of enzymes. Like the hormones, the enzymes are proteins whose amino acid sequences are specified by the blueprint of bases in DNA. Thus, the instructions for making hormones

Table 1.2 Hormones Classified into Families by Structural Similarities

HYPOTHALAMIC NEUROHORMONES
oxytocin, arginine vasopressin, lysine vasopressin, vasotocin, mesotocin, isotocin, glumitocin, valitocin, aspartocin

HYPOPHYSIOTROPIC NEUROHORMONES
somatostatin, CRH, TRH, LRH, MIF, MRF, GRH

GI HORMONES AND RELATED MOLECULES
secretin, glucagon, gastric inhibitory peptide, vasoactive intestinal peptide, cholecystokinin, gastrin, caerulein, bombesin

MELANOTROPINS
ACTH, α-MSH, β-MSH, lipotropin, endorphins, enkephalins

INSULIN-LIKE HORMONES
insulin, somatomedins, insulin-like growth factors, relaxin, multiplication-stimulating activity

PROLACTIN-LIKE HORMONES
growth hormone, prolactin, placental lactogen

IODINATED AMINES
thyroxine, triiodothyronine, monoiodotyrosine, diiodotyrosine

INDOLEAMINES
melatonin, serotonin, auxin

STEROIDS
testosterone, estrogen, progesterone, cortisol, aldosterone, ecdysone

GLYCOPROTEIN HORMONES
FSH, LH, TSH, HCG

CATECHOLAMINES
epinephrine, norepinephrine, dopamine

OTHER HORMONES
prostaglandins, inhibin, müllerian regression factor, parathyroid hormone, calcitonin, angiotensin

are in the genes. The ability to make hormones and the exact sequences of amino acids in these hormones is, therefore, inherited.

To find a specific gene or to make its peptide product, such as a hormone, the structure of the peptide hormone must first be worked out. Fortunately for endocrinologists, the sequencing of the amino acids of most peptide hormones has already been accomplished. The nucleotide sequence of the DNA for the hormone can be deduced from the amino acid sequence of the protein. The DNA can be produced by chemical synthesis, or it can come from chromosomal DNA, or it can be DNA produced by reverse transcription.

Recombinant methods promise mass production of polypeptide hormones that were previously only available in miniscule quantities obtained from living organisms, their dead carcasses, their blood, or their urine. This means that hormones will now be more available for clinical use. The first hormone that was made using recombi-

nant techniques was somatostatin.[8] Gertz and Baxter discuss how protein hormones can be produced:

...sequences that encode the desired proteins must be inserted in the regions of plasmids downstream from bacterial regulatory sequences. The region would include a promoter; the sequences encoding a ribosomal binding site; and an AUG codon, which codes for methionine and is necessary in mRNA to initiate translation. The bacterial regulatory sequences are responsible for directing the synthesis of the desired proteins [hormones]. By this method of direct expression, the synthesized proteins [hormones] can frequently be obtained in yields that represent several percent of the total bacterial proteins.[9]

They also discuss an alternative approach,

Table 1.3 Hormones are Present in Minute Amounts

Molecules	mM
glucose	5.
cholesterol	5.
albumin	0.7
antibodies	0.09
high-density lipoprotein	0.013
thyroxine	0.00009
testosterone	0.00002
insulin	0.00000005

Concentrations of some hormones (thyroxine, testosterone, and insulin) along with some other organic molecules show the concept that hormones are present in "minute amounts" in human blood. Data from Gorbman, A.; Dickhoff, W.; Vigna, S.; Clark, N.; Ralph, C. Comparative Endocrinology. New York: John Wiley & Sons; 1983; page 26.

used for human insulin and ß-endorphin, which involves cleavage of the protein hormone from a fusion (hybrid) protein. The use of recombinant DNA to make insulin is illustrated in Figure 1.6.

Because some endocrine disorders are present in families from one generation to the next, they are believed to be genetic in origin. Sometimes, the etiology is clearcut; for example, congenital adrenal hyperplasia may be due to inherited inability to synthesize specific adrenal enzymes. Abnormal DNA coding (due to mutations, deletions, insertions, or a missing gene) for the sequence of a particular hormone or its receptor is the culprit. In other cases, the genetic cause is not so clearcut; it appears that what is inherited is a susceptibility to developing a disease. Some examples of endocrine diseases with a genetic component are: type II diabetes mellitus, dwarfism, testicular feminization, pseudohypoparathyroidism, congenital adrenal hyperplasia, and multiple endocrine neoplasia syndromes.

An individual person's DNA can be used for diagnosis of genetic disorders. The diagnosis is possible even before the symptoms of the disorder appear. Real hope of repairing genetic disorders is the subject of genetic engineering. The idea would be to insert genes for normal hormone production. For example, an insulin gene would be placed in a diabetic to repair the insulin deficiency. Does this seem impossible? Methods already exist to place DNA into cells. The DNA can be injected into the cell nucleus, or plasmid cDNA can be sent by electroporation. Cells will consume DNA calcium phosphate precipitates. Viruses and bacteria can be used to deliver cDNA to target cells.

METHODS OF ANATOMY AND HISTOLOGY

Finding the exact locations of hormones in cells has been accomplished with **histochemistry**. Histochemical techniques include dye staining, autoradiography using radioactive compounds, microscopy with fluorescent agents, and immunohistochemistry with antibodies. In immunohistochemistry, a tissue is exposed to antibodies "raised" using a hormone as the antigen; the antibodies bind to sites on the tissue and indicate the location of a hormone. In autoradiography, an organism or a

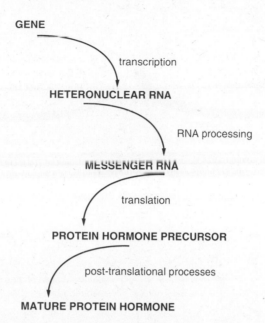

GENE

transcription

HETERONUCLEAR RNA

RNA processing

MESSENGER RNA

translation

PROTEIN HORMONE PRECURSOR

post-translational processes

MATURE PROTEIN HORMONE

Figure 1.5 The diagram shows the flow of information from the genes (DNA) in the nucleus to the assembly of proteins at the ribosomes in the cytoplasm. Redrawn, with permission, after Chin, W. Hormonal regulation of gene expression. In DeGroot, L.J., editor. Endocrinology. Philadelphia: W. B. Saunders Co.; 1989; p. 7.

tissue is labelled with a radioactive molecule (e.g., a radioactive isotope of a hormone). A tissue section is coated with photographic film, exposed, and developed. The radioactivity exposes the film. When the film is developed, peppery black speckles in the photographic film superimposed on the microscopic section make it possible to locate the radioactive molecules to learn where hormones act.

METHODS OF CHEMISTRY

Using **isotopic labelling**, especially radioactive isotopes, it is possible to follow the paths of hormones around the body and to identify hormone targets. A "labelled" hormone is injected, and some time later its distribution in the organs and cells is assessed. Places where the hormone localizes, or **binds**, are suspected of being **targets** and having receptors, or sites where the hormone attaches.

The methods used to measure hormones are collectively called **hormone assays**. The assays may be conducted using living target organs *in vivo* or *in vitro,* in which case the assays are

called **bioassays**. Units based on bioassays are arbitrary; that is, they depend on the bioassay, and they refer to the amount of a physiological response. Such units are usually designated **International Units** (I.U., IU, or U.). They do not designate weights (as do grams and milligrams) though their equivalent in weight may be known. In addition to bioassays, it is possible, and nowadays more common, to measure some hormones with physical or chemical tests.

Radioimmunoassays use the principle of competitive protein binding. In competitive protein binding, a molecule of hormone competes for reactive binding sites on a protein antibody. Reagents include antibodies for hormones and radioactive isotopes. Radioimmunoassays (RIAs) have made it possible to measure small quantities of hormones.

Most hormones can now be measured absolutely and expressed in terms of grams or in terms of moles (the formula weight calculated from the atomic weight and expressed in grams). Usually hormone amounts are expressed per unit volume of fluid or per unit weight of tissue. Some-

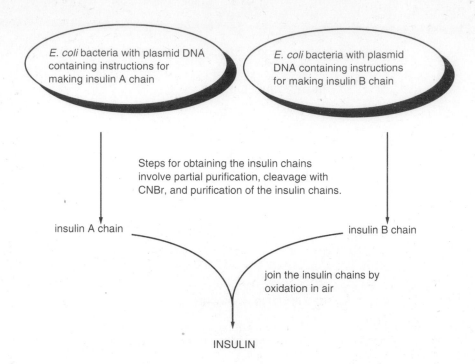

Figure 1.6 The production of insulin by the use of bacteria is shown. The insulin chains are made as part of a larger precursor protein, β-galactosidase. The insulin chains are severed from the precursor protein and joined by oxidation. Itakura, K.; Hirose, T.; Crea, R.; Riggs, A. Expression in *Escherichia coli* of a chemically synthesized gene for the hormone somatostatin. Science 198: 1056–1062; 1977.

times, hormones in the serum of the blood are given as "mg%," which means milligrams of hormone per 100 milliliters (or cubic centimeters) of serum. Now infrequently, hormone concentrations are expressed as "titers" (grams of hormone per cubic milliliter of solution) because of the titration methodology used to measure chemicals.

The technique used to recover hormones is called **extraction**. Hormones are extracted from homogenates of the glands that synthesized them, from blood, or from urine. Once an extract is obtained, the hormones are further isolated by chemical purification. New hormones are still being extracted.

METHODS OF PHYSIOLOGY

When a gland is removed by excision or surgery or amputation, a word used to describe the removal is **ablation**. Ablation has been one of the most common experimental techniques used to try to determine the function of a gland. Ablation of a gland that produces a stimulatory hormone usually leads to regression (decreased size) or inactivity of its target(s). Ablation of an endocrine gland(s) is sometimes referred to informally as "glandectomy," or "ectomies." Informal abbreviations use "X" to indicate gland removal; for example, PitX indicates pituitary removal.

The initial breakthroughs in endocrinology, discoveries of a gland's functions, were often achieved with ablation. But there are other means of interfering with a gland's formal function. It can be destroyed by a disease. It can be missing for hereditary reasons. It can be destroyed by chemicals (e.g., the chemical alloxan causes diabetes by destroying pancreatic islets). A gland can be

Table 1.4 Biological Variability and Common Statistics Used in Endocrinology

	Noon nmol/gland/hr	Midnight nmol/gland/hr
data	2016, 2284, 2779, 1450, 2091, 1965	47764, 54093, 47213, 50228, 58217, 27015
mean	2097	47422
maximum	2779	58217
minimum	1450	27015
standard deviation (SD)	434	10821
standard error	177	4417

The table shows N-acetyltransferase activity in the pineal gland. Enzyme activity was measured by supplying pineal homogenate with radioactive substrate precursors and measuring the products that were produced. Endocrine graphs normally show the means and vertical lines that indicate plus one and minus standard error. The data are for eight-week-old chicks (N = 6 per group) raised and maintained in LD12:12 with lights-on at 0600. Binkley, S.; MacBride, S.; Klein, D.; Ralph, C. Pineal enzymes: Regulation of avian melatonin synthesis. Science 181: 273–275; 1973.

damaged by antibody-antigen reactions using immunochemicals. Such studies provide clues to the function of the gland and its hormones.

The endocrinology of a gland and its hormones can be studied in the entire living animal or human being, in which case the study is said to take place *in vivo*. Alternatively, the gland or its cells or its hormones or its target cells can be studied in a situation where they are removed from the living organism, or *in vitro*. The *in vitro* studies have the advantage that conclusions can be made about one step at a time. It is possible, however, to obtain an *in vitro* response that would not occur in the whole organism. *In vivo* experiments are required to examine the multiple effects of hormone action and complex regulation.

A common experiment in endocrinology is to ablate a gland, to inject a suspect hormone, and to observe the consequences. This is called a **hormone replacement** experiment. Hormone replacement therapy is also used clinically. A well known example is the use of estrogen replacement therapy after menopause or hysterectomy.

The endocrine glands can sometimes be studied by transplanting endocrine tissues. **Transplants** can be made by moving an endocrine gland from its normal location to another part of the same individual's body (autotransplantation, homotransplantation). Or, an endocrine gland can be transplanted from a donor organism to a recipient organism (heterotransplantation). Destinations for transplanted tissues have commonly included the capsule of the kidney and the anterior chamber of the eye. The progress of transplants (e.g., of the ovary or the pineal) placed in the anterior chamber of the eye can be inspected visually and the transplants have a lower rate of rejection in the eye location.

Evidence for hormone action includes: (i) ablation of the source gland abolishes the response, (ii) blocking blood flow abolishes the response, (iii) blood is the route of transport, (iv) target denervation does not affect the response, (v) physiological doses of purified hormone produces a normal response.

STATISTICS

Endocrinologists, like other scientists, use statistics to decide whether or not an observed effect is real. In measuring hormones, there is a considerable amount of biological variability (Table 1.4).

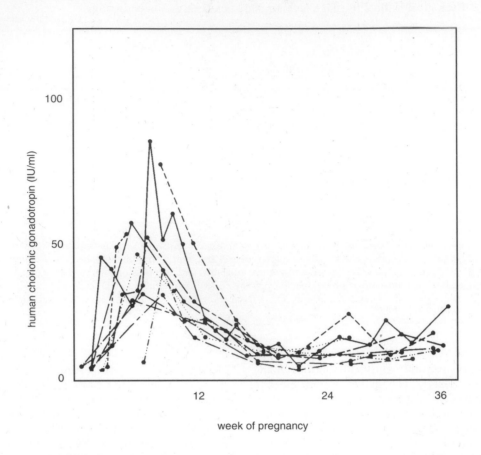

week of pregnancy

Figure 1.7 The graphs illustrate individual biological variation in a hormone. Plasma human chorionic gonadotropin (HCG), a hormone of pregnancy, is shown for eight women throughout gestation. Modified, with permission. Vaitukaitis, J. Human chorionic gonadotropin. In Fuchs, F.; Klopper, A., editors. Endocrinology of Pregnancy, Second Edition. New York: Harper & Row; 1977; p. 67.

For example, if levels of the hormone, HCG, are compared in eight different pregnant women, there is considerable variation. Nonetheless, there is a general pattern that can be easily seen in the graph—HCG is present during pregnancy and there is more HCG during the first three months of pregnancy (Figure 1.7). Other good examples of natural individual variation can be found in this book in the length of the human female menstrual cycle and in the levels of testosterone.

Endocrine data may be given as individual numbers, or, more routinely, as **means** or averages for a group. Variation may be indicated by the range (maximum and minimum) of values, or by calculation of a standard deviation (SD) or **standard error** of the mean (SEM). The variation may be indicated by drawing vertical lines representing these values. Standard errors are shown on some graphs in this book (e.g., for the melanotropin rhythm or the pineal N-acetyltransferase rhythm). Endocrinologists make use of statistical tests, for example Student's **t-test**, to test statistical "significance." Statistical significance is expressed with "p," or **probability**, values. The usual standard is to consider $p < 0.05$ to indicate a statistically significant difference.

Table 1.5 Interchangeability of Hormones Among Vertebrate Species

More species-specific	Less species-specific
high molecular weight hormones: proteins, polypeptides, glycoproteins	low molecular weight hormones: steroids, amines

RHYTHMS

In studying endocrinology, it is often part of the experiment to make environmental manipulations. These manipulations may involve the ambient temperature, the light-dark cycle, or the presence of social cues from other individuals. Even when environmental parameters are not changed as part of an experiment, it is usual to specify them as part of the conditions under which the experimental organisms were housed.

Most hormones have now been found to have daily and/or seasonal cycles or **rhythms**. A cycle can be one fluctuation; a rhythm implies more than one fluctuation, or repeated cycles. In order to properly interpret the quantity of a hormone in a sample, it may often be necessary to know at what time of day the sample was taken, what stage of the reproductive cycle the sample was removed, and what month of the year the sample was acquired.[10] The highest value of a cycle is its peak or maximum; the lowest value of a cycle is its nadir or minimum.

The duration of light in a 24-hour light-dark cycle is called the **photoperiod**. A common photoperiod used with rats is designated LD14:10—fourteen hours of light in alternation with ten hours of dark. Photoperiod is of particular relevance to the subject of endocrinology because it is used in controlling seasonal breeding.

SPECIES SPECIFICITY

Another generality involves the degree of species specificity (Table 1.5). Some hormones are less species specific, they act in most organisms in which they are found. These hormones are invariably small molecules, the steroid and amine hormones, with simple structures.

For example, the steroid testosterone has the same structure in all species—rat testosterone is identical to human testosterone. Testosterone is not species specific. That is, testosterone obtained from rats will act in humans just like human testosterone. Other hormones are more species specific. Species-specific hormones are often polypeptides or proteins. These hormones vary in structure and biological activity from one species to another. For example, there may be variation in the sequence of amino acids between growth hormone from whales and growth hormone from humans. So growth hormone of whales, for example, does not stimulate growth in humans. Monkey growth hormone, on the other hand, is more similar to the growth hormone of humans and can stimulate growth in humans.

HIERARCHIES

Some of the endocrine glands can be arranged in **"endocrine hierarchies."** In hierarchies, hormones can be organized by function and interaction (Figure 1.8). In this method of classifying hormones, the hormones are assigned to groups by their participation in regulation. In making the classification, each set of glands and hormones are listed in functional sequences, or hierarchies.

In the generalized hierarchical model, brain regions and the pineal gland regulate the hypothalamus. The hypothalamus secretes hormones that control the pituitary gland. Other hormones secreted in turn by the pituitary gland control the gonads and the adrenal glands and the thyroid gland.

The hierarchical endocrine arrangement produces a powerful regulatory tool. A tiny signal perceived by the brain can, with synthesis or release of just a few molecules, be converted to an enormous effect. This is because there is multiplica-

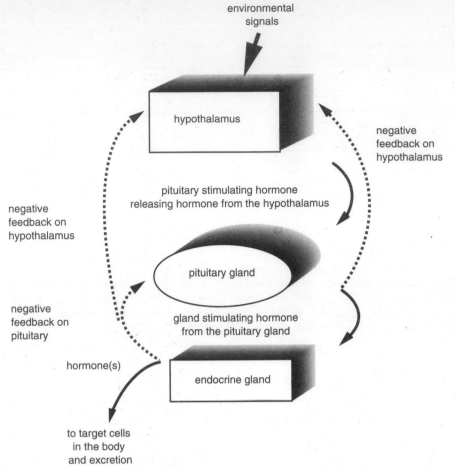

environmental
signals

hypothalamus

negative
feedback on
hypothalamus

negative
feedback on
hypothalamus

pituitary stimulating hormone
releasing hormone from the hypothalamus

pituitary gland

negative
feedback on
pituitary

gland stimulating hormone
from the pituitary gland

hormone(s)

endocrine gland

to target cells
in the body
and excretion

Figure 1.8 The figure shows a generalized model of an endocrine hierarchy with feedback (dotted lines). Hierarchy and feedback are involved in regulation of endocrine glands. In the hierarchy, each gland is driven by signals (downward-pointing arrows). Feedback, usually negative, by the final hormones is used to stop synthesis (upward-pointing arrows). A shorter feedback loop can also occur between the pituitary gland and the hypothalamus. Environmental signals are perceived by sensory organs and influence the endocrine system via neural signals of the brain to the hypothalamus. The general model shown involves the hypothalamus, the pituitary gland, and an endocrine gland. Note that three (or more) hormones are involved.

tion of the strength of the signal, or amplification, at each step. In endocrinology, **amplification** occurs three independent ways–in the hierarchies, in the steroid mechanism of action, and in the cyclic AMP mechanism of action.

Why have an endocrine system to carry chemical messages if you already have a perfectly good nervous system? There are at least two possible reasons. First, the time scale of endocrine responses is much slower than the speed of neural responses, usually less than 24 hours. Second, the hormones make use of the circulatory system to send the same signal to many parts of the body at the same time.

SET POINT REGULATION

Neurosecretory cells in the hypothalamus may themselves be sensitive to various kinds of

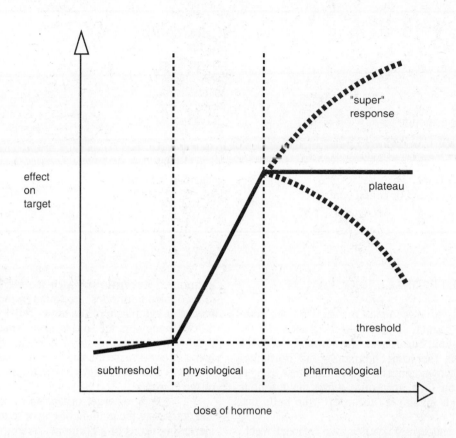

effect on target

"super" response

plateau

threshold

subthreshold | physiological | pharmacological

dose of hormone

Figure 1.9 The graph illustrates a dose-response curve. A physiological dose is above the threshold in the range of the "normal" response. Physiological doses fall in the effective range. In the physiological range the response is proportional to the dose. Standard curves for bioassays can be made in the physiological range. Subthreshold doses are too low to produce an effect. Pharmacological doses are those in excess of normal. Pharmacological doses may produce an abnormal stimulation, inhibition, or no additional effect.

signals. In the hypothalamus, scientists have shown that some cells are directly sensitive to temperature, circulating levels of glucose, or salt concentration in the blood. Where such sensitive cells have been found, "set point regulation" has been proposed. The idea is that a group of cells work very much like "thermostats" to achieve a desired level of something (e.g., body temperature). The setting can be increased or decreased. The cells are sensitive to increases or decreases in temperature in their immediate environment.

For example, if the temperature of the blood bathing the cells is too high, the cells set off an endocrine sequence via the thyroid hierarchy whose end result lowers the body temperature. Similarly, if the temperature is too low, the cells trigger endocrine events that raise body temperature. Set point regulation has been invoked as part of the schemes of regulation for the thyroid (blood temperature detection by a **thermostat**), for growth hormone (blood glucose detection by a **glucostat**), and for antidiuretic hormones (blood salt concentration detected by an **osmostat**).

Table 1.6 General Topics Applicable to Most Endocrine Glands

HISTORY	**HORMONES**
	structure
ANATOMY	nomenclature
location	biosynthesis
histology	metabolism
embryology	secretion
comparative anatomy	assays
innervation	
vascularization	**FUNCTION**
	normal physiology
REGULATION	mechanism of action
feedback system and/or neural control	rhythms
	disorders

NEGATIVE FEEDBACK REGULATION

Negative feedback mechanisms are common in the regulatory schemes for glands and the targets of their hormones. In negative feedback mechanisms (servomechanisms), the hormones control their own concentrations. A signal triggers the secretion of a hormone; when the hormone reaches high levels, it "turns off" the cells that secrete it.

In endocrinology, negative feedback mechanisms are sometimes classified as long loop or short loop. In **short loop feedback** mechanisms, the hormone feeds back on the gland that stimulated its production (or secretion, or release) in the first place. For example, growth hormone from the anterior pituitary turns off the secretion of growth hormone releasing hormone in the hypothalamus. In **long loop feedback** mechanisms, a hormone feeds even further back on a gland still higher in its hierarchy. For example, thyroid hormone feeds back on the hypothalamus which secretes thyroid-stimulating hormone releasing hormone.

TARGETS AND RECEPTORS

The organ, tissue, or cells upon which a hormone(s) acts is called its **target.** The uterus is an organ that is a target of the hormone estrogen. In some cases, a hormone may have more than one target and a target can respond to more than one hormone. **Receptors,** which the target cells use to recognize hormones, are found in the cell membranes or cytoplasm of the target cells. Because of this, the receptors are said to have "specificity" for the hormone they recognize. The factors that increase or decrease the production or secretion of a hormone from its gland constitute the **regulation** of the hormone.

Using a target organ, an endocrinologist can determine the amount of response to a series of increasing doses of a hormone. A graph of the results is called a **dose-response curve** (Figure 1.9). Very low doses of the hormone may produce no detectable response at all from the target; such low doses are said to be **subthreshold.** Once a sufficiently large dose is given to produce a response, the dose is considered to have reached the **threshold** and to be in the **physiological** range. In the physiological range the response of the target cells is proportional to the dose of the hormone. Hormones in blood may be free or bound to other molecules, and the free form is believed responsible for the hormone's activity (the **free hormone hypothesis**).[11] Because the response is proportional to the dose, the physiological range can be used to make **standard curves** for bioassays of hormone amounts. The idea of a physiological range has even broader implications and usages. The amounts of hormones that can be found normally *in vivo* are called the "physiological" concentrations. Still larger doses of hormone may produce one of three abnormal, or **pharmacological**,

Table 1.7   Types of Hormones and Embryonic Origins

Layers	Type of hormone	Organs derived from layer	Subcellular generalities
ectoderm	peptides, proteins, amines, catecholamines	skin, central nervous system, pineal, pituitary, adrenal medulla	endoplasmic reticulum well developed, granular, rough
endoderm	proteins, peptides, iodinated amines	digestive lining, liver, pancreas, thyroid, parathyroid, thymus, lungs	endoplasmic reticulum well developed, granular, rough
mesoderm	steroids	muscles, skeleton, reproductive system, adrenal cortex	endoplasmic reticulum in whorls, smooth

responses. First, the target may respond with a larger than normal response, or a **super** response, to a high dose of hormone. Second, the response may level off to a **plateau** so that higher doses of hormone do not produce more than the maximal response of the target. Third, high doses of hormone beyond the physiological range may actually inhibit the response of the target.

Hormones can act in a variety of ways. They can **stimulate** a response of the target. They can **inhibit** something the target is doing. Two hormones can oppose, or **antagonize**, the action of each other. And, two or more hormones can act in concert upon a single target, in which case they are said to **synergize** each other.

MECHANISMS OF ACTION

A scientific objective for endocrinologists is to explain the fundamental way a hormone acts in terms of chemical reactions. Such explanations are called **mechanisms of action.** Fortunately for endocrine students, the mechanisms of action fall into two main categories, a type of mechanism of action for steroid and thyroid hormones (Lepri's "roid" mechanisms of action), and a type of mecha-

nism of action for protein and amine hormones (Lepri's non-"roid" mechanisms of action.)

SEMASIOLOGY

Endocrinologists challenge the beginning endocrine student by giving more than one name and abbreviation to a single hormone. That means that it is necessary not only to learn a hormone's name and spelling, but also its aliases. For example, one hormone of the thyroid gland is called "thyroid hormone," aka "thyroxine," or it can be abbreviated—"T_4" (tee-four).

Some glands are listed in dictionaries only as adjectives (thus you write pineal gland, thyroid gland, or pituitary gland) while others are listed as nouns (thus you can say ovary, pancreas, or testes but you don't write "ovary gland"). In practice, especially in verbal speech, most of the glands are commonly referred to as nouns (e.g., the pituitary), even though they remain adjectives in some dictionaries. Words that are capitalized in endocrinology usually derive from the name of a person (e.g., islets of Langerhans or Leydig cells are named after people, but chromaffin cells are named by staining properties).

The author, whose research was done with a tiny bit of tissue most esoterically called the epiphysis cerebri, fell innocently into these semantic arguments: should the structure be called the pineal body, the pineal organ, the pineal gland, or simply, the pineal? The endocrinology teacher can provide little help other than to put forth the alternatives. The author is, of course, guilty of participating in these arguments by objecting to the nonsense of abbreviating the short name "melatonin" to M, MT, or MEL (melatonin is the name of the hormone secreted by the pineal).

Endocrinologists have a multiplicity of spellings for some words. The word that denotes sexual heat (or rut) is spelled four ways: "estrous" (adjective, also spelled "oestrous"), "estrus" (noun, also spelled "oestrus").

The language used to describe glands and hormones is indicative of status. If a structure is referred to as a "body" rather than a "gland," it usually means the author or his reviewers did not accept the structure as an endocrine gland. If a molecule is referred to as a "hormone" then it has been accorded that status by endocrinologists. But, if a molecule is only referred to as a "factor," then some uncertainty still remains as to whether the molecule is a true hormone. Historical changes in status of a hormone or gland can also be discerned by observing the amounts of space devoted to a gland and its hormone in endocrinology textbooks!

HISTORY

McCann traces the history of endocrinology to antiquity and Aristotle's association of effects of castration with masculine behavior in boars, Galen's idea that animal spirits were secreted into the nose and from the pituitary gland, and Descartes' association of the pineal gland with the very soul. Credit for the first endocrine experiment is generally given to Berthold[12] who castrated roosters which then had smaller combs and crowed less; transplanting testes into the castrated roosters restored these signs of masculinity.[13] The last endocrine gland discovered was the parathyroid, which was discovered in 1891 by Gley. Schafer and George Oliver in 1894 in England showed that extracts of the adrenal gland medulla had physiological effects on muscles, heart, and arteries.[14] The active principle, epinephrine (adrenalin) was identified shortly after by Americans J. J. Abel and A. C. Crawford. The experimental basis for the science of endocrinology was thus developed within the last hundred years.

ORGANIZING ENDOCRINOLOGY

The general aspects of each endocrine gland can be organized (Table 1.6). The history of the science of the gland can be told. The gross anatomy of a gland—its location, size, and appearance to the naked eye—can be described. The appearance of the cells of the gland can be revealed using microscopes and the stains of histology. The anatomical development of the gland can be traced by describing the gland's embryology.

A useful generalization is that the chemical nature of the hormones of a gland is a consequence of the gland's embryological origin (Table 1.7). Glands that develop from the embryonic layers endoderm and ectoderm (pituitary, pineal, thyroid, pancreas, hypothalamus) make amine and protein hormones. Glands that develop from the embryonic layer mesoderm (adrenal cortex, ovary, testis) are usually paired and they make steroid hormones.

An endocrine system can be summarized. The central feature is a gland that synthesizes hormones and secretes them. The gland is regulated by signals (nerve signals, hormones from other glands, hormone feedback from itself). The hormones secreted by the gland travel in the blood to targets (cells, tissues, organs). The targets recognize the hormones because the target cells possess receptor molecules that are specific for the hormones. The targets respond to the hormones by increasing or decreasing their own characteristic functions. The hormone signals are ended by inactivation of the hormones.

REFERENCES

1.   Webster's New Universal Unabridged Dictionary. New York: Simon & Schuster; 1979.
2.   Hoerr, N.L.; Osol, A.; editors. Blakiston's New Gould Medical Dictionary, Second Edition. McGraw-Hill Book Co., Inc.; 1956; p. 558.
3.   Ganong, W.F. Neuroendocrinology. In Greenspan, F.S., editor. Basic and Clinical Endocrinology, Third Edition. Norwalk, CT: Appleton & Lange; 1991; p. 66.
4.   Stagg, R. B.; Fletcher, W. H. The hormone-

induced regulation of contact-dependent cell-cell communication by phosphorylation. Endocrine Reviews 11: 302; 1990.

5. Loewenstein, W. R. Intercellular communication. Scientific American 222: 79–86; 1970.

6. Neutra, M.; Leblond, M.N. The Golgi apparatus. Scientific American 220: 100–107; 1969.

7. Tuomanen, E. Breaching the blood-brain barrier. Scientific American 268: 80–84; 1993.

8. Itakura, K.; Hirose, T.; Crea, R.; Riggs, A.; Heyneker, H. L.; Bolivar, F.; Boyer, H. Expression in *Escherichia coli* of a chemically synthesized gene for the hormone somatostatin. Science 198: 1056–1062; 1977.

9. Gertz, B.J.; Baxter, J.D. Gene expression and recombinant DNA in endocrinology and metabolism. In Greenspan, F.S., Forsham, P.H., editors. Basic and Clinical Endocrinology, Second Edition. East Norwalk, CT: Lange Medical Publications; 1986; p. 670.

10. Binkley, S. Wrist activity in a woman: Daily, weekly, menstrual, lunar, annual cycles? Phys. Behav. 52: 411–421; 1992.

11. Ekins, R. Measurement of free hormones in blood. Endocrine Reviews 11: 5; 1990.

12. Berthold, A. A. Transplantation der Hoden. Arch. Anat. Physiol. Wiss. Med. 16: 42–46; 1949.

13. McCann, S.M., editor. Endocrinology: People and Ideas. Bethesda, MD: American Physiological Society; 1988; p. v–vi.

14. Rasmussen, H., editor. Cell Communication in Health and Disease. New York: W. H. Freeman and Company; 1991; p. viii.

CHAPTER 2

Receptors, Mechanisms of Action, and Prostaglandins

Hormones and their targets recognize each other with receptors that are located in the targets. Peptide and amine hormones use receptors on the outsides of the target cell membranes. Second messengers (e.g., cyclic AMP synthesized in the cell membrane by the enzyme adenyl cyclase) relay the hormone signal to the interior of the cell. The second messenger causes the cell to respond to a hormone signal by initiating a cascade of reactions, enzyme activations, inside the cell. In contrast, steroid and thyroid hormone receptors are inside the cell in the cytoplasm. The target cells transcribe DNA into mRNA, which in turn is translated to produce proteins characteristic of the target cell. Prostaglandins are included in this chapter because they are synthesized in the cell membrane and sometimes oppose cyclic AMP.

OVERVIEW

In the last twenty-five years, the mechanisms by which hormones act on their targets has been a subject of vigorous research with the result that many mechanisms of action for hormones are now known.

Hormone binding studies were used to identify target locations in organisms. A consequence of the principle that hormones bind to their own specific targets led to the concept that target organs possessed receptors for their hormones.

Studies of the interaction of hormones with target cells led to the discovery of two general types of mechanisms of action.

In the first type of mechanism of action, used by hydrophilic peptide and amine hormones which don't readily diffuse into cells (Lepri's non-"roid" mechanism of action), the hormone binds to the cell membrane. The hormone receptors reside in the cell membrane. The interaction of the hormone and the cell is carried out by an intermediary in the cytoplasm, a second messenger, which is a small molecule (e.g., cyclic nucleotides and inositol triphosphate). The second messengers lead to enzyme activations/inactivations and to calcium ion movements which carry out the target cell response.

In the second general type of mechanism of action, used by lipophilic steroids which readily penetrate cell membranes and by thyroid hormones (Lepri's "roid" mechanism of action), the hormone enters the cell and binds to cytoplasmic receptors located in the cytoplasm. Hormone-receptor complexes stimulate the nuclear production of new mRNA and the cell makes new proteins which may be secreted proteins, enzymes for reactions, or structural proteins.

Cell membranes also contain the precursors for a group of chemical messengers named "prostaglandins" which sometimes oppose second messenger action. They are therefore included in this chapter.

RECEPTORS

Target cells must have ways of recognizing the hormones to which they respond. Once radioactive forms of hormones were available, it was possible to demonstrate specific "binding" of hormones to their targets. That is, more radioactive tagged hormone was found in targets than in non-targets. The specificity is due to receptors possessed by the target organs. The receptors account for the observed binding of hormones to target tissues.

Receptors are proteins. The receptors are thought of as having one or more **binding sites** per receptor. The molecules, or hormones, that bind to them are called ligands. Molecules (i.e., of hormone) compete for binding sites (i.e., on protein receptors). Any molecule that binds to a receptor can compete; the fewer different kinds of molecules that can bind, the more specific the binding is said to be.

AFFINITY

The term **affinity**, as used in chemistry, refers to that force by which atoms of certain elements combine and remain combined.

In endocrinology, there is affinity between a receptor and its hormone whose amount can be described. The affinity constant, K_d, is the concentration of free hormone at which half the receptors are saturated. The kinetics of hormone-receptor are usually represented graphically (Figure 2.1).

Nonspecific binding has low affinity and high capacity—hormones may have nonspecific binding with many proteins. Specific binding, characteristic of hormone interaction with their receptors, has high affinity and relatively low capacity. The number of binding sites are estimated by subtracting nonspecific or nonsaturable binding from total binding.

Scatchard plots illustrate the kinetics of free hormone concentration [H] and receptor [R] interaction when they form a hormone-receptor complex [HR]. k_1 is the rate constant for the association of the hormone and its receptor; k_2 is the rate constant for the dissociation of the hormone and its receptor. At equilibrium the rates are equal. The quantity K_d is the equilibrium dissociation constant. K_d is a measure of the affinity between the receptor and the hormone. When the receptors have combined with all the hormone molecules that they can, the receptors are said to have reached the "binding capacity" or to be "saturated."

It is assumed that hormones act at low concentrations (10^{-8} to 10^{-10} M) so that their receptors must have high binding affinity. For example, a $K_d = 10^{-3}$ M would indicate weak bind-

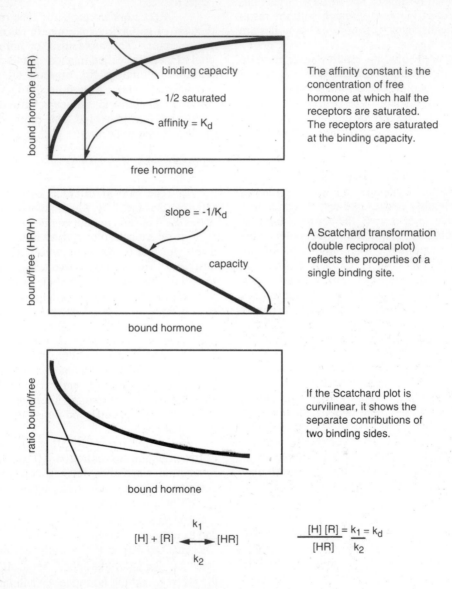

The affinity constant is the concentration of free hormone at which half the receptors are saturated. The receptors are saturated at the binding capacity.

A Scatchard transformation (double reciprocal plot) reflects the properties of a single binding site.

If the Scatchard plot is curvilinear, it shows the separate contributions of two binding sides.

Figure 2.1 The graphs represent kinetics of binding of hormone to its receptor. [H] = concentration of free hormone. [R] = concentration of receptor. [HR] = concentration of hormone receptor complexes. k values = rate constants. Redrawn, after Williams, J.A. Mechanisms in hormone secretion, action, and response. In Greenspan, F., editor. Basic & Clinical Endocrinology, Third Edition. Norwalk, Connecticut: Appleton & Lange; 1991; p. 8.

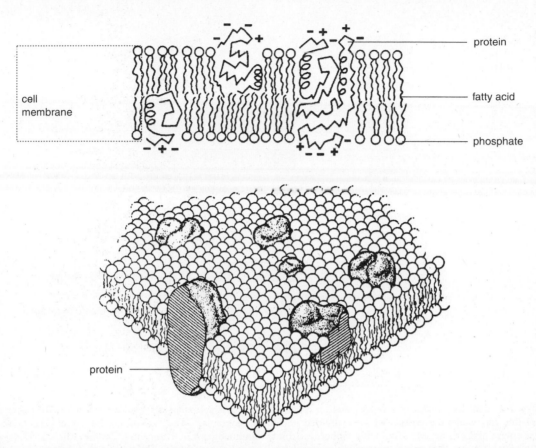

Figure 2.2 The drawings show the classical fluid mosaic membrane model of the structure of cell membranes in two (upper) and three (lower) dimensions. Two layers of phospholipids form a lipid bilayer. Circles (hydrophilic, polar, phosphate groups) attached to wavy lines (hydrophobic, nonpolar, fatty acid chains) designate phospholipids (phosphatidylcholine and phosphatidylethanolamine). Proteins (represented by long jagged and coiled lines) are embedded in, or bridge, the membrane. The proteins carry electrical charges on their ends and the coils represent an alpha helical structure characteristic of proteins. In the lower representation, the proteins are shown as irregular globules. Modified, with permission, from Singer, S.J.; Nicolson, G.L. The fluid mosaic model of the structure of cell membranes. Science 175: 720; 1972.

ing, whereas $K_d = 10^{-8}$ or 10^{-10} would indicate strong specific binding appropriate for hormones. Demonstration of specific binding is considered to be a defining characteristic of a hormone receptor interaction. As mentioned, there is also binding that occurs more generally between molecules and proteins, where the binding affinity is low, that is called nonspecific binding.

Simple systems have only one receptor site; but more complex systems may have multiple receptor sites. Whether there is more than one receptor can be decided based on whether the Scatchard plot is linear (one receptor) or curvilinear (more than one receptor).

There is a limited **capacity** whether or not there is more than one receptor. That is, binding activity of a receptor (or receptors) can be **saturated**, or used up, by its hormone. We can visualize this as the receptor(s) having a number of receptor "sites;" each site binds a molecule; the sites can be filled up (e.g., by hormone molecules).

RECEPTOR STRUCTURE

Cells have internal and external boundaries that are called "membranes." Thus the cell is

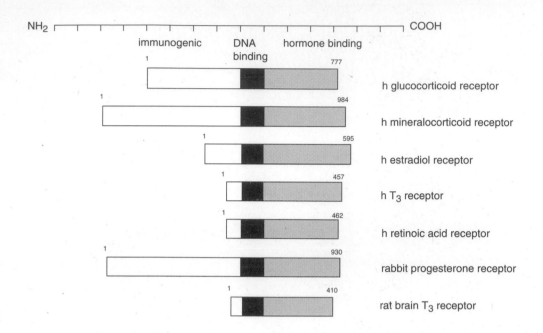

Figure 2.3 The figure shows a representation of the family to which steroid receptors belong. The upper horizontal line represents the protein which is divided into three "domains." The domain on the left is variable among the receptors and can be identified with antibodies so it is "immunogenic." The central domain binds DNA and has zinc binding fingers that are characteristic of regulatory proteins that bind to DNA. On the right is the domain that binds steroids. The numbers over the lines represent the numbers of amino acid (with 1 on the left) in the receptor. Redrawn, with permission. West, J.B. Physiological Basis of Medical Practice, Twelfth Edition. Baltimore: Williams & Wilkins; 1991; p. 790.

surrounded by a bilayer that is 7.5 nanometers thick. This membrane is called the **cell membrane** or plasma membrane or plasmalemma. Inside cells, there are other membranes surrounding the nucleus of the cell, and organelles possess membranes as well.

Cell membranes of cells that have nuclei are composed of protein and lipid—phospholipids, phosphatidylcholine and phosphatidylethanolamine and their complexes with fatty acids, cholesterol, or steroids. Water is involved in maintaining the integrity of membranes. The lipids' phosphate head is water soluble (hydrophilic, polar) and the tail ends are insoluble in water (hydrophobic, nonpolar). The lipids thus line up with their head ends facing water that is inside and outside the cell. Their insoluble tails end up inside the membrane

forming a lipid bilayer (Figure 2.2).

Some proteins are "embedded" in the lipid bilayers of membranes. The proteins are on the outside surface of the membrane, on the inside surface of the membrane, or traverse the membrane. Some of the proteins are glycoproteins (containing carbohydrates) and other proteins are lipoproteins (containing lipid). The proteins provide structure, pump ions across membranes, form channels for ions, catalyze reactions (enzymes), and serve as receptors.

The membranes are dynamic. The proteins can move about and the movement may involve microtubules and microfilaments.[1] New proteins are introduced or old proteins discarded from the membranes. The membrane proteins vary among cells and in the organelles and are

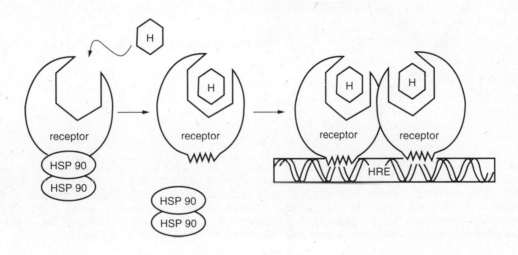

Figure 2.4 (Upper) Zinc fingers are binding regions of transcription factor proteins which attach to the promotor segment of DNA. They are found in the family of molecules that include the steroid receptors. (Lower) The figure shows a model of interaction of steroid receptor with HSP 90 (heat shock protein). On the left is shown the inactive complex of receptor and two HSP molecules. The hormone (H) causes dissociation of the receptor from the HSP 90 which activates the receptor. Next, on the right, the hormone-receptor complex dimers bind to specific hormone response elements (HRE) on DNA. Redrawn, with permission. Carson-Jurica, M.A.; Schrader,W.T.; O'Malley, B. Steroid receptor family: Structure and functions. Endocrine Reviews 11: 201–219; 1990.

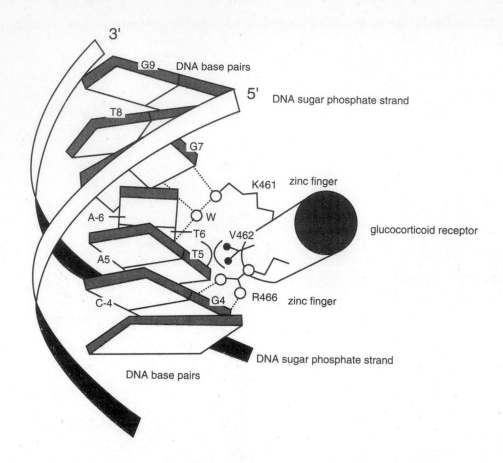

Figure 2.5 The model shows an example of interaction of a DNA-binding domain and a receptor for glucocorticoids. The first alpha helix of the nucleic acid, DNA, is on the left and constitutes the major groove of the GRE (glucocorticoid response element) half-site. In direct contact, on the right, is represented the GR (glucocorticoid receptor), bound by zinc fingers. Reprinted, with permission. Luisi, B.F.; Xu, W.X.; Otwinowski, Z.; Freedman, L.P.; Yamamoto, K.R.; Sigler, P.B. Crystallographic analysis of the interaction of the glucocorticoid receptor with DNA. Nature 352: 497–505; 1991; ©Macmillan Magazines Ltd.

responsible for cell differences.

In the case of hormone target cells, the receptor proteins, which may be glycoproteins, are referred to simply as the receptors. The receptors are different on different target cells. This makes it possible for a specific hormone and a specific target cell to recognize each other.

As mentioned, the hormone (or other substance) that binds to a receptor is called the ligand. Molecules that imitate a ligand's biological activity and bind to its receptor are **agonists**; molecules

that bind to a receptor but prevent biological activity of the natural hormone are called **antagonists**. A cell can have more than one kind of receptor, permitting it to respond to more than one hormone.

The structures of some receptors have been identified. For example, the amino acid sequence of the beta receptor for catecholamines has been worked out. It is similar to an amino acid sequence worked out for the retinal pigment rhodopsin.

Other identified receptors belong to the

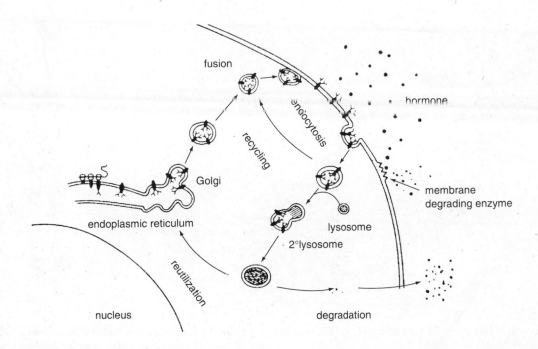

Figure 2.6 A general model for the life cycle of the hormone receptor is shown. Rough endoplasmic reticulum is the site for the synthesis of the membrane receptors. The Golgi apparatus is the site at which glycosylation occurs and the receptors are inserted in membrane with membrane fusion. The receptors bind hormone, aggregate, and are internalized by either coated or noncoated pits. An endosome containing the hormone-receptor complex fuses with lysosomes which degrade the hormone. The receptor is degraded or recycled to the membrane. Reproduced, with permission, C.R. Kahn. Membrane receptors for peptide hormones. In DeGroot, L.J., editor. Endocrinology. Philadelphia, PA: W. B. Saunders Co., Harcourt Brace Jovanovich, Inc.; 1989; p. 43.

"steroid receptor family" and include receptors for glucocorticoid, mineralocorticoid, estrogen, androgen, progesterone, and 1,25-dihydroxyvitamin D_3. There are receptors with structures similar to steroid receptors for thyroxine and retinoic acid (Figure 2.3)[2] The receptors possess a cysteine-rich region, or domain, which binds DNA and they may have a ligand-binding domain near the carbon terminal. The cysteines in the DNA-binding region form complexes with zinc ions called "zinc fingers."

Until they are associated with hormones, receptors are "inactive." Proteins have been proposed for involvement in the inactivation mechanism because isolated receptors were unable to bind DNA. One possible protein is the heat shock protein (HSP 90) which has been found complexed with steroid receptors. Adding a hormone dissociates the HSP-90 receptor complexes so that the receptors can be activated to bind

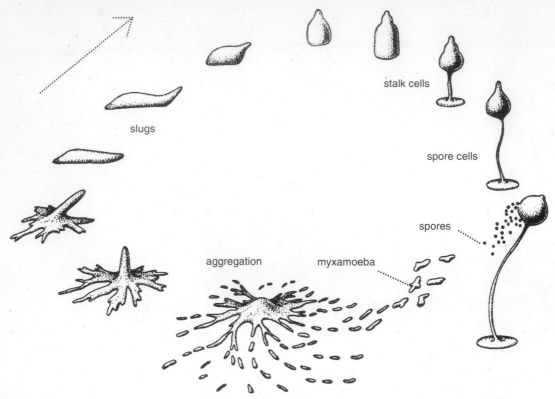

stalk cells

slugs

spore cells

spores

aggregation   myxamoeba

Figure 2.7 Life cycle of a slime mold. The spores shed form mature fruiting bodies called myxamoebae. When the good supply is reduced, the myxamoebae aggregate until a slug, or migrating pseudoplasmodium, is formed. When the slug stops moving, it forms a fruiting body to release more spores. Cyclic AMP functions as an attractant during the aggregation of the myxamoebae. Redrawn with permission, after Gilbert, S.F. Developmental Biology, Second Edition. Sunderland, MA: Sinauer Associates, Inc.; 1988, p. 22.

with DNA (Figure 2.4).

The interaction of the DNA and receptors has been modeled (Figure 2.5).[3] Luisi[4] and colleagues describe the interaction of the glucocorticoid receptor with DNA:

> Two crystal structures of the glucocorticoid receptor DNA-binding domain complexed with DNA are reported. The domain has a globular fold which contains two Zn-nucleated substructures of distinct conformation and function. When it binds DNA, the domain dimerizes, placing the subunits in adjacent major grooves. In one complex, the DNA has the symmetrical consensus target sequence; in the second, the central spacing between the target's half-sites is larger by one base pair. This results in one

subunit interacting specifically with the consensus target half-site and the other nonspecifically with a noncognate element. The DNA-induced dimer fixes the separation of the subunits' recognition surfaces so that the spacing between the half-sites becomes a critical feature of the target sequence's identity.

REGULATION OF RECEPTORS

Receptors can be regulated. Changes in the receptor numbers of target tissues alters their responsiveness to hormone signals. Increasing the numbers of receptors (per target cell or per target organ) is called **up regulation**; up regulation increases the sensitivity of cells to hormones. Low hormone levels can cause up regulation.

Decreasing the numbers of receptors in the cell surface is called **down regulation**. Down regulation makes the cells less sensitive to hormones. High hormone levels can cause down regulation.

Up regulation can be achieved by recycling receptors (and membrane) and by *de novo* synthesis of receptors.

How can down regulation be accomplished? Where do the receptors go? Any process that reduces the numbers of receptors can be considered as contributing to down regulation, but when insulin binds to its receptor, the hormone-receptor complex becomes "internalized"—that is, it goes inside the cell cytoplasm. This mechanism for internalization of receptors is called receptor-mediated endocytosis of hormone-receptor complexes. Receptor-mediated endocytosis can result in the loss of receptors on the cell surface and thus provides a mechanism for down regulation.

RECEPTOR-MEDIATED ENDOCYTOSIS

Receptor-mediated endocytosis is a process for down regulation that involves special coated pits (Figure 2.6). Some of the ligand receptors are in the **coated pits** on plasma membranes; the pits can be seen with a microscope. Coated pits, which can account for 2% of cell surface area, are made of a fibrous protein called "clathrin," and receptors cluster there. When the ligand binds to the receptor, it triggers endocytosis. A lateral movement of the cell membrane occurs so that the receptors end up aggregated in the coated pits. A vesicle forms when the pit pinches off. Hormones and receptors engulfed in such vesicles are internalized. Some vesicles have walls made up of clathrin, a polypeptide that forms a protein lattice. Some of these vesicles made from coated pits have walls and are, logically, called "coated vesicles."

Ligand internalization occurs when the hormone-receptor complex is taken into the cell. Ligand internalization may explain why peptide hormone receptors and peptide hormones have been found inside cells. Ligand internalization also makes it possible for a peptide hormone to have continued long-term action, or to bind to a receptor on an organelle. So a hormone could have both a rapid effect by binding to a receptor and a delayed effect by ligand internalization.

Receptor mediated endocytocis may function in internalization of low density lipids, insulin, epidermal growth factor, and nerve growth factor. Some of the vesicles fuse with lysozomes whose digestive enzymes dispose of the peptide hormones. Receptor-mediated endocytocis thus provides one means for down regulation. However, the purpose of the endocytocis is not just to inactivate peptide hormones and to destroy receptor complexes—receptor bound hormone molecules also produce actions within the target cell after being internalized.

Receptor-mediated endocytocis is distinguished from two other kinds of endocytocis. In **phagocytosis** (cell eating), the cell engulfs a large particle such as a bacterium. In **pinocytosis** (cell drinking), the cell surrounds a droplet of the liquid extracellular medium and anything dissolved in the liquid to form a vesicle about 0.1 micrometer in diameter. Cell drinking is nonspecific. Receptor-mediated endocytocis is specific because the receptors are membrane proteins that have binding sites that fit a particular ligand (e.g., a hormone) which is a protein or small particle.

Receptor-mediated endocytocis of hormone complexes can be seen as a subset of the way that receptors in general can bring proteins and particles into cells. Other examples are proteins in the yolk of insect and bird eggs, antibodies (from the mother's blood) in fetal cells lining the yolk sac, cholesterol bearing LDL receptors, and hormones and other proteins that deliver signals to cells. Receptor-mediated endocytosis can be very rapid as described by Dautry-Varsat and Lodish[5] for the transferrin (a carrier protein that binds iron ions) receptor:

> On the average it takes four minutes for a transferrin receptor on the surface to bind to a ferrotransferrin ligand. The ferrotransferrin-receptor complex is internalized in about five minutes. It takes another seven minutes for the iron to dissociate from the transferrin and the apotransferrin-receptor complex to return to the surface, after which the apotransferrin is released from the receptor in only 16 seconds. The total elapsed time is about 16 minutes.

Table 2.1 Intracellular Messengers and Their Chemical Messengers[6]

CYCLIC AMP	CALCIUM ION-DIACYLGLYCEROL
adrenocorticotropin	acetylcholine
ß-adrenergic catecholamines	α-adrenergic catecholamines
calcitonin	angiotensin
follicle-stimulating hormone	cholecystokinin
glucagon	gastrin
luteinizing hormone	oxytocin
parathyroid hormone	vasopressin
secretin	luteinizing hormone-releasing hormone
thyroid-stimulating hormone	thyroid-stimulating hormone-releasing hormone
vasopressin	
acetylcholine	
α-adrenergic catecholamines	
dopamine	
opiate peptides	
somatostatin	
	TYROSINE KINASE
CYCLIC GMP	epidermal growth factor
atrial natriuretic peptide	insulin
	insulin-like growth factor

COOPERATIVITY

Yet another means of regulation, besides up and down regulation, exists in the possibility of modulating the affinity of receptors. Hormone binding can affect subsequent binding of other receptors on the cells. The effects of a hormone on receptor binding are collectively referred to as "cooperativity." If affinity of receptors is increased by a hormone, the binding is called "positive cooperativity," and the cells are sensitized to the hormone. If the affinity of receptors is decreased by the hormone, the binding is called "negative cooperativity"; the cells are desensitized to the hormone. If the hormone does not change affinity of its receptors, the binding is noncooperative.

SPARE RECEPTORS

Cells give maximum biological responses when only a few receptors, perhaps only 1%, are occupied. The remaining receptors are called "spare receptors." Aren't spare receptors superfluous? The extra receptors may be present to increase sensitivity to low hormone concentrations. But some cells give larger responses when there is more hormone, so the spare receptors may be present to permit a graded response.

SOCIAL AMOEBAE

A remarkable (or maybe unremarkable!) organism played a role in the elucidation of the cyclic AMP involvement in hormone mechanisms of action. A slime mold, one of the Acrasiales, lives out its life cycle in the soil (Figure 2.7. In some ways, it looks and acts like human white blood cells (leukocytes). The slime mold amoebae consume bacteria by eating them in a process called endocytosis. When the amoebae run out of food, they aggregate in colonies of 100,000 cells. The properties of the whole (aggregate amoebae, the "slug") is greater than the sum of its parts (individual amoebae). The slug can crawl, it is attracted to heat, it is attracted to light, and it has

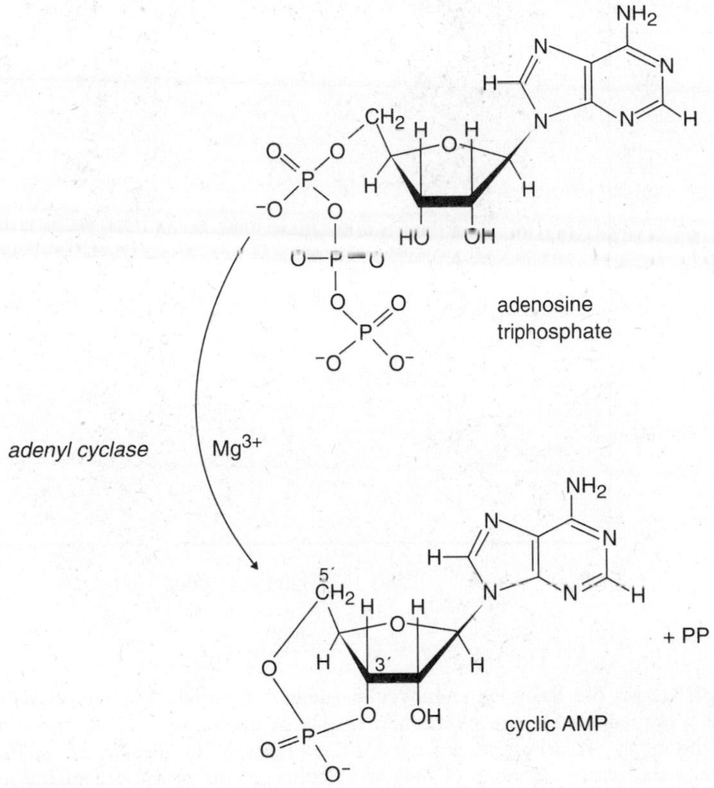

Figure 2.8 Cyclic AMP is synthesized from ATP (adenosine triphosphate) by removing two phosphate groups and enclosing a ring. Adenyl cyclase catalyzed the formation of cyclic AMP. Cyclic AMP is inactivated (not shown) by phosphodiesterase which breaks the ring by hydrolysis, producing inactive product, 5'adenosine monophosphate (5'AMP). Modified, with permission, Devlin, T.M. Textbook of Biochemistry. New York: John Wiley & Sons; 1982; p. 205.

a head end. Its purpose seems to be to find a propitious location for formation and dissemination of its reproductive spores. When it finds such a location, its appearance changes. The amoebae reorganize to form a stalk and spores, and the spores disperse to start new generations of amoebae.

Of interest to endocrinology are the mechanics of the aggregation process. Experimentally, the amoebae were attracted, even through a semipermeable membrane. In a stream of water, the downstream amoebae aggregated. This led

Bonner to reject temperature and electricity as explanations, and instead, to hypothesize that a small molecule was involved in the attraction. He says: "I favored the idea of a chemical, and I gave the unidentified attractant the name acrasin because the proper name of the cellular slime molds is Acrasiales, and also because in Edmund Spenser's Faerie Queene there is a witch named Acrasia who attracted men and transformed them into beasts."[7]

Problems in isolating the attractant made it appear that the acrasin rapidly disappeared. It was

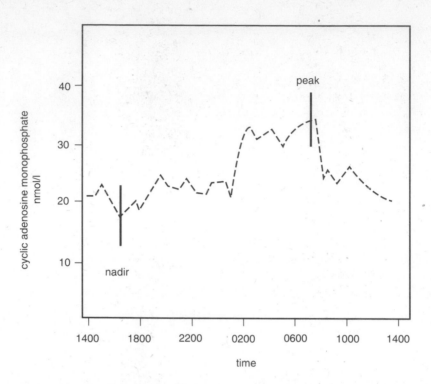

Figure 2.9 The graph shows the daily cycle in cyclic adenosine monophosphate concentration in six normal humans. Cyclic AMP was measured in the glomerular filtrate of the kidney. Error bars (vertical lines) represent the standard errors of the mean. Redrawn, after Logue, F.C.; Fraser, W.D.; Reilly, St. J.; Besastall, G.H. The circadian rhythm of intact parathyroid hormone (1–84) and nephrogenous cyclic adenosine monophosphate in normal men. Journal of Endocrinology 121: R1–R3; 1989.

possible to collect the attractant by freezing water from aggregation centers. It was further possible to stabilize the acrasin by shaking the water with methanol. Another investigator, Shaffer, collected the acrasin by painting amoebae on the outside of a sausage casing; water dripped through the inside of the casing, collected the acrasin, and it was stable.

Using amoebae attraction as a bioassay, scientists Konijn and Barkley were able to show that a compound known as cyclic AMP attracted slime mold. Only 10 picograms (10^{-11} grams) were needed. The reason that the cyclic AMP appeared to be unstable was that the amoebae produced phosphodiesterase, an enzyme that breaks down cyclic AMP. In short, the amoebae were using cyclic AMP as a pheromone to aggregate.

SECOND MESSENGER HYPOTHESIS, CYCLIC AMP

Cyclic AMP is a main character in the endocrinology of vertebrates as well as in the behavior of slime molds.

In the second messenger hypothesis, or, since the hypothesis is well supported by evidence, the second messenger mechanism, an amine or peptide hormone is the first messenger (Table 2.1).[8] The first messenger arrives in the blood at the target cell membrane where it interacts with a specific receptor. The interaction activates an enzyme, adenyl cyclase, a process which has been named transduction. The activation of adenyl cyclase produces an intracellular increase in **cyclic AMP** (Figure 2.8) which acts as an intracellular second messenger.

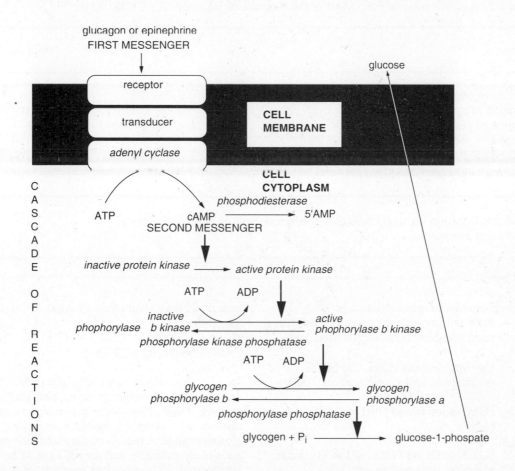

Figure 2.10 The diagram illustrates the classical cascade of reactions in the second messenger hypothesis where the hormone, glucagon (or epinephrine), is the first messenger and cyclic AMP is the second messenger.

The amazing thing about the second messenger concept is that it is a common mechanism for the action of a multitude of extracellular signals on cells. The hormones or first messengers are many, the cyclic AMP systems of their targets are similar, and the responses of their targets are diverse.

Cyclic AMP was discovered by Sutherland and Rall in 1958.[9]   Cyclic AMP (cAMP, cyclic 3'5' AMP, cyclic adenylic acid, cyclic adenosine 3'5'-monophosphate, 3'5'-cyclic adenosine monophosphate) is synthesized from ATP (adenosine triphosphate). The enzyme, **adenyl cyclase** (adenylate cyclase) catalyzes the reaction. Maximal effects of hormones are not additive,

which implies that when several hormones can affect a cell via cAMP, they do so by using the same population of adenyl cyclase molecules.

Most hormones have daily cycles. Those hormones that act via cAMP mechanisms should produce cAMP daily cycles in their target cells (Figure 2.9).

PHOSPHODIESTERASE

Cyclic AMP is inactivated by **phosphodiesterase** (PDE), which converts cyclic AMP to 5'AMP (5' adenosine monophosphate). The phosphodiesterase opens the cyclic ring. There are several different forms, or isoenzymes, of

Table 2.2 Amplification in Four Steps of the Cascade of Reactions for Cyclic AMP[10,11] ·

Reaction	Amplification
activation of adenylate cyclase in response to a hormone	
production of cyclic AMP	10^2
activation of protein kinase	
activation of phosphorylase kinase	10^2
activation of phosphorylase	10^2
production of glucose from glycogen	10^2
overall amplification—a single molecule of hormone may be able to release 10^8 molecules of glucose	10^8

phosphodiesterase in mammalian cells.

Five subfamilies of phosphodiesterases and their regulators have been characterized:

(i) Ca^{++}/calmodulin PDEs, CaM-PDE (muscarinic cholinergic agonists, LRH);

(ii)   cGMP-stimulated PDEs, cGS-PDE (ANF);

(iii)   cGMP-inhibited PDEs, cGI-PDE (insulin, glucagon, dexamethasone);

(iv)   cAMP-specific PDEs, cAMP-PDE (FSH, PGE_1, TSH, ß-adrenergic agonists); and

(v)   cGMP-specific PDEs, cGMP-PDE (light).

A hypothetical structure has been proposed for cyclic nucleotide phosphodiesterases. The molecule is proteinaceous with three regions, or domains. A regulatory domain at the N terminus has binding sites for cyclic GMP and calmodulin. A catalytic domain has about 270 amino acids and is similar among species. A C terminus domain has unknown function. Conti and colleagues suggest that the multiple forms of phosphodiesterases and their accompanying regulation provide a means of altering the time of cyclic nucleotide persistence: "By virtue of the multiple forms involved in this regulation, the changes in rate of cyclic nuceotide

hydrolysis may span over a period of minutes to days."[12]

CASCADE OF REACTIONS

One of the most appealing ideas in endocrinology is the concept of a **"cascade"** of re-**actions**. Most of the steps that make up a cascade involve activation of inactive enzymes. The response can be achieved quickly since the proteins are already available and do not have to be newly synthesized. The classical example of a second messenger and a cascade of reactions is the action of glucagon and epinephrine on liver cells that causes the liver cells to produce glucose from glycogen (Figure 2.10).

The cascade mechanism may first seem unnecessarily complex, but it permits **ampli-fication** (Table 2.2). Amplification can be demonstrated with the effect of glucagon on a liver cell: hundred-fold amplifications achieved by activation of four enzymes (adenyl cyclase activation, protein kinase activation, phosphorylase kinase activation, and phosphorylase) mean that one molecule of glucagon can release at least 10^8 molecules of glucose.[13] Thus, a small signal, just a few molecules of glucagon interacting with liver cell receptors, is amplified to a large result, the release of a profusion of molecules of glucose into the blood.

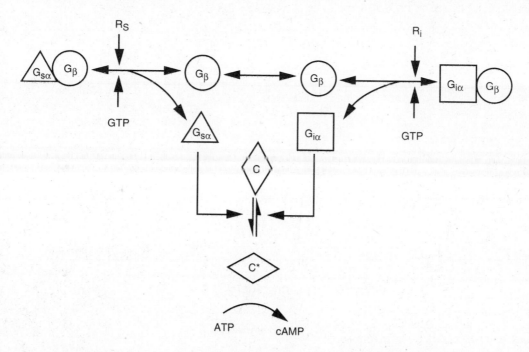

Figure 2.11 The diagram shows a model for transduction in the cell membrane. Left: A stimulatory hormone (not shown) is recognized by receptor R_s; GTP and R_s dissociate the subunits ($G_{s\alpha}$ and G_β) of the nucleotide regulatory (G) protein ; the $G_{s\alpha}$ subunit activates adenyl cyclase (C); cyclic AMP (cAMP) is produced. Right: A different and inhibitory hormone (not shown) is recognized by a different receptor (R_i); GTP and R_i dissociate the subunits ($G_{i\alpha}$ and G_β) of the nucleotide regulatory (G) protein with the same beta subunit (G_β) , but a different, and inhibitory, alpha subunit ($G_{i\alpha}$); the alpha subunit ($G_{i\alpha}$) inactivates adenyl cyclase. Reproduced, with permission. Gilman, A. G proteins and dual control of adenylate cyclase. Cell 36: 577–579; 1984.

TRANSDUCTION

When peptide hormones bind to their receptors, they increase the activity of enzymes. The mechanism for the receptor-enzyme activation process is called transduction (Figure 2.11). In the current view of this interaction, a **mobile receptor model**, there are two steps that follow in a sort of domino activation effect.

First, the hormone occupies the receptor protein and causes a change in the shape (conformation) of the receptor protein. The altered receptor protein then activates a **regulatory protein** in the cell membrane (e.g., guanyl nucleotide regulatory protein, GTPase) and the two proteins form a **regulatory unit**. The regulatory unit can bind GTP (obtained from inside the cell). The activated regulatory protein dissociates from the receptor.

Second, the activated regulatory protein and the enzyme adenyl cyclase interact so that adenyl cyclase is activated. Adenyl cyclase can then convert ATP to cyclic AMP. To deactivate the **catalytic unit** of the regulatory protein and the adenyl cyclase, the GTP is hydrolyzed to yield GDP, and this permits the regulatory protein to dissociate from the catalytic unit.

The regulatory proteins involved in transduction are from a family of **G proteins**. The G proteins are involved in the activation of adenyl cyclase, the inhibition of adenyl cyclase, regulation of potassium and calcium

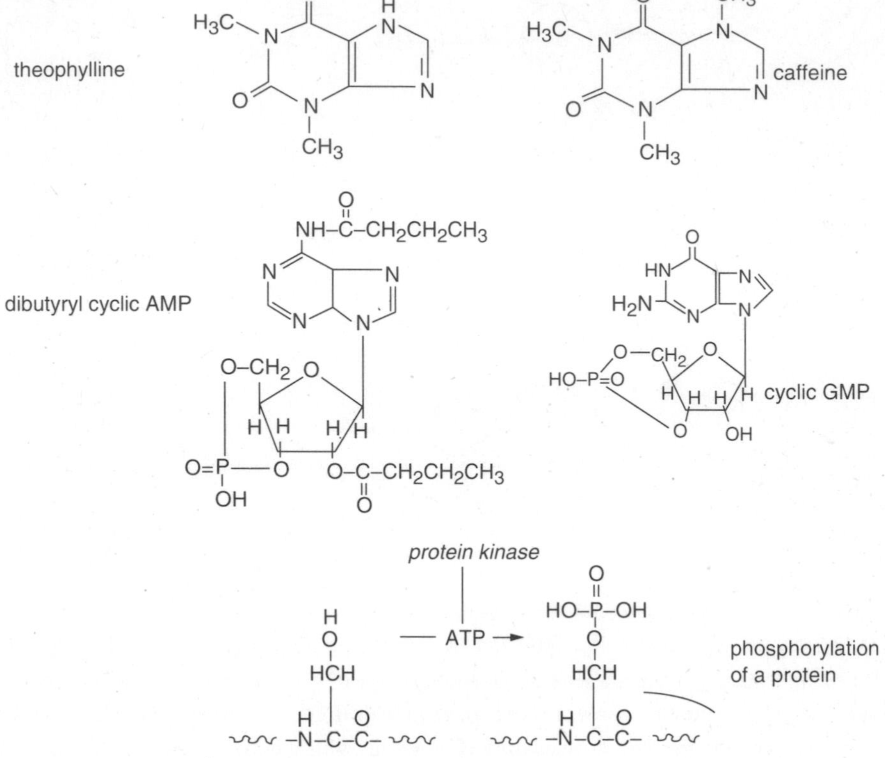

Figure 2.12 Phosphodiesterase blockers (theophylline, caffeine), a cyclic AMP analog (dibutyryl cyclic AMP), cyclic GMP, and phosphorylation of a protein are shown. Redrawn, with permission, Hadley, M.E. Endocrinology, Third Edition. Englewood Cliffs, NJ: Prentice Hall; 1992; pp. 72, 75, 76, 92.

ion channels, and senses (vision, smell). The G proteins have beta and gamma subunits that are alike, and they have alpha subunits that are different from one another.

One of the G proteins stimulates adenylate cyclase (designated G_s). A second inhibits adenyl cyclase (designated G_i). The two proteins have identical beta subunits and differing (s = stimulatory, i = inhibitory) alpha subunits. Another regulatory protein (designated G_p) activates phospholipase C. A fourth (transducin) links rhodopsin to phosphodiesterase. The G proteins allow for the possibility of interaction of two different receptors in the cell membrane to affect one adenyl cyclase.

CYCLIC AMP ASSAYS, ANALOGS, AND BLOCKERS

Attraction of the social amoebae provides a bioassay for cyclic AMP. Amoebae in a saline droplet are placed on an agar plate. A water droplet with the test substance is placed nearby. Attraction of amoebae out of their water droplet is a positive test for cyclic AMP. But it is not an easy assay. The agar must be just so rigid, the amoebae may migrate without a test substance, and the amoebae

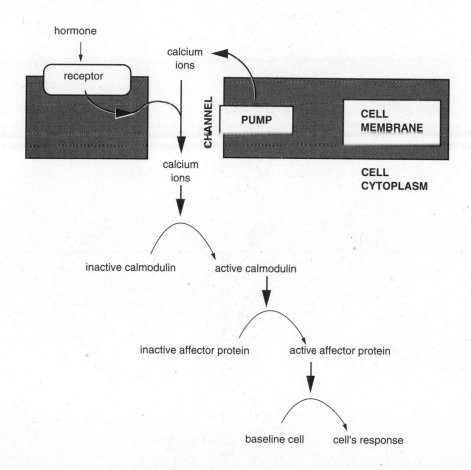

Figure 2.13 The diagram is a simplified representation of calcium ion movements and calmodulin participation in cell function. In this representation, the hormone interacts with a receptor, permitting calcium ions to enter the cytosol to function in affector protein (enzyme) activation.

must be exactly at the right stage of development. Easier, if less appealing, assays for cyclic AMP include enzyme assays, radioimmunoassays, electrophoretic assays, chromatographic assays, and binding assays.

Adenyl cyclase can be measured by determining the cyclic AMP production from radiolabelled precursors. Phosphodiesterase can be studied by measuring the 5'AMP production with 5'-nucleotidase.

Synthetic analogs of cyclic AMP (dibu-tyryl cAMP, 8-bromo cyclic AMP) have been created with more or less potency than cyclic AMP. Dibutyryl cyclic AMP (DB-cAMP) has the experimental advantage that it penetrates cell membranes more readily than cyclic AMP (Figure 2.12).

There are a group of chemicals, the "methyl xanthines," that inhibit phosphodiesterase. By preventing the breakdown of cyclic AMP, these chemicals potentiate or mimic hormones that use cyclic AMP mechanisms.

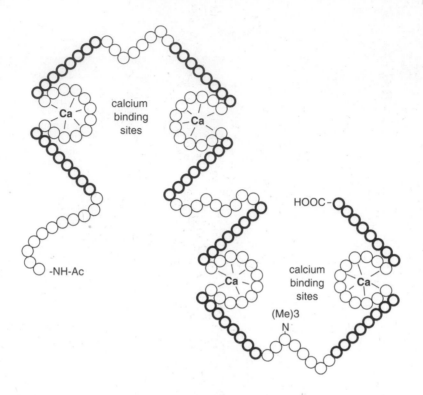

Figure 2.14 The structure of calmodulin (CDR) is illustrated. Calmodulin is a polypeptide with 148 amino acid residues represented here by circles. Calmodulin functions as an intracellular calcium receptor. It has four calcium binding sites (marked Ca) and it is structurally similar to troponin C found in muscle. Only seven amino acids differ when calmodulin from vertebrates is compared with calmodulin of marine coelenterates. Binding of calcium causes a conformational change in the calmodulin. Modified, with permission, after Klee, C.B.; Crouch, T.H.; Richman, P.G. Calmodulin. Annual Review of Biochemistry 49: 489–515; 1980.

Methylxanthines include theophylline, caffeine, and the synthetic 1-methyl-3-isobutylxanthine.

CYCLIC GMP

In the same way that cyclic AMP is made, cyclic GMP (cyclic guanosine monophosphate) is synthesized from GTP (guanosine triphosphate) with an enzyme named guanylate cyclase and catabolized with phosphodiesterase. In a manner similar to cyclic AMP, **cyclic GMP** can act as a second messenger. In some tissues, for example muscle, the two second messengers have opposite roles.

There is an appealing hypothesis about the opposing actions of cyclic AMP and cyclic GMP called the **yin yang hypothesis**. In this hypothesis, the two nucleotides have contrasting actions where cells have bimodal responses. But examples supporting this attractive hypothesis are sparse. Cyclic AMP causes smooth muscle relaxation and cyclic GMP causes smooth muscle

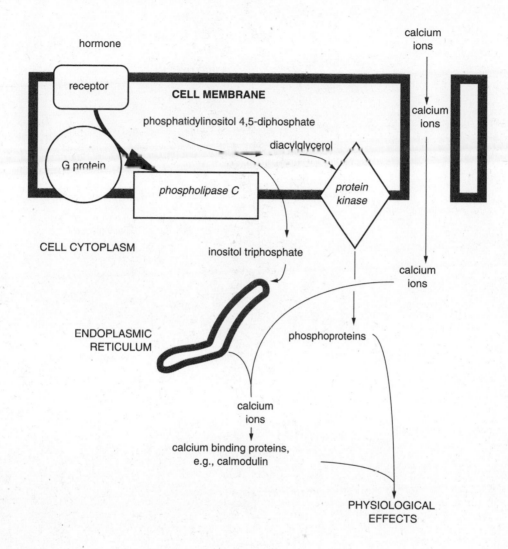

Figure 2.15 A hormone hypothetically activates phospholipase C, resulting in an increase in calcium in the cells via calmodulin.

contraction. The concentrations of the two cyclic nucleotides, cyclic AMP and cyclic GMP, vary inversely. In another example in nerve, cyclic GMP has a role in depolarization and cyclic AMP plays a role in hyperpolarization. Cyclic GMP increases are usually accompanied by a parallel rise in calcium ion which may activate a cytoplasmic form of guanylate cyclase.

CALCIUM AND CALMODULIN

Calcium ion has been considered to be an intracellular messenger (Figure 2.13). Calcium ion may work together with cAMP because calcium relates to the enzymes responsible for cAMP synthesis and destruction (adenyl cyclase

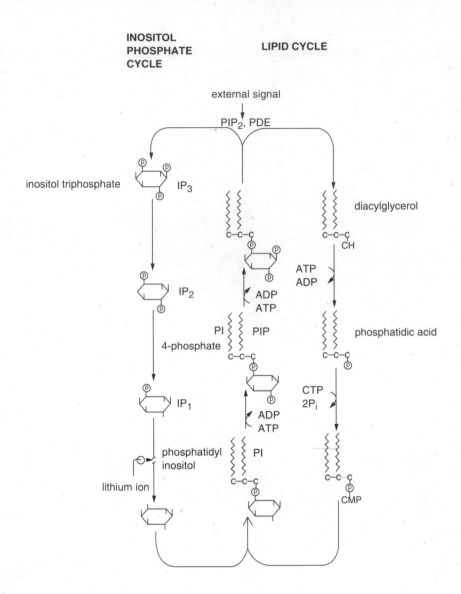

Figure 2.16 The relationships of inositol and diacylglycerol is shown by the inositol-lipid cycles. The enzyme PIP_2 phosphodiesterase, which breaks PIP_2 into diglycerol (DG) and IP_3, is controlled by external signals (top). ATP and CTP supply inorganic phosphate for the cycles. Lithium ions block the pathway. Modified, with permission, Berridge, M.J. The molecular basis of communication within the cell. In Rasmussen, H. Cell Communication in Health and Disease. New York: W.H. Freeman, Co.; 1991; p. 46.

and phosphodiesterase). Minute flows of calcium ion, acting transiently as go-betweens, convey signals from the cell surface to the inside of the cell. The concentration of calcium ions in fluid outside the cell is 10,000 times the concentration of calcium ions in the cytosol. The gradient is maintained by balancing calcium ion influx (calcium ion leakage into the cell) with calcium ion efflux (calcium ion driven out of the cell by a membrane-bound "pump"). A signal at the cell's surface (voltage change due to transmitter, receptor interaction with hormone or neurotransmitter) causes channels in the plasma membrane to open. Calcium and other ions flow in two to four times as fast. The calcium acts as an intracellular messenger. Calcium plays such roles in the secretion of hormones, secretion of neurotransmitters, secretion of digestive enzymes, cardiac and skeletal muscle contraction, intestinal water and salt transport, and regulation of liver glycogen.

The calcium attaches to calcium-binding proteins. The calcium-calcium binding protein complexes interact with other cell proteins causing the cells to alter their functions. The calcium-binding proteins (**calmodulin**, troponin C, and calcimedin) are found in cells of plants, invertebrates, and mammals. Calmodulin is found in the cytosol of all nucleated (eukaryotic) cells. Calmodulin is a single chain of 148 amino acids, with molecular weight 16,700 Daltons. Negatively charged carboxylate (COO-) side chains on glutamate or aspartate amino acids give it the ability to bind calcium ion.

Calmodulin functions as an intracellular calcium receptor and its structure has been identified (Figure 2.14). Calmodulin (calcium-dependent regulatory protein, CDR) forms a complex with calcium ions. The calmodulin-calcium complex activates enzymes by binding to them. Some enzymes activated by calmodulin include adenyl cyclase, phosphodiesterase, myosin light chain kinase, phospholipase A_2, calcium dependent ATPase, NAD kinase, calcium dependent protein kinase, and phosphorylase kinase.

Calcium binding proteins also participate in movement of chromosomes during mitosis, microtubule disassembly, muscle contraction, maintenance of intracellular calcium levels, and glycogen breakdown. According to Cheung,[14] calmodulin has a multiplicity of roles:

Calmodulin, then, has a double set of functions: it not only transmits calcium's message to receptor enzymes but also modulates the intracellular concentration of the ion.....Having sensed the arrival of calcium and thereby been activated to stimulate an enyzme, calmodulin proceeds to turn on the pump that rids the cell of unneeded calcium.

The calcium signal is short lived, or transient (i.e., finished within ten minutes). In order to achieve the more sustained secretion of hormones (i.e., for periods more than half an hour), an enzyme that functions as a "transducer," has been proposed.

Cheung suggests that the relationships of hormones, calcium, and cyclic nucleotides have to do with time—hormones act over minutes to hours or weeks; cyclic AMP acts in the seconds to minutes time range; and calcium functions in the millisecond range.

KINASES

Protein kinases in general are enzymes that are inside cells and which phosphorylate proteins. By phosphorylation, they change the proteins' configuration, which alters their activity.

Some endocrine target cells secrete their hormones via activation of **protein kinase C** (PKC) which is a family of calcium phospholipid dependent protein kinases (Figure 2.15). Endocrine targets that use protein kinase C include adrenal cells (catecholamines, aldosterone), pancreatic beta cells (insulin), pituitary cells (GH, LH, PRO, TSH), parathyroid cells (PTH), and testis Leydig cells (steroids). Nonendocrine tissues also use protein kinase C and they include exocrine pancreas amylase secretion, parotid gland amylase and mucin secretion, lung alveolar cell surfactant secretion, neuromuscular junctions acetylcholine secretion, caudate nucleus acetylcholine secretion, platelet thromboxane synthesis, neutrophil superoxide generation, mast cell release of histamine, and lymphocyte activation of T and B cells.[15]

Some hormones (e.g., epidermal growth factor) act through a receptor that acts like a tyrosine kinase. The tyrosine kinase phosphorylates proteins.

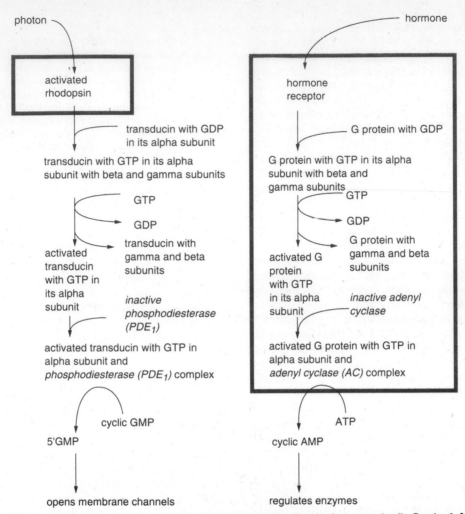

Figure 2.17 The diagram shows similarities that may exist in two "excitation cascades." On the left is a model by which the retina responds to light using 5'GMP; on the right is a very similar sequence of events for the production of cyclic AMP in response to a hormone signal. The rectangles enclose events of the cell membrane.

PHOSPHOINOSITIDES

Phosphoinositides are another group of molecules that also can function as second messengers (Figure 2.16). **Inositol triphosphate** and **diacylglycerol (DAG)** and **arachidonic acid** (precursor of prostaglandins, prostacyclins, thromboxanes, and leukotrienes) are messenger molecules that are liberated from phosphoinositides in response to hormones and their agonists Angiotensin II uses such a mechanism. The sequence of events in the mechanism may be as follows: (i)

the hormone binds to a membrane receptor. (ii) Via a G protein, the hormone activates **phospholipase C (PLC)**. (iii) Phospholipase C hydrolyzes phosphoinositol diphosphate (PIP_2, also called bisphosphate), which is found in cell membranes, to produce diacylglycerol (DAG) and inositol triphosphate (IP_3). (iv) Inositol triphosphate (also called trisphosphate) releases calcium ions from the endoplasmic reticulum. (v) The calcium ions bind to calcium-binding proteins to produce physiological effects in the cell. Meanwhile, at the

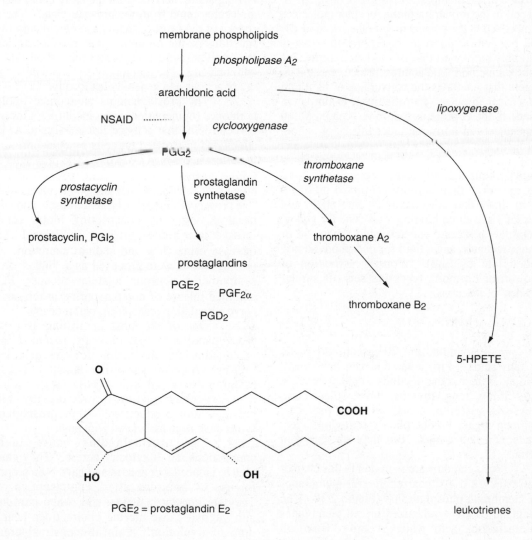

Figure 2.18 Synthesis of prostaglandins from cell membrane phospholipids is shown. NSAIDs are non-steroidal anti-inflammatory drugs (aspirin, indomethacin) that inhibit cyclooxygenase. The letters PG- in an abbreviation indicate a prostaglandin. 5-HPETE is 5-hydroperoxyeicosatetraenoic acid. The structure of one prostaglandin, PGE_2, is shown in the lower left.

cell membrane, diacylglycerol activates protein kinase C in the cell membrane, causing the production of phosphoproteins which also have physiological effects.

HORMONE ACTION AND VISION

Remarkable parallels have been found between the hormone action and vision (Figure 2.17).[16] First, the important receptor molecules are in membranes. The rhodopsin molecule is embedded in the membrane of the disk organelle of a rod cell in the retina; hormone receptor molecules are embedded in the plasma membrane. Second, the visual pigment, rhodopsin, has a structure that is remarkably similar to that of the beta receptor for catecholamine hormone actions. Third, transducin, a protein that mediates the conversion of light into an electrical impulse (transduction), is similar in structure to the G proteins that have been proposed as transducers in hormone mechanisms of action. Transducin and G proteins both have three subunits (signal-coupling proteins have similar beta subunits, about half the same sequences in their alpha subunits), their activity is "turned off" by a built-in timer that converts GTP into GDP, and they each have three binding sites (one for guanyl nucleotides, a second for activated rhodopsin or hormone receptor, and a third for phosphodiesterase or adenylate cyclase). Fourth, activation of rhodopsin or hormone receptors sets off similar "cascades" of reactions.

PROSTAGLANDINS

Prostaglandins are 20-carbon carboxylic acid "fatty acids." Prostaglandins have been found in prostate, semen, renal medulla, seminal vesicles, uterine lining, lung, thymus, brain, spinal cord, kidney, iris, placenta, menstrual fluid, pancreas, blue-green algae, higher plants, sea whips, gorgonians, and soft corals. But they are absent in bacteria.

Prostaglandins are included in this chapter because they are synthesized in cell membranes from membrane phospholipids (Figure 2.18. The prostaglandins are synthesized in cell membranes from arachidonic acid, which is derived from cell membrane phospholipids. Prostaglandin synthetase converts cyclic endoperoxide intermediates (PGG_2, PGH_2) into prostaglandins, and prostacyclin synthetase converts the intermediates to prostacyclin. The family of compounds to which the prostaglandins belong are the **eicosanoids**. Eicosanoids, which are derivatives of arachidonic acid, also include the thromboxane and leukotrienes. Molecules of the family activate membrane nucleotide cyclases such as adenyl cyclase (PGE_2, PGI_2) or guanylate cyclase (TXA_2, $PGF_{2\alpha}$).

In 1930, Lieb and Kurzroik noticed that semen contracted uterine strips. The name, prostaglandin, derives from the early belief that the molecules came from the prostate gland. The discovery of the prostaglandins and elucidation of the functions of the hormones met early obstacles in the small amounts present and their short (90-second) half-life. The hormones have a bewildering array of actions and generally act locally.

The prostaglandins antagonize lipolytic hormones (epinephrine, norepinephrine, glucagon, corticotropin) that activate lipase. Cyclic AMP is stimulated in isolated fat cells by epinephrine, but the effect is blocked by PGE_1. The prostaglandins inhibit gastric secretion (acid, pepsin) and this effect prevented duodenal and peptic ulcers in rats. The prostaglandins relax bronchi muscle and widen nasal passages by constricting blood vessels. Infused into kidney arteries, PGE_1 and PGA_1 increase urine flow and sodium excretion. The prostaglandins were proposed as a "brake" on the sympathetic nervous system because PGE_2 inhibited release of norepinephrine in response to nerve stimulation (cat spleen, rabbit heart).

One of the most interesting aspects of prostaglandins is that they are included in an explanation for the action for the pain killer aspirin. Aspirin, and other nonsteroidal anti-inflammatory drugs (NSAIDs) inhibit cyclooxygenase activity and thereby block prostaglandin production. High prostaglandin levels have been associated with pain.

The prostaglandins cause uterine contractions, an "oxytocic" action. They can be used to induce labor at term and have been proposed for use as "morning after" contraceptive pills. They are present in semen and, when introduced into vagina, cause uterine contractions near the time of ovulation. Painful menstrual cramps (dysmenorrhea) occur in 30–50% of women. The cramps are accompanied by two to three times normal levels of prostaglandin in the menstrual fluid. The cramping is relieved by drugs that inhibit prostaglandin synthesis (ibuprofen, indomethacin, mefenamic acid, naproxen-sodium, aspirin).

CYTOPLASMIC RECEPTORS FOR STEROIDS AND THYROID HORMONES

In contrast to the cell membrane receptors for amine and peptide hormones, the receptors for

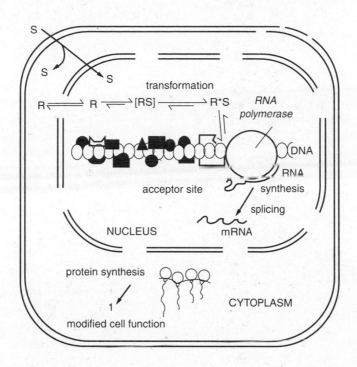

Figure 2.19 The diagram illustrates the mechanism of action for steroid hormones. S = steroid; R = receptor; a section of DNA (e.g., glucocorticoid regulatory element or GRE in the glucocorticoid mechanism of action) is represented, presumably, with various interacting molecules (blackened). Redrawn, with permission, Walters, M.R. Steroid hormone receptors and the nucleus. Endocrine Reviews 6:512–543, 1985; p. 532.

steroid hormones and thyroid hormones are not located in the cell membrane. Instead the receptors are located in the cell cytoplasm (Figure 2.19) and cell nucleus (Figure 2.20). These receptors and their hormones carry out their functions by acting on genes to alter the production of proteins. Chin[17] describes this "hormonal regulation of gene expression:"

> ....the major effect of hormones [on gene expression] is exerted at the transcriptional level. Clearly, modulation of gene activity by altering transcriptional rates of genes can significantly alter the amount of protein ultimately produced in a cell by determining, in a major way, the level of functional mRNA in the cytoplasm.

Chin also describes potential sites of hormonal regulation of gene expression. The sites for regulation include events of transcription (initiation, elongation, termination), heteronuclear RNA (alternative RNA splicing, degradation), mRNA metabolism and extranuclear transport, events of translation (initiation, elongation, termination), posttranslation events (alternative protein processing, noncovalent events such as folding of the protein, covalent events such as phosphorylation and glycosylation, degradation), storage, and secretion. Of these events, all of which may be affected by hormones, Chin singles out the **transcriptional initiation** as the key event.

The general model for the mechanism action of steroids was developed studying effects of estrogen on rat uteri and effects of progesterone on chick oviducts.[18,19,20,21] The model has the following sequence: (i) The lipid soluble steroids

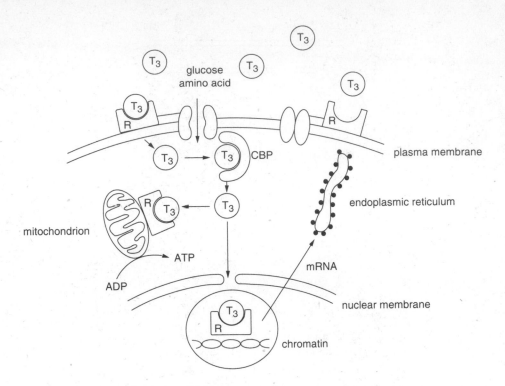

Figure 2.20 The diagram illustrates the mechanism of action for thyroid hormones. T_3 = triiodothyronine, a thyroid hormone; R = receptor protein; CBP = cytoplasmic binding proteins. Redrawn, with permission, Williams, J. A. Mechanisms of hormone secretion and action. In Greenspan, F., editor. Basic and Clinical Endocrinology. Norwalk, CN: Appleton & Lange, p. 18.

enter the cell; the mechanism is assumed to be diffusion. (ii) Inside the cell, the steroids bind to receptor proteins. (iii) The steroid-receptor complex migrates (translocation) to the cell nucleus. In older models the steroid-receptor complex was also believed to change form (transformation) during the migration. In more recent models, the steroid may be transferred from one receptor to another. (iv) Inside the cell nucleus, the steroid-receptor complex interacts with chromosomal proteins. (v) Chromatin binding of the steroid-receptor complex causes derepression of a DNA sequence and increased messenger RNA synthesis (transcription). (vi) The new mRNA exits the cell nucleus, enters the endoplasmic reticulum, and serves as a template for the construction of new proteins from amino acids (translation). Alternatively, it is possible that there are receptor sites for hormones in the nucleus itself.

Specificity occurs in the receptor protein, the chromosomal proteins, the DNA sequence, the mRNA synthesized, and the final protein produced. In other words, the hormone causes the cell to produce one or more specific proteins. Usually the protein that is produced is characteristic of the target cell (e.g., actin and myosin in uterine muscle). Receptor specificity determines which hormones a given cell responds to even though the same hormones may enter all cells. The receptor for estrogen in uterine cells is named estrophilin.

Amplification occurs in the cytoplasmic receptor mechanisms because more than one mRNA molecule can be transcribed from the derepressed DNA and more than one protein molecule can be translated from each mRNA molecule.

The responses mediated by intracellular receptors are generally thought of as being slower

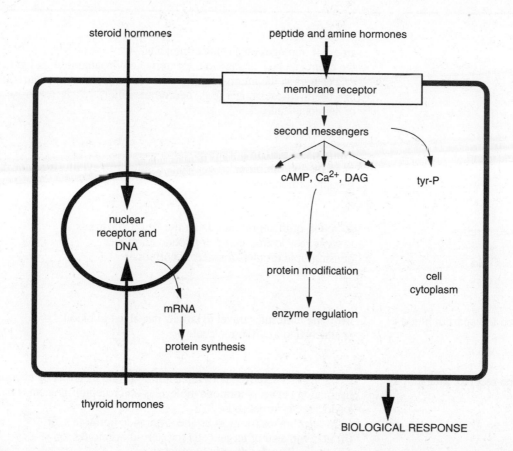

Figure 2.21 A simplified overall diagram of a "target" cell showing various pathways through which different types of hormones act upon a cell to achieve their function which is to produce new proteins (enzymes) or to regulate enzymes, and, in the end, to stimulate or inhibit the biological response of the cell. The large rectangle represents the cell membrane; the circle represents the cell nucleus. Redrawn, with permission, after a model in West, J.B., editor. Physiological Basis of Medical Practice, Twelfth Edition. Baltimore: Williams & Wilkins; 1991; p. 784.

(taking hours or days) than those that use membrane receptors (taking seconds or minutes).

CRITERIA FOR DISTINGUISHING BETWEEN CYCLIC AMP AND STEROID MECHANISMS OF ACTION

There are criteria for distinguishing between the cyclic AMP and steroid types of mechanisms of action. Criteria that must be satisfied to propose a cyclic AMP mechanism of action include: (i) The hormone (first messenger) raises cyclic AMP in the target cells. (ii) Theophylline (which blocks phosphodiesterase) mimics the action of the hormone. (iii) Cyclic AMP mimetics (DBcAMP) imitate the action of the hormone. (iv) The temporal sequence should be increased in cyclic AMP, then increased protein phosphorylation, and finally the cellular response. (v) The hormone should stimulate adenyl cyclase. Moreover, it is

Table 2.3 Generalized Sequence of Endocrine Events

signal	an event impinges on an endocrine gland— the event can be a change in the external environment (e.g., light), or a change in the internal environment (e.g., glucose concentration), or a chemical messenger (e.g., neurotransmitter), or hormone feedback
endocrine gland	synthesis of protein hormones, or activation/inhibition of enzymes resulting in synthesis of amine or steroid hormone molecules
hormone secretion	secretion of the hormones using the Golgi apparatus to form vesicles for amine or peptide hormones or using lipid droplets for steroid hormones
hormone transport in blood	hormone molecules travel to targets dissolved in blood or attached to a carrier molecule
hormone-receptor interaction	recognition is achieved between a hormone and its target by chemical interaction between hormone molecules and receptor molecules that are located in target cells: (i) in membranes for most amine or peptide hormones, or (ii) in cytoplasm of target cells for steroid hormones, or (iii) the nucleus for thyroid hormones
target response	initiation of a cascade of reactions in the target cells via a second messenger for most peptide or amine hormones, or stimulation of protein synthesis in the target cells for steroid hormones and thyroid hormones— the response of the target cell is characteristic of the target cell (e.g., synthesis of glucose or another hormone)

not necessary for the hormone to penetrate the cell membrane to cause its biological action.

On the other hand, to meet criteria for steroid mechanism of action, it is important that the hormone first enter the cell. A temporal sequence of events should then commence if the hormone is stimulatory: increase in RNA polymerase, increase in RNA, increase in protein synthesis.

SEQUENCE OF ENDOCRINE FUNCTION

The plethora of endocrine phenomena described in these introductory chapters can at first seem overwhelming. However, they can all be fitted into a rather simple framework (Figure 2.21, Table 2.3) in which a gland responds to a signal by secreting its particular hormone which is carried by the blood to a target organ where the hormone exerts its action with cyclic nucleotides or receptors that interact with DNA using zinc fingers.[22]

DISEASES INVOLVING RECEPTORS AND MECHANISMS OF ACTION

Sometimes cell communication fails and disease results. There are some disorders in which receptors, eicosanoids, and mechanisms of action have been assigned roles. Some examples include cholera, Grave's disease, myasthenia gravis, and dysmenorrhea.

Vibrio cholerae, the pathogen that causes **cholera**, secretes cholera toxin which binds to receptor sites on cells lining the small intestine. They bind to guanyl nucleotide regulatory protein. The binding is irreversible and leads to constant cyclic AMP production with abnormal water and electrolytes as a consequence.

In **Grave's disease**, hyperthyroidism is caused by an immunoglobulin called thyrotropin-stimulating antibody (TSAb) which occupies the thyrotropin receptors and causes excess thyroid hormone production.

The presence of antibodies to cholinergic receptors is considered an "autoimmune" disease, **myasthenia gravis**. Antibodies to receptors for acetylcholine block neuromuscular junction function, which, in turn, causes muscle dysfunction.

Dysmenorrhea, menstrual cramping, involves high prostaglandins. Thus, menstrual cramps can be treated with NSAIDs which inhibit prostaglandin synthesis.

REFERENCES

1. Getzenberg, R.H.; Pienta, K.J.; Coffey, D. The tissue matrix: Cell dynamics and hormone action. Endocrine Reviews 11: 399; 1990.
2. Carson-Jurica, M.A.; Schrader, W.T.; O'Malley, B. Steroid receptor family: Structure and functions. Endocrine Reviews 11: 201–204; 1990.
3. Freedman, L.P. Anatomy of steroid receptor zinc finger region. Endocrine Reviews 13: 129–145; 1992.
4. Luisi, B.F.; Xu, W.X.; Otwinowski, Z.; Freedman, L.P.; Yamamoto, K.R.; Sigler, P.B. Crystallographic analysis of the interaction of the glucocorticoid receptor with DNA. Nature 352: 497–505; 1991.
5. Dautry-Varsat, A.; Lodish, H.F. How receptors bring proteins and particles into cells. In Rasmussen, H., editor. Cell Communication in Health and Disease. New York: W. H. Freeman and Company; 1991; pp. 90–101 (or Scientific American, May, 1984).
6. Williams, J.D. Mechanisms of hormone secretion and action. In Greenspan, F.S., editor. Basic and Clinical Endocrinology, Third Edition. Norwalk: CT: Appleton & Lange; 1991; p. 11.
7. Bonner, J.T. Hormones in social amoebae and mammals. Scientific American 220: 78–91; 1969.
8. Greenspan, F.; Forsham, P., editors. Basic and Clinical Endocrinology, Los Altos, CA: Lange Medical Publications; 1986.
9. Sutherland, E. Studies on the mechanism of hormone action. Science 177: 401–408; 1972.
10. Turner, J.T.; Bagnara, J.T. General Endocrinology, Sixth Edition. Philadelphia: W. B. Saunders; 1976; p. 310.
11. Goldberg, N.D. Cyclic nucleotides and cell function. Hospital Practice May:127; 1974.
12. Conti, M.; Catherine Jin, S.-L.; Monaco, L.; Repaske, D.R.; Sinnen, J.V. Hormonal regulation of cyclic nucleotide phosphodiesterases. Endocrine Reviews 12: 218–234; 1991.
13. Goldberg, N.D. Op. cit.
14. Cheung, W.Y. Calmodulin. In Rasmussen, H., editor. Cell Communication in Health and Disease, New York: W. H. Freeman and Company; 1991; pp. 51–65 (or Scientific American, June 1982).
15. Ganong, W. Review of Medical Physiology, Thirteenth Edition. Norwalk, CT: Appleton & Lange; 1987.
16. Stryer, L. The molecules of visual excitation. In Rasmussen, H., editor. Cell Communication in Health and Disease. New York: W. H. Freeman and Company; 1991; pp. 76–89 (or Scientific American, July, 1987).

17. Chin, W. W. Hormonal regulation of gene expression.   In Degroot, L. J., editor. Endocrinology. Philadelphia: W. B. Saunders Co.; 1989, pp. 8–15.

18. O'Malley, B. W.; Means, A.R. Female steroid hormones and target cell nuclei. Science 183: 610–620; 1974.

19. Jensen, E.V; E.R. DeSombre. Estrogen-receptor interactions. Science 182: 126–134; 1973.

20. Hamilton,T. Control by estrogen of genetic transcription. Science 161: 649–661; 1968.

21. O'Malley, B.W.; Schrader, W.T.. Receptors of steroid hormones. Scientific American, 234 (February), p. 32–43; 1976.

22. Rhodes, D.; Klug, A. Zinc fingers. Scientific American 268 (February): 56–65; 1993.

SECTION II

AMINE AND PEPTIDE HORMONES FROM GLANDS IN THE HEAD: HYPOTHALAMUS, PITUITARY, AND PINEAL

Neuroendocrinology comprises a subtopic of endocrinology and deals, generally, with the hormones that are made in the hypothalamus of the brain or in the glands, the pituitary and pineal, which are anatomically connected to the brain by short stalks. The principal brain hormones are synthesized in the hypothalamus. The hormones of the pituitary control other endocrine glands, and this is why the pituitary gland was called the "master gland." The pineal gland has been linked especially to those functions that involve environmental lighting and circadian rhythms.

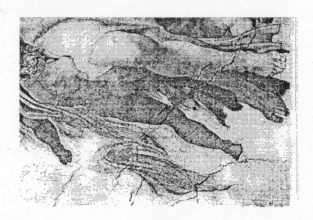

CHAPTER 3

Hypophysiotropic Neurohormones

A part of the brain, the hypothalamus, functions as an endocrine gland whose hormones control the pituitary gland (the hypophyseotropic neurohormones) and a family of nonapeptide hormones (the hypothalamic neurohormones). The pituitary is in many ways slave of and conduit for the hypothalamus. Each of the endocrine hierarchies in which the hypothalamus is a participant will be discussed in separate chapters. The nonapeptide hormones, such as oxytocin and vasopressin, will be further covered in their own chapter and the chapters on reproduction.

ANATOMY

The hypothalamus is a part of the brain that lies at its base (Figures 3.1 and 3.2). The hypothalamus is connected to the pituitary gland by a stalk, the infundibulum. The hormones of the hypothalamus are all peptides ranging from the smallest which has 3 amino acid residues to the largest which has almost 45 amino acid residues.

The hypothalamus has been subdivided by scientists into a number of subregions, or nuclei (Figure 3.3). The nuclei are collections of brain cells. The use of the terms "nuclei" or "nucleus" or "nuclear area" to refer to a collection of brain cells is not to be confused with the use of the word "nucleus" to refer to the nucleus of a cell. Unfortunately, in endocrinology, decisions as to the meaning of the words—nuclear, nuclei, nucleus— have to be made in the context of the word use. Some of the regions of the hypothalamus that are of particular interest to endocrinologists are named the supraoptic nucleus, the paraventricular nucleus, and the suprachiasmatic nucleus.

Unmyelinated nerve fibers impinge upon the regions of the hypothalamus. Those fibers carrying incoming information are afferent neural pathways, and those fibers carrying signals away from the hypothalamus are efferent pathways. Many areas of the brain communicate with the hypothalamus with tracts of nerve fibers. Some parts of the brain that exchange information with the hypothalamus include: fornix, stria terminalis, serotonergic neurons, adrenergic neurons, and the periventricular system. Some communicating tracts (bundles of nerve fibers) are medial forebrain bundle, dorsal and ventral noradrenergic bundles, retinohypothalamic fibers, thalamohypothalamic fibers, and pallidohypothalamic fibers. Efferent pathways include the hypothalamohypophyseal tract. Tracts are named for the regions they connect (e.g., retinohypothalamic fibers connect the retina and hypothalamus, the hypothalamohypophyseal tract connects the hypothalamus with the pituitary gland).

NEUROVASCULAR HYPOTHESIS

The idea that nerve cells of the hypothalamus make neurohormones that are transported down nerve fibers to the median eminence where they are released into the blood and transported via the portal vessels to act on the adenohypophysis is the "neurovascular hypothesis" (Figure 3.4).[1] The hormones of the hypothalamus fit the classic idea of **neurosecretion**—neurohormones, hormones made by nerve cells, are secreted into the blood. All of the hypothalamic hormones are neurohormones, and they all meet the definition of hormones in that they are ultimately transported by blood. The hypothalamic hormones are secreted in two neurohemal organs—the median eminence and the posterior pituitary.

The hypophysiotropic neurohormones of the hypothalamus control the hormones of the anterior pituitary gland. Neurosecretory cells of the hypothalamus secrete some neurohormones in the median eminence which in turn target another endocrine gland, the pituitary gland, causing it to release or to retain its hormones. This is the relationship of the hypophysiotropic neurohormones of the hypothalamus to the anterior pituitary hormones.

Neurohormones of the hypothalamus can be secreted into a storage cell in the posterior pituitary; the posterior pituitary subsequently resecretes the neurohormones into the blood. Or, neurohormones of the hypothalamus may be secreted directly into the blood in the posterior pituitary gland, bypassing the storage cell

The relationship of the hypothalamus to the pituitary gland is of great importance to the organism because it provides a means by which the endocrine system can make appropriate responses to changes in the organism's environment. As stated by William Ganong:

> The nervous system receives information about changes in the internal and external environment from the sense organs. It brings about adjustments to these changes through effector mechanisms that include not only somatic movement but also changes in the rate at which hormones are secreted.[2]

NOMENCLATURE

The hypothalamic hormones can be divided into two groups: the hypothalamic neurohormones and the hypophysiotropic (alternately spelled hypophyseotropic) neurohormones (Table 3.1).

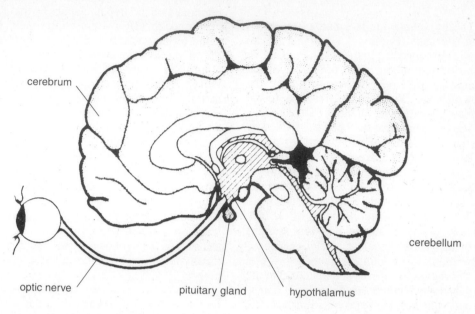

cerebrum

cerebellum

optic nerve

pituitary gland

hypothalamus

Figure 3.1 The sketch shows the location of the hypothalamus in relation to the pituitary gland and other parts of the brain. Modified, with permission, Fregly, M.; Luttge, W. Human Endocrinology: An Interactive Text. New York: Elsevier Biomedical; 1982, p. 32.

The first group of hormones is the structural family of peptide hormones (with eight, or nine, amino acid residues) that are synthesized in the supraoptic and paraventricular nuclei of the hypothalamus. Most of the fibers from the paraventricular nucleus end in the median eminence; most of the fibers from the supraoptic nucleus end in the posterior lobe of the pituitary. To reach the posterior lobe, **hypothalamic neurohormones** descend the hypothalamohypophysial tract. The word "tract" refers to a bundle or collection of nerve fibers. Oxytocin and vasopressin are the names of two hormones in this group. This group of hormones participates in first level organization where one gland (the hypothalamus) secretes one hormone (oxytocin) which travels to its target. The hormones are sometimes called the hypophysial (-eal) neurohormones.

The second group of hormones, the **hypophysiotropic neurohormones**, is also synthesized in the hypothalamus, but they are secreted into the portal system capillaries of the median eminence. Their targets are cells just a short distance away in the adenohypophysis. The

hypophysiotropic neurohormones that have been identified are thyroid-stimulating hormone-releasing hormone, luteinizing hormone-releasing hormone, somatostatin, corticotropin-releasing hormone, growth hormone-releasing hormone, and dopamine. The hypophysiotropic neurohormones participate in second and third level organization; they are the molecules that carry stimulating and inhibiting messages from the hypothalamus to the adenohypophysis.

In the older literature, it is common to see the hypophysiotropic neurohormones referred to as "factors" instead of as "hormones," especially before their structure was known. Thus, the hypophysiotropic neurohormones are sometimes encountered abbreviated with an "F" instead of an "H." TSH-releasing hormone (TRH) was once called TSH-releasing factor (TRF).

There is an embarrassing shortage of releasing hormones for the gonadotropins. So far, only one releasing hormone has been identified, luteinizing hormone-releasing hormone (LRH) which is also called gonadotropin-releasing hormone (GnRH). A follicle-stimulating hormone

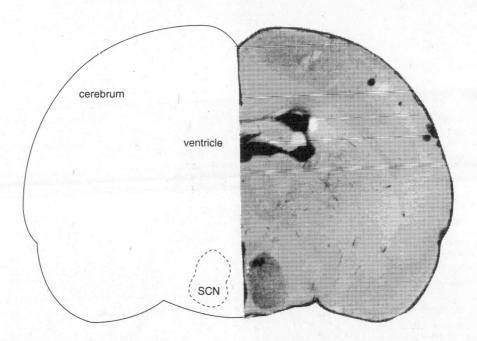

Figure 3.2 The figure shows a section through a rodent brain showing the location of the hypothalamus. The sketch on the left shows a diagrammatic representation of one half of the brain; on the right is a photomicrograph of the other half of the brain. In this section, one of the hypothalamic nuclei, the suprachiasmatic nucleus (SCN) in the hypothalamus can clearly be seen as a darker region (the SCN is the location of the circadian biological clock in mammals and some other species). Modified, with permission. S. Binkley. The Pineal: Endocrine and Nonendocrine Function. Englewood Cliffs, NJ: Prentice Hall; 1988; p. 21.

releasing hormone has yet to be found and identified. However, FSH and LH often appear in the blood independently, so two mechanisms are required for their regulation, but endocrinologists have only provided one releasing hormone which requires further explanation.

CHEMISTRY

Six hypophysiotropic peptide and amine hormones of the hypothalamus have been identified and their structures determined (TRH, LRH, somatostatin, CRH, GRH, dopamine). The hormones of the hypothalamus are peptides and polypeptides (Figure 3.5) except for one small molecule, an amine named dopamine.

The hypothalamus produces a family of nonapeptide (nine amino acid) hormones which in-

cludes **oxytocin**. The active forms of the nonapeptide hormones all have a disulfide bond connecting the two cysteine amino acid residues. Their chemistry is considered further in the chapter on vasopressin and oxytocin.

Disulfide bonds are present in the hypothalamic neurohormones and in somatostatin. The disulfide bonds connect two cysteine amino acid residues in the peptide (and then are sometimes called cystine). Counting cystine as one amino acid versus counting two cysteines accounts for some discrepancies in reporting numbers of amino acid residues.

HYPOPHYSIOTROPIC NEUROHORMONES

The principal function of the hypophysiotropic neurohormones is to stimulate the

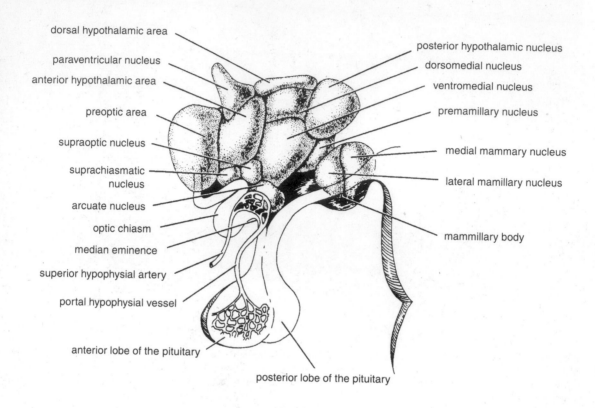

dorsal hypothalamic area

paraventricular nucleus

anterior hypothalamic area

preoptic area

supraoptic nucleus

suprachiasmatic nucleus

arcuate nucleus

optic chiasm

median eminence

superior hypophysial artery

portal hypophysial vessel

anterior lobe of the pituitary

posterior hypothalamic nucleus

dorsomedial nucleus

ventromedial nucleus

premamillary nucleus

medial mammary nucleus

lateral mamillary nucleus

mammillary body

posterior lobe of the pituitary

Figure 3.3 The diagram represents the human hypothalamic nuclei, pituitary gland, and associated structures. Some representations, as this one, show the anterior pituitary to the left. The anterior pituitary is comprised of the pars distalis and pars tuberalis. Modified, with permission, Ganong, W. Review of Medical Physiology, Fourteenth Edition, Norwalk, CT: Appleton & Lange; 1989; p. 192.

release, or inhibit the release, of hormones of the anterior pituitary gland (Table 3.2).

The peptide hormone **TRH** (thyrotropin-releasing hormone) causes the pituitary gland to release thyroid-stimulating hormone. So the hypothalamic hormone is considered to be a releasing hormone, and it is named thyroid-stimulating hormone-releasing hormone. TRH was the first hypophysiotropic neurohormone whose chemical formula was identified as a three amino acid peptide. The identification required a formidable effort and is one of the great historical feats of endocrinology. The hormone was originally extracted by two groups using two million pig brains or five million sheep brains. Seven tons of hypothalami were used to get one milligram of pure TRH. The cell bodies that synthesize TRH are located in the paraventricular and dorsomedial nuclei and neighboring regions. TRH is secreted in the medial portion of the external layer of the median eminence. TRH also stimulates prolactin release.

The peptide hormone **LRH** (luteinizing hormone-releasing hormone) has ten amino acid residues. LRH releases FSH and LH from the pituitary gland. It is uncertain whether there is yet an

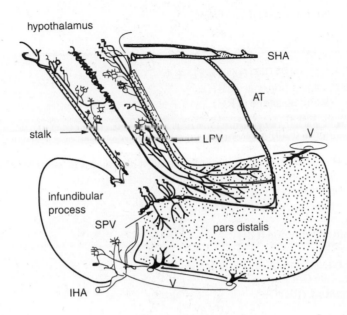

Figure 3.4 The diagram illustrates the vascular arrangements of the ventral hypothalamus, the infundibular stalk and process, and the pars distalis of the human hypophysis cerebri. SHA, superior hypophysial artery; IHA, inferior hypophysial artery; LPV, long portal vessels; SPV, short portal vessels; AT, trabecular artery; V, hypophysial veins draining into local venus dural sinuses. The portal veins receive hormones in the upper complex's tufted and coiled capillaries and discharge the hormones into the pars distalis below. In this figure the anterior pituitary is shown on the right; the anterior pituitary is comprised of the pars distalis and pars tuberalis. Reproduced, with permission, Warwick, R.; Williams, P., editors. Gray's Anatomy, 35th British Edition. Philadelphia: W. B. Saunders Co.; 1973; p. 137.

FRH that is separable from LRH, and it is possible that LRH serves both LH- and FSH-releasing functions The cell bodies of the neurosecretory cells that secrete LRH are located in the preoptic and arcuate nuclei and regions of the hypothalamus that are between the two nuclei. The development of LRH neurons is curious: LRH neurons migrate during development from the medial side of the olfactory placode into the brain,[3] which has clinical implications (Kallman's syndrome links LRH deficiency, hypogonadism and anosmia[4]). LRH is secreted in the lateral regions of the median eminence. LRH may provoke calcium ion oscillations in pituitary gonadotropin-secreting cells.[5] In proposing a

model for second messengers for the mechanism of action of LRH, Naor writes:

> ...after [LRH] binding to its specific receptors, [LRH] stimulates phosphoinositide turnover, mobilizes Ca^{2+}, activates protein kinase C (PKC), and induces arachidonic acid (AA) release. The production of multiple second messenger molecules is responsible for gonadotropin release and synthesis.[6]

The hormone **somatostatin**[7] has 14 amino acid residues, that is, it is a tetradecapeptide. Somatostatin inhibits the release of growth

Table 3.1 Hormones of the Hypothalamus

HYPOTHALAMIC NEUROHORMONES
oxytocin (OT, OXY)
vasopressin, antidiuretic hormone (ADH)

HYPOPHYSIOTROPIC NEUROHORMONES
corticotropic hormone-releasing hormone (CRH)
thyrotropic hormone-releasing hormone (TRH)
  TSH-releasing hormone
luteinizing hormone-releasing hormone (LRH)
  gonadotropin-releasing hormone (GnRH)
  luteinizing hormone follicle-stimulating hormone-releasing hormone (LH-FSH RH)
  follicle-stimulating hormone-releasing hormone (FSH-RH)
growth hormone-releasing hormone (GRH, hpGRF)
  somatotropin-releasing hormone (SRH)
  somatocrinin
growth hormone-inhibiting hormone (GIH)
  somatostatin (SS)
  somatotropin release-inhibiting hormone (SRIH)
prolactin-releasing hormone (PRH)
prolactin-inhibiting hormone (PIH)
  dopamine
melanophore-stimulating hormone-releasing hormone (MRF)
  serotonin
melanophore-stimulating hormone-inhibiting hormone (MIH, MRIH)

The table lists eleven hypothalamic hormones, their abbreviations, and their other names (indented). The hormones are sometimes abbreviated with F (for factor) instead of H (for hormone). A distinct FSH-RH has been elusive and may not exist.

hormone from the anterior pituitary gland. The anterior periventricular nuclei above the optic chiasm contain the neurons that secrete somatostatin. Somatostatin is secreted in the median eminence. Somatostatin also inhibits TSH secretion, has peripheral function, and is secreted peripherally (e.g., by the pancreas; somatostatin inhibits glucose-stimulated secretions of the pancreas).[8]

The polypeptide hormone **CRH** (corticotropin-releasing hormone) has 41 amino acid residues. Plasma CRH in individual normal subjects ranges 0.9–22 pmol/liter; there are varied reports as to factors associated with blood or hypothalamus CRH level changes (higher in women, increased during pregnancy, increased with age, evening peak).[9] CRH causes the adenohypophysis to release ACTH. CRH was the first neurohypophysiotropic neurohormone to be hypothesized on the basis of experimentation, but its structure was not discovered until after TRH had already been identified. CRH-secreting cells are found in the anterior paraventricular nuclei and CRH is secreted in the median eminence. CRH also stimulates secretion of beta lipotropin which is made from the same precursor as ACTH. The hypothalamic nonapeptide, vasopressin, and the hormone angiotensin also stimulate ACTH secretion. CRH, like many other hormones, has a daily cycle (Figure 3.6).

The polypeptide hormone **GRH** (growth hormone-releasing hormone) has 43 amino acid residues. GRH causes the pituitary gland to release growth hormone. The cell bodies that make GRH are located in the arcuate nuclei and GRH is secreted in the median eminence. A GRH

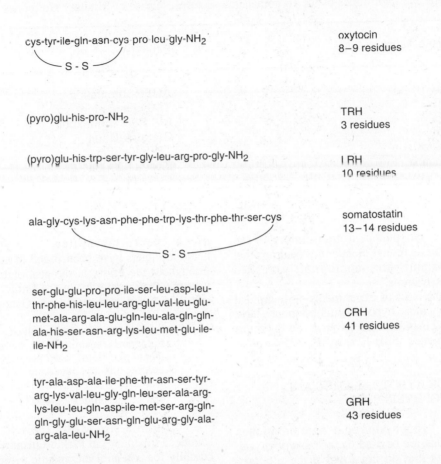

cys-tyr-ile-gln-asn-cys pro leu gly-NH$_2$ oxytocin
     S - S   8–9 residues

(pyro)glu-his-pro-NH$_2$ TRH
     3 residues

(pyro)glu-his-trp-ser-tyr-gly-leu-arg-pro-gly-NH$_2$ LRH
     10 residues

ala-gly-cys-lys-asn-phe-phe-trp-lys-thr-phe-thr-ser-cys   somatostatin
     S - S   13–14 residues

ser-glu-glu-pro-pro-ile-ser-leu-asp-leu-
thr-phe-his-leu-leu-arg-glu-val-leu-glu-
met-ala-arg-ala-glu-gln-leu-ala-gln-gln-
ala-his-ser-asn-arg-lys-leu-met-glu-ile-
ile-NH$_2$ CRH
     41 residues

tyr-ala-asp-ala-ile-phe-thr-asn-ser-tyr-
arg-lys-val-leu-gly-gln-leu-ser-ala-arg-
lys-leu-leu-gln-asp-ile-met-ser-arg-gln-
gln-gly-glu-ser-asn-gln-glu-arg-gly-ala-
arg-ala-leu-NH$_2$ GRH
     43 residues

Figure 3.5 The amino acid sequences of the structures of peptide hypothalamic neurohormones are shown. For the larger molecules, the amino acid residues are arrayed in rows of ten amino acid residues. Dopamine and serotonin are amines, not peptides, and are not shown in the figure.

that is a 44-amino-acid residue peptide, with similarities to gut peptides glucagon and secretin, was isolated from human pancreatic tumor tissue. Pancreatic somatocrinin is similar to putative hypothalamic somatocrinin.

The amine, **dopamine**, is classified chemically with epinephrine and norepinephrine as a catecholamine. Dopamine inhibits the pituitary gland from releasing prolactin, so dopamine is a prolactin-inhibiting hormone (PIH). Dissociation of dopamine from its D$_2$ receptors on pituitary cells that make prolactin may be the signal for prolactin secretion.[10] Dopamine may also stimulate growth hormone secretion. The dopamine comes from tuberoinfundibular neurons which originate in the arcuate nuclei and which terminate in the lateral median eminence (the tuberoinfundibular dopaminergic system). This is not the only system in the brain involving dopamine. The nigrostriatal system regulates movement; disruption of function of the system is a cause of Parkinson's disease. There is a mesocortical dopaminergic system whose action on the brain may be disrupted in schizophrenia. Dopamine is also found in the adrenal medulla and adrenergic neurons where it is a precursor of epinephrine and norepinephrine. Dopamine is a neurotransmitter in sympathetic ganglia, carotid body, in brain, and in interneurons. It

Table 3.2 Hormones of the Hypothalamus Control Release of Pituitary Hormones

Hypothalamus	Pituitary
CRH	ACTH stimulation
TRH	TSH stimulation
LRH	LH, FSH stimulation
GRH	GH stimulation
somatostatin	GH inhibition
dopamine	PRO inhibition

is one of the synaptic neurotransmitters in the retina and inhibits retinal melatonin. Neurons that secrete dopamine are, appropriately, called "dopaminergic neurons."

On the basis of experiments or theoretical considerations, more hypothalamic hormones have been supposed than have been found. So the status of these hormones (FSH-RH, MRF, PRH) is less certain.

BEYOND THE HYPOTHALAMUS AND ADENOHYPOPHYSIS

The hypophysiotropic neurohormones have effects that are beyond the adenohypophysis, that is, effects that do not involve the pituitary gland. The neurohormones have other targets besides the pituitary gland. They have also been implicated in the control of behavior.[11] Some, such as somatostatin, are synthesized in other places as well as in the hypothalamus. For example, LRH injections cause lordosis behavior in rats given priming doses of reproductive steroids. Female rats normally arch their backs in response when stroked and this is called lordosis. The lordosis response is part of the rats' normal sexual behavior repertoire.

Somatostatin directly inhibits insulin release from the pancreas, but it comes from many sources including the pancreatic D cells which can secrete somatostatin themselves. Various parts of the brain also secrete somatostatin as a neurotransmitter. Somatostatin has been suggested for involvement in causing psychological depression.

In fact, somatostatin is not the only hypophysiotropic neurohormone that may be synthesized outside the hypothalamus and function

as a neurotransmitter. Hypothalamic neurohormones have been found in nerve endings throughout the brain, in the gastrointestinal tract, in sympathetic ganglia, in the brain stem, in the spinal cord, and in invertebrates. Ganong suggests:

> ...when the pituitary evolved, existing neurotransmitters or neurohormones (or both) were preempted to become the hypothalamic hormones secreted by or involved in the regulation of the pituitary gland.[12]

A role for MIF-I (prolyl-leucylglycinamide, a tripeptide) in Parkinsonism was a subject of study for potential therapeutic value because it relieved symptoms (tremors, rigidity of the body, and abnormal lack of movement) and augmented the stimulatory effects of dopa. In pursuing this line, investigators believed that Parkinsonism was due to dopamine absence because of degeneration of neurons in the caudate nucleus of the brain.

FUNCTION AND BIOASSAYS

Even when the pituitary was still called the "master gland," there was evidence that the pituitary was controlled by factors beyond itself. The pituitary's anatomical connection to the brain via a stalk was a priori evidence for a functional relationship of the brain and pituitary gland. Manipulations of the brain (with electrical stimulation, electrical lesions, surgery, sexual behavior, implantation of drugs or hormones) all changed pituitary function. Transplanting pituitary glands from their

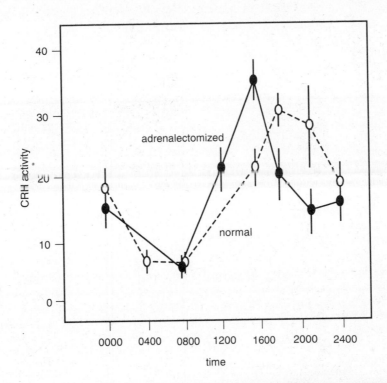

Figure 3.6 The graph shows daily cycles of CRF activity in male rats. The points represent mean activities (N = 6–11) and the vertical lines represent standard errors of the mean. Adrenalectomy advanced the timing of the daily peak. Redrawn, after Hiroshige, T.; Wada, S. Modulation of CRF activity in the rat hypothalamus. In Aschoff, J.; Ceresa, F.; Halberg, F., editors. Chronobiological Aspects of Endocrinology. Stuttgart and New York: F. K. Schattauer Verlag; 1974; p. 52.

normal sites to a kidney capsule location changed pituitary secretory function which implied that the pituitary gland's normal connections and location were functionally important. Pituitary stalk section changed pituitary function if foil was interposed to prevent regeneration of portal vessels.

When a hypothalamus was placed *in vitro* with a pituitary gland, prolactin production was inhibited. This type of finding provided bases for bioassays for detection of the hypophysiotropic neurohormones (Figure 3.7). For example, rat pituitary glands were used for *in vitro* bioassays. The pituitary glands were taken from rats and sliced in half to get hemipituitaries. One hemipituitary served as control, the other as experimental. The hemipituitaries were placed in culture medium in individual culture dishes. The test substance (i. e., an extract containing a hypothalamic hormone) was added to one hemipituitary; control solution with only the diluent was added to the other pituitary. A pituitary hormone was assayed in the culture medium of both control and experimental dishes. If the hormone increased in the test dish compared to the control, it was evidence for the presence of a release factor. If a hormone decreased compared to the control, that was evidence for the presence of a release-inhibiting factor. The bioassay derived from the method of proving that the hypothalamus secretions controlled the pituitary gland secretion. Schally discussed his critical experiment with Saffran in his Nobel lecture:

> Using isolated rat anterior pituitary fragments, we devised a test system for measuring the release of ACTH. . . I still recall our exaltation when we found that hypothalamic or neurohy-

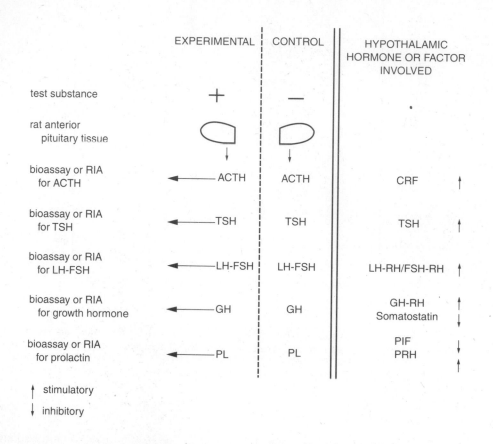

Figure 3.7 The hypophysiotropic hormone assays make use of the secretion of pituitary hormones from rat hemipituitaries. The figure is a representation of *in vitro* tests for assay of hypothalamic hormones that release or inhibit hormones of the anterior pituitary. To do a test for a single sample, a rat pituitary is cut in half; the two halves are "hemipituitaries." The hemipituitaries are cultured in separate dishes. The test substance is added to the culture medium. The "experimental" test substance, which may contain the hormone for which the bioassay is being done, is represented under the heading "Hypothalamic hormone or factor involved." The hemipituitaries secrete pituitary hormones—if a hypophysiotropic neurohormone is present, then the secretion of pituitary hormone is changed. The investigator measures pituitary hormone secreted into the culture media. The actual pituitary hormone whose secretion from hemipituitaries is measured is determined with RIA and is listed on the left. The control is a hemipituitary that does not receive the test substance but receives the diluent. The result is the increase or decrease in the pituitary hormone when the experimental is compared with the control. If the result is zero, or no effect, then no hypophysiotropic hormone activity is present. If the result is > 0, then the pituitary hormone is stimulated and the hypophysiotropic release factor activity is present. If the result is < 0, then the pituitary hormone is inhibited, and hypophysiotropic inhibiting factor activity is present. Reproduced, with permission, Schally, A. B. Aspects of hypothalamic regulation of the pituitary gland. Science 202: 18–28; 1978.

pophysial extracts added to the anterior pituitary tissue caused an unequivocal increase in the release of ACTH. We 'knew' then that we had done it, that we had demonstrated experimentally for the first time the existence of a substance that stimulated the release of ACTH. We named this substance corticotropin-releasing factor (CRF).[13]

REGULATION OF THE HYPOTHALAMUS

The afferent neural pathways to the hypothalamus themselves provide evidence that hypothalamic neurosecretion is regulated by the brain.

Neurotransmitters secreted by the afferent neurons alter the pituitary hormones by affecting the release and inhibiting hormones. As mentioned, dopamine controls prolactin. Norepinephrine stimulates secretion of FSH, LH, GH, and TSH and decreases ACTH, oxytocin and vasopressin. The norepinephrine is probably secreted from the nucleus which receives afferent fibers from the baroreceptors in the arteries, but there are also adrenergic fibers projecting to the hypothalamus from the locus ceruleus. Serotonin increases prolactin secretion, possibly via a PRH. The serotonin neurons have cell bodies in the raphe nuclei in the midbrain, pons, and medulla. The fibers also project to the suprachiasmatic nuclei which are involved in controlling hormone daily rhythms. Opioid peptides, possibly acting as neurotransmitters, inhibit ACTH, LH, and vasopressin secretion and they may stimulate prolactin. Vasoactive intestinal peptide (VIP), which is high in cortical brain, may be released in the hypothalamus and median eminence; intraventricular administration of VIP increases plasma prolactin. Prostaglandins increase LRH in portal blood; the midcycle surge of LH that is provoked by LRH can be abolished in rats with drugs (i.e., aspirin or indomethacin) which inhibit prostaglandin synthesis.[14]

Hormones of other glands control the hypothalamus and affect the brain. The hormones from the pituitary gland and from the glands controlled by the pituitary (gonads, adrenal, thyroid) can control the hypothalamus by negative feedback with both long and short loops. The hypothalamus has receptors for the pineal hormone melatonin.

Hypotheses have also been put forward that cells of hypothalamic regions are themselves directly sensitive to their immediate environments. Regional heating and cooling of the hypothalamus has proved that the brain is temperature sensitive, and a brain **"thermostat"** has been proposed for involvement with the thyroid in control of body temperature. The brain is sensitive to blood salt concentrations, so an **"osmostat"** has been proposed to participate with antidiuretic hormone in the regulation of salt and water balance. The brain is sensitive to blood glucose levels, so a **"glucostat"** has been hypothesized (glucostatic hypothesis) in the regulation of blood sugar with growth hormone and other hormones.

The hypothalamus receives fibers directly from the retina by a separate tract that is distinct from the optic nerve. The tract, the **retinohypothalamic tract**, conveys light information to the suprachiasmatic nuclei of the hypothalamus.[15] The light information is in turn conveyed to the pineal gland where it participates in regulation of the production of the pineal hormone melatonin. The suprachiasmatic nucleus is hypothesized to be a circadian oscillator involved in the synchronization of circadian rhythms that occur in hormones and other physiological variables.

Thus regulation of the hypothalamus is complex involving input from chemicals (e.g., neurochemicals, hormones), physiological variables (e.g., temperature, salt, sugar), and nerves (e.g., neural and retinohypothalamic tracts). However, these multiple inputs provide a remarkable adaptive system by which the environment and behavior and the body's own physiology can influence the hypothalamus which in turn can make appropriate adjustments with the endocrine system.

HYPOTHALAMUS AND RHYTHMS

The hypothalamus, in particular the suprachiasmatic nuclei, is the circadian rhythm oscillator, the biological clock responsible for generating daily cycle in mammals and some other vertebrates. Most hormones have daily cycles which, presumably, derive their rhythms from the pacemaker in the hypothalamus.

If the hypothalamus controls daily rhythms in the hormones of other glands, we would expect hypothalamic hormones to be rhythmic. As mentioned above, there is a rhythm in CRF activity in the median eminence of rats. The rhythm is phase shifted, but not abolished by adrenalectomy, so that the rhythm is not controlled by a feedback

Table 3.3 Neuropeptides Localized in Hypothalamus and Behavior

Peptide	Behavior
TRH	general arousal, modulates affective disorders
somatostatin	decreases general arousal, grooming behavior, feeding
LRH	induces sexual behavior
CRH	decreases feeding, increases locomotor activity, inhibits sexual behavior
GRH	increases feeding
vasopressin	improves attention and memory, increases alertness
oxytocin	influences sexual behavior, suckling behavior
ACTH 4-10, MSH	improves attention, memory, learning
MIF	decreases Parkinsonism tremor, modulates affective disorders
opioid peptides	analgesia, modifies learning, decreases sexual arousal
neurotensin	decreases feeding, hypothermia, modulates autonomic function
bombesin	decreases feeding and temperature, increases grooming
neuropeptide Y	increases feeding
cholecystokinin	decreases feeding
vasoactive intestinal peptide	decreases feeding
calcitonin	decreases feeding
angiotensin II	increases water intake, increases blood pressure
atrial natriuretic factor	visceral/autonomic function
delta sleep-inducing peptide	induces sleep

The behavior column lists observed behaviors (induced when a particular peptide was infused into the hypothalamus of an experimental animal). Modified, with permission, after Moss, R.L.; Dudley, C.A.; Gosnell, B.A. Behavior and the hypothalamus. In DeGroot, L.J., editor. Endocrinology. Philadelphia: W.B. Saunders; 1989; p. 257.

relationship between the hypothalamus and the adrenal gland.

Pulsatile signals may be crucial to the functioning of some hormones of the hypothalamus. If LRH is administered at a rate of 1 pulse/hour, LH is secreted. But 5 pulses/hour suppresses LH secretion. Reducing the rate to one pulse per 3 hours diminished LH but increased FSH. If the dose was increased to 1 μg/10 min, FSH secretion was suppressed. Thus, fine adjustments of dose and rate of pulses of administration determine the gonadotropin profile that is secreted in response to LRH and can provide an explanation for how one gonadotropin (LRH) can control two pituitary hormones (LH and FSH).[16]

HYPOTHALAMUS AND BEHAVIOR

Moss and coworkers summarize the functions of the hypothalamus:

....the hypothalamus also provides an important interface between the brain, pituitary gland and periphery. It is not surprising then, that the hypothalamus plays a critical role in the regulation of diverse and dynamic physiological and behavioral processes such as visceral/autonomic function, thermoregulation, endocrine function, water metabolism/electrolyte balance, food and water intake, sleep-wake cycle, circadian rhythms, emotional behavior, and reproductive processes and behavior.[17]

Table 3.3 lists hypothalamic neuropeptides and their associated behavior. Feeding behavior and "satiety" sites are in the medial and lateral regions of the hypothalamus. Scientists know this because lesions in the ventromedial region of the hypothalamus produce obesity and overeating. In contrast, lesions in the lateral hypothalamus cause aphagia (undereating) and adipsia (underdrinking). Experimentally, lesions can be made electrically, with knife cuts, or with chemicals (e.g., 6-hydroxydopamine, a neurotoxin that destroys catecholaminergic cells). Moreover, localized hypothalamic injections of peptides alter food intake. CRH, neurotensin, CCK, calcitonin, and bombesin reduce food intake. Opioid peptides and neuropeptide Y increase food intake. Effects of injected substances depend on the exact location of the injection site. Norepinephrine, epinephrine, and GABA increase food intake if they are injected into the paraventricular nucleus of the hypothalamus. Norepinephrine, epinephrine, dopamine, or GABA decrease food intake if they are injected into the lateral perifornical area. Neurons in the hypothalamus change their firing rates in response to direct applications of glucose, free fatty acids, or insulin. In other words, the hypothalamus can sense the "energy status" of the body by detecting the substances the blood brings to its cells. The hypothalmus then can send signals which make appropriate adjustments in feeding behavior.

Male and female sexual behavior are also associated with neural sites in the hypothalamus. Research with the sexual receptivity response of the female rat (lordosis, arching the back) has shown that a key hypothalamic secretion, LRH, is the signal. If LRH is infused into the areas of the hypothalamus known to be involved in sexual behavior, lordotic activity increases but other behaviors are not affected.

Sites controlling thirst and drinking are found in the lateral hypothalamus, circumventricular organs, and preoptic areas. Sleep is controlled by the reticular formation of the brain stem which has neural connections with the posterior hypothalmus/mammillary bodies. The hypothalamus is part of the limbic system which determines the emotional, aggressive, defensive, and drive aspects of behavior. MIF-I and TRH improve the rigidity and tremors of patients suffering from Parkinson's disease, and somatostatin and TRH have been suggested as having roles in depression.[18]

In summary, the hypothalamic regulatory hormones (the hypophysiotropic neurohormones) that control the release of pituitary hormones were originally thought to include at least nine hormones and perhaps as many as ten hormones—CRH, TRH, LH-RH, FSH-RH, GH-RH, GIH, PIF, PRF, MIF, and MRF.[19] The hypothalamus also makes a family of nonapeptide hormones which include vasopressin and oxytocin.

REFERENCES

1. Guillemin, R.; Burgus, R. The hormones of the hypothalamus. Scientific American 227: 24–33; 1972.

2. Ganong, W. Review of Medical Physiology, Thirteenth Edition. Norwalk, CT: Appleton & Lange; 1987; pp. 203–204.

3. Schwanzel-Fukuda, M.; Jorgenson, K.L.; Bergen, H.T.; Weesner, G.D.; Pfaff, D.W. Biology of normal lutenizing hormone-releasing hormone neurons during and after their migration from olfactory placode. Endocrine Reviews 13: 623–634; 1992.

4. Crowley, W.F.; Jameson, J.L. Clinical Counterpoint: Gonadotropin-releasing hormone deficiency: Perspectives from clinical investigation. Endocrine Reviews 13: 635–640; 1992.

5. Stojilkovic, S.S.; Catt, K.J. Calcium oscillations in anterior pituitary cells. Endocrine Reviews 13: 256–280; 1992.

6. Naor, Z. Signal transduction mechanisms of Ca^{2+} mobilizing hormones: The case of gonadotropin-releasing hormone. Endocrine Reviews 11: 326–353; 1990.

7. Vale, W.; Brazeau, P.; Rivier, C.; Brown, M.; Boss, B.; Rivier, J.; Burgus, R.; Ling, N.; Guillemin, R. Somatostatin. Rec. Prog. Horm. Res. 31: 366–397; 1975.

8. Bonora, E.; Moghetti, P.; Zancanrao, C.; Cigolini, M.; Querena, M.; Cacciatori, V.; Zenere, M.; Corgnati, A.; Muggeo, M. Normal inhibition by somatostatin of glucose-stimulated B cell secretion in obese subjects. Horm. Metab. Res. 22: 584–588; 1990.

9. Orth, D. N. Corticotropin-releasing hormone in humans. Endocrine Reviews 13: 164–191; 1992.

10.   Martinez de la Escalera, G.; Weiner, R. Dissociation of dopamine from its receptor as a signal in the pleiotropic hypothalamic regulation of prolactin secretion. Endocrine Reviews 13: 241–255; 1992.

11.   Marx, J.L. Learning and behavior II: The hypothalamic peptides. Science 190: 544–545; 1975.

12.   Ganong, W. Neuroendocrinology. In Greenspan, F.; Forsham, P., editors. Basic and Clinical Endocrinology, Second Edition. East Norwalk, CT: Appleton & Lange; 1986; p. 36.

13.   Schally, A. V. Aspects of hypothalamic regulation of the pituitary gland. Science 202: 18–28; 1978.

14.   Mishell, D.R.; Davajan, V. Infertility, Contraception, and Reproductive Endocrinology. Oradell, NJ: Medical Economics Books; 1986; pp. 13–14.

15.   Moore, R. Y.; Klein, D. Visual pathways and the central neural control of a circadian rhythm in pineal serotonin N-acetyltransferase. Brain Research 71: 17–33; 1974.

16.   Mishell, D.R., V. Davajan. Op. cit. p. 26.

17.   Moss, R.L.; Dudley, C.A.; Gosnell, B.A. Behavior and the hypothalamus. In L. J. DeGroot, editor. Endocrinology. Philadelphia: W. B. Saunders; 1989; pp. 254–263.

18.   Marx, J.L. Learning and behavior II: The hypothalamic peptides. Science 190: 544–545; 1975.

19.   Schally, A.V.; Arimura, A.; Kastin, A.J. Hypothalamic regulatory hormones. Science 179: 341–350; 1973.

CHAPTER 4

Pituitary Anatomy and Hierarchies

The pituitary gland, or pituitary, is central in the organization of most of vertebrate endocrinology. The pituitary and hypothalamus are "main characters" in any endocrinology book. In this chapter the focus is on the anatomy and a brief overview of the pituitary hormones, their nomenclature, and their general chemistry. The pituitary provides an example of correlation between fine anatomy and hormones. The hypothalamus, pituitary, and each of their hormones will be discussed again in their own chapters and in chapters having to do with the pineal gland, ovaries, testes, adrenal glands, and thyroid gland.

PITUITARY RELATIONSHIP TO BRAIN AND HYPOTHALAMUS

The hypothalamus and pituitary gland are functionally and anatomically related. The functional relationship is recorded for all to see in their anatomical relationship (Figures 4.1 and 4.2). The hypothalamus lies at the center and bottom of the brain. The pituitary gland lies below the hypothalamus, and thus, directly inferior to the brain. Indeed the pituitary has another name, **hypophysis cerebri**, which means "lying under" the brain. The hypothalamus is connected with the pituitary gland by a stalk, the **infundibulum**. The part of the hypothalamus, where the infundibulum attaches, is posterior to the optic chiasm, and is called the **median eminence**.

NOMENCLATURE OF THE HORMONES OF THE PITUITARY

The anterior pituitary gland makes six hormones (growth hormone, adrenocorticotropin, thyroid-stimulating hormone, prolactin, follicle-stimulating hormone, luteinizing hormone). The intermediate lobe makes one more hormone, melanophore-stimulating hormone. The various names and abbreviations for these hormones are listed in Table 4.1. The seven hormones are discussed in more depth in other chapters where their biochemistry and function is explained in detail.

The hormones of the pituitary gland are all peptides or proteins or they are glycoproteins—they all contain chains of amino acids. They share features in their nomenclature, roles in hierarchies, and chemistry.

Each of the hormones of the anterior pituitary gland and the intermediate lobe of the pituitary gland has several abbreviations and names. The hormones are named for the site of hormone synthesis or the functions of the hormones. Some authors use the ending -*phin* instead of -*pin*, and -*phic* instead of -*pic*. Other endocrinologists insert hyphens between some of the words in the names. The reasons for the multiplicity of names and abbreviations are usually historic and not intentionally diabolical—several hormones were named on the basis of function and then were found to have a common chemical structure. For example, we find both corticotropin and corticotrophin used for the hormone abbreviated ACTH.

The pituitary hormones are all regulated in hierarchical schemes which include the hypothalamus and the pituitary. Hierarchies, and the amplification which they achieve, were discussed in the first chapter. The pars nervosa is viewed as a neurohemal organ because oxytocin (and other peptide hormones) made in the hypothalamus are stored and released into the blood in the pars nervosa.

BRIEF SURVEY OF PITUITARY HORMONES

The hormones of the pituitary gland are described in detail in other chapters, but a brief survey is included here to provide an overview.

Growth hormone and **prolactin** are proteins with nearly 200 amino acids belonging to the hormone structure family, prolactin-like hormones discussed in the first chapter. The secretion of these hormones is regulated by releasing and inhibiting peptides (somatostatin, GRH) or amines secreted by the hypothalamus (PIH or dopamine) and transported to the pituitary gland by the blood. Growth hormone and prolactin act on target cells throughout the body. Another name for growth hormone (somatotropin) derives from the word "soma" which means the entire body except for the germ cells. The name prolactin derives from the Latin word "*lac*" for milk.

FSH (follicle-stimulating hormone), LH (luteinizing hormone), and TSH (thyroid-stimulating hormone) are glycoproteins with about 100–200 amino acids belonging to the glycoprotein LH-like hormone family. These hormones are controlled by releasing peptides (LRH, LH-releasing hormone; TRH, TSH-releasing hormone) secreted by the hypothalamus and transported to the pituitary gland by the blood. The targets of FSH, LH, and TSH are other glands. TSH stimulates the thyroid gland to produce its hormones. A name for TSH, thyrotropin, derives from this function. FSH and LH act upon the gonads, the testes, and the ovaries. FSH and LH are two of a number of "gonadotropins" which are grouped for their action on the gonads.

ACTH (adrenocorticotropic hormone) is a peptide hormone with 39 amino acids. It belongs to the family of melanotropins. ACTH is controlled by a releasing peptide (CRH, ACTH-releasing hormone) secreted by the hypothalamus and transported to the pituitary gland by the blood. A principal target of ACTH is the cortex of the

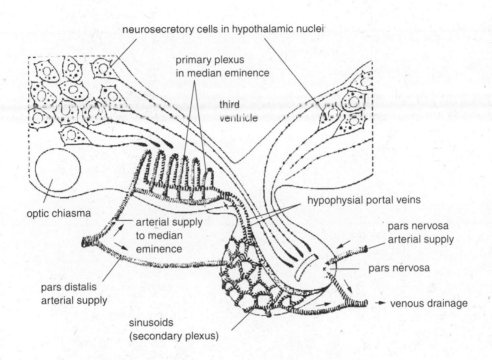

neurosecretory cells in hypothalamic nuclei

primary plexus
in median eminence

third
ventricle

hypophysial portal veins

optic chiasma

arterial supply
to median
eminence

pars nervosa
arterial supply

pars nervosa

pars distalis
arterial supply

venous drainage

sinusoids
(secondary plexus)

Figure 4.1 The drawing shows the pituitary gland suspended below the hypothalamus by a stalk, the infundibulum. This diagram emphasizes the blood supply to the anterior and posterior lobes. Notice the portal veins that carry blood from the median eminence of the hypothalamus to the pars distalis. The pituitary gland lies in a pocket of bone called the sella turcica (not shown). The neurosecretory cells in the hypothalamus are the sources of hormones (oxytocin, vasopressin, releasing and inhibiting hormones). Redrawn, with permission. Turner, C.D.; Bagnara, J.T. General Endocrinology, Sixth Edition. Philadelphia: W.B. Saunders Co.; 1976; p. 30.

adrenal gland. ACTH stimulates the adrenal gland to produce glucocorticoid steroid hormones and that is why another name for ACTH is corticotropin.

MSH (melanophore-stimulating hormone) is a peptide synthesized from the same precursor as ACTH and the opioid hormones, and it also belongs to the family of melanotropins. MSH may be controlled by peptide hormones and/or serotonin. Some of the targets of MSH are the pigmented cells containing melanin, such as the melanophores, that are found in amphibian skin. The function involving melanin is the reason that the MSH hormones are also called the melanotropins.

The posterior pituitary does not synthesize hormones. Instead, nonapeptide (nine amino acid residue) hormones that are synthesized by the hypothalamus descend a nerve fiber tract of the infundibulum to be secreted in the posterior pituitary. The hypothalamic hormones secreted in the posterior pituitary belong to the antidiuretic family of hormones. Oxytocin and vasopressin are names of two of these hormones.

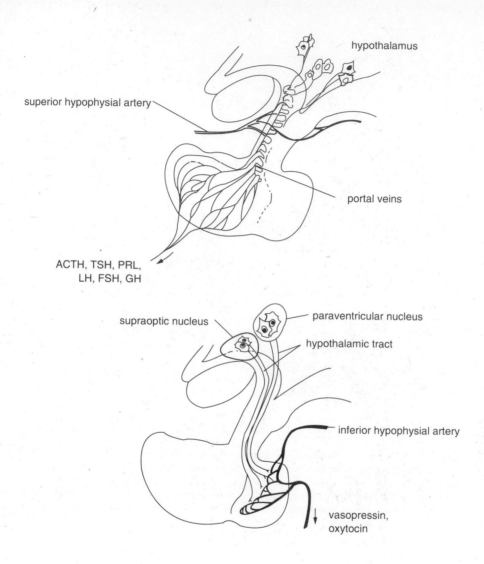

hypothalamus

superior hypophysial artery

portal veins

ACTH, TSH, PRL,
LH, FSH, GH

supraoptic nucleus

paraventricular nucleus

hypothalamic tract

inferior hypophysial artery

vasopressin,
oxytocin

Figure 4.2 The diagrams show connections between the hypothalamus and the pituitary gland. The upper diagram shows the vascular connections between the hypothalamus and the anterior pituitary. Neurosecretory cells in the hypothalamus make releasing and inhibiting hormones which they secrete into the capillary bed in the median eminence. The releasing and inhibiting hormones travel in the blood flowing in from the superior hypophysial artery via the portal veins to the anterior pituitary. In the anterior pituitary, the release and inhibiting hormones control the secretion of the pituitary hormones (ACTH, TSH, PRL, LH, FSH, GH). The lower diagram shows the neural connections of the hypothalamus and the posterior pituitary. Neurosecretory cell bodies in the hypothalamic nuclei make oxytocin and vasopressin hormones which travel down the axons of the neurosecretory cells to the posterior pituitary. In the posterior pituitary, oxytocin and vasopressin are released into the blood flowing from the inferior hypophysial artery. Modified, with permission, Guillemin, R.; Burgus, R. The hormones of the hypothalamus. Scientific American 227: 24–33; 1972.

Table 4.1 Names, Chemical Nature, and Abbreviations for Hormones Made by the Pituitary Gland

---

growth hormone, GH
191 amino-acid polypeptide, MW 21,500

somatotropin, STH
human growth hormone, HGH, hGH

prolactin, PRO, PRL, PL
198 amino acids, MW 22,000

lactogenic hormone
luteotropin, LTH
mammotropin
lactogenic hormone
galactin

luteinizing hormone, LH
89 and 115 amino acid subunits, MW 29,000

interstitial cell–stimulating hormone, ICSH
lutropin

follicle-stimulating hormone, FSH
89 and 115 amino acid subunits, MW29,000

follitropin

thyroid-stimulating hormone, TSH
89 and 112 amino acid subunits, MW28,000

thyrotropin

adrenocorticotropic hormone, ACTH
39 amino acids, MW4,500

corticotropic hormone
corticotropin
adrenocorticotropin

melanophore-stimulating hormone, MSH
alpha 13, beta 18, and gamma 12
amino acid residues

intermedin
melanocyte-stimulating hormone
melanotropin

ACTH and MSH are synthesized from a larger precursor molecule, proopiomelanocortin (POMC) with over 200 amino acid residues and MW31,000. The anterior pituitary also secretes ß-liptropin and ß-endorphin derived from POMC. There are three forms of MSH that share a common heptapeptide with ACTH. The alpha subunits of LH, FSH, and TSH are the same.

GROSS ANATOMY

The pituitary gland nests below the hypothalamus in a pocket of the sphenoid bone called the sella turcica, the "Turk's saddle." Vesalius named the gland in the sixteenth century. Based on location of the gland, he thought that the gland secreted pituita, which was the name for the mucus found in the throat and the nasal fluid. The cavernous sinuses are separated from the sides of the pituitary gland by dural membranes. Surgical removal of the pituitary gland is called **hypophysectomy**. Depending on the species, hypophysectomy can be done through the roof of the mouth, through the ear, or through the nose (e.g., to remove adenomas or for experimentation).

In the human, the pituitary gland is about 15x10x6 mm in size and it weighs 500–800 mg. It is about the size of the tip of the human small finger. Size of the pituitary gland varies in response to changing physiology. For example, the gland is larger in women than in men and the size doubles during pregnancy. Pituitary size changes have provided clues for physiologists seeking its function. Factors that influence pituitary size, and which are therefore clues to its function, include: puberty, castration, thyroidectomy, age, dwarfism or gigantism, seasonal breeding, brooding, gender, and environmental light.

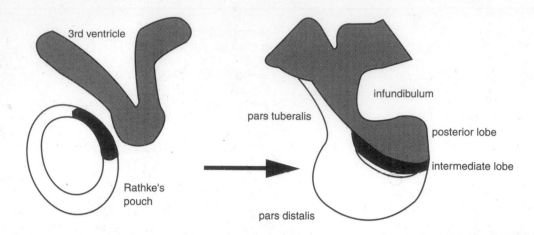

Figure 4.3 The pituitary gland develops from the embryonic layers that form the brain and the mouth. Rathke's pouch of the stomodeum (oral ectoderm, epithelial tissue) pushes upward and meets the infundibulum of the diencephalon (ectoderm, nervous tissue) and gives rise to pars distalis, pars tuberalis, and pars intermedia (fusion region). Neuroectoderm gives rise to the pars nervosa, infundibulum, and the median eminence. [1]

DEVELOPMENT

The pituitary gland has two embryological origins (Figure 4.3). Part of the gland, the pars nervosa, develops from neural ectoderm as a downward projection, the infundibulum, from the brain. Other parts of the gland, pars intermedia and pars distalis, arise from **Rathke's pouch** and are derived from surface ectoderm evaginating from the oral epithelium. When the pituitary forms during development, it comes from the brain and the mouth. Rathke's pouch of the stomodeum (ectoderm) pushes upward and meets the infundibulum of the diencephalon (ectoderm). In other words, the roof of the pharynx or primitive mouth grows up to meet a downgrowth from the floor of the forebrain. The pars intermedia, pars tuberalis, and pars distalis come from Rathke's pouch. The posterior lobe and the infundibulum come from the diencephalon. The lumen of Rathke's pouch becomes the residual cleft. The intermediate lobe forms from the cells of Rathke's pouch where the adenohypophysis meets the neurohypophysis.

The histology and functions of the adeno- and neurohypophysis are related to their embryology. Since Rathke's pouch comes from the epithe-lium, the cells of the adenohypophysis are characteristic of glandular epithelium—many cells, little intercellular space with little connective tissue. The tissue of the neurohypophysis is, in contrast, basically nervous tissue with glial supporting cells and axons.

PARTS OF THE PITUITARY GLAND

The pituitary gland has been divided into parts by several different methods depending on its histology, its development, and the viewpoint of the beholder (Table 4.2). In yet another classification (not shown),[2] the posterior lobe is equivalent to the pars nervosa, and the neurointermediate lobe includes the pars intermedia and posterior lobe.

ADENOHYPOPHYSIS HISTOLOGY

The different regions of the pituitary can be readily distinguished in photomicrographs (light microscopy, Figure 4.4).

The cells of the pituitary pars distalis have been classified histologically and matched with the hormones secreted (Table 4.3). The idea was that each hormone was synthesized by a separate cell

Table 4.2 Equivalent Parts of the Pituitary Gland in Four Nomenclatures

1	2	3	4
adenohypophysis	lobus glandularis	pars distalis	anterior lobe
adenohypophysis	lobus glandularis	pars tuberalis	anterior lobe
adenohypophysis	lobus glandularis	pars intermedia (intermediate lobe)	posterior lobe
neurohypophysis	lobus nervosa (pars nervosa)	processus infundibuli	posterior lobe
neurohypophysis	infundibulum (neural stalk)	infundibular stem	hypothalamus
neurohypophysis	infundibulum (neural stalk)	median eminence of tuber cinereum	hypothalamus

type: a one-hormone-made-by-one-cell-type hypothesis. Moreover, the chemical nature of the hormones secreted is also associated with the cell type. Using increasingly advanced histological techniques (electron microscopy, cytohistochemistry, autoradiography, and now, immunocytohistochemistry) it has been possible to discern at least five types of cells. The task of assigning cell types is complicated by the fact that the appearances of the cells may change as they proceed with their normal functions. Physiological events (pregnancy, lactation, brooding, seasonal breeding, thyroidectomy, castration, excess adrenal glucocorticoid hormone) correlate with changes in the morphology of the pituitary cells.

The cell types of the pituitary gland were originally classified by their staining properties. **Chromophobes** are the cells that do not stain. **Chromophils** are the cells that do take up stain and the chromophils comprise 50% of the cells in the pituitary gland. The chromophils are further subdivided into the cells that take up basic stains, the **basophils** (10% of the cells of the gland), and the cells that take up acidic stains, the **acidophils** (the remaining 40% of the cells). Now, immunochemistry provides better and more accurate ways of classifying the cells.

The subcategories of the basophilic and acidophilic cell types are named by the hormones synthesized (corticotrops secrete corticotropin). The cell names end in *-troph* (implying a growth function) in some endocrine writings, but in others the cell names in *-trope* or *-trop* (denoting a cell containing a substance that produces changes). Granule sizes, measured from electron micrographs, have been used in the identification of the cells. Granule numbers may change as hormones are synthesized, stored, and secreted.

Acidophils make the protein hormones, growth hormone and prolactin. Basophils make the glycoprotein gonadotrophins and thyroid-stimulating hormone. Acidophils or chromophobes make the polypeptide hormones, MSH and ACTH.

The numbers of chromophobes decline with age to 25% of the cells in the pituitary gland. Because the cells don't stain, they are described as being "agranular," however, granules have been found with electron microscopy. One idea about the chromophobes is that they are "stem" cells, undifferentiated progenitors of the secretory chromophils. Another suggestion is that they produce hormones that remain to be identified (e.g., ovarian growth factor, androgen-stimulating hormone, aldosterone-stimulating factor). The cells of the

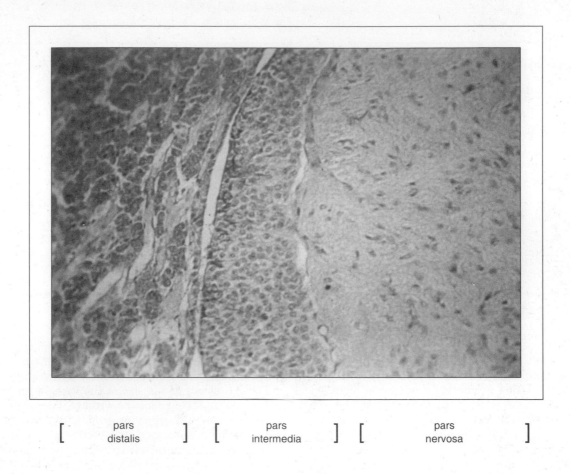

[pars distalis   ]   [pars intermedia   ]   [pars nervosa   ]

Figure 4.4 The kitten pituitary gland showing the three regions of the gland. Humans would not have such a distinct pars intermedia. The figure is a photograph made by the author from a transparency of a histological section. With permission, Eichler, V.B. Histology of the Endocrine System. Slide set #617, Educational Images, Ltd., Lyons Falls, NY; 1982.

pars intermedia and corticotrops are sometimes described as being chromophobic.

Somatotrops comprise 4–10% of the net weight of the anterior pituitary. They are acidophilic. Hematoxylin and eosin or orange G can be used to stain somatotrops.[3] Granule sizes are variously reported to have diameters of 300 to 400 nanometers (millimicrons). The somatotrops are thought to make the protein hormone growth hormone. A deficiency of acidophils correlates with dwarfism.

Mammotrops are also called **lactotrops** and are believed to make the protein hormone prolactin. The mammotrops stain with orange G. During pregnancy, the number of mammotrops increase dramatically. The proliferation of the mammotrops accounts for the two-fold increase in pituitary gland size seen in pregnant women.

The number of mammotrops is also high during lactation in mammals. Suppressed secretion is accompanied by increased prominence of lysosomes in the cells. When birds are nesting, or brooding, their normal acidophils and basophils almost disappear. The glands become predominated by a cell type, **broody cells**, which may secrete prolactin. The names—mammotrop, lactotrop—derive from the word "mamma" for breast and the word "lac" for milk.

The **gonadotrops** are basophils that stain with PAS (periodic acid Schiff reagent). The gonadotrops and their hormones, the gonadotropins, are named for their influence on the gonads (ovaries and testes). The periodic acid-Schiff (PAS) reaction identifies their glycoprotein secretions. There may be two kinds of gonadotrops. FSH gonadotrops have slightly smaller granules and they have more prominent rough endoplasmic reticulum and Golgi. LH gonadotrops (luteotrops) are characterized by slightly larger granules, by less extensive Golgi, and by polar accumulation of granules near the periphery of cells. Most gonadotrops probably secrete both glycoprotein hormones, FSH and LH, but some gonadotrop subpopulations containing only one of the gonadotropins have been identified. The gonadotrops may be a heterogeneous population of changing cells that can synthesize and store either or both of the hormones. In Klinefelter's syndrome and in Turner's syndrome, where there is primary gonad failure, the gonadotrops hypertrophy and the pituitary gland enlarges. Following castration or with aging, "signet ring cells," probably derived from the basophilic gonadotrops, continue to secrete FSH and LH. During puberty, degranulation of the gonadotrops is observed. Environmental light causes degranulation of basophils in birds.

Thyrotrops, like gonadotrops, are basophilic cells and their glycoprotein hormone, TSH, is revealed by a positive periodic acid-Schiff (PAS) reaction or aldehyde fuchsin. The thyrotrops are named for their function in the regulation of the secretion of the thyroid glands. The thyrotrops are the smallest of the pituitary cell types; they have flattened nuclei and the smallest granules. After thyroidectomy, or in primary thyroid failure, the pituitary gland may enlarge because basophil thyrotrops hypertrophy and become amphophils (thyroidectomy cells, T cells). The amphophils have a characteristic appearance and secrete TSH.

The **corticotrops** secrete the peptide hormone that regulates the adrenal cortex, corticotropin or ACTH, and the corticotrops secrete related peptide lipotropins, LPH, and endorphins. Embryologically, the cells originate from the intermediate lobe. These APUD (amine precursor uptake and decarboxylation) cells stain with PAS. The granule sizes are variously reported as large (360 nm) or small (50-200). ACTH controls the secretion of the glucocorticoid hormones of the adrenal cortex. When the adrenal cortex makes excess glucocorticoid, or when excess glucocorticoid is administered, the corticotrops lose granules and hyalinization of the microtubules takes place (Crooke's hyaline degeneration).

Melanotrops are polygonal cells of the pars intermedia that are similar to corticotrops. The cells are named for their role in regulating the pigment, melanin. Pars intermedia cells that stain with lead hematoxylin produce polypeptide hormones such as MSH. Other pars intermedia cells are positive for periodic acid-Schiff reactions. Melanotrops also stain with aldehyde fuchsin and are APUD cells.

NEUROHYPOPHYSIS HISTOLOGY

The histology of the posterior pituitary gland is simpler than that of the anterior pituitary. The bulk of the posterior lobe (pars nervosa) consists of the axonal endings of processes that come from cells in the hypothalamus. The axons are processes of neurosecretory neurons whose cell bodies are located in nuclei of the hypothalamus called the **supraoptic** and **paraventricular nuclei**. The endings, which may be organized into rodlike palisades, are closely associated with blood vessels. Thus the peptide hormones that are released into the neurohypophysis (e.g., oxytocin, vasopressin) are hormones of the hypothalamus. The posterior pituitary acts as a "**neurohemal organ**."

There are some cells called **pituicytes** which are connective tissue cells of the nervous system (modified astroglia, stellate cells containing fat globules). Originally, these cells were thought to be the source of the peptide hormones now known to be synthesized in cell bodies of the neurosecretory cells of the hypothalamus. Noncellular accumulations of stainable material seen with the light microscope may be neurosecretory material and have been called **Herring bodies**; they are thought to be dilated axonal endings with accumulations of secretory material.

Table 4.3 Cell Types and Hormones Synthesized[4,5,6,7]

Cell type	Hormone	Staining reaction	Granule diameters (nm)
somatotrop	GH	acidophilic	300–400
mammotrop	PRO	acidophilic	550–700
FSH gonadotrop	FSH	basophilic	about 200
LH gonadotrop	LH	basophilic	200–250
thyrotrop	TSH	basophilic	50–150
corticotrop	ACTH	basophilic	350–400
melanotrop	MSH	basophilic	–

INNERVATION

The adenohypophysis is typical of endocrine glands in that innervation does not play a major role in its regulation. The pars distalis of most species is regulated by other hormones. However, in teleost fishes there are neuronal elements that may affect the pars distalis.

In contrast, innervation plays a major role for the endocrinology of the neurohypophysis. The innervation of the neurohypophysis consists of the endings of the hypothalamic neurosecretory cells whose cell bodies reside in the paraventricular nuclei (PVN) and supraoptic nuclei (SON). The axons reach the pituitary by the hypothalamic-hypophysial tract which courses the infundibum. Thus the hormones are made in the cell bodies in the hypothalamus but are secreted by nerve terminals in the neurohypophysis.

The pars intermedia may be regulated by neurohormones like the anterior pituitary. But in some species there is direct innervation of the pars intermedia from the hypothalamus. In amphibians and in some mammals, a plexus surrounds the cells of the pars intermedia and regulates MSH secretion. The innervating cells are catecholaminergic (catecholamines are epinephrine, norepinephrine and dopamine) and neurosecretory. For example, in the skate, aminergic and peptidergic neurons originate in the preoptic nucleus and the postoptic nucleus of the hypothalamus. Their aminergic fiber tracts innervate the pars intermedia where the catecholamine neurons synapse with melanotrops. The processes of the neurosecretory neurons (tuberohypophysial innervation) follow a neurosecretory tract that ends at the border of the pars nervosa (where its function is unknown) and pars intermedia (where it inhibits MSH secretion).

VASCULARIZATION

Since the main idea of endocrinology is that hormones are chemical messengers carried from one place to another by the bloodstream, the vascularization of every gland is an important consideration in studying the function of the gland. Most endocrine glands are highly vascularized, that is, they have a rich blood supply.

The blood supply for the anterior pituitary is unique because it has a special system of portal vessels. Blood originating from the internal carotid artery enters the region at the superior aspect of the infundibulum and median eminence via the superior hypophysial artery. The blood proceeds to the primary plexus of capillaries located on the surface of, and looping into, the median eminence of the hypothalamus. Here, the hypothalmic neurosecretory cells secrete hypothalamic hypophysiotropic hormones into the blood. The capillaries are drained by the sinusoidal **portal hypophysial vessels** (portal veins) which descend the pituitary stalk and end in a capillary bed of the adenohypophysis. The capillary beds and portal vessels that connect the hypothalamus and the anterior pituitary gland are called the hypothalamic-hypophysial portal system. The portal system provides a very direct route for neurohormones of the hypothalamus to reach the anterior pituitary targets. Generally, the hypophysial neurohormones release (or inhibit the release of) the hormones of the anterior pituitary.

The intermediate lobe may also receive hormone signals from the hypothalamus via the hypophysial portal vessels. Arguments are still in progress over the possibility of a hypothalamic melanostatin, a role for serotonin, or a role for dopamine in regulating the release of MSH.

The veins of the pituitary gland drain to dural venous sinuses located between the layers of the dura mater or into the veins of the basosphenoid bone.

COMPARATIVE ANATOMY

The structure of the pituitary gland varies among species of vertebrates (Figure 4.5). The main variation is in the pars intermedia. The extent to which the adenohypophysis contacts the neurohypophysis during development determines the size of the pars intermedia.

In birds, the two developing structures remain separated so that birds lack a distinct pars intermedia and MSH. Cells with an origin similar to the pars intermedia may be in the anterior pituitary gland. In humans, the pars intermedia is present in the developing embryo and fetus, but it regresses and may be absent in the adult. So the pars intermedia is sometimes anatomically absent (adult humans, whales, dolphins, elephants, armadillos, birds).

On the other hand, the pars intermedia is particularly prominent in vertebrates that are able to change their skin color to blend with the color of their backgrounds (such as the lizard, *Anolis carolinensis*). Well developed pars intermedia are found in cyclostomes, amphibians, reptiles, and most mammals. Teleost and elasmobranch fishes have melanotrops that are continuous with other pars distalis cells. The term "neurointermediate lobe" refers collectively to the pars nervosa and pars intermedia which are inseparable in some vertebrates.

REGULATION OF THE ANTERIOR PITUITARY GLAND

Regulation of the anterior pituitary gland is accomplished by the neurohormones of the hypothalamus that are transmitted to the anterior pituitary via the hypophysial portal vessels.

Some of the anterior pituitary hormones, those with short loop feedback and second order levels of organization, are regulated by two hormones of the hypothalamus and a set point mecha-nism. The hypothalamus contains neurosecretory cells that have set points for local stimuli (blood glucose, blood salts). They adjust pituitary hormone production by secreting a **releasing hormone** to increase pituitary hormone secretion or by secreting a **release-inhibiting hormone** to decrease pituitary hormone secretion. The hypothalamus makes releasing and inhibiting hormones for growth hormone (GH) and prolactin (PL).

Other anterior pituitary hormones, those with long loop feedback and third order organization, are regulated by one hormone of the hypothalamus, a releasing hormone. Hormones of the thyroid gland, gonads, and adrenal glands inhibit their own release by acting on the hypothalamus and/or pituitary (negative feedback) to stop the pituitary from secreting stimulatory hormones: TSH, LH, FSH, ACTH

The possibility of interactions—paracrine and autocrine interactions—among the cells that constitute the anterior pituitary gland has been studied using improved cell separation techniques, methods of molecular biology, and other new techniques. Some of the paracrine factors that have been suggested are activin, inhibin, angiotensin, angiotensinogen, follistatin, LRH, TRH, interleukin, endothelin, galanin, vasoactive intestinal peptide, neurotensin, neuropeptide Y, substance P, acetylcholine, and growth hormone. Some of these are hormones, some are neurotransmitters, and some are other substances. Follistatin (activin-binding protein) is a protein made in some anterior pituitary cells that acts on pituitary cells and decreases secretion of FSH and gene expression. The paracrine factors increase or decrease hormone secretion of pituitary cells, or they cause other effects such as changes in appearance or immunoreactivity of the cells.[8]

Anterior pituitary cells have 10–500 nM calcium ion $[Ca^{2+}]_i$ oscillations with frequencies ranging from two to ten minutes. Intracellular calcium signals are believed to be important for the control of cellular activities including excitability, exocytosis, contraction, growth, differentiation, and division. The VSCC (voltage-sensitive calcium channels) and other calcium channels provide the mechanism for the generation of the calcium ion oscillations. Increases in $[Ca^{2+}]_i$ are associated with activation of the secretory responses in anterior pituitary cells.[9]

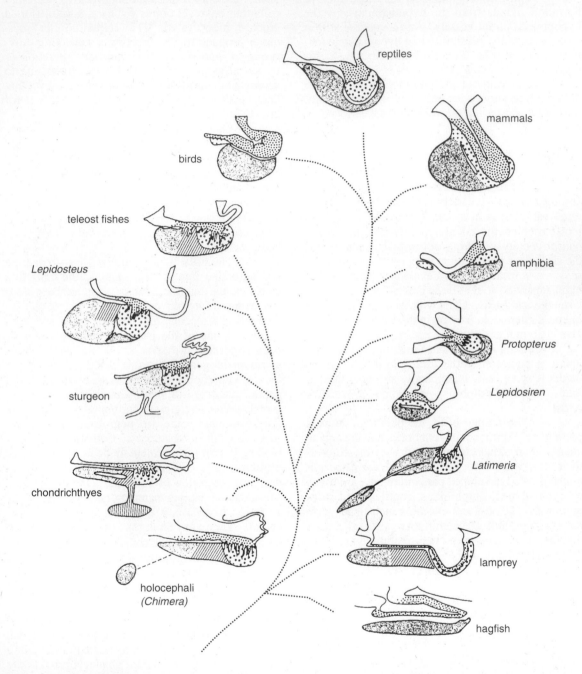

Figure 4.5 The illustration shows the variable nature of the comparative anatomy of the pituitary gland. The diagram shows a "phylogenetic tree" in which the pituitary glands of vertebrate groups are shown in sagittal section. Fine stippling and cross hatching designate areas of pars distalis; open circles, pars intermedia; plus signs, pars tuberalis; coarse dots, neurohypophysis. Modified, with permission, Gorbman, A.; Dickhoff, W.; Vigna, S.R.; Clark, N.B.; Ralph, C.L. Comparative Endocrinology. New York: John Wiley & Sons; 1983; p. 62.

Table 4.4 Endocrine Hierarchies

THYROID HIERARCHY
Hypothalamus
TSH-stimulating hormone (TRH)
Anterior pituitary gland
thyroid-stimulating hormone (TSH)
Thyroid
thyroxine, triiodothyronine

GONADS HIERARCHY
Hypothalamus
gonadotropin-releasing hormone (GnRH, LRH)
Anterior pituitary gland
luteinizing hormone LH
follicle-stimulating hormone (FSH)
Gonads (Ovaries and Testes)
estrogen, testosterone

INTERMEDIN HIERARCHY
Hypothalamus
MSH-releasing factor (MRF)
serotonin
Anterior pituitary gland
melanophore-stimulating hormone (MSH)

GROWTH HORMONE HIERARCHY
Hypothalamus
growth hormone-releasing hormone
somatostatin
Anterior pituitary gland
growth hormone (GH)

PROLACTIN HIERARCHY
Hypothalamus
prolactin-releasing hormone (PRH)
prolactin-inhibiting hormone (PIH, dopamine)
Anterior pituitary gland
prolactin (PRL)

ADRENAL HIERARCHY
Hypothalamus
corticotropin-releasing hormone (CRF)
Anterior pituitary gland
adrenocorticotropic hormone (ACTH)
Adrenal gland
glucocorticoids

PITUITARY HIERARCHIES

The pituitary was originally viewed as a "master gland" because of the early discoveries that the pituitary gland controlled the endeavors of other glands (the thyroid gland, gonads, and adrenal glands). However, the pituitary suffered loss in status when it was discovered to be the conduit or slave of hormones of the hypothalamus.

Because the pituitary gland is controlled by the hypothalamus, and the hypothalamus is part of the brain, a route is provided for external information from the organism's environment, perceived by the brain, to influence the endocrine system. The hypothalamus integrates both external and internal information.

The pituitary gland functions in many of the major "hierarchies" that constitute the endocrine system (Table 4.4). Further details of pituitary function will be supplied with the individual glands and hormones that compose the hierarchies that include the pituitary gland.

However masterful (mistressful?), the pituitary gland has not escaped the pens of novelists. In a metabolic discussion of good versus evil, Tom Robbins imagines a movie about the reaction to that slimy villain Cholesterol:

> "The film might begin on a stormy night in the central nervous system. Alarmed, the ever-watchful pituitary gland dispatches a couple of trusted hormones with a message for the adrenals. Even though it's all downstream, the going is rough because of boulders of white sugar and passageways dangerously narrowed due to atherosclerosis."[10]

REFERENCES

1 Telford, I.; Bridgman, C.F. Introduction to Functional Histology. New York: Harper & Row; 1990; p. 433.

2. Hadley, M.E. Endocrinology, Sixth Edition, Englewood Cliffs, NJ: Prentice Hall; 1988; p. 86.

3. Telford, I., Op. cit. p. 445.

4. Findling, J.W.; Tyrrell, J.B. Anterior pituitary and somatomedins: I. Anterior pituitary. In Greenspan, F.S.; Forsham, P.H., editors. Basic and Clinical Endocrinology, Second Edition. Los Altos, CA: Lange Medical Publications; 1986; p. 45.

5. Turner, C.D.; Bagnara, J.T. General Endocrinology, Sixth Edition. Philadelphia: W.B. Saunders Co.; 1976; p. 82.

6. Norman, G.; Litwack, G. Hormones. Orlando, FL: Academic Press; 1987; pp. 184–185.

7. Telford, I., Op cit. page 437–438.

8. Schwartz, J.; Cherny, R. Intercellular communication within the anterior pituitary influencing the secretion of hypophysial hormones. Endocrine Reviews 13: 453–475; 1992.

9. Stojilkovic, S.S.; Catt, K.J. Calcium oscillations in anterior pituitary cells. Endocrine Reviews 13: 256–280; 1992.

10. Tom Robbins. Even Cowgirls Get the Blues. New York: Bantam Books; 1976; p. 317.

CHAPTER 5

Vasopressin and Oxytocin

The hypothalamic neurohormones are a group of nonapeptides. Two of the hormones in the group are vasopressin and oxytocin. They are synthesized in the hypothalamus and secreted into the blood in the posterior pituitary gland. Vasopressin is also discussed in chapters including other hormones that affect water balance (e.g., mineralocorticoids, angiotensin, and atrial natriuretic peptide). Oytocin is considered in more detail in the chapters on female reproduction.

ANATOMY

The **neurosecretory cell bodies** that make the nonapeptide hormones, collectively called the hypothalamic neurohormones, or neurohypophysial neurohormones, are in the hypothalamus. The nonapeptide hormones were formerly thought to be made in the posterior pituitary gland and were (and still are) sometimes referred to as "posterior pituitary hormones." But the hormones are only secreted by the posterior pituitary.

The nonapeptide hormones are synthesized in the large, magnocellular neurons of the **supraoptic nuclei** (SON) and **paraventricular nuclei** (PVN) of the hypothalamus. Their projections mainly emanate to the pituitary. Smaller, parvicellular neurons found in the suprachiasmatic and paraventricular nuclei also synthesize arginine vasopressin (AVP), and their diffuse projections distribute widely to other locations including the median eminence, nucleus of the solitary tract, dorsal motor nucleus of the vagus, spinal cord, and the choroid plexus. There are some cells in other locations that may be able to synthesize oxytocin and vasopressin (suprachiasmatic nuclei, gonads, adrenal cortex, thymus). So, a given nonapeptide hormone may be synthesized in several places: AVP, for example, is synthesized in the supraoptic nuclei, the paraventricular nuclei, and the suprachiasmatic nuclei.[1,2,3]

The neurosecretory cells that make neurohormones are quite respectable as neurons because they can generate and conduct action potentials. Normally the vasopressin neurons are at rest, but when a signal is received from environmental stimuli (e.g., bleeding), the neurons first increase firing rate and then attain a pattern of phasic bursting (about two bursts a minute of high-frequency discharge in alternation with electrical quiescence).[4]

A **hypothalamoneurohypophysial nerve tract** of the axonal processes of the neurosecretory cells descends the infundibulum and terminates in the posterior pituitary gland. The fibers are fine, unmyelinated fibers that descend in thick networks. The nerve tract has 100,000 fibers in humans. The fibers are characterized anatomically by the presence of 1 to 50 micrometer swellings. This is the principal pathway for the vasopressinergic neuronal projections, but there are others that project to the median eminence, the organus vasculosum, forebrain, brain stem, and spinal cord.

The **posterior pituitary** thus consists mainly of the neurosecretory cell terminals, or nerve endings, of the neurosecretory cells of the hypothalamus. Release of the hormones is a consequence of action potentials traveling down the neurosecretory cell axons.

The hormones are released by exocytosis which requires calcium. Secretory granules are present in the posterior pituitary and stain so as to be readily visible with light microscopy. The granules are called **Herring bodies**.

There are only a few cells, called **pituicytes**, in the posterior pituitary gland. They are branching cells with endings on vascular sinusoids between nerve endings of the neurosecretory cells. Their function is not settled, but they are probably glial cells (neuroglia) and may act like the central nervous system cells which are thought to perform support functions for neurons. Previously, the pituicytes were sometimes viewed as storage cells upon which the neurosecretory cells terminated.

The pituitary weighs about 600 mg in adult humans, of which 20% is the posterior lobe.

CHEMISTRY

The family of hypothalamic neurohormones includes oxytocin and vasopressins (Figure 5.1). The members of the family are nonapeptides. They all have six amino acids linked into a ring by a disulfide bond, and they possess "tails" consisting of three amino acid tails.

One function attributed to hormones secreted at the posterior pituitary gland is water retention, mainly viewed as control of renal (kidney) water excretion. For this reason, endocrinologists proposed and named antidiuretic hormone (ADH). Antidiuretic "hormone" is three molecules collectively called vasopressins: arginine vasopressin, lysine vasopressin, 4-ser-lys-vasopressin. Scientists reporting in the literature have used ADH or vasopressin, depending on what they were measuring (e.g., antidiuretic activity or amount of a hormone) so ADH does not always equal vasopressin(s).

The structures of oxytocin and vasopressin were determined and synthesized by du Vigneaud in 1953. The synthesis was of general biological and medical significance because oxytocin and vasopressin were the first peptides to be synthesized.[5]

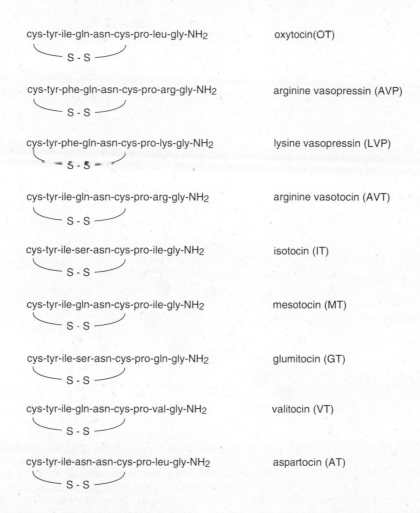

cys-tyr-ile-gln-asn-cys-pro-leu-gly-NH$_2$ S - S	oxytocin(OT)
cys-tyr-phe-gln-asn-cys-pro-arg-gly-NH$_2$ S - S	arginine vasopressin (AVP)
cys-tyr-phe-gln-asn-cys-pro-lys-gly-NH$_2$ S - S	lysine vasopressin (LVP)
cys-tyr-ile-gln-asn-cys-pro-arg-gly-NH$_2$ S - S	arginine vasotocin (AVT)
cys-tyr-ile-ser-asn-cys-pro-ile-gly-NH$_2$ S - S	isotocin (IT)
cys-tyr-ile-gln-asn-cys-pro-ile-gly-NH$_2$ S - S	mesotocin (MT)
cys-tyr-ile-ser-asn-cys-pro-gln-gly-NH$_2$ S - S	glumitocin (GT)
cys-tyr-ile-gln-asn-cys-pro-val-gly-NH$_2$ S - S	valitocin (VT)
cys-tyr-ile-asn-asn-cys-pro-leu-gly-NH$_2$ S - S	aspartocin (AT)

Figure 5.1 Structures of the nonapeptide hormones.

The disulfide bonds in oxytocin and vasopressin are necessary for activity. When the bonds are broken, and the sulfur groups are reduced to sulfhydryl (-SH) groups, the hormones lose their biological activity.

SYNTHESIS OF PEPTIDE HORMONES

The general pattern (Figures 5.2, 5.3) for peptide (or polypeptide, or protein) synthesis as follows: The nucleotide sequence in DNA provides the genetic code for synthesis of another nucleic acid, RNA. The process takes place in the cell nucleus and is called transcription. At the ribosomes in the endoplasmic reticulum in the cytoplasm, a protein is synthesized from amino acids according to the code provided by the RNA in a process called translation.

In hormone synthesis, the completed protein is called the **preprohormone**. The prohormone contains extra sequences of amino acids (e.g., the signal peptide) beyond those in the ultimate hormone. Some of these pieces are cleaved off, leaving a **prohormone**. The prohormone may undergo changes (e.g., folding or formation of disulfide bonds). The prohormone molecule may

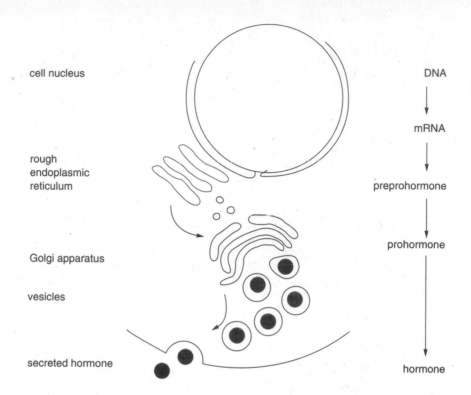

Figure 5.2 The left side of the diagram lists the cell structures where protein hormone synthesis and secretion takes place; the right side represents the molecular changes. In the cell nucleus (circle), genes code the sequence of messenger RNA (mRNA); the synthesis of RNA using the DNA code is transcription. mRNA determines the sequence of amino acids which are linked by peptide bonds to make the protein preprohormone in the endoplasmic reticulum. Vesicles transport the preprohormone to the Golgi apparatus where it is converted to the prohormone. The Golgi packages polypeptide hormones into secretory granules which release the hormone through the cell membrane by exocytosis.

even be the prohormone for several hormones, as is the case for proopiomelanocortin. The prohormone is found in the lumen of the endoplasmic reticulum.

The prohormone moves by vesicular transport (involving microtubules, disrupted by colchicine) to the Golgi apparatus (or region) where it is interred in vesicles or granules. The prohormones undergo further modification (terminal glycosylation and conversion to hormones) in the Golgi. Finally secretory granules are formed which contain the hormones along with ATP, calcium, dopamine, proteins, etc. The secretory granules are stored in cell cytoplasm and are released at the cell membrane by the process of exocytosis.

BIOSYNTHESIS OF HYPOTHALAMIC NONAPEPTIDES

The synthesis of the hypothalamic nonapeptides illustrates generally the involvement of large precursor molecules (prehormones or prepro- hormones) that is typical of the synthesis of many peptides.

The nonapeptides are associated with larger molecules. The larger molecule associated with va-

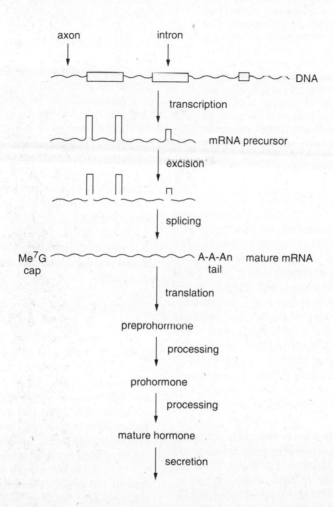

Figure 5.3 The diagram illustrates the biosynthesis of protein hormones. The genetic information is in the DNA. A messenger RNA precursor is produced from the DNA by transcription from which the intervening sequences (introns) are removed and the protein coding sequences (exons) are spliced together to form mature messenger RNA. Messenger RNA is translated into protein, often into a protein that is larger than the final, circulating hormone. The "pre" sequence is a signal or leader sequence characterizing secretory proteins. The sequence, after specifying the directional synthesis of the protein in the inside of the membrane of the endoplasmic reticulum, is removed. The remaining prohormone is transferred to the Golgi complex where it is further converted by proteolysis and packaged into secretory granules. Reproduced, with permission. West, W. B., editor. Physiological Basis of Medical Practice, 12th Edition. Baltimore: Williams & Wilkins; 1992; p. 791.

sopressin was named **neurophysin (Np)**. Neurophysin was first thought to be a carrier protein for the hormone. The larger molecules, found in the posterior pituitary gland and in the pineal gland, were originally grouped as the "neurophysins" as described by Reinharz and coworkers:[6]

> The pituitary neurophysins consist of cysteine-rich proteins which are believed to function as carriers for the

neuropeptides vasopressin and oxytocin. These peptides are synthesized in the supraoptic and paraventricular nuclei of the hypothalamus and are transported by rapid axoplasmic transport to the neurohypophysis...[E]ach hormone (vasopressin and oxytocin) and its specific neurophysin are derived from a large precursor molecule. The principal function of neurophysins, cleaved from precursor during maturation of the secretory granules, appears to be the stabilization of the hormones.

Now, it is believed that the hormone and the larger molecule, neurophysin, are associated with one another because they are synthesized together as parts of a larger precursor molecule. The precursor for arginine vasopressin, prepro-pressophysin, is 145 amino acids consisting of a signal peptide, arginine vasopressin, and a glycosylated moiety. The oxytocin precursor, prepro-oxyphysin, consists of the signal peptide and oxytocin (no glycosylated moiety). Oxytocin and vasopressin have different neurophysins; oxytocin is associated with neurophysin I; vasopressin is associated with neurophysin II. The prehormones, prepro-pressophysin and prepro-oxyphysin, lose their leader sequences in the endoplasmic reticulum (Figure 5.4).[7]

The precursor travels the axons from the synthesizing cell bodies in the hypothalamus to the posterior pituitary. It takes 1.5 hours from the time of synthesis to the release of arginine vasopressin in the blood. The neurophysin-nonapeptide complexes are cleaved as they travel down the axons of the neurosecretory cells using axoplasmic flow. The secretory storage granules contain free nonapeptide and neurophysin and uncleaved precursors. Herring bodies are found in the posterior pituitary gland and are thought to consist of neurosecretory material. Both arginine vasopressin and neurophysin are secreted.

The metabolism of a nonapeptide such as vasopressin is rapid. The hormones are inactivated in the liver and kidneys. The half-life for antidiuretic hormone is short, only 5–18 minutes. The half-life for oxytocin is even shorter, 3 minutes. A typical circulating nonapeptide value is 2 pg/ml vasopressin in human plasma. AVP is not bound to protein in the circulation as are some other hormones, but it is associated with the platelets.

COMPARATIVE BIOCHEMISTRY

Certain nonapeptides are characteristic of particular vertebrate groups. Glumitocin, valitocin, and aspargtocin are in the cartilaginous fishes (rays and sharks). Mesotocin is distributed more widely in birds, reptiles, amphibians, and lungfish. Isotocin is characteristic of bony fishes. Lysine vasopressin is found in the suiformes (pigs), peccaries, wart hogs, and hippopotami. Arginine vasopressin is found in mammals except for the domestic pigs. Oxytocin is a mammalian nonapeptide. Arginine vasotocin has the widest distribution; it is found in birds, reptiles, amphibians, and fish. Because of the comparative distribution, Acher proposed that arginine vasotocin (AVT) is the ancestral peptide.[8]

EVOLUTION OF PEPTIDE HORMONES

Amino acid substitutions at positions 3, 4, and 8 account for the structural differences among the nonapeptide hormones (Figure 5.5). The substitutions can be explained by single nucleotide changes in the genetic code. Ingenious schemes describing the evolution of peptide hormones have been formulated based on the distribution of nonapeptides among vertebrate groups and the structures of the hormones.

First, in making a scheme, the distribution of the peptides among species is considered with respect to the evolution of the species. Second, scheme-making uses the assumption that some of the molecules can be derived by single amino acid substitution from an ancestral molecule and subsequent secondary amino acid substitution to get the remaining molecules (similarity in amino acid sequence means evolutionary proximity). Third, the schemes minimize the number of genetic code mutations that would be required for the hormones to evolve. Fourth, the schemes are supported by evidence that arginine vasotocin is the ancestral molecule. Arginine vasotocin presents itself as a likely candidate for an ancestral molecule for three reasons: (i) it has a wide distribution in vertebrates, (ii) it differs from some of the nonapeptides by only one amino acid (oxytocin, arginine vasopressin, mesotocin), and (iii) it is present in fetal mammals.

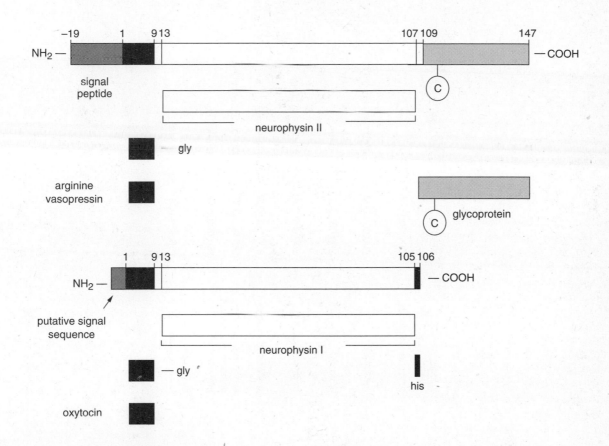

Figure 5.4 The diagram illustrates the synthesis of vasopressin (upper) and oxytocin (lower). Following the pattern for the synthesis of protein hormones, oxytocin and vasopressin (VP) are synthesized from large prepro-hormone precursor proteins. The numbers represent the numbers of amino acids beginning with 1 at the N-terminal of the hormones, oxytocin or vasopressin. Prepro-pressophysin has a signal peptide (amino acids 1 to 19) and a glycoprotein moiety. Prepro-oxyphysin lacks a glycoprotein moiety. Redrawn, with permission. Ivell, R.; Schmale, H.; Richter, D. Vasopressin and oxytocin precursors as models of preprohormones. Neuroendocrinology 37: 235; 1983.

ANTIDIURETIC EFFECTS

The first function assigned to the peptide hormones released in the neurohypophysis is the **antidiuretic effect**. The word "diuresis" means increased production of urine. Drugs that cause increased urine production are therefore known as diuretics. A hormone that prevents the production of urine is called an antidiuretic hormone. So **antidiuretic hormone, ADH**, causes water reten-tion by acting on a target involved in water balance, for example, the kidney. The peptides that have the most ADH activity include the vaso-pressins (arginine vasopressin, lysine vasopressin, 4-ser-lys-vasopressin) and arginine vasotocin (Table 5.1).

ADH increases the permeability of the collecting ducts of the kidney (Figure 5.6). This means the water comes out of the urine collecting ducts and into the interstitium of the renal pyra-

AMINO ACID SEQUENCE	NAME	YEARS	OCCURRENCE
cys-tyr-ileu-gln-asn-cys-pro-arg-gly	arginine vasotocin	500,000,000	all
cys-tyr-ileu-gln-asn-cys-pro-ileu-gly	mesotocin	400,000,000	birds, reptiles, amphibians, fishes
cys-tyr-ileu-ser-asn-cys-pro-arg-gly	isotocin	300,000,000	fishes
cys-tyr-ileu-gln-asn-cys-pro-leu-gly	oxytocin	200,000,000	mammals, birds
cys-tyr-phe-gln-asn-cys-pro-arg-gly	arginine vasopressin	200,000,000	mammals
cys-tyr-phe-gln-asn-cys-pro-lys-gly	lysine vasopressin valitocin, aspartocin from oxytocin?	180,000,000	hippo, pig, wart hog
		180,000,000	sharks, rays
	glumitocin from isotocin	180,000,000	sharks, rays

Table 5.1 Neurohypophysial Hormone Activities

	Rat uterus	Chicken blood pressure	Rabbit mammary gland	Rat antidiuresis	Rat blood pressure
oxytocin	450	450	450	5.00	5.00
ichthyotocin	150	320	300	0.18	0.06
arginine vasopressin	16	60	65	400.00	400.00
lysine vasopressin	5	40	60	250.00	270.00
arginine vasotocin	115	285	210	250.00	245.00
mesotocin	291	502	330	1.10	6.30

The numbers represent activity of hormone (IU/micromole) compared for five different bioassays. Frieden, E.; Lipner, H. Biochemical Endocrinology of the Vertebrates. Englewood Cliffs, N.J.: Prentice Hall; 1973; p. 45.

mids. The water retention by the kidney decreases the urine volume and makes the urine more concentrated. In the absence of ADH, the water remains in the collecting ducts, the urine excreted is dilute, and the urine volume is great.

In the average adult human, 2600 ml water are lost per 24 hours: 1500 ml are lost in the urine, 500 ml are lost via the skin, 400 ml are lost via respiration through the lungs, and 100 ml are excreted in the feces. So the urine represents the greatest water loss. Consider the water filtered into the proximal tubules of the human kidney (100%). 20% of the water enters the distal convoluted tubules. In the absence of ADH, 8% of the water is reabsorbed into the kidney, 12% of the water is lost in the urine (15 ml/min), and urine osmolarity is 30–60 mmol/l. With maximal ADH (10–12 pg/ml), 19% of the water is reabsorbed and only 1% is lost in the urine (1 ml/min), and urine osmolarity is 1200–1400 mmol/l.[9]

ADH in humans, as in most mammals, is usually arginine vasopressin (AVP) and may be referred to as "vasopressin." In human subjects with normal ADH, urine excretion is 2 liters/day.

However, in a human without ADH, urine excretion increases to 4–12 liters per day. In mammals then, ADH secretion causes the production of concentrated urine, and ADH deficiency results in dilute urine (Figure 5.7).

Desert animals are more interesting. A kangaroo rat, a desert species, produces 50 milliunits/day of ADH and can concentrate urine five times as much as a dog, a nondesert species, which produces only 6 milliunits/day of ADH. The neural lobe of the pituitary gland of a kangaroo rat is larger than that of a laboratory rat and has more ADH. When kangaroo rats are dehydrated (e.g., by injection of NaCl), osmiophilic neurosecretory material of the neural lobes is lost and is replaced by large clear vesicles.

The skin and bladder join the kidney as ADH targets in some species. Bentley described the urinary toad bladder preparation used to study antidiuretic activity in vitro:

> Two lobes of the urinary bladder of the toad *Bufo marinus* were prepared. . . . Each lobe was dissected and tied to the end of a piece of Pyrex

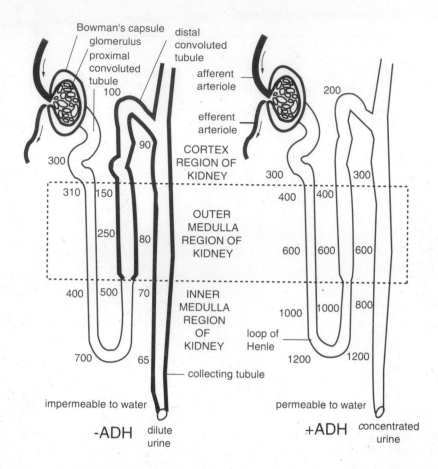

Figure 5.6 Diagram of two nephrons of the kidney. Blood from the afferent arteriole enters a knot of capillaries (glomerulus), is filtered, and exits the efferent arteriole. Urine is formed in the Bowman's capsule, tubules, and collecting duct. In an ingenious mechanism, called the "countercurrent multiplier," the nephron makes use of parallel tubes with fluid flowing in opposite directions to concentrate urine. The numbers represent concentrations of urine in milliosmols (mosm) in the tubules. Higher numbers represent more concentrated solutions; lower numbers represent more dilute solutions. The numbers shown on the left nephron represent production of dilute urine in the absence of ADH. Heavy lines show parts of the nephron that are impermeable to water in the absence of ADH. When ADH acts, as on the right, water from the collecting tubules exits the collecting ducts into the interstitial tissue because of the high concentration of salt in the interstitial fluid, and the urine becomes more concentrated. Compare the concentrations in the loop of Henle and the collecting duct. Modified, with permission. Tortora, G.J.; Anagnostakos, N.P. Principles of Anatomy and Physiology, Sixth Edition. New York: Harper & Row; 1990; p. 842.

glass tubing that had been pushed through the centre of a rubber stopper. Gain or loss of water was measured by weighing the tubing, attached bladder and contents . . . . The bladder was filled with 1.5 ml of the

required solution through the piece of glass tubing to which it was attached and immersed in a test tube filled with 30 ml of . . . Ringer's solution which was aerated with an aquarium aerator. The whole unit

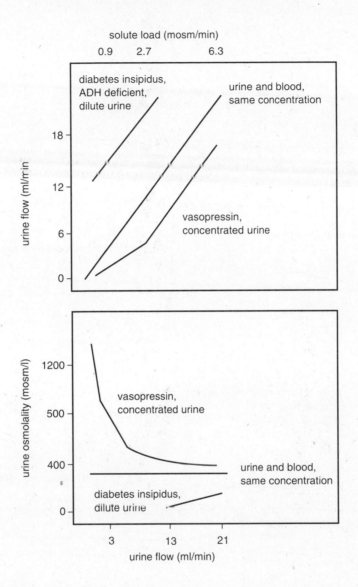

Figure 5.7 Graphs illustrate the relationship of vasopressin (antidiuretic hormone) and urine formation and concentration. Modified, with permission, Berliner, R.W.; Giebisch, G.; Brobeck, J.R., editors. Best and Taylor's Physiological Basis of Medical Practice, Ninth Edition. Williams & Wilkins; 1979.

was placed in a bath kept at 25°C. . . One lobe of the toad bladder was used for the experimental treatment and the other lobe as a control. . . . [W]ater always moved through the bladder wall towards the fluid of higher osmotic pressure.[10]

In the presence of 1 mu/ml vasopressin (Pitressin®), the toad bladder changed 113 mg; the control without vasopressin changed only 4.3 mg. Water moves across the membranes of the toad bladder by osmosis. In the presence of vasopressin, water moves outward five times faster than it moves inward.

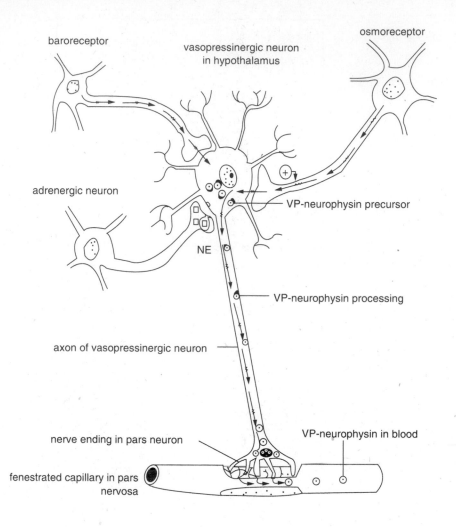

Figure 5.8 The figure shows four neurons and a blood vessel to illustrate a model for vasopressin formation and secretion into the blood. Neurons (baroreceptor, osmoreceptor, and adrenergic) have axons that terminate at and synapse with the vasopressinergic neuron. The baroreceptors (in carotid sinus, aortic arch, left atrium) are activated by fright or pain; the osmoreceptors respond to plasma osmolality; the adrenergic neurons respond to pain, fright, adrenal insufficiency, cardiac failure, hypoxia, alarm reactions, and stress by releasing norepineprhine at their axon terminals. Signals from these neurons stimulate the vasopressinergic neuron. The vasopressin cell body synthesizes prepro-pressophysin. Prepropressophysin loses its leader sequences in the cell body. Vasopressin-neurophysin complexes descend the axon by axoplasmic flow. The VP-neurophysin complexes are secreted through fenestrations in capillaries into the blood as it circulates through the pars nervosa. In another viewpoint, not shown, the VP-neurophysin complex is stored before entering into the blood. Modified, with permission. Lincoln, D. The posterior pituitary. In Austin, C.R.; Short, R.V., editors. Reproduction in Mammals, Book III. Hormonal Control of Reproduction, Second Edition. New York: Cambridge University Press; 1984; pp. 21–50.

Table 5.2 Factors That Alter Vasopressin Secretion[11,12]

Increase secretion	Decrease secretion
increase plasma osmotic pressure	decrease plasma osmotic pressure
decrease ECF volume	increase ECF volume
pain	alcohol
emotion	butorphanol (opioid antagonist)
stress	oxilorphan
exercise	
nausea and vomiting	
standing	
morphine	
nicotine	
barbiturates	
chlorpropamide (oral glucose lowering sulfonylurea)	
clofibrate (lowers serum lipids)	
carbamazepine (anticonvulsant and analgesic)	
angiotensin II	

Frogs can use their skins to exchange water with their environments.[13] If an anuran (frog or toad) is placed in water, its weight will increase if it is injected with peptides from the neurohypophysis. This weight increase in response to peptides (e.g., vasotocin) is called the **Brunn effect**. In causing the Brunn effect, the hormones act to prevent water loss by the kidneys, they increase water uptake through the skin, and they provoke water absorption from the urinary bladder.

REGULATION OF NONAPEPTIDES

Regulation of secretion of antidiuretic hormones, such as vasopressin, is by a set point mechanism. The set point mechanism makes use of **osmoreceptor** cells (Figure 5.8). The osmoreceptor cells, which respond to plasma osmolality (or cerebrospinal fluid sodium), are believed to be located in the anterior hypothalamus in a circumventricular organ (organum vasculosum of the lamina terminalis).

Osmoreceptors respond to changes in osmolality as small as 1%. Normal plasma osmolality is 290 mosm/l and it is maintained in the narrow range of 280–295 mmol/kg. Vasopressin comes into play when the osmolality rises. Vasopressin secretion increases, and neurosecretory cell firing rate increases, beginning at 285 mosm/kg.

Blood osmolality is the major regulator of AVP secretion but modest changes in blood volume may alter the response.[14] Pain is also associated with vasopressin secretion which implies that it responds to neural signals, and angiotensin increases ADH secretion which implies that it can be regulated by hormones.

Oxytocin is subject to neurochemical regulation.[15] Oxytocin is regulated by afferent neural signals from touch receptors in the breast (e.g., during nursing), uterus (e.g., during parturition), and genitalia (e.g., during sexual activity). Estrogen increases effects of oxytocin on smooth muscle and uterus. Oxytocin levels are also altered by the same factors that affect vasopressin. Oxytocin changes in response to norepinephrine, dopamine,

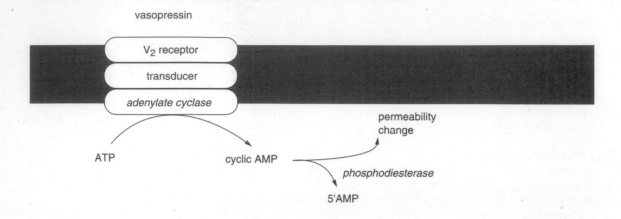

Figure 5.9 Vasopressin stimulates the activity of the enzyme adenylate cyclase in the cell membranes of its target tissues (e.g., of the cells of the collecting ducts in the kidney). In turn, the increase in adenylate cyclase activity produces more cyclic AMP from ATP. The increase cAMP causes a permeability change so that water can penetrate the cell membrane more easily, as if pores in the membrane were enlarged. The vasopressin stimulation is stopped by another enzyme, phosphodiesterase, which breaks down the cyclic AMP to for 5'AMP.

serotonin, acetylcholine, glutamate, γ-aminobutyric acid, vasoactive intestinal peptide, angiotensin II, cholecystokinin, enkephalin, ß-endorphin, and corticotropin-releasing factor.

OSMOREGULATION

So what happens in osmoregulation? If concentrated saline (hypertonic salt solution, e.g., 855 mmol/l) is infused, plasma osmolality increases, plasma AVP increases from below detectable levels to up to 20 pmol/l, antidiuresis ensues and urine concentration increases. Maximum antidiuresis is attained at about 295 mmol/kg with plasma AVP about 5 pmol/l; increasing the osmolality further results in dehydration. In healthy people, thirst osmoreceptors are stimulated at about 298 mmol/kg, drinking ensues, and dehydration is reversed or prevented. Drinking large volumes of fluid suppresses AVP secretion (e.g., to <0.5 pmol/l) and the kidney can excrete 15–10 liters of urine per 24 hours.[16]

A number of factors can increase or decrease vasopressin secretion (Table 5.2). One of these factors is cigarette smoking which, in 30 minutes, increases vasopressin neurophysin more than three-fold.[17]

Baylis[18] describes the history of our understanding of the working of hormones in antidiuresis:

Our understanding of the mechanisms that regulate water balance in mammals began [in 1947] with the classic studies of Professor E.B. Verney and his colleagues in Cambridge, England. In a series of experiments on conscious, trained dogs with permanent exteriorized carotid arteries to allow rapid injections of solutions into the cerebral circulation, Verney demonstrated that hypertonic solutions of sodium chloride, sucrose and glucose caused antidiuresis; observations which formed the basis of the concept of the 'osmoreceptor'. Verney proposed that cells within the central nervous system altered their volume thus regulating the release of an antidiuretic hormone which acted upon the kidney. The results of subsequent experiments [by Jewell and Verney in 1957] suggested that these osmotically sensitive cells were located in the anterior hypothalamus.

Antidiuretic hormone functions with other hormones (aldosterone, ACTH, glucocorticoids, angiotensin) in the regulation of water balance.

MECHANISM OF ACTION

The mechanism of action of ADH activity is a cyclic nucleotide (cyclic AMP) mechanism, and it involves the idea of a **pore size theory** (Figure 5.9). There are 0.4 nm diameter channels in the membranes of the lumens of the cells of the collecting ducts (peritubular sides). The interaction of vasopressin with receptors on the membranes stimulates adenylate cyclase. The resulting increase in cyclic AMP leads to a sequence of events which increases diffusion of water through the membrane. Amphibian skin and bladder were useful target tissues for studying the mechanisms of action for antidiuretic hormones because they could be observed in vitro. Receptors (V_2 receptors in the nephrons on the blood side of the tubular cells in the thick ascending limb of Henle and the collecting duct) have been found for the ADH activity.

VASOPRESSOR EFFECT

Vasopressin is named for effects on blood pressure. There are several vasopressins (e.g., arginine vasopressin and lysine vasopressin). Usually, the term "vasopressin" by itself refers to arginine vasopressin or to the biological activity of the nonapeptides on blood pressure. Despite the name vasopressin, which implies a role for the pituitary in blood pressure control, removing the pituitary gland does not result in a decrease in blood pressure. However, at large (possibly pharmacological) doses, some of the nonapeptides cause contraction of smooth muscle in the walls of blood vessels, increase the vascular reactions to catecholamines, and cause peripheral vasoconstriction. All of these actions would have the effect of raising blood pressure. In turn, low pressure receptors in the great veins, atria, and pulmonary blood vessels respond to low blood pressure and are associated with an increase in vasopressin secretion.

Hypotension (low blood pressure) and hypovolemia (low blood volume), which can be caused by bleeding, increase vasopressin secretion. Vasopressin can increase to over 100 pg/ml when blood volume drops during hemorrhage (bleeding). Blood volume must be reduced at least 10% to increase antidiuretic activity or plasma immunoreactive AVP concentrations. Blood pressure decreases of 5% or more can raise AVP; a 40% reduction of baseline blood pressure causes AVP to rise to 100 pmol/l. Baylis[19] suggests that the 5–10% daily decreases in blood pressure in resting individuals at night might stimulate AVP production and explain the antidiuresis that occurs during sleep.

Low pressure "baroreceptors" are found in the left atrium and the great veins of the chest and these baroreceptors can detect changes in blood volume. High pressure baroreceptors are found in the aortic arch and the carotid blood vessels. There are V_1 receptors for the vasoconstrictor effects of vasopressin in the blood vessels, brain, and glomerular mesangial cells which may work using PIP_2 (phosphatidylinositol 4,5-diphosphate) and calcium without activation of adenylate cyclase.

The blood pressure effects can, however, be confusing. In birds, vasopressin has the opposite effect to its action in mammals. In birds, vasopressin acts as a depressor, that is, it lowers blood pressure. The effects of AVP on blood pressure invite consideration of the possibility that AVP plays a role in causing high blood pressure (essential hypertension) in human beings. But, although there is some animal experimental evidence for this idea, the evidence has so far not pointed to a principle role of AVP in causing essential hypertension in people.

OXYTOCIC EFFECT

The oxytocic effect is the contraction of the smooth muscle of the uterus. This effect is observed mainly on the pregnant uterus where oxytocin probably participates in the initiation of labor and the process of parturition (birth).

Oxytocin may facilitate sperm transport in the nonpregnant uterus. In some species, the act of coitus results in oxytocin secretion which in turn causes uterine contractions which may be involved in the movement of sperm. So the uterus is a target of oxytocin.

The breasts are also targets of oxytocin. Touch receptors around the nipples responding to

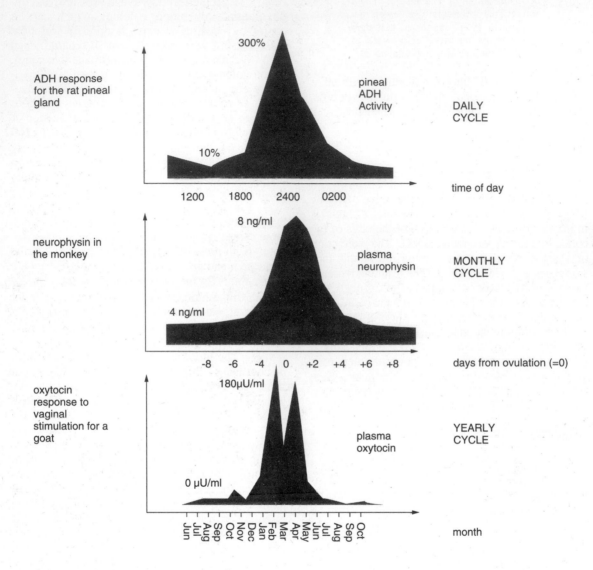

Figure 5.10 The figure shows rhythms in the system of neurohypophysial neurohormones. The numbers on the graph are approximate peak and nadir values. Both the vertical and horizontal axes have different units because the data came from different sources for different responses. Drawn by the author from data in Konig, A.; Meyer, A. The effect of continuous illumination on the circadian rhythm of the antidiuretic activity of the rat pineal. J. Interdiscipl. Cycle Res. 2: 255–262; 1971. Robinson, A.G.; Ferin, M.; Zimmerman, E.A. Neurophysin secretion in monkeys: Emphasis on the hypothalamic response to estrogen and ovarian events. J. Clin. Endocrinol. Metab. 44: 330; 1976. Roberts, J.S. Seasonal variations in the reflexive release of oxytocin and in the effect of estradiol on the reflex in goats. Endocrinology 89; 1029; 1971.

suckling send neural signals to the paraventricular and supraoptic nuclei. The oxytocin neurons of the hypothalamus secrete oxytocin from the posterior pituitary, and the oxytocin causes contraction of the myoepithelial cells surrounding the mammary alveoli. As a consequence of the contractions, the duct ejects the milk. The neuroendocrine (neurohumoral) reflex involving the nipple and oxytocin is called **milk ejection** (also called milk letdown, the suckling reflex, or the galactogenic effect). The reflex can become a conditioned reflex so that a crying infant or the arrival of feeding time initiates milk ejection.

There is some reason to believe that oxytocin plays a role in the physiology of orgasm. Plasma oxytocin baseline levels were 1.1 ± 0.2 pmol/l in eight men. Masturbation caused an increase in the plasma oxytocin to 4.1 ± 1.1 pmol/l during orgasm. The increase was blocked by the drug, naloxone, which also potentiates oxytocin release in response to vaginocervical stimulation in goats.[20]

OTHER ACTIONS

Vasopressin has other actions—it slows the heart rate and it suppresses release of renin from the kidneys. Vasopressin acts on the brain where it enhances passive avoidance behavior. Vasopressin also acts on the adenohypophysis where it causes ACTH release (acting as a CRH). Vasopressin releases TSH from pituitary cells *in vitro*.[21]

The gastrointestinal hormone cholecystokinin (CCK), which has been implicated in feeding behavior, increases oxytocin. Ablation of the paraventricular nucleus which makes oxytocin results in overeating and obesity in rats suggesting that oxytocin plays a role in feeding behavior.

Vasotocin may be involved in reproductive behavior. The clasping behavior of amphibians is called amplexus. Amplectic clasping is a response of male newts to intraventricular injections of arginine vasotocin (AVT). Elevated AVT has been associated with oviposition in marine turtles and may be involved in the motility of the oviduct in reptiles.

Other behaviors as well may be affected by vasopressin. People were asked to count different kinds of rare tone pips. The subjects' auditory event-related potentials were measured. A synthetic vasopressin (experimental) or placebo (control) was administered intranasally. The synthetic vasopressin altered the auditory event-related potentials. The authors suggested that the changes resulted from a "general excitatory effect of [synthetic vasopressin] on cortical activity."[22] In another test of the same substance, subjects were presented with 15 words; synthetic vasopressin did not change the total number of recalled words, but did alter the memory performance in terms of the serial position of the words.[23] Vasopressin, administered as 12–16 USP units per day in a nasal spray, has been suggested as a smart drug "necessary for imprinting new information in your memory" and is supposed to work within seconds.[24]

BIOASSAYS, INTERNATIONAL UNITS, CYCLES

Bioassays illustrate the overlap in function that is due to similarities among the nonapeptide hormones. Bioassays also illustrate the differences in relative potencies of the nonapeptide hormones for various effects. However, today, radioimmunoassays would be used to measure the nonapeptide hormones. The use of a diversity of units can be confusing. But there is a good reason for exercising caution in converting units to a standard form—the measurements were made using different assays and the assays may have not detected the same thing.

The **isolated rat uterus** provides an *in vitro* bioassay for oxytocic activity. Female rats are pretreated with estrogen for three days or are used during estrus when their estrogen levels are high. The rat uteri are removed and incubated at 28–30 °C in a bathing solution. Contractions of the rat uteri measure the activity of hormone. The **chicken blood pressure** assays vascular activity *in vivo*. Blood pressure reduction in the chicken's cannulated ischiatic artery is measured. The **rabbit mammary gland** assay utilizes the rabbit's milk duct *in vivo*. Volume or pressure is measured in the cannulated milk duct in response to hormone. The **rat antidiuresis** assay measures vasopressin *in vivo* by determination of the rate of urine formation in hydrated rats (e.g., given a measured oral dose of water). The **rat blood pressure** assay makes use of measurement of elevated blood pressure in rats in response to doses of hormone *in vivo*. Typically, to do these assays, a standard curve of measurements is constructed using standard doses of pure hormone. Then, the response to an unknown is compared with the standard curve.

International units were used to measure nonapeptides. For these peptides, 1 I.U. was equal to the amount of pituitary hormone contained in 0.5 mg of acetone-dried pituitary powder. Absolute equivalents were established later.

Table 5.3 Some Causes of Syndrome of Inappropriate ADH Secretion (SIADH)

MALIGNANT TUMORS
carcinoma of lung, pancreas, duodenum, prostate
thymoma
mesothelioma
Ewing's tumor

NEUROLOGICAL DISEASE
meningo-encephalitis
brain tumor
subarachnoid hemorrhage
Guillian-Barre syndrome
cerebral and cerebellar atrophy
Shy-Drager syndrome
hydrocephalus
brain abcess

LUNG DISEASE
pneumonia
tuberculosis
cystic fibrosis
empyema
asthma
pneumothorax

DRUGS
vasopressin, oxytocin
vinblastine, vincristine
chlorpropamide
thiazide diuretics
clofibrate
phenothiazines
MAO inhibitors
tricyclic antidepressants
carbamazepine
nicotine

ENDOCRINE DISORDERS
hypothyroidism
adrenal insufficiency

MISCELLANEOUS
porphyria
psychosis
idiopathic

Modified, with permission. Baylis, P.H.; Thompson, C.J. Osmoregulation of vasopressin secretion and thirst in health and disease. Clinical Endocrinology 29: 459–576; 1988; p. 562.

1 mg synthetic oxytocin
= 450 I.U. oxytocic potency

1 I.U. oxytocic potency
= 2.2 micrograms synthetic oxytocin

1 mg synthetic arginine vasopressin
= 400 I.U. pressor potency

1 I.U. pressor or antidiuretic activity
= 2.5 micrograms synthetic arginine vasopressin

The peptide hormones of the ADH family have a wide array of rhythms–seasonal rhythms, monthly rhythms, and daily rhythms (Figure 5.10). For example, there are daily rhythms of vasopressin and oxytocin and neurophysin in the retinas and Harderian glands of rats; rat pineal glands have a rhythm of vasopressin.[25] Neurophysin correlates with the reproductive cycle in monkeys with peak neurophysin correlating with peak estrogen and LH levels. Oxytocin responses to vaginal stimulation showed a seasonal rhythm in a goat with peak levels from January to May.

DIABETES INSIPIDUS AND SIADH

Often, in associating diseases with endocrine function, there are diseases that can be linked to a deficiency of hormone secretion (hyposecretion) and other diseases that can be attributed to hormone excess (hypersecretion). In the case of antidiuretic hormones, a disease of deficiency is diabetes insipidus and a disease of excess is SIADH.

There is a syndrome in humans named **diabetes insipidus.** The syndrome is characterized by copious urine production (polyuria) during both day and night. If the thirst mechanism is functional, there is a concomitant intake of large amounts of fluid (polydipsia) which the victims use to maintain water balance. Disease processes (e.g., neoplastic or vascular lesions, trauma) in the hypothalamic nuclei, the hypothalamohypophysial tract, or the posterior pituitary gland can cause the vasopressin deficiency. Kidney failure to respond to vasopressin is another cause of diabetes insipidus. If the sense of thirst is damaged, then the suffering individual becomes dehydrated because of insufficient fluid intake. Diabetes insipidus may be hereditary. There is an animal model for diabetes insipidus; a strain of rats exists that cannot synthesize arginine vasopressin. The rats drink 80% of their body weight each day and excrete 70% of their body weight each day as urine. The rats are called the Brattleboro strain of rats. The Brattleboro rats have hereditary hypothalamic diabetes insipidus.[26] Early treatments for deficiency of the antidiuretic nonapeptides used pituitary powder administered as "snuff." Treatments of diabetes insipidus have included vasopressin injections, vasopressin administration by intranasal spray, intranasal desmopressin acetate (DDAVP, a synthetic vasopressin analog), and other drugs. The reason for the intranasal route is that, because the hormones are peptides, they would be degraded by digestive enzymes after oral administration.

Disorders with excess vasopressin have been collectively named **syndrome of inappropriate secretion of vasopressin**, or SIADH. Hyponatremia (low blood sodium) is a characteristic of SIADH. High AVP, from tumors or the posterior pituitary, may cause SIADH. Symptoms vary in severity but can include lethargy, apathy, anorexia, confusion, muscle cramps, disorientation, seizures, coma, or death. SIADH has been treated with fluid restriction, diuretics, and intravenous 5% saline. There are a number of conditions associated with SIADH (Table 5.3).

REFERENCES

1. Baylis, P.H. Vasopressin and its neurophysin. In L. DeGroot, editor. Endocrinology, Second Edition. Philadelphia: W. B. Saunders, Co.; 1989.

2. Baylis, P.H.; Thompson, C.J. Osmoregulation of vasopressin secretion and thirst in health and disease. Clinical Endocrinology 29: 549–576; 1988.

3. Baylis, P.H. Osmoregulation and control of vasopressin secretion in healthy humans. Am. J. Physiol. 253: R671–R678; 1987.

4. Wakerly, J.B. Hypothalamic neurosecretory function: Insights from electrophysiological studies of the magnocellular nuclei. IBRO News 4: 15; 1985.

5. Freidinger, R.M.; Hirschmann, R.; Veber, D.F. Titanium (III) as a selective reducing agent for nitroarginyl peptides: Synthesis of arginine vasotocin. Journal of Organic Chemistry 43: 4800–4803; 1978.

6. Reinharz, A. C.; Klein, M.; Offord, R.E.; Vallotton, M.B. Similarity of pituitary and pineal human oxytocin neurophysins indicated by peptide mapping after radioactive alkylation and proteolysis. Neuroendocrinology 41: 224–229; 1985.

7. Hope, D.B.; Pickup, J.C. Neurophysins. In E. Knobil; Sawyer, W. H., editors. Handbook of Physiology, Endocrinology, Section 7, Volume IV, Part 1. Washington D.C.: American Physiological Society; 1974; pp. 173–189.

8. Acher, R. Chemistry of the neurohypophysial hormones: An example of molecular evolution. In Knobil, E.; Sawyer, W. H., editors. Handbook of Physiology, Endocrinology, Section 7, Volume IV, Part 1. Washington, D.C.: American Physiological Society; 1974; pp. 119–130.

9. Hawker, R. Notebook of Medical Physiology: Endocrinology. New York: Churchill Livingstone; 1978; p. 21.

10. Bentley, P.J. Directional differences in the permeability to water of the isolated urinary bladder of the toad, *Bufo marinus*. J. Endocrin. 22: 95–100; 1961.

11. Ganong, W. Review of Medical Physiology, Fourteenth Edition. Norwalk, CT: Appleton & Lange; p. 203.

12. Physicians' Desk Reference. Montvale, NJ: Medical Economics Data; 1993.

13. Adolph, E.F. Exchanges of water in the frog. Amer. J. Physiol. 115: 200–240; 1936.

14. Dunn, F.L.; Brennan, T.J.; Nelson, A.E.; Robertson, G.L. The role of blood osmolality and volume in regulating vasopressin secretion in the rat. J. Clin. Invest. 52: 3212–3219; 1973.

15. Crowley, W.R.; W. E. Armstrong. Neurochemical regulation of oxytocin secretion in lactation. Endocrine Reviews 13: 33–65; 1992.

16. Baylis, P.H. Vasopressin and its Neurophysin. In DeGroot, L., editor. Endocrinology,

Second Edition. Philadelphia: W. B. Saunders; ; 1989.

17. Robinson, A.G. Neurophysins and their physiologic significance. Hosp. Pract. 12: 57–63; 1977.

18. Baylis, P.H.; Thompson, C.J. Osmoregulation of vasopressin secretion and thirst in health and disease. Clinical Endocrinology 29: 549–576; 1988.

19. Baylis, P.H. Vasopressin and its Neurophysin. In L. DeGroot, editor. Endocrinology, Second Edition. Philadelphia: W. B. Saunders; 1989.

20. Murphy, M.R.; Checkley, S.A.; Seckl, J.R.; Lightman, S.L. Naloxone inhibits oxytocin release at orgasm in man. J. Clin. Endo. Metab. 71: 1056–1058; 1990.

21. Lumpkin, M.D.; Samson, W.K.; McCann; S. Arginine vasopressin as a thyrotropin-releasing hormone. Science 239: 1070; 1987.

22. Pietrowsky, R.; Born, J.; Fehm-Wolfsdorf, G.; Fehm, H.L. The influence of a vasopressin-analogue (DGAVP) on event-related potentials in a stimulus mismatch paradigm. Biological Psychology 23: 239–250; 1989.

23. Pietrowsky, R.; Fehm-Wolfsdorf, G.; Born, J.; Fehm, H.L. Effects of DGAVP on verbal memory. Peptides 9: 1361–1366; 1989.

24. Dean, W.; Morgenthaler, J. Smart Drugs and Nutrients. Santa Cruz, CA: B&J Publications; 1990; p. 143.

25. Gauquelin, G.; Gharib, C.; Chaemmaghami, F.; Allevard, A.; Cherbal, F.; Geelen, G.; Bouzeghrane, F.; Legros, J. A day/night rhythm of vasopressin and oxytocin in rat retina, pineal, and Harderian gland. Peptides 9: 289–293; 1988.

26. Valtin, H.; Sokol, H.; Sunde, D. Genetic approaches to the study of regulation and actions of vasopressin. Rec. Prog. Horm. Res. 31: 447–486; 1975.

CHAPTER 6

Growth Hormone from the Anterior Pituitary

Growth hormone is a hormone of the anterior pituitary gland. As its name indicates, it functions in causing growth working with somatomedins. Other hormones, for example, thyroid hormone, act synergistically with growth hormone to promote growth. Growth hormone also functions in the regulation of proteins, fats, and carbohydrates.

HISTORY AND NOMENCLATURE

In 200 A.D., Galen is credited with noticing the pituitary gland. By the seventeenth century, early thinkers knew it was not the source of nasal secretions (pituita, for which the pituitary was named), but they thought the gland was vestigial. In 1864, an Italian named Verga associated acromegaly with pituitary secretion, and in 1886 Pierre Marie observed that the pituitary gland enlarges in acromegaly. So, it was realized quite early that the pituitary gland had something to do with growth.

The hormone to which the growth function of the pituitary has been ascribed is called growth hormone (GH). It is also called somatotropin (STH). Human growth hormone has its own abbreviation, HGH (hGH).

GH CHEMISTRY

Growth hormone is a protein (Figure 6.1). The molecular weight of growth hormone is about 21,500. Human growth hormone has 191 amino acids.[1] It has two disulfide bonds. A variant of GH has a 17-amino acid deletion. GH is synthesized from pre-growth hormone which has 217 amino acids.

The structure of growth hormone is similar to the structures of prolactin and placental lactogen. Prolactin has 199 amino acids and three disulfide bonds. Placental lactogen (human chorionic somatomammotropin, hCS) differs from growth hormone by only 29 amino acids.

Sequences of amino acid residues in growth hormone, the primary structure, differ from one species to another (Table 6.1). Growth hormones from different species vary in their chemical properties. For example, isoelectric points range from 4.9 to 6.8.

There are also variations in the sequences of amino acid residues that compose GH within an individual. This variation, **heterogeneity**, in the peptide hormone has implications for the chemical properties of GH, the measurement of GH with antibodies, and the biological activity of GH.

The variations in the structures of GH are reflected in the variability of interactions with antibodies to GH. Antibodies to GH do not cross react equally with the growth hormones of all species. For example, if rabbit anti-bGH (antibody to bovine growth hormone, bGH) is mixed with ovine

GH (oGH), the antibody reacts with the hormone, there is a cross reaction, and a precipitate is formed. On the other hand, rabbit anti-bGH does not cross react with human growth hormone.

Primate growth hormone works in humans and monkeys, but the only growth hormone that works in guinea pigs is guinea pig growth hormone (Table 6.2). The reason that bGH does not work in humans is that it fails to bind to the human growth hormone receptor.

ANAPHYLACTIC SHOCK

When one species cannot tolerate growth hormone from another species, an immune response ensues and **anaphylactic shock** is possible. Anaphylaxis is an acute, even explosive, reaction which usually occurs in a previously sensitized person 1–15 minutes after subsequent exposure to the antigen. The systemic reaction is characterized by symptoms—smooth muscle spasm, capillary dilatation, glandular secretion, changes in vessel permeability, respiratory distress, wheezing, coughing, sneezing, throbbing in the ears, seizures, vomiting, abdominal cramps, incontinence, generalized flush, hives or rash, itching, arrhythmias, and cardiogenic shock—that are due to the fixation of a specific antibody in certain tissues. The response can be quite serious and may even result in death. Turner and Bagnara wrote:

> Ovine STH is highly antigenic in the guinea pig; when this hormone is given to recipients previously sensitized to the same preparation, 90 to 100 percent of the animals die from anaphylactic shock.[2]

GH-BINDING PROTEIN

Originally, it was thought that growth hormone circulated as a free molecule. But more recent data have been used to argue for protein carrier molecules with high affinity for growth hormone (GH-BP, growth hormone binding proteins).[3] A binding protein has a region identical to the extra-cellular domain of the growth hormone receptor (GHR).

GH-BP decreases the metabolic clearance rate of GH. About 40–45% of the circulating 22K GH is complexed with GH-BP. GH-BP is low in the human fetus and newborn, rises in childhood,

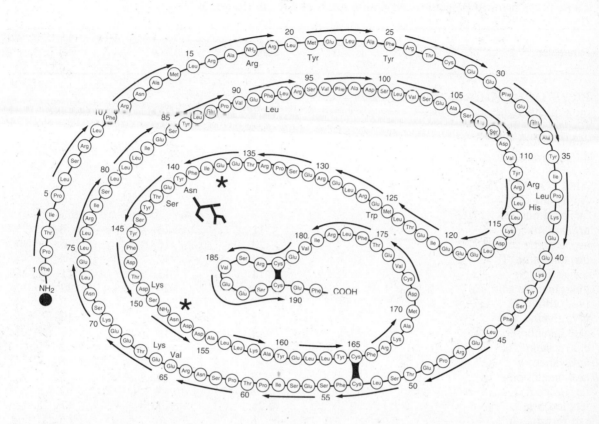

Figure 6.1 The structure of hGH is shown. Two disulfide bonds (not shown) are present in the molecule. Baumann, G. Growth hormone heterogeneity: Genes, isohormones, variants, and binding proteins. Endocrine Reviews 69: 424–449; 1991.

and stays constant in human adults. Individual differences are great and there is no gender difference. Similar GH-BPs have been found in rabbits, pigs, and pregnant rodents but very little has been found in serum of cows and sheep.

The binding protein amounts are regulated by GH and by testosterone.

GENETICS AND EVOLUTION OF GH

A hypothesis for the evolution of the family of hormones related to growth hormone starts with a common ancestral gene, then genes for prolactin and somatotropin, finally evolution of the somatotropin gene for placental lactogen. In birds, growth hormone and prolactin may not be distinct hormones.

Such hypothesizing about peptide hormone evolution and heterogenity may be clarified by discovery of the gene loci that are responsible for the production of multiple forms of related hormones such as Baumann[4] describes for the GH locus.

Table 6.1 Chemical Properties and Amino Acids of Growth Hormones

Parameter	Human	Cow	Rat
PHYSIOCHEMICAL PROPERTIES			
molecular weight	21500	45000	46000
isoelectric point, pH	4.90	6.80	–
sedimentation coefficient	2.18	3.19	3.21
diffusion coefficient	8.88	7.23	–
AMINO ACIDS			
lys, lysine, K	9	11	10
his, histidine, H	3	3	3
arg, arginine, R	11	13	8
asp, aspartic acid, D	20	16	16
thr, threonine, T	10	12	7
ser, serine, S	18	13	11
glu, glutamic acid, E	26	24	22
pro, proline, P	8	6	8
gly, glycine, G	8	10	10
ala, alanine, A	7	15	13
cys, cysteine, C	4	4	2
val, valine, V	7	6	8
met, methionine, M	3	4	3
ile, isoleucine, I	8	7	7
leu, leucine, L	26	27	17
tyr, tyrosine, Y	8	6	5
phe, phenylalanine, F	13	13	8
try, tryptophan, W	1	1	–

The physical properties and numbers of amino acids in the growth hormones are given for three species. For some organisms, there are several of these lists with differing numbers because more than one form of growth hormone has been found. Wilhelmi, A.E. Chemistry of growth hormone. Handbook of Physiology, Endocrinology, Volume 4, Part 2; 1974; p. 59; Frieden, E.H.; Lipner, H. Biochemical Endocrinology of the Vertebrates. Englewood Cliffs, NJ: Prentice Hall; 1971; p. 22. Cow and rat GH are now believed to have MW of about 22,000.

The locus for the family containing growth hormone has been found on chromosome 17 in humans and consists of five genes: a gene for pituitary hGH (hGH-1), three genes for growth hormones that are expressed by placenta (hGH-2, hCS-1, hCS-2), and a pseudogene (hCS-5).[5,6]

BIOASSAYS

Growth hormone can be measured with radioimmunoassays (RIA) developed by Glick and Greenwood in 1964. For diagnoses, HGH can be measured in human plasma with RIA. A problem with the RIAs is that they do not always measure biological activity. Inconsistencies between RIA

Table 6.2   Growth Hormone Activity Among Species

Source	Stimulates Growth in Recipient				
	Humans	Monkeys	Rats	Birds	Fish
humans	yes	yes	yes		yes
monkeys	yes	yes	yes		yes
whales	no		yes		
pigs	no	no	yes	no	yes
sheep	no		yes		yes
cows	no	no	yes	yes	yes
birds			yes	yes	
amphibia			yes		
reptiles			yes		
fish			no		yes

The table shows the ability of growth hormone from one species to act in another. Sources of hormone are listed vertically on the left; recipients of hormone are listed horizontally across the top. Modified, with permission, Ganong, W. F. Review of Medical Physiology, Fourteenth Edition. Norwalk, CT: Appleton & Lange; 1989, p. 342; and Colin Scanes, personal communication).

and bioassays can occur when biological activity and antigenicity use different sites of recognition on the hormone molecule.

There are bioassays used in the past for growth hormone which were based on its growth promoting properties and utilized the responses of target tissues

The tibia test is a bioassay that makes use of the leg bones of either rats or mice. Growth hormone (or unknowns) are injected into a hypophysectomized (pitx) animal. The width of the cartilage plate, the epiphyseal cartilage of the tibia, is measured. The width increases in response to growth hormone (Figure 6.2).

Another way to measure growth hormone involves female rats. Female rats usually grow to a weight of 250 grams, while male rats grow much larger and attain double the weights of the female, approximately 500 grams. It is possible to artificially increase the weight of female rats once they have stopped growing by administration of growth hormone. So the bioassay involves injection of growth hormone or unknowns.

Another bioassay uses immature animals. The pituitary glands are removed from the animals (hypophysectomy, pitx) to remove the animals' own source of growth hormone. Growth hormone, or unknowns, are injected into the animals followed by measurements of their body weights. Growth hormone doses of 10 micrograms per day produce an impressive 1 gram per day increase in the body weight.

REGULATION

Regulation of growth hormone involves the interplay among (i) hormone feedback, releasing and inhibiting factors (somatocrinin, GRH, GHRF; and somatostatin, GIH, SRIF, SRIH, SS), (ii) set point regulation for sugar (glucostat), (iii) and neurotransmitters (catecholamines). The hypothalamus (Figure 6.3) controls anterior pituitary secretion of growth hormone with a growth hormone-inhibiting hormone (somatostatin) and a growth hormone-releasing hormone (GRH, somatocrinin).

Structures of the hypophysiotropic neuro-

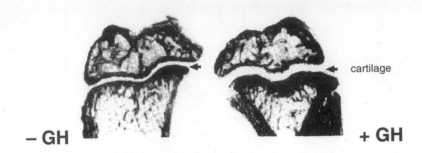

Figure 6.2 The figure illustrates the "tibia test." In a tibia test, growth hormone is administered to a hypophysectomized rat (or mouse) for four days. Increase in the width of the cartilage is evidence of growth hormone. The figure is a computer scan made by the author of a photograph. Modified, with permission. Evans, H.M., et al. Bioassay of pituitary growth hormone. Endocrinology 32: 14; 1943.

hormones, SS and GRH, are known. Somatostatin has 14 amino acid residues and a disulfide bond; GRH is a polypeptide with 40–44 amino acids. SS and GRH may interact regulating each other.

Growth hormone stimulates liver somatomedins. Somatomedins influence target tissues and feed back negatively on the pituitary GH secretion and stimulate somatostatin secretion by the hypothalamus (Figure 6.4).

Growth hormone also appears to have direct actions on target cells (e.g., stem cell chondrocytes that are in the epiphyseal growth plate of bones).

A hypothalamic glucostat may influence growth hormone. The glucostatic cells form a satiety center in the ventromedial nucleus of the hypothalamus. Electrical stimulation of the nucleus causes growth hormone release. Blood sugar may directly affect GH secretion by affecting ventromedial nucleus secretion of GRH, or it may have indirect effects by causing the brain to send signals via adrenergic neurons that in turn stimulate the arcuate nucleus of the hypothalamus to secrete GRH.

GH secretion is amplified by gonadal steroids during the pubertal growth spurt.[7,8]

INSULIN-LIKE GROWTH FACTORS

Originally, it was thought that growth hormone achieved its actions directly. Subsequently, it was thought that insulin-like growth factors mediated the growth-promoting action of growth hormone. Common characteristics among somatomedins include cell mitosis in chondrocytes, osteoblasts, and other extraskeletal cells; insulin-like action; plasma level regulated by GH; plasma source liver; and protein carrier transport in the blood.

IGF-I (insulin-like growth factor I, somatomedin C, SM-C, sulfation factor, basic human somatomedin) is one of the polypeptide growth factors made by the liver (Figure 6.5). The hormone activity, growth promotion, is now attributed to a number of different molecules that are structurally similar to the hormones insulin and relaxin.

IGF-I increases cartilage formation (chondrogenesis) and stimulates protein, fat, and glycogen formation. IGF-I has 70 amino acids and it is synthesized from a precursor molecule, preproIGF-I with 130 amino acids. IGF-I is necessary for an individual to grow to normal stature. In human children, somatomedin levels increase from about 0.5 U/ml at two years of age to 1.0 U/ml by eight years of age.

IGF-II (insulin-like growth factor-II, multiplication-stimulating activity or MSA, somatomedin, neutral human somatomedin SM-A) may function to promote fetal growth. IGF-II has 67 amino acids and it is synthesized from preproIGF-II which has 180 amino acids. Growth hormone is less important to the regulation of IGF-II which is synthesized in a variety of tissues.

Binding proteins in the plasma prolong

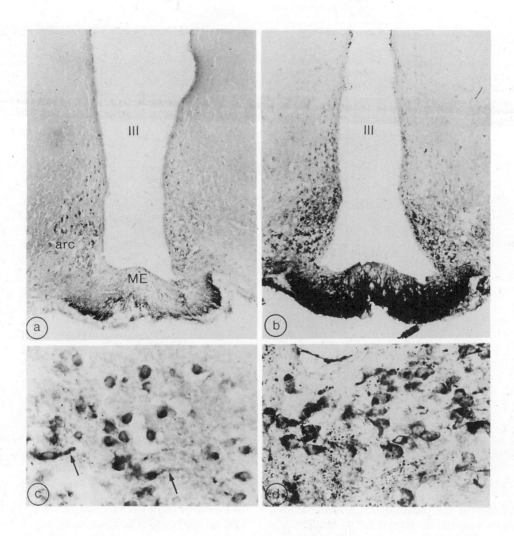

Figure 6.3 The figure shows immunohistochemistry of coronal sections of rat brains with the arcuate nuclei (arc) and the distribution of GRF (black). The control rat (a,c) was injected with water; the experimental rat (b,d) was injected with cysteamine which increases the labelling. The sections were immunostained for GRF which concentrated in the terminals of neurons of the arcuate nucleus and the median eminence. The extent of staining was increased by cysteamine indicating an increase in GRF retention in arcuate neurons. At the same time, cysteamine depleted somatostatin and plasma GH. The results are evidence that somatostatin regulates brain GRF. Reproduced, with permission. Tannenbaum, G.S.; McCarthy, G.F.; Zeitler, P.; Beaudet, A. Cysteamine-induced enhancement of growth hormone-releasing factor (GRF) immunoreactivity in arcuate neurons: Morphological evidence for putative somatostatin/GRF interactions with the hypothalamus. Endocrinology 127: 2551–2560; 1990.

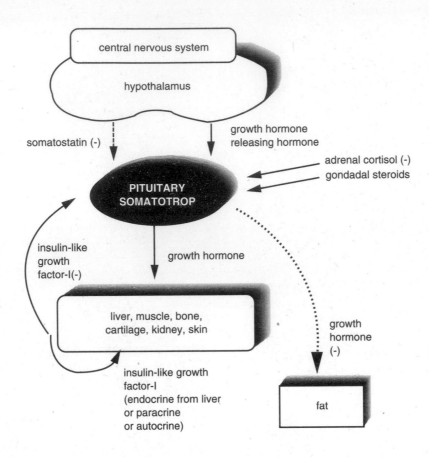

Figure 6.4 The diagram shows a scheme for hormonal regulation of growth hormone. A glucostat in the hypothalamus and neurotransmitters may also participate in the regulation of growth hormone.[9]

the half-life of the insulin-like growth factors. Four to six insulin-like growth factor binding proteins (IGFBP) have been suggested which bind IGF-I and IGF-II.[10,11]

Feedback by insulin-like growth factors on the hypothalamus and pituitary provide mechanism for the regulation of growth hormone.

Insulin-like growth factors, or somatomedins, are also made by other tissues (fibroblasts, myoblasts, chondrocytes, osteoblasts, bone, brain, gastrointestinal epithelium, kidney, some fetal cells, some tumor cells). Spencer makes the suggestion: "Local production of somatomedins may be very important physiologically in that they may act in a autocrine or paracrine fashion, in contrast to circulating somatomedins, which act in an endocrine fashion."[12] If one of an animal's two tibia is locally injected with growth hormone, the cartilage width increases, but the width does not increase in the other, uninjected, tibia. Now this is interpreted as growth hormone stimulation of somatomedin production by the cartilage which in turn causes the cartilage to widen.

OTHER GROWTH FACTORS

Growth hormone and insulin-like growth-factors are among the plethora of polypeptide

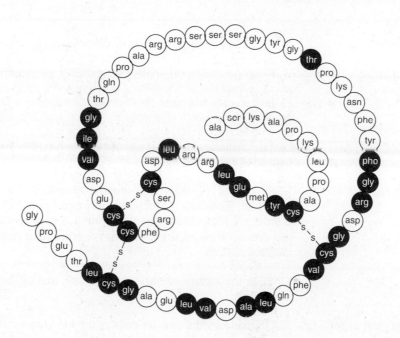

Figure 6.5 The structure of insulin-like growth factor I is shown. It has 70 amino acids (three-letter abbreviations) and three disulfide (-S-S-) bonds. The hormone is similar in structure to insulin (shared amino acids are blackened) and the hormone relaxin. Modified, with permission. Humbel, R.E.; Rinderknecht, E. From NSILA to IGF (1963-1967). Giordano, G.; Van Wyk, J.J.; Minuto, F., editors. Somatomedins and Growth. London: Academic Press; 1979; pp. 61–75.

hormones and factors (Table 6.3) involved in growth. Growth is a complex case of synergism.

Thyroid hormones play a major role in growth. Thyroid deficiency in humans results in retardation of both growth and mental function. Prolactin, not surprisingly because of its similarity to growth hormone, also promotes growth. It is especially important for development and growth of the mammary glands. Placental lactogen, made in the placenta, may have a role in promoting growth of the fetus. The thymus gland makes polypeptides, which cause lymphocytes to differentiate and proliferate. Some of the thymus polypeptides are called thymosin, thymopoietin, serum thymic factor, and thymic humoral factor. The pancreas and its hormone, insulin, is involved in growth.

There are growth-inhibiting, as well as growth-promoting, factors. Various tissues make a group of local hormones that inhibit cell prolif-

eration or growth called the "chalones."

There are still other substances, not all of which are peptides, that affect growth. Androgens, from the gonads and the adrenal, spur growth especially at puberty. Adrenal cortex hormones have a permissive action on growth.

Growth is not only initiated, it must also be stopped. During puberty, androgens and estrogens cause the epiphyses to close, and once this occurs, height increases cease.

GROWTH

Animal experiments provided a clear early picture of a dramatic role of the pituitary gland in growth. For example, the pituitary gland was removed from a 2.7-kg immature rhesus monkey. Two years later it still weighed 2.7-kg. The control monkey weighing 2.9 kg was permitted to mature normally and it weighed 8.4 kg two years later.

Table 6.3 Some Examples of Growth Factors

nerve growth factor	NGF, causes sympathetic neurite orientation and growth.[13]
epidermal growth factor	EGF (urogastrone), originally isolated from submandibular glands of mice, is responsible for epithelial cell mitosis. EGF is a peptide with 53 amino acids and three disulfide bonds and is in a family of peptide growth factors which also includes TGFα, amphiregulin, and vaccinia growth factor. EGF is abundant in mouse urine (3000 ng/ml) and human prostatic fluid (280 ng/ml), and is found in lesser amounts in human blood (<0.01 ng/ml).
fibroblast growth factors	FGFs are polypeptides with about 140 amino acids. They act on cells that have neural, mesenchmal, and epithelial embryological origins. Widespread tissue distribution, wide species distribution, and conservation of structure imply a primordial role.[14] The FGFs enhance mitosis.
erythropoietin	EP from the kidney stimulates production and differentiation of red blood cells.
platelet-derived growth factor	PDGF made by the platelet cells in the blood causes smooth muscle growth in the blood vessels.

Similarly, when rats were hypophysectomized at 4 weeks of age (weight 72 grams), they grew less than controls, so that at 10-months old the hypophysectomized rats weighed 81 grams but the control rats with intact pituitary glands tilted the laboratory balance at 465 grams. A hormone was suspected in causing growth because pituitary extracts produced growth in experimental animals such as dogs.

Growth hormone is anabolic and growth promoting. But, as mentioned, it does not act alone. Adequate nutrition and a host of other growth-promoting substances such as the somatomedins are required for full and normal growth to take place.

Growth of the fetus does not depend on growth hormone. Rapid growth continues in infants. Children who have illnesses may exhibit "catch-up" growth that can be four times normal. Growth hormone and somatomedins may be responsible for growth during childhood. Thyroid hormone is also necessary for normal growth and mental maturation. The growth spurt at puberty may be attributed to anabolic androgens from the testes and the adrenals acting in synergism with growth hormone and somatomedins.

AMOUNTS AND RHYTHMS

Data showing GH values and responses to exercise, fasting, and age appear in Table 6.4. In addition, Williams[15] gives the circulating level of GH as 1.8 ng/ml for men and 5.6 ng/ml for boys. Norman and Litwack[16] write that growth hormone circulates at levels greater than 3 ng/ml and that the total daily output is 1–4 mg. Other stimuli increase or decrease the secretion of growth hormone.

There is a pronounced daily rhythm in human growth hormone which may mean that reported measurements of GH need re-evaluation. Peak growth hormone activity is a nocturnal surge in the first nightly episode of paradoxical sleep which occurs in the first three hours during a

Table 6.4 GRH, Growth Hormone, and Somatomedins in Humans[17,18,19,20,21,22]

GRH (GH-RH)	
half-life	50 minutes
GROWTH HORMONE (GH)	
half-life	20–50 minutes
secretion rate, healthy adults	400 µg/day = 18.6 nmol/day
secretion rate, young adolescents	700 µgs/day = 32.5 nmol/day
BLOOD GROWTH HORMONE (GH)	
fasting at rest, male	< 5 ng/ml, SI < 233 pmol/l
children, after exercise	> 10 ng/ml, SI > 465 pmol/l
male, after exercise or glucose load	> 10 ng/ml, SI > 465 pmol/l
female	up to 30 ng/ml, SI 0–1395 pmol/l
female, after glucose load	< 5 ng/ml, SI < 233 pmol/l
adult human	3.2 ng/ml
exercising, adult human	17–53 ng/ml
children	12 ng/ml
SOMATOMEDIN C, CIRCULATING	
somatomedin C, prepubertal	0.08–2.8 u./ml
somatomedin C, during puberty	0.9–5.9 u./ml
somatomedin C, adult males	0.34–1.9 u./ml
somatomedin C, adult females	0.45–2.2 u./ml
adult serum somatomedins	0.4–2 u./ml (1 unit about 200 ng of SM-C)
SERUM IMMUNOREACTIVE IGF-I	
normal adults	about 200 ng/ml
acromegalics	about 750 ng/ml
hypopituitary dwarfs	near 0 ng/ml
pigmies	about 80 ng/ml

Several values are given from different sources to show the differences reported in the literature and standard tables. SI (Systeme International) units have been used in the international literature for years; for somatomedin C, u. = SI arbitrary units. Paradoxically, sources routinely report that fasting raises GH and then show data for GH with low values. No indication of time of day was given in the sources for these values.

night's sleep (Figure 6.6). Sleep has been divided into two stages based on EEG activity. In paradoxical sleep, the electroencephalogram (EEG, the electrical activity recorded from the scalp) has similarities to the waking electroencephalogram despite the fact that it takes the largest stimuli to wake a person from sleep; that's why it is "paradoxical." Paradoxical sleep (PS, dream sleep, REM sleep, rapid eye movement sleep) alternates with slow wave sleep (SWS) during the night with a cycle about 90 minutes in length. The nocturnal surge accounts for 70% of growth hormone secretion. In acromegaly, secretion of growth hormone is still episodic, but the characteristic nocturnal surge is lost.

GH secretion in humans is mainly during the first 90 minutes of sleep. In rats, STH is secreted every 3.3 hours—an ultradian rhythm.[23] The GRF and SRIF are secreted tonically, a steady state release, from the hypothalamus into the

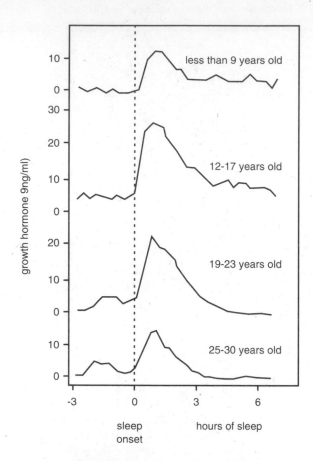

Figure 6.6 Growth hormone rises in human males at the time of sleep onset. Growth hormone increases from values less than 5 ng/ml to a peak of about 25 ng/ml between one and two hours after sleep onset. The graphs represent averages for four age groups (N = 6–21 males per graph). After data in Parker, D.C.; Rossman, L.G.; Kripke, D.F.; Gibson, W.; Wilson, K. Rhythmicities in human growth hormone concentrations in plasma. In Krieger, D.T., editor. Endocrine Rhythms. New York: Raven Press; 1979; p. 163.

hypophysial portal blood. An additional 3- to 4-h rhythmic surge of GRF and SRIF account for the ultradian rhythm in GH secretion.[24]

Growth hormone increases osteocalcin (Oc). Osteocalcin is also called bone Gla protein (BGP). Osteocalcin is synthesized by bone cells (osteoblasts). Levels of serum osteocalcin correlate with bone mineralization. Osteocalcin exhibits a rhythm in which night levels in serum are 30–50% higher than day levels (Figure 6.7)[25] and peak levels are found in children during times of rapid growth.[26]

METABOLISM

Other functions of growth hormone have to do with metabolism. Growth hormone regulates proteins, fats, and carbohydrates; in turn, GH is regulated by intake of protein, free fatty acids, and glucose as well as other factors (Table 6.5).

Growth hormone increases protein synthesis. That is, growth hormone causes protein anabolism. Going along with the increase in protein

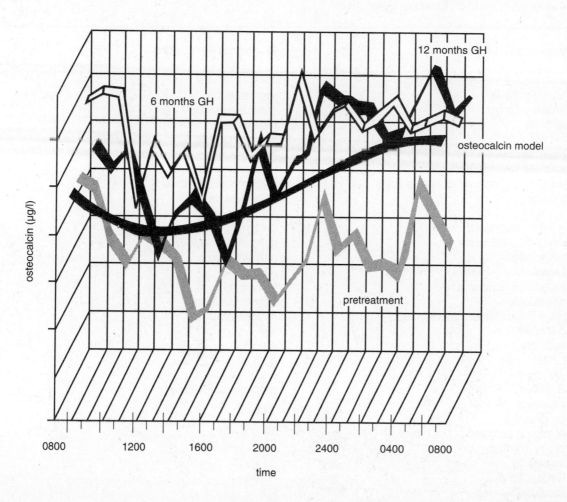

Figure 6.7 The graphs show the rhythms in osteocalcin. The graphs represent mean osteocalcin patterns except for the black line which is the investigators' osteocalcin "model" rhythm from healthy young adults. The four "experimental" subjects suffered from ISS (idiopathic short stature). Pretreatment subjects (lowest graph) represent pretreatment short stature controls. Graphs are shown for subjects after six and twelve months of growth hormone therapy. The authors concluded that GH increased osteocalcin by altering osteocalcin circadian rhythms. Growth rate increased by more than 35%. Modified, with permission. Markowitz, M.E.; Dimartino-Nardi, J.; Gasparini, F.; Fishman, K.; Rosen, J.; Saenger, P. Effects of growth hormone therapy on circadian osteocalcin rhythms in idiopathic short stature. J. Clin. Endocrinol. Metab. 69; 420–425; 1989.

synthesis are decreases in urine nitrogen, retention of amino acids by the kidney, increased serum protein, and decreased blood amino acids. Growth hormone is regulated by proteins. Growth hormone is released by eating a protein meal, but, paradoxically, it is also increased by malnutrition.

Growth hormone causes fat mobilization.

GH increases the levels of circulating free fatty acids (FFAs). The effect, which can be observed as increased ketone bodies, is facilitated by steroid hormones. The mobilization of fat, which takes several hours, provides a source of energy under conditions of stress, fasting, or hypoglycemia. Elevated concentrations of free fatty acids (FFA) in

Table 6.5 Growth Hormone Alterations

Increased GH secretion	Decreased GH secretion
hypoglycemia	somatostatin
2-deoxyglucose	growth hormone
exercise	progesterone
fasting	glucocorticoids
protein meal	phentolamine
infusion of arginine	α-adrenergic antagonists
infusion of some other amino acids	β-adrenergic agonists
glucagon	isoproterenol
pyrogen	serotonin antagonists
lysine vasopressin	methysergide
psychological stress	dopamine antagonists
sleep onset	phenothiazine
L-dopa	obesity
α-adrenergic agonists	acromegaly
apomorphine	hypothyroidism
other dopamine receptor agonists	hyperthyroidism
estrogens	REM sleep
androgens	glucose
GRH	cortisol
ACTH	free fatty acids
α-MSH	medroxyprogesterone
clonidine	
propranolol	
serotonin precursors	
bromocriptine	
muscimol	
GABA agonists	
anorexia nervosa	
starvation	
renal failure	
hypophysiotropic neurohormones	

the blood stream reduce responsiveness of the hypothalamus-pituitary to hypoglycemia or arginine infusion.

Growth hormone affects carbohydrate metabolism. When early scientists removed the pancreas from a dog, the dog became diabetic and had sugar in its urine. However, when they subsequently removed the pituitary from the dog, the dog became less diabetic. The result is explained by the fact that growth hormone raises blood sugar (GH causes hyperglycemia, or high blood sugar). In this regard, GH has the opposite effect to the hormone from the pancreas, insulin (insulin lowers blood sugar). Increase in blood sugar is known as the **diabetogenic effect** of growth hormone. Growth hormone also decreases glucose utilization, the **antiinsulin effect**. In hypophysectomized subjects, growth hormone increases muscle glycogen, the **glycostatic effect**. Permanent diabetes mellitus (a disease of insulin insufficiency) is caused by long term growth hormone because it destroys the beta cells of the pancreas by overworking them.

Glucose, in turn, regulates GH. Oral or intravenous glucose administration lowers GH; hypoglycemia (low blood sugar) stimulates the release of GH.

MECHANISM OF ACTION

The targets of growth hormone are tissues in general. First, GH was believed to act directly on many tissues such as fat cells. Second, growth hormone was thought to act via somatomedins produced by the liver or by target cells. For example, injections of growth hormone into proximal tibial epiphysis stimulates IGF-I production by cartilage cells and thereby increases cartilage width. A dual effector theory of somatotropin action involves the growth hormone stimulation of responsiveness to IGF-I.

There is a linear protein receptor for growth hormone in cell membranes. The receptors are like the hormones in that they form a gene family. Primate growth hormones bind to both PRL and GH receptors (GHR), which agrees with functional information that the GH affects growth and, like prolactin, is lactogenic.[27]

Kelly and coworkers write about the status of knowledge of the mechanism of action of prolactin and growth hormone:

> Very little is known about the mechanism of action of PRL and GH. The events that are responsible for the transfer of the hormoneal stimulation inside the cell, which occur after the interaction of these hormones with the receptors, remain, for the most part, unknown. No clear second messenger for either of these hormones has yet been identified.[28]

DWARFISM

Several disorders are associated with the growth-promoting function ascribed to growth hormone and the hormones of the growth hormone-regulating system. Disorders involving too little growth hormone (**hyposecretion**) are found. Abnormal pituitary secretions can be caused by tumors or have no obvious etiology (idiopathic hypopituitarism).

The disorder of hypopituitarism, too little production of pituitary hormones, has been associated with short stature, or dwarfism (Figure 6.8). Anatomical evidence that the pituitary growth hormone is involved is found in the observation that short stature is sometimes accompanied by abnormal somatotrops in the pituitary gland. General Tom Thumb, actually Charles S. Stratton, who rose to the height of three feet two inches, probably suffered from pituitary dwarfism due to one or more inherited recessive genes which resulted in a failure to produce growth hormone.[29] He married a shorter woman, Lavinia Warren, who was only two feet eight inches tall. In panhypopituitarism, where all the pituitary hormones are deficient, there are symptoms involving all the pituitary hormone systems.

The short stature disorders (e.g., ISS, idiopathic short stature) can be due to deficiencies in growth hormone from the pituitary gland, but it can also be caused by insufficient GRH or IGF-I or by other causes. Laron dwarfism results when there is enough growth hormone but its targets' responses, such as liver production of somatomedin, are diminished due to missing or abnormal growth hormone receptor and a circulating binding protein.

Interestingly, in the pigmies of Africa, GH and IGF-I are normal relative to non-pygmies in the same area, before puberty, but the pigmies fail to show the IGF-I increase and concomitant growth spurt at puberty. Low GH-BP has been found in pygmies. Low GH-BP is also associated with Laron dwarfism, liver cirrhosis, uremia, and insulin-dependent diabetes.

There are also disorders of short stature involving the thyroid (cretinism) and the gonads (XO chromosomal pattern). The phrase "constitutional delayed growth" is used to denote short stature with no known cause.

Anorexia nervosa patients have abnormal pituitary function tests and usually exhibit increased growth hormone.

GIGANTISM

Disorders involving too much growth hormone secretion (**hypersecretion**) are also found. When hyperpituitarism occurs before adult growth is completed, especially during early childhood before the closure of the epiphyses, a disorder characterized by abnormal large skeletal growth, called pituitary gigantism, can occur. Both bone length and bone width increase. The resulting legendary individual can be seven or eight feet tall.

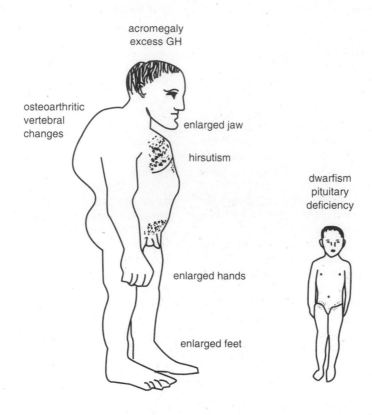

acromegaly
excess GH

osteoarthritic
vertebral
changes

enlarged jaw

hirsutism

dwarfism
pituitary
deficiency

enlarged hands

enlarged feet

Figure 6.8 The sketches show the symptoms of acromegaly (left) and dwarfism (right). The dwarf due to pituitary hyposecretion is only 35 inches tall at eight years old compared to normal height of 55 inches. But the proportions of a pituitary dwarf are those of a normal boy. The acromegalic, due to excess growth hormone secretion after growth has stopped, has characteristic symptoms which include visual field alterations and breast development with lactation. Redrawn, after sketches in Ganong, W. Review of Medical Physiology, Fourteenth Edition. Norwalk, CT: Appleton & Lange; 1989; p. 343; and Wilkins, L. The Diagnosis and Treatment of Endocrine Disorders in Childhood and Adolescence, Third Edition. Springfield, IL: Thomas; 1966.

Gigantism was associated with enlargement of the pituitary gland.

Skeletons from individuals with gigantism can be found in medical museums such as the Royal College of Surgeon's in London. There is an unsavory story about an Irish giant named O'Brien who lived in London. According to the story, an anatomist was particularly interested in securing O'Brien's eight-foot-tall skeleton upon his death. The anatomist or his servant stalked the giant. The giant noticed this unusual interest and set forth orders to have his corpse watched until it could be buried at sea in a lead casket. But, at O'Brien's demise in 1783 at age 22, body snatchers, promised ten times the going rate for corpses, provided drink to the mourning guards, and substituted stones for the corpse in the casket which was subsequently "buried" in the Irish sea. The anatomist was in possession of the skeleton. Sir Arthur Keith and Harvey Cushing subsequently published a diagnosis (growth hormone producing pituitary adenoma) for O'Brien. Hypogonadism is often associated with gigantism so that not only is excess growth initiated, but the mechanisms to stop the growth are not properly in place.

The inquisitive person need not travel to England in search of giant skeletons. The Mutter Museum of medical curiosities in Philadelphia houses the skeleton of the "American Giant" in an enormous glass case. Towering seven and a half feet tall, the giant was from Kentucky. Its skeleton was purchased in 1877 from Professor de Foote for $50.00. The giant has an enlarged sella turcica which indicates a pituitary tumor.

ACROMEGALY

Excess growth hormone can also occur after closure of the epiphyses. The term "acromegaly," from Greek words meaning large extremities, is used to denote this disorder. Symptoms of overgrowth of bone particularly affect the mandible and skull so that the result is protrusion of the jaw (prognathism, overbite, separated teeth). The face coarsens, the hands widen, the fingers become broad, the feet enlarge, and the skin thickens. Sweating increases, women may have excessive hair, and the breasts may produce milk. Joint pain accompanies erosion of the articulating surfaces. Internal organs, such as the lungs, liver, heart, and kidneys enlarge as well. Other symptoms of excess growth hormone include fatigue, photophobia, hypertension, enlarged heart, and kidney stones.

Excess growth hormone was involved in the plot of a work of fiction, *Creature*, by John Saul:

Jeff was still barely recognizable as having once been human. Indeed, it was still possible to recognize his blue eyes peering out from their sunken sockets. His face was twisted now, and his jaw had grown heavier. His teeth, protruding from his mouth, had forced themselves out of alignment as they grew, and now he could no longer close his mouth at all. His shoulders had broadened grotesquely, and at the ends of his arms, which now hung below his knees, his hands

had grown into massive clubs.[30]

PROLACTIN, SYNERGISM, AND OTHER FUNCTIONS

As noted, the structure of growth hormone has similarities to prolactin, so growth hormone has prolactin-like effects.

Growth hormone has other functions. Growth hormone stimulates the thymic lymphocytes. In addition, growth hormone can act synergistically with the other "trophic" hormones of the anterior pituitary gland: ACTH, FSH, LH, and TSH. ACTH and GH act together to repair the cortex of adrenalectomized animals. Thyroid hormone and growth hormone act together to produce both growth and maturation. Growth hormone improves the appearance of the gonads. Growth hormone can enhance the growth-promoting effects of cancer-causing agents (carcinogens); removing the pituitary suppresses responses to carcinogens.

AGING

There are some elusive paradoxes in the story of growth hormone. For example, from studies of hypophysectomy and hormone replacement, GH appears to control growth, yet the differences in GH secretion during growth versus adults is not as striking as might be expected. Explanations for the paradox are increased GH at night during the teen growth spurt, and synergism with sex steroids. Thyroid hormone is also necessary for growth and the acquisition of full adulthood.

Growth, as measured by height increase, stops because androgens and estrogens stop linear growth (height increases) by causing epiphyseal closure—the epiphyses fuse in the long bones.

Perhaps the GH paradox may also arise partially because growth has generally been assessed in humans by measuring height in males, a fact that is reflected in the graphs in most physiology and endocrinology books. Adults do grow; they stop growing taller, but they gain weight (Parisians' weights increase from 68 kg at age 25 to 77 kg at age 45, followed by a decline to 63 kg at age 75).[31] Lean body mass falls from 60 kg in the mid-twenties to 48 kg in 75-80 year old men.[32] In aging, there are gender differences and there is a change from protein to fat production. Perhaps the drop in weight in seniors occurs when growth hormone declines. A broader definition of growth that includes weight and fat might provide a more satisfactory correlation of growth with growth hormone.

A great deal of excitement has surrounded the function of GH in adults. Some of the effects of aging, as mentioned, are decreases in GH secretion and serum IGFs, decreases in protein synthesis, decreases in percent of lean body and bone masses, and increases in fat. The implication is that administration of GRH, GH, or IGFs might retard or reverse some of the physical consequences of aging in humans.[33] An increased risk of leukemia has been a worry for those using growth hormone to treat aging.[34]

HGH REPLACEMENT THERAPY

Pituitary dwarfism can be treated in children with 2 IU of growth hormone on alternate days. Increased availability of growth hormone by modern production techniques using molecular biology raise issues of whether, and when, it is appropriate to treat children with short stature with growth hormone to attain the goal of increasing their heights.[35]

Originally growth hormone for clinical use was scarce. Human growth hormone constitutes 4–10% of the dry weight of the human pituitary gland. There are 5–10 mg of growth hormone per human pituitary gland.[36] It is possible to isolate 2 mg of growth hormone per kg of human pituitary. But the hormone obtained in this way is precious; it takes 2.5 mg/week to treat pituitary dwarfism in a child—the initial treatment was 2 mg of GH three times a week. More recent regimens involve an injection at bedtime in keeping with the knowledge of the GH daily rhythm. Treatment options were severely limited by the small supply of GH. Now, however, biosynthetic growth hormone produced by recombinant techniques (r-hGH) is available. This means that the supply for clinical use is potentially unlimited and the preparation is free of pituitary contaminants, so the options have widened.[37]

Concern has accompanied the use of growth hormone by athletes (not an approved use), especially weight lifters, for the purposes of achieving body weight and/or height increases. Use of GH produces undesirable side effects (symptoms normally associated with acromegaly and diabetes).

AGRICULTURE

Bovine growth hormone (bST, bovine somatotropin; or bGH) has been produced with genetic engineering techniques using a bacteria, *E. coli*. GH increases milk production by 14%.[38]

The question of whether GH administration to cows will result in GH in milk as been studied. The administration of bST to dairy cows increased the bST blood levels (from 0 to 2.0 ng/ml), the milk bST levels (from 0.5 to 3 ng/ml, but only with twenty-five times the recommended bST dose), the blood somatomedin level (from 50 to 100 ng/ml), and the milk somatomedin (up to twofold).[39] Since bST and IGF-I should not be orally active in humans because they are digested, promotors of the treatment of cows with bST believe that its use in dairy cows will not be harmful to humans.[40] Certainly the use of exogenous GH to increase feed efficiency in pigs or to reduce fat in livestock has enormous commercial implications.

REFERENCES

1. Findling, J.W.; Tyrrell, J.B. Anterior pituitary and somatomedins: I. Anterior pituitary. In Greenspan, F.; Forsham, P., editors. Basic and Clinical Endocrinology, Second Edition. East Norwalk, CT: Appleton & Lange;1987; p. 84.

2 Turner, C.D.; J. T. Bagnara. General Endocrinology, Sixth Edition. Philadelphia, PA: W. B. Saunders; 1976; p. 100.

3. Baumann, G. Growth hormone·heterogenity: Genes, isohormones, variants, and binding proteins. Endocrine Reviews 12: 424–449; 1991.

4. Baumann, G. Ibid..

5 Kerrigan, J.R.; Rogol, A.D. The impact of gonadal steroid hormone action on growth hormone secretion during childhood and adolescence. Endocrine Reviews 13: 281–298; 1992, p. 282.

6. Walker, W.H.; Fitzpatrick, S.L; Barrera-Saldana, H.A.; Resendez-Preez, D.; Saunders, G.F. The human placental lactogen genes: Structure, function, evolution and transcriptional regulation. Endocrine Reviews 12: 316–328; 1991.

7. Kerrigan, J.R.; Rogol, A.D. The impact of gonadal steroid hormone action on growth hormone

secretion during childhood and adolescence. Endocrine Reviews 13: 281–298; 1992.

8. Wehrenberg, W.B.; Giustina, A. Mechanisms and pathways of gonadal steroid modulation of growth hormone secretion. Endocrine Reviews 13: 299–308; 1992.

9. Corpas, E.; Harman, S.M.; Blackman, M.R. Human growth hormone and human aging. Endocrine Reviews 14; 20–39; 1993; p. 21.

10. Otto, J., Jorgensen, I. Human growth hormone replacement therapy: Pharmacological and clinical aspects. Endocrine Reviews 12: 189–207; 1991.

11. Kerrigan, J.R.; Rogol, A.D. Op. cit.; p. 283.

12. Spencer, E. M. Somatomedins. In Greenspan, F.; Forsham, P., editors. Basic and Clinical Endocrinology, Third Edition. East Norwalk, CT: Appleton & Lange;1991; p. 137.

13. Fisher, D.A.; Lakshmanan, J. Metabolism and effects of epidermal growth factor and related growth factors in mammals. Endocrine Reviews 11: 418–442; 1990.

14. Hadley, M.E. Endocrinology, Third Edition. Prentice-Hall, Englewood Cliffs, NJ; 1992; p. 322.

15. Daughaday, W. H. The adenohypophysis. In Williams, R., editor. Textbook of Endocrinology, Philadelphia, PA: W. B. Saunders; 1987; p. 90–91.

16. Norman, A.; Litwack, G. Hormones. Orlando, FL: Academic Press; 1987; p. 205.

17. Findling, J.W.; Tyrrell, J.B. Op. cit.; p. 85, 86.

18. Norman, A.; Litwack, G. Op. cit.; p. 205.

19. Spencer, E. M. Op. cit. p. 135.

20. Berkow, R. The Merck Manual of Diagnosis and Therapy Volume 1: General Medicine, Sixteenth Edition, Merck & Co: Rahway, NJ; 1992; pp. 1428–1430.

21. Zapf, J.; Walter, H.; Froesch, E.R. Radioimmunological determination of insulin-like growth factors I and II in normal subjects and patients with growth disorders and extrapancreatic tumor hypoglycemia. J. Clin. Invest. 68: 1321–1330; 1981.

22. Merimee, T.; Thomas, J.; Zapf, J.; Froesch, R. Dwarfism in the pigmy: An isolated deficiency of insulin-like growth factor I. The New England Journal of Medicine 305: 965–968; 1981.

23. Tannenbaum, G.S. Somatostatin as a physiological regulator of pulsatile growth hormone secretion. Horm. Res. 29: 70–74; 1988.

24. Tannenbaum, G.S.; N. Ling. The interrelationship of growth hormone (GH)-releasing factor and somatostatin in generation of the ultradian rhythm of GH secretion. Endocrinology 115: 1952–1957; 1984.

25. Markowitz, M.E.; Dimartino-Nardi, J.; Gasparini, F.; Fishman, K.; Rosen, J. F.; Saenger, P. Effects of growth hormone therapy on circadian osteocalcin rhythms in idiopathic short stature. J. Clin. Endocrinol. Metab. 69: 420–425; 1989.

26. Johansen, J.S.; Giwercman, A.; Hartwell, D.; et al. Serum bone Gla-protein as a marker of bone growth in children and adolescents: Correlation with age, height, serum insulin-like growth factor I, and serum testosterone. J. Clin. Endocrinol. Metab. 67: 273–278; 1988.

27. Kelly, P.A., Djiane, J.; Postel-Vinay, M.; Edery, M. The prolactin/growth hormone receptor family. Endocrine Reviews 12: 235–251; 1991.

28. Kelly, P.A., Djiane, J.; Postel-Vinay, M.; Edery, M. Ibid. p. 235.

29. McKusick, V.A.; Rimoin, D.L. General Tom Thumb and other midgets. Scientific American (July) 217: 102–110; 1967.

30. Saul, J. Creature. Bantam: New York; 1989; p. 295.

31. Arking, R. Biology of Aging. Prentice Hall: Englewood Cliffs, NJ; 1991; page 56.

32. Abrams, W.B.; Berkow, R., editors. The Merck Manual of Geriatrics. Merck Sharp & Dohme Research Laboratories, Rahway, NJ; 1990; p. 4.

33. Corpas, E.; Harman, S.M.; Blackman, M.R. Op. cit.; pp. 20–39.

34. Fradkin, J.; Mills, J.L.; Schonberger, L.B.; Wysowski, D.K.; Thomson, R.; Durako, S.J.; Robison, L.L. Risk of leukemia after treatment with pituitary growth hormone. JAMA 270: 2829–2832; 1993.

35. Fradkin, J.; Schonberger, LB.; Mills, J.L.; Gunn, W.J.; Piper, J.M.; Wysowski, D.K.; Thomson, R.; Durako, S.; Brown, P. Creutzfeldt-Jakob disease in pituitary growth hormone recipients in the United States. JAMA 265: 880–884; 1991.

36. Hadley, M.E. Op. cit.; page 106.

37. Jorgensen, J.O.L. Op. cit.; pp. 189–207.

38. Grossman, C.J. Genetic engineering and the use of bovine somatotropin. JAMA 264: 1028; 1990.

39. Daughaday, W.; Barbano, D. Bovine somatotropin supplementation of dairy cows. JAMA

264: 1003–1005; 1990.
40. Elmer-Dewitt, P. Udder insanity. Time, May 17, 1993; p. 52.

CHAPTER 7

Melanotropins and the Intermediate Pituitary

The polypeptide hormones derived from the precursor, pro-opiomelanocortin (MSH, ACTH, ß-LPH) function to change skin color, control the adrenal cortex, and alter fat metabolism. A dramatic and simple demonstration of the power of hormones is to expose a piece of green skin from the lizard *Anolis carolinensis* to homogenate of rat pituitary glands. In a few minutes, the piece of green skin turns first to dark brown and then to black. If you watch the color response using a light microscope, it is even more dramatic with a kaleidoscope of iridescent pink and blue and brown colored organelles in motion. Because the functions of the melanotropins in color change occur in lower vertebrates, they are a main subject of comparative endocrinology. Pigment movement is not only affected by the hormones that come from pro-opiomelanocortin, it is also altered by melatonin and catecholamines.

MELANOTROPINS

"Melanotropins" collectively refers to the group of five polypeptide hormones that affect color changes in the skin of amphibians. The chemically related group includes three melanophore-stimulating hormones (alpha, beta, and gamma MSH), a hormone that stimulates the adrenal cortex (ACTH), and a hormone that causes fat to break down (ß-LPH). Other molecules, also related chemically to the melanotropins, are molecules that may act as internal natural "morphine" (endorphins, enkephalins).

The hormone that has the most potency in changing skin color for which the group of hormones is named is melanotropin. There are three molecular subgroups called "MSH"—alpha, beta, gamma—which differ from each other in the amino acid sequences but which have a similar sequence of seven amino acids.

BIOSYNTHESIS AND CHEMISTRY

The melanotropins are polypeptide hormones. The biosynthesis of the melanotropins is typical of hormones composed of amino acids. There is a large precursor molecule (MW28,500) now called "pro-opiomelanocortin" (POMC). Previously, portions of pro-opiomelanocortin were called big ACTH, proACTH, and preproACTH. Synthesis of melanotropins is completed by proteolytic cleavage of pro-opiomelanocortin (Figure 7.1). Cleavage locations are marked by successively smaller fragments at pairs of basic amino acids (-lys-arg-, -lys-lys-, -arg-arg-). Pro-opiomelanocortin is also synthesized in the hypothalamus, lungs, gastrointestinal tract, and placenta.

The hormone for which the group was named is **melanophore-stimulating hormone** (MSH). Alpha-MSH (α-MSH) has 13 amino acids; beta-MSH (ß-MSH) has 18 amino acids (Figure 7.2); and gamma-MSH (γ-MSH) has 12 amino acids. MSH has other names: melanotropin, melanocyte-stimulating hormone, and intermedin. Melanocyte-stimulating hormone is used when the hormone is referred to in mammals. MSH is usually the hormone most commonly associated with the intermediate lobe of the pituitary gland. MSH is also found in the arcuate nucleus of the hypothalamus.

The hormone that stimulates the adrenal cortex is **corticotropin** (ACTH). ACTH has 39 amino acids (MW 4500). ACTH, adrenal cortex-stimulating hormone, is also called adrenocorticotropin and adrenal corticotrophic hormone. ACTH is the prohormone for α-MSH.

Beta-lipotropin (ß-LPH) is a lypolytic hormone, that is, the hormone "mobilizes fat" or causes fat to break down. ß-LPH has 91 amino acids and MW 11,200. Beta-lipotropin serves as the prohormone for a smaller peptide, gamma-lipotropin.

A peptide called **corticotropin-like-intermediate lobe peptide** (CLIP) consists of amino acids 18-39 of ACTH. No function has been found for CLIP.

Melanotropins have a **common heptapeptide**. Amino acids 3–9 are all the same (-met-glu-his-phe-arg-trp-gly-) in α-MSH, β-MSH, and ACTH; the sequence (-met-*gly*-his-phe-arg-trp-gly-) comprises amino acids 3–9 in γ-MSH. The amino acid sequence of α-MSH varies among mammals, sharks, and salmon. The amino acid sequence of β-MSH also varies among vertebrates (e.g., ox, sheep, pig, horse, camel, monkey, shark, and salmon).

There are some molecules derived from pro-opiomelanocortin that are not melanotropins. The prohormone, ß-lipotropin, is the precursor for **ß-endorphin**. Beta-endorphin has 31 amino acids and MW 4000. **Met-enkephalin** is a peptide with only 5 amino acids; the same sequence of five amino acids is also found at the N-terminal of β-endorphin.

The order in which the biosynthesis proceeds is yet a matter of conjecture. Hadley says about this: "It is unclear whether in the pars intermedia ACTH is first enzymatically released from pro-opiomelanocortin to yield α-MSH and CLIP or whether the two peptides are liberated directly from pro-opiomelanocortin."[1]

Most of the peptides derived from pro-opiomelanocortin are glycosylated at the N-terminal. The polysaccharide moiety is responsible for basophilic staining of corticotrophs and differences in reported molecular weights.[2]

ASSAYS

The peptide hormones of the melanotropin family can be measured with radioimmunoassays. However, there are classic bioassays that were used to measure the melanotropins in early investigations.

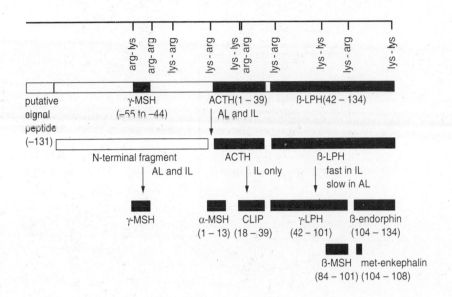

Figure 7.1 The diagram represents the derivation of melanotropic hormones and related molecules from a large precursor molecule (pro-opiomelanocortin, upper two lines). The numbers represent amino acid residues that make up the fragments. The positive numbered amino acids read from the N terminal of ACTH toward the C-terminal portion of the precursor. The fragments are produced by proteolytic cleavage at lys-arg and other basic amino acid residues (locations shown on upper line). AL = anterior lobe; IL = intermediate lobe. Reproduced, with permission. Ganong, W. Review of Medical Physiology, Fourteenth Edition. Norwalk, CN: Appleton & Lange; 1989; p. 340.

Melanophore-stimulating activity was measured by observations of darkening of the skin in the physiological skin color change. The skin darkening is dramatically rapid, it takes only about five minutes. It is easily visible to the naked eye as a change from pale to dark (in the case of tadpoles) or green to brown (in the case of lizards). Bioassays can be done *in vivo* (e.g., with tadpoles) or *in vitro* (e.g., with amphibian or lizard skin) by adding MSH, unknowns, or pituitary extracts to the bathing medium.

A typical bioassay for MSH is based on the reflectance of amphibian skin (*Xenopus laevis*, the African clawed frog or toad). If the frogs are hypophysectomized, the skin becomes twice as sensitive. Amounts of MSH can be expressed in several kinds of units:

1 I.U. MSH activity
= 0.5 mg MSH
= 1.33 x 10^4 Shizume Units

Shizume units are named after their creator. Skin color can easily be assessed by using a "melanophore index." The melanophores are dark cells that are observed in fresh or fixed tissue using a light microscope and scoring with a standard scale (Figure 7.3). It is also possible to assess the skin color by measuring light reflectance or transmission through the skin. The author used light transmission and image analysis (microdensitometry) to quantify color in fixed *Xenopus* tadpoles. The tadpoles with dispersed melanosomes in their melanophores transmitted less

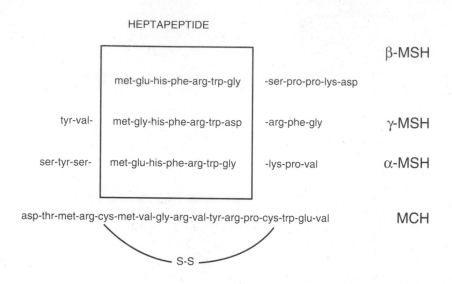

HEPTAPEPTIDE

				β-MSH
	met-glu-his-phe-arg-trp-gly	-ser-pro-pro-lys-asp		
tyr-val-	met-gly-his-phe-arg-trp-asp	-arg-phe-gly		γ-MSH
ser-tyr-ser-	met-glu-his-phe-arg-trp-gly	-lys-pro-val		α-MSH

asp-thr-met-arg-cys-met-val-gly-arg-val-tyr-arg-pro-cys-trp-glu-val   MCH

S-S

Figure 7.2 The amino acid sequences for the peptide hormones of the intermediate lobe are shown from top to bottom: three melanophore-stimulating hormones (MSHs) and one melanophore-concentrating hormone (MCH). The box encloses the heptapeptide that is common to beta and gamma MSHs, ACTH, and (with the exception of one amino acid), alpha MSH. The heptapeptide may be essential for biological activity. There are related fragment analogs for the 17-amino acid residue MCH (not shown).

light (31 ± SEM 2 arbitrary units) than the tadpoles with punctate melanophores (44 ± SEM 2 arbitrary units).[3]

In other bioassays, lipolytic activity is measured with the rabbit fat pad, and corticotropic activity is measured as stimulation of the adrenal cortex.

PARS INTERMEDIA

The anatomy, the cellular origins of pituitary hormones, the vasculature, and the innervation involved in secretion of the melanotropins and regulation of the pars intermedia are difficult to decipher because of variations from one species to another. The clinical endocrinologist may have little use for this variability, but comparative endocrinologists look for clues to function in the varia-

tion. Interspecies variation in the appearance of a gland is a signal that the gland functions in environmental adaptation (to light, to temperature, or to water).

The pars intermedia (zona intermedia, intermediate lobe) is not even present in all vertebrates. It is visibly absent as a separate layer in birds, some mammals (cetaceans, the whales and dolphins), and the human adult. The pituitary gland of the human fetus does have an intermediate layer which becomes rudimentary as development proceeds.

Some birds, which appear not to have a separate pars intermedia, may still have the MSH-secreting cells that are dispersed among the cells of the pars distalis. Moreover, in fishes (elasmobranchs, teleosts) MSH-secreting cells are continuous with other cells of the pars distalis but

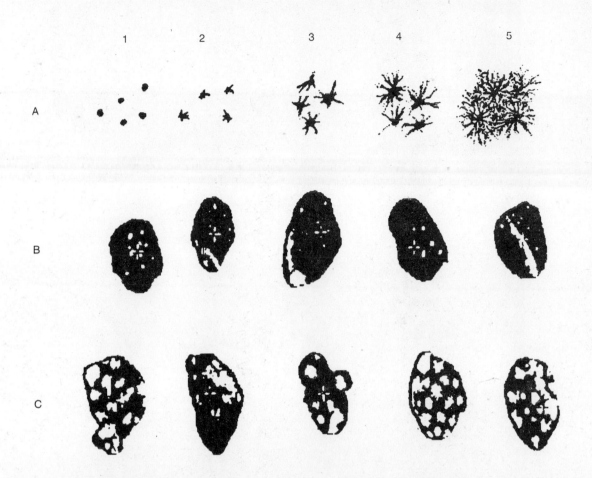

Figure 7.3 The figure shows how skin color can be quantified using a melanophore index or densitometry images. (A) The melanophore index is used to assign numerical values on the basis of the dispersion of melanosomes in melanophores. There are sketches of four melanophores that appear black for index 1 (punctate melanophores), indices 2-4, and index 5 (dispersed melanophores). (B) Densitometry images of fields of skin from five tadpoles with punctate melanophores. (C) Densitometry images of fields of skin from five tadpoles with dispersed melanophores (melanophores appear white in a negative image of a skin field). The indices are redrawn, with permission, after Hadley, M.E. Endocrinology, Second Edition. Englewood Cliffs, NJ; 1988; page 169. The densitometry images are reproduced, with permission, from Binkley, S.; Mosher, K.; Rubin, F.; White, B. *Xenopus* tadpole melanophores are controlled by dark and light and melatonin without influence of time of day. Journal of Pineal Research 5: 87–97; 1988.

they are situated along the caudal perimeter of the pars distalis. In four-footed animals, the pars intermedia is inseparable from the pars nervosa. In this last case, the part of the pituitary has been referred to by the collective name of the neurointermediate lobe.

Animals that can change color to blend with their surroundings have a large pars intermedia which is evidence for the function of the pars intermedia in color change. *Anolis carolinensis*, the so-called Florida chameleon, has served children as pets and provided investigators an outstanding example of biological color change. During the daytime, an *Anolis* lizard is bright green when it is hot

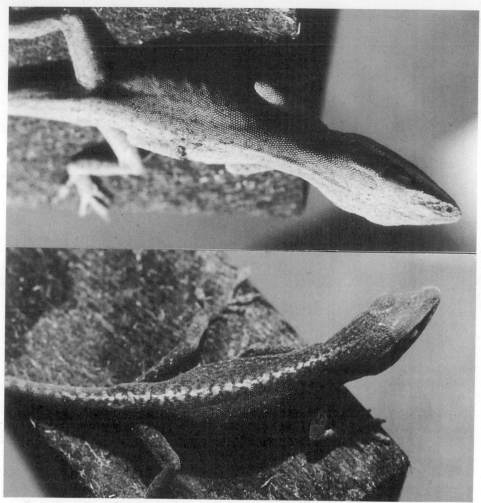

Figure 7.4 Color change in the lizard *Anolis carolinensis,* or Florida chameleon, is illustrated by computer scans of photographs. On the left, a dark brown lizard is posed wearing the brown color typical of light-time on a black substrate. On the right, a green lizard has donned the pale color that would occur on a white substrate in the daytime or at night in darkness or (as here) when warmed and stressed by handling. The illustration does not show background adaptation; the lizards were posed briefly on wood blocks for their portraits. Photographs by author.

or the background is white; *Anolis* turns very dark brown if it is chilled or placed on a black background (Figure 7.4).

    If the intermediate lobe's appearance has anything to do with its function, then a role for the pars intermedia in water and electrolyte balance is likely. Dehydration affects the size of the intermediate lobe. The intermediate lobe cells hypertrophy when rats are injected with saline or are dehydrated. Table 7.1 summarizes the cellular sources of melanotropins.

    The vascularization of the intermediate lobe is unusual among endocrine glands which usually have a rich blood supply. There is very little vasculature, the pars intermedia is avascular, when compared to other endocrine glands. Perryman and Bagnara proposed an extravascular means of transfer which could provide a route for secretions.[4]

    The pars intermedia and the neurointermediate lobe (lizards), like the pars distalis, may have no hypothalamic nerve terminals. However, the pars intermedia of some other species do receive

Table 7.1 Cell Sources of Melanotropins and Related Molecules

Cells	Organisms	Hormones
pars intermedia PIPbH cells	teleost fishes	MSH
pars intermedia PIPAS cells	teleost fishes	?
melanotrops	cyclostomes amphibians, reptiles most mammals	MSH
melanotrops	human	α-MSH CLIP γ-LPH β-Endorphin
corticotrops	vertebrates	pro-opiomelanocortin ACTH β-lipotropin endorphins γ-MSH

PIPbH cells stain with lead hematoxylin. PIPAS cells stain with periodic acid-shiff. The teleost PIPAS cell secretory product has not been identified, but the cells control the darkening response of fish on black backgrounds. In human adults, the intermediate lobe is rudimentary and neither alpha or beta MSH appear to be secreted. Basophilic cells of intermediate lobe origin and chromophobes have also been suggested as possible corticotrops.

neural endings from cells in the hypothalamus. The endings appear to be both neurosecretory and adrenergic. The adrenergic endings form a plexus around the secretory cells.

CHROMATOPHORES, ORGANELLES, PIGMENTS

Melanophore-stimulating hormone (MSH) is named for its function in causing melanophores to darken in color. Melanophores are one subcategory of pigmented cells, the chromatophores. Three types of chromatophores—melanophores, iridophores, xanthophores—constitute a **dermal chromatophore unit**. The unit is re-sponsible for the rapid pale-to-dark or green-to-brown color change. Understanding color changes can be difficult if the terms light and dark are used to refer to the background, the light from the sky, and the color of the animals. Chromatophores develop from neural crest. They migrate all over the body. Chromatophores have been found in various membranes: skin, peritoneum, meninges, and walls of blood vessels.

Dermal **melanophores** are cells with nerve-like projections, or processes, that are sometimes arranged basket-like around other pigment cells, the iridophores. The melanophores contain, and are named for the brown pigment, **melanin**, which the cells synthesize from the amino acid, tyrosine. There are brown or black melanins (eumelanins) and there are red or light colored melanins (phaeomelanins) which color fur. Melanin is synthesized from tyrosine in a sequence of steps with dopa and quinones as intermediates; the enzyme tyrosinase participates in melanin synthesis. During biosynthesis, the melanin is sequestered onto a corncob-like scaffolding of organelles called **melanosomes**. To accomplish rapid color changes in minutes, the organelles are simply rearranged. The pigment amount does not change in the rapid color change.

Iridophores contain crystals of purines (guanine, hypoxanthine, adenine, uric acid) in organelles called "reflecting platelets." The reflecting platelets are arranged in "stacks." Their orientation can be altered to make the skin more or less reflective. Iridophores are found in the skin of poikilotherms ("cold blooded" animals: the reptiles, amphibians, and fish) and in bird irises.

Xanthophores and **erythrophores** are cells containing yellow, orange, and red pigments. The cells are only found in poikilotherms. The pigments are carotenoids (contained in vesicles) and pteridines (in organelles composed of a series of concentric lamellae called pterinosomes).

Epidermal melanocytes release pigmented melanosomes at their dendritic processes into surrounding cells to color hair and feathers and to tan skin. Melanin that is "secreted" in this way is called **cytocrine melanin**. A melanocyte and its associated cells can be thought of as an epidermal melanin unit.

PHYSIOLOGICAL COLOR CHANGE

The rapid color change that takes place in minutes in poikilotherms during background adaptation has been called physiological color change. Physiological color change does not require increased melanin synthesis, it is achieved by melanosome rearrangement (Figure 7.5). It is different than morphological color change which takes place over a period of days and involves the synthesis of more melanin. In background adaptation, physiological color change is both quick and dramatic.

On a black background, the melanosomes **disperse** throughout the melanophore into its basketlike processes. The effect of spreading the melanosome is to color the entire cell. Because of the arrangement of the cells in the dermal chromatophore unit, the melanosomes in the processes

block light reflection by the iridophores, further enhancing the effect. Collectively, the cells with dispersed melanosomes are responsible for brown-black skin color. The platelets in the iridophores orient perpendicularly (to the surface of the skin), enhancing still further the skin blackening effect. MSH causes the melanosomes to disperse.

On a white background, the melanosomes **aggregate** into a clump. The melanophores are described as being punctate. Most of the cytoplasm of the melanophore is transparent in this condition. The iridophores are not masked by pigment in the basket-like processes of the melanophores, and they orient their platelets horizontally (parallel to the skin surface). The collective effect is to make the skin pale colored. Young *Xenopus* tadpoles with punctate melanophores, for example, are almost transparent and their internal organs can clearly be seen. In the absence of MSH, the melanosomes aggregate.

To darken the color of the skin requires centrifugal movement of melanosomes to achieve dispersion of the melanosomes in the melanophores. To lighten the color of the skin requires centripetal movement of melanosomes to achieve aggregation of the melanosomes in the melanophores. The likely candidates for moving the melanosomes about are cytoskeletal elements: microtubules and microfilaments. However, these structures are not found in all melanophores.

Chromatophores have been used as "model" systems to study movement in cells. McNiven and Porter write:

Teleost chromatophores have proven valuable in the study of the cytomatrix and its involvement in intracellular transport. These cells, which move their pigment rapidly, can be isolated from the scales of fish and maintained in culture for several days. Their transport activity can be followed with the light microscope and recorded by cinematography. Individual pigment granules can be seen moving radially toward the cell center in aggregation, then back toward the cortices during dispersion. These two motions are different. In aggregation, the granules move smoothly and rapidly (5–10 mm/s), reminding one of the behavior of chromosomes during anaphase. In

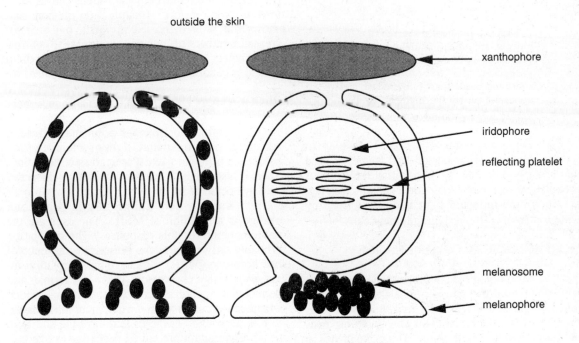

outside the skin

xanthophore

iridophore

reflecting platelet

melanosome

melanophore

inside the skin

DARK SKIN
dispersed melanosomes,
MSH,
black background
daytime

PALE SKIN
punctate melanophore,
no MSH,
white background in daytime
any background at night

Figure 7.5 Two-dimensional sketches of two dermal chromatophore units in the skin illustrate physiological color change. The three kinds of cells are all chromatophores (melanophores, iridophores, xanthophores). The organelles are the melanosomes (which can disperse or aggregate) and the reflecting platelets (which can orient).

dispersion, which takes twice as long as aggregation, the granules move haltingly, first out (orthograde) and then back (retrograde). This saltatory motion continues throughout dispersion but ceases suddenly at the onset of the next aggregation. . . .All the fish chromatophores . . . possess a similar internal organization. A highly structural centrosome complex consisting of a centriole pair and surrounding stratified layers of dense material occupies the cell center. Thousands of microtubules nucleate from this structure and extend outward, organizing the pigment into linear columns. . . . the structure of the surrounding cytoplasm is . . . wispy flocculent material [that is] a three-dimensional latticework of fine filaments or trabeculae (2–6 nm in diameter) that suspend the pigment. . . .With the pigment dispersed, the filaments are thin and delicate in appearance, as if extended. Upon aggregation, the trabeculae become short and beaded, as if contracted, and appear to clump the pigment together during aggregation.[5]

Other pigment cells come into play to produce the various shades of gold, taupe, and red that color poikilotherms. In addition, green color is explained by the phenomenon Tyndall scattering, in which blue-reflected light is colored green by yellow pigments in overlying pigment cells.[6]

MORPHOLOGICAL COLOR CHANGE

Morphological color change is the process where increased melanin is synthesized. It takes a much longer time (weeks) for morphological color changes. Morphological color change is responsible for mammalian hair color. The melanocytes in hair skin are clustered around the hair follicles (follicular melanocytes). Melanocytes synthesize melanin which colors the hair. MSH and steroids stimulate melanin pigmentation together or sequentially. The follicular melanocytes produce variously colored melanins, so the hairs can be complexly colored with black, brown, and white bands.

Some mammals, especially those exposed to snowy winter environments, change hair color with season (varying hare, *Lepus americanus*). Most of these animals exchange a brownish summer coat for a white winter coat on an annual basis which seems to have adaptive significance in providing protective color camouflage. MSH appears to be involved in the white-to-brown coat changes of weasels and Siberian hamsters. Experimentally, sensitivity of mammalian melanocytes to MSH can be shown with yellow mice. Injecting MSH into a mouse makes new hair grow in dark colored.[7]

Some animals also change color when they are in breeding condition, the "nuptial coloration." The changes associated with reproduction may involve other hormones, such as testosterone. For example, testosterone injections cause sparrow bills to turn black, and male sparrows also have black bills during the breeding season.

Morphological color changes can be induced with background. Maintaining frogs for long periods of time on black backgrounds causes them to turn darker colors. Examination of their skin shows not only increased pigment, but also increased numbers of melanophores. MSH controls the response. Melanoblasts proliferate and exhibit cytodifferentiation in response to MSH *in vitro*.

REGULATION OF COLOR CHANGE

Rapid color changes occur in response to substrate, environmental lighting, temperature, stress, and behavior (sexual or aggressive behavior). There is also a daily cycle of color change characterized by nocturnal pallor.

Background adaptation through color change is a function of MSH. The eyes are the photoreceptor for this response. The adaptation probably only requires the presence or absence of one hormone (MSH). Background adaptation involves all the chromatophores—epidermal and dermal melanophores and iridophores. Background adaptation occurs later in development than adaptation to darkness. Tadpoles that have the ability to background adapt are called secondary stage tadpoles. If the tadpoles are moved to the light at night, the light depresses melatonin and the tadpoles will then darken in response to the black background.

Adaptation to darkness, that is the lack of light (e.g., at night), is quite different. Many poikilotherms show nocturnal pallor. This is true, for example, of *Xenopus* tadpoles, *Anolis* lizards, and many varieties of tropical fish. At night, the dermal melanophores blanch, or become punctate. MSH is low at night, but night-time blanching may be mediated by melatonin (from the pineal gland and/or the eyes). Only the dermal melanophores respond to melatonin. Night-time pallor is a capability of very young, primary stage tadpoles, which cannot adapt to background. The rhythm of nocturnal blanching is a true circadian rhythm in *Anolis*, it persists in constant dark with a period length of about 24 hours.[8] In achieving these actions, melatonin, during the night, might act two ways: on the chromatophores and by inhibition of MSH. A bihumoral hypothesis, involving both melatonin (produced at night) and MSH (produced in the day), accounts for the rhythmic change in color. The **pineal gland** generates en-

Table 7.2 Control of MSH Secretion by Melanotrops[9]

Secretion increased by	Secretion decreased by
thyrotropin-releasing hormone (TRH)	dopamine (DA)
corticotropin-releasing hormone (CRH)	epinephrine (E)
serotonin (5-HT)	norepinephrine (NE)
5-hydroxytryptamine	ergot alkaloids
MRFs	dopamine receptor agonists
	gamma amino butyric acid (GABA)
	neuropeptide Y (NPY)
	MIFs

dogenous daily cycles of melatonin secretion that persist in constant darkness, but the rhythm had not yet developed in very young tadpoles; in very young tadpoles the melatonin appeared to be controlled by the presence of light or dark. Light acting on the pineal does not necessarily require the eyes for this effect. Astonishingly, the animals have extraretinal light perception for the response. While pineal glands of some species have photoreceptor-like organelles, even blind, pinealectomized animals can detect light so that there must be yet other sites of light perception.

Extraretinal light perception has been demonstrated in fish, reptiles, amphibians, and birds. The presence of extraretinal light perception in developing mammals is disputed, but it is not a capability of adult mammals. Extraretinal light perception function has been demonstrated for light sensitive phenomena including synchronization of circadian rhythms, seasonal breeding, color change in poikilotherms, and feeding behavior in fish. The pineal may itself detect light as the pineal glands of some species, such as chickens, respond directly to light *in vitro*.[10] However, investigators have shown that there is extraretinal light perception based on photoreceptors that are neither in the retina nor the pineal; the investigators believe these other photoreceptors might be located in the brain.

The chromatophores of some fish and reptiles have innervation. Moreover, isolated tails of *Xenopus* tadpoles respond directly to light.

Skin color changes have potential for a role in behavioral **thermoregulation**. The skin color changes in response to temperature. *Anolis* that are held under a warming lamp turn green, which should reflect radiation, irrespective of their background. *Anolis* that are chilled on ice turn dark brown irrespective of their background. The fact that temperature affects color provokes the attractive idea that the animals turn brown when they are cold to absorb more light to raise their temperature, and that the animals turn green or pale when they are hot to reflect more light to lower their temperatures. Body temperature in *Anolis* did not change when the lizards changed color (Binkley, unpublished), so, if this attractive idea has any validity, the animals must detect miniscule changes in temperature to which they adjust rapidly so that they maintain relatively constant internal body temperature. Nonetheless, the possibility that color change and MSH affect body temperature lingers, even in mammals. Alpha-MSH and ACTH injected into rabbit cerebral ventricles produce hyperthermia, and both hormones localize in anterior preoptic hypothalamic nuclei important in temperature regulation. In addition, temperature extremes may directly affect the cellular components that move the melanosomes.

An organism that turns pale in response to stress is said to be displaying "**excitement pallor**." Rapid color changes can also be evoked by "stress." Handling or chasing *Anolis carolinensis* (e.g., to recover them when they escape their cages) causes the lizards to change color. This phenomenon, which may involve darkening or lightening and changes of the color pattern, is probably not mediated by MSH. It is likely that it is mediated by the adrenal glands. Injections of adrenergic agents such as epinephrine into an *Anolis* evokes a stress color pattern (bright green color, black stripe down the back, black speckles over the body, and blackening of a patch of skin behind the eye). The colorful pattern, which epinephrine provoked in four minutes, was also described for *Anolis* preparing for combat.

What color, then, is an *Anolis*? A hierarchical model for the control of color change in a poikilotherm such as *Anolis* has been proposed. In the model the factors determining skin color are ranked: (i) temperature > (ii) stress > (iii) background > (iv) rhythm. The hypothesis permits determination of a lizard's color this way: (i) The poikilothermic lizard can't do much about temperature extremes which override its hormonal and behavioral mechanisms. (ii) In times of stress (e.g., threat from a predator) it follows the rule, change color and run. The effect of epinephrine from the adrenal gland is stronger than the effects of background or time of day. (iii) If there is no immediate danger, the lizard uses MSH to adapt to background (color camouflage) to avoid being seen by predators (e.g., birds). MSH exerts its effects in the light during the daytime when melatonin is absent. (iv) Finally, when darkness descends, the lizard can't see the background to adapt, the predators can't see the lizard, so, unless it is very cold, the lizard's circadian rhythm of melatonin comes into play and nocturnal pallor results.[11]

HUMAN PIGMENTATION

The melanin-containing cells in humans are called melanocytes and MSH is called "melanocyte-stimulating hormone." As mentioned, in adult humans, the pars intermedia is rudimentary and neither alpha nor beta MSH is present in the pituitary or secreted.

Human melanocytes synthesize melanin and contain melanosomes. The melanosomes are transferred to keratinocytes (skin cells), some of which surround hair follicles. In addition to responsibility for hair color, melanocytes are responsible for suntanning. But, since MSH is supposed to be absent in humans, it is not claimed to have a role in suntanning, and it is possible that the skin cells are directly stimulated by sunlight to produce more melanin.

Despite the fact that MSH is apparently not a hormone in adult humans, injections of MSH into darkly pigmented individuals visibly increases skin pigmentation in a few days.[12]

Moreover, MSH may have a role in pregnancy. The nipples and areolae darken during pregnancy.

> The MSH-like activity of the blood and urine is increased during pregnancy, and indeed, the frog skin bioassay for MSH was originally designed to measure an elevation of the hormone as an index for predicting pregnancy in the human...[MSH during pregnancy] might be of fetal origin as the fetal, but not the adult, pituitary is thought to produce a melanotropin [or MSH] might be synthesized by the pars intermedia of the pregnant female.[13]

Thus, it is possible that MSH comes from the pars intermedia of pregnant females, but it is more intriguing to speculate that the activity originates with the fetus.[14] The fetus after all does have a visible pars intermedia, and, if MSH plays a role in pigment cell formation and activity, then that role may take place during fetal development. However, darkening is also caused by steroids, and, since they rise during pregnancy, they may account for the changes in pigmentation.

Pigmentation is an inherited characteristic. Melanocytes might be directly activated by light, possibly by stimulation of formation of cholecalciferol (vitamin D).

Several diseases involve changes in pigmentation. Clinical endocrinologists attribute some of the changes to alterations in ACTH which has melanotropin activity. For example, a symptom of a disease of the adrenal, Addison's disease, is darkened skin, and Addison's sufferers have high ACTH levels. A symptom of hypopituitarism is abnormal pallor.

Some other diseases with skin color abnormalities appear to be due to disorders of melanin synthesis. For example, albinos lack genes necessary for melanin synthesis. Another genetic disorder is piebaldism where some areas of skin lack melanin because the melanocyte precursor cells do not migrate from neural crest to some areas of the skin during development. In vitiligo, which also is characterized by differences in skin color patches, the melanin loss appears after birth.

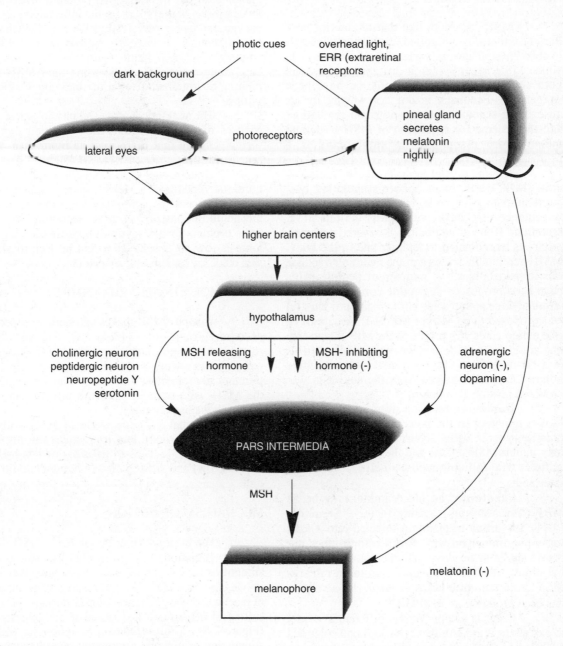

Figure 7.6 A generalized scheme for the regulation of physiological color change. The hypothalamus may regulate the pars intermedia with neurons or hormones. Eyes and/or extraretinal light perception may convey information about the light from above to the pineal gland. The pineal generates a rhythm of melatonin (peak at night) and may also affect higher brain centers, hypothalamus, and pars intermedia. As drawn, the melanosomes are aggregated at night in the dark because of melatonin and dispersed in the day in the light on a dark background because of MSH. The scheme is probably more complex since melatonin is made and secreted by the retinas and melatonin from this source most likely targets the hypothalamus, possibly via a retinohypothalmic tract.

REGULATION OF MSH

MSH secretion, like that of anterior pituitary hormones, is controlled by the hypothalamus (Table 7.2). There is variability in the ways in which MSH is controlled in different species, and both neural and hormonal regulation have been suggested. Feedback is not noteworthy for its absence in schemes for melanotropin regulation; and the scheme for regulation of MSH in dermal melanophore dispersion in amphibians is a neuroendocrine reflex.

A hypophysial neurohormone, melanostatin (MIF, MIH, melanophore-stimulating hormone-inhibiting hormone) has been sought. There is evidence that the hypothalamus inhibits MSH secretion. If the infundibulum is severed or the pituitary is transplanted to another site in the body, MSH secretion increases and the neurointermediate lobe hypertrophies. A number of peptide MIFs have been proposed. A peptide containing the C-terminal three amino acids of oxytocin (pro-leu-gly) was proposed to be MIF or MRIH-I. A peptide of five amino acids was proposed for MIF-II (pro-his-phe-arg-gly). Tocinoic acid was suggested as MIF-II (cys-tyr-ile-gln-asn-cys, connected with a disulfide bond). An MRF derived from tocinoic acid was proposed (cys-tyr-ile-gln-asn).

Dopamine released from aminergic neurons originating in the postoptic nucleus inhibits pars intermedia cells. **Neuropeptide Y** (NPY) may inhibit MSH release and the inhibition may be indirect via folliculo-stellate cells of the pars intermedia. [15]

Serotonin, an indoleamine, may be an MRF (melanotropin-releasing factor). Serotonin (5HT, 5-hydroxy tryptamine) injected into *Anolis* turns the animal brown. But serotonin does not brown the skin *in vitro*. Thus serotonin may act by stimulating MSH release. Serotonin releases MSH from hemipituitaries *in vitro*. So serotonin has been proposed as an MRH.[16]

There is a upper retinal differential model to explain how animals detect background color and adapt using their hormones. The idea is that when an animal sits on a black background, the retina will have very little light reflected to its upper aspect, which it can discriminate from the greater light from the overhead light source, and secretes MSH in response. However, there is still a matter of the sequence of events between the retina of the eye and the neurointermediate lobe of the pituitary gland. Perhaps the retinohypothalamic tract provides a direct neural route for the information about background that is perceived by the eye to reach the hypothalamus. There, the signals could inhibit aminergic and peptidergic neurons of the postoptic and preoptic nuclei from releasing their MSH-inhibiting neurotransmitters at the individual melanotrops.

The anatomical array and physiological responses of diverse species are so varied that it seems possible that there may be more than one scheme for the regulation of MSH (Figure 7.6).

There is even a possible role for the pineal hormone melatonin. Melatonin reverses the *in vitro* response of hemipituitary MSH to serotonin; melatonin inhibits *in vitro* MSH secretion. This is not a problem in the daytime, because then melatonin is low so that MSH would be free to alter skin color for background adaptation.

MSH AMOUNTS AND RHYTHMS

Xenopus MSH makes appropriate responses to background color (Table 7.3). Plasma MSH rose in the amphibians on a black background compared to a gray or white background. In the pituitary, the opposite was seen. The idea is that the MSH was secreted from the pituitary in response to the background.

Rats have a daily cycle of MSH with a peak in the afternoon and low values during the night (Figure 7.7). Thus MSH is high when melatonin is low, and MSH is low when melatonin is high.

MECHANISM OF ACTION

The mechanism of action for α-MSH dispersing melanosomes in melanophores is a straightforward second messenger mechanism involving cyclic AMP. The end result of the cascade of reactions is the activation of melanofilaments resulting in centrifugal migration of melanophores (Figure 7.8). The mechanism of action for MSH stimulation of melanin production by melanocytes likewise involves cyclic AMP. In the proposed mechanism, the cascade of reactions initiates transcription and translation to increase synthesis of the enzyme tyrosinase.[17]

Melanophores are particularly useful for experimental generation of models for receptors, stimulators, and inhibitors. The melanophores can

Table 7.3 MSH in Background-Adapted *Xenopus*

	Background		
	White	Gray	Black
total pituitary MSH content (ng)	73	68	11
plasma MSH concentration (pg/ml)	22	62	107
MSH clearance (ng/day)	1.6	4.5	29
rate of turnover of pituitary content (days)	46	15	0.4

Alpha MSH was measured with radioimmunoassay in adult African clawed toads. The animals were adapted to illuminated backgrounds for one week. The data are from Wilson, J.F; Morgan, M.A. Alpha-melanotropin-like substances in the pituitary and plasma of *Xenopus laevis* in relation to colour change responses. Gen. Comp. Endocrinol. 38: 172–182, 1979.

be worked with *in vitro* using pieces of skin or cultures of cells. Substances are easily tested by adding them to the culture medium, then observing their effects on pigment migration or biochemicals in the skin or cells. Such studies produce a model of a melanophore with various receptors in its cell membrane which respond specifically to catecholamines, MSH, or acetylcholine and of a melanophore that can be influenced by other molecules that penetrate the cell membrane.

RECEPTORS AND PHARMACOLOGY

Because the melanophores can be studied *in vitro* in cell cultures, or, even more simply, in isolated pieces of amphibian or reptile skin, they are ideally suited for studying hormone receptors and pharmacological actions.

Pituitary extract turns skin dark *in vitro*, evidence for MSH action on melanophores (Figure 7.9). The melanotropic action of MSH (and also ACTH) is dependent on calcium ions so a calcium requirement is a characteristic of MSH receptors. The initial event in MSH mechanisms of action is that MSH, the first messenger, binds to the melanophore or melanocyte cell membrane at receptor sites that are specific for MSH (MSH receptors). Binding activates an enzyme localized in the cell membrane, adenylate cyclase, which results in the production of the second messenger molecule,

cyclic AMP. Analogs of cyclic AMP, such as dibutyryl cyclic AMP (DB-cyclic AMP) darken lizard skin. The second messenger does not require calcium for melanosome movement.[18] The calcium requirement appears to be specific to receptors.

The adrenergic agents, or catecholamines, epinephrine and norepinephrine also change skin color. Skin darkening seems to utilize a beta adrenergic receptor with cyclic AMP as a second messenger. Blockading the beta receptor does not affect the response to MSH, and cells that do not respond to MSH have beta receptors, so the beta receptor is distinct from the MSH receptor. The catecholamines darken without requiring calcium.

Catecholamines can also lighten the color of amphibian skin. The response is mediated by alpha receptors. The action of catecholamines on a particular melanophore is determined by the ratio of alpha to beta receptors on that melanophore. This makes it possible to achieve darkening of some melanophores at the same time that others lighten rendering complex changes in coloration. The overall action of catecholamines on the melanophores of a species depends on the array of alpha and beta receptors in that species.

Melatonin, an indoleamine, antagonizes MSH, and pineal extracts lighten the color of melanophores. Heward and Hadley[19] characterized a melatonin receptor for frog skin melanophores.

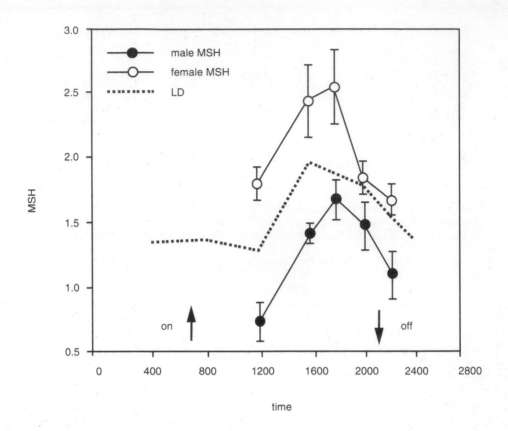

Figure 7.7 The graphs plot pituitary MSH content at different times of the day in male and female rats (N = 8). The pituitary MSH was measured with a frog bioassay and the units on the y-axis are micrograms/pituitary gland ± error bars representing SEM. The dashed lines show the rhythm in a light-dark cycle (LD). The rats were housed in LD14:10 with lights on at 0700 (upward-pointing arrow) and lights out were at 2100 (downward-pointing arrow). Drawn by the author from data in Tilders, F. J. H.; Smelik, P. G. A diurnal rhythm in melanocyte-stimulating hormone content of the rat pituitary gland and its independence from the pineal gland. Neuroendocrinology 17: 296–308; 1975.

Melatonin might achieve its action by stimulating guanylate cyclase and a cGMP second messenger to achieve the melanosome aggregation. The possibility exists that melatonin achieves its effects on skin color by directly controlling melanophores and/or by influencing the secretion of pituitary hormones.

Methylxanthines (theophylline, caffeine) darken lizard skin. The methylxanthines inhibit the enzyme, phosphodiesterase, which normally inacti-vates cyclic AMP by converting it to 5'AMP. So the likely mechanism for methylxanthine darkening of melanophores is that they cause an accumulation of cyclic AMP which in turn causes dispersion.

N-ethylmaleimide is a sulfhydryl reactive chemical that darkens lizard skin. Its mechanism is unknown, but its inhibitory action is evidence that free sulfhydryl groups, -SH, may be necessary for melanosome dispersion.

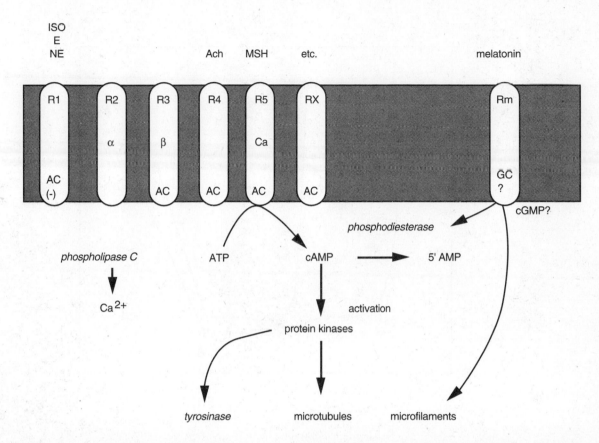

Figure 7.8 The multiple receptor model for melanophore responses incorporates several ideas. Hormones (MSH, melatonin, epinephrine = E) in the blood and neurotransmitters from nerve endings (acetylcholine = ACh; norepinephrine = NE) or injected drugs (isoproterenol = ISO) impinge on a hypothetical melanophore cell membrane that is studded with several kinds of receptors. NE, E, ISO interact with alpha receptors (e.g., to produce excitement pallor) which increase intracellular calcium by activating phospholipase C or by inhibiting adenylate cyclase. MSH interacts with a calcium dependent receptor; NE, E, ISO also act with a beta receptor—the interactions increase adenylate cyclase (AC) so that cyclic AMP (cAMP) is produced. Cyclic AMP activates protein kinases which stimulate tyrosinase to increase melanin formation and microtubules to disperse melanophores. Melatonin, via its own receptor, aggregates melanosomes, via guanylate cyclase (GC) and cyclic GMP (cGMP).

Colchicine darkens frog skins *in vitro*. Colchicine is a poison that inhibits microtubule assembly by binding with tubulin, the protein subunit of microtubules. Cytochalasin B lightens skin. Cytochalasin B interferes with microfilament function. The fact that the two drugs, which alter the cytoskeleton, affect melanophores is evidence that the cytoskeleton is involved in melanosome movements.

Prostaglandins disperse melanosomes in the melanophores of fish and amphibians and may therefore participate in color change.

MELANIN-CONCENTRATING HORMONE

A hormone of the pituitary gland has been proposed for fish which has the opposite effect to melanotropins. The hormone, dubbed melanin-concentrating hormone (MCH) causes aggregation of melanosomes in melanophores and thereby

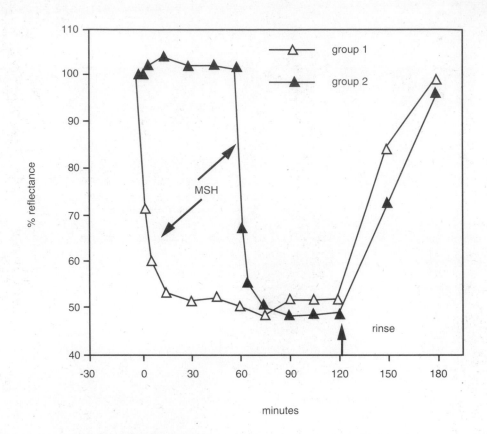

Figure 7.9 *Anolis* skin pieces (N = 8) were cultured *in vitro*. At time zero, MSH was added to the skin pieces in group 1; at time 60 minutes, MSH was added to the skin pieces in group 2; at time 120 minutes, all the pieces were rinsed several times with Ringer solution. Green colored skin has a high % reflectance; brown colored skin has a low % reflectance. The time for skin color darkening was about five minutes; skin color lightening time exceeded 60 minutes. The data are regraphed by the author from Bagnara, J.T.; Hadley, M.E. Chromatophores and Color Change. Englewood Cliffs, NJ: Prentice-Hall; 1973.

lightens the skin color. The primary structure has been identified as a cyclic heptadecapeptide (17 amino acids) and synthetic peptides containing amino acids 5–14 (-cys-met-val-gly-arg-val-try-arg-pro-cys-) were agonists. In bioassays using eel skin, as little as 10^{-12} M MCH causes aggregation. When MCH was tested in frogs, toads, and lizards, however, it caused melanophore dispersion. It has also been suggested that MCH might function as a hypophysiotropic hormone inhibiting MSH and ACTH secretion.

OTHER ACTIONS OF MSH

The actions of MSH are not limited to stimulation of dispersion in melanophores and melanin synthesis.

The products derived from pro-opiomelanocortin appear to vary with state of life. Alpha MSH and CLIP are secreted in fetal primates, but ACTH predominates in adults. The fetal MSH may stimulate a fetal adrenal zone which involutes at birth. Moreover, MSH may stimulate adrenal aldosterone secretion.

MSII has growth promoting properties in fetal rats and stimulated GH in human children.

Behavioral effects of melanotropins have been observed in animals and humans: longer attention span, arousal, motivation increases, memory retention, augmented learning ability.

Effects of MSH and ACTH have been observed in studies of nerve cells or muscle cells *in vitro*. The hormones increase the changes in action potentials and reduce fatigue due to the stress of repeated stimulation.[20]

Turner lists yet other extrapigmentary functions of MSH:

> ...thyrotropic action, hypocalcemic action, aqueous flare response, positive chronotrophic action, action on monosynaptic potentials, induction of stretching and yawning, action on knifefish electrical discharge, hypersensitivity in mice, actions on conditioned reflexes, and electroencephalographic actions.[21]

REFERENCES

1. Hadley, M. E. Endocrinology, Second Edition. Englewood Cliffs, NJ: Prentice Hall; 1988; p. 162.

2. Frohman, L.A. Diseases of the anterior pituitary, Chapter 7. In Felig, P. et al., editors. Endocrinology and Metabolism. McGraw-Hill, New York; 1981; pp. 151–231.

3. Binkley, S.; Mosher, K.; Rubin, F.; White, B. *Xenopus* tadpole melanophores are controlled by dark and light and melatonin without influence of time of day. Journal of Pineal Research 5: 87–97; 1988.

4. Perryman, E.K.; Bagnara, J.T. Extravascular transfer within the anuran pars intermedia. Cell. Tiss. Res. 193: 297–313; 1978.

5. McNiven, M.A.; Porter, K. Chromatophores—Models for studying cytomatrix translocations. J. Cell Biol. 99, 153s–158s; 1984.

6. J.T. Bagnara; Hadley, M.E. Chromatophores and Color Change. Englewood Cliffs, NJ: Prentice-Hall; 1973.

7. Geschwind, I.; Museby, R.; Nishioka, R. The effect of melanocyte-stimulating hormone on coat color in the mouse. Rec. Prog. Horm. Res. 28: 91–130; 1972.

8. Binkley, S.; Reilly, K.; Hermida, V.; Mosher, K. Circadian rhythm of color change in *Anolis carolinensis*: Reconsideration of regulation, especially the role of melatonin in dark-time pallor. Pineal Research Reviews 5: 133–151; 1987.

9. Hadley, M. E. Endocrinology, Third Edition. Englewood Cliffs, NJ: Prentice Hall; 1992; p. 185.

10. Binkley, S.; Riebman, J.; Reilly, K. The pineal gland: A biological clock *in vitro*. Science 202: 1198–1201; 1978

11. Binkley, S.; Reilly, K.; Hermida, V.; Mosher, K. Op. cit., pp. 133–151.

12. Pawelek, J.M.; and A.M. Korner. The biosynthesis of mammalian melanin. Amer. Sci. 70: 136–145; 1982.

13. Hadley, M.E. Third Edition, Op. cit. p. 190.

14. Shizume, K.; Lerner, A.; Fitzpatrick, T. *In vitro* bioassay for the melanocyte stimulating hormone. Endocrinology 54: 553–560; 1954.

15. Hadley, M. E. Third Edition, p. 185.

16. Thornton, B.; Geschwind, I. Evidence that serotonin may be a melanocyte-stimulating hormone-releasing factor in the lizard, *Anolis carolinensis*. Gen. Comp. Endocrinol. 26: 346–353; 1975.

17. Hadley, M. E. Second Edition, Op. cit., p. 177.

18. Veseley, D.L.; Hadley, M.E. Ionic requirements for melanophore stimulating hormone (MSH) action on melanophores. Comp. Biochem. Physiol. 62A: 501–508; 1979.

19. Heward, C.; Hadley, M.E. Structure-activity relationships of melatonin and related indoleamines. Life Sciences 17: 1167–1178; 1975.

20. Strand, F.L. The influence of hormones on the nervous system. Bioscience 25: 568–577; 1975.

21. Turner, C.D.; Bagnara, J. Endocrinology, Sixth Edition. W. B. Saunders: Philadelphia, PA; 1976; p. 154.

CHAPTER 8

Melatonin and the Pineal and Retina

Functions of the pineal gland and its hormone, melatonin, which is synthesized in the dark at night, include roles in skin color change, seasonal reproduction, regulation of circadian rhythms, and photoreception. Rhythmic melatonin synthesis was also discovered in the retinas of the eyes of many species. The finding that the retina could synthesize melatonin rhythmically, like the pineal, explains negative results of pinealectomy. The pineal gland has served as a model system for studying the catecholamine mechanism of action and for studies of oscillating cells; and the pineal rhythms and their regulation by light provoked interest in the study of hormone rhythms of other glands.

DESCARTES

The function of the pineal gland was unknown for so long that the pineal was subject of a mythology. Perhaps the mystery was heightened by the fact that the pineal gland assumes a central location in the human head. During the Renaissance, notions of science, philosophy, and art were not as separated as they are today. Descartes (1596–1650), for example, mulled both the mysteries of the soul and the pineal gland (Figure 8.1) and concluded, in what one reviewer called an "inspired sophistry," that there was a connection about which he wrote:

> ...although the soul is joined to the whole body, there is yet in that a certain part in which it exercises its functions more particularly than in all the others; and it is usually believed that this part is the brain...but...the soul exercises its functions immediately [in] a certain very small gland which is situated in the middle of its substance and so suspended above the duct whereby the animal spirits in its anterior cavities have communication with those in the posterior, that the slightest movements which take place in it may alter very greatly the course of these spirits...[1]

PINEAL GLAND

Another name for the pineal gland is the epiphysis cerebri which designates a location lying over the brain. The pineal gland has also been referred to as pineal or pineal body. Pineal is pronounced pine-eel (long i) by pinealogists who associate the word with its origin—the pineal was named by Galen (A.D. 130–200) for its pine-cone shape in humans. The name is also sometimes pronounced pin-eel (short i).

Pineal function is one of the subjects included in neuroendocrinology. Wurtman, Axelrod, and Kelly[2] refer to the pineal gland as a neuroendocrine transducer. A neuroendocrine transducer converts a neural signal to an endocrine signal. Neuroendocrinology also includes the hypothalamus-pituitary system. The hypothalamus, neural controlled function of the pituitary gland, and the adrenal gland also meet the definition of neuroendocrine transducers.

ANATOMY

The pineal gland is a single organ located in the head (Figures 8.2 and 8.3) However, it is one of the glands whose exact location and shape vary from one species to the next. The pineal gland may have its main portion located just beneath the skull at the juncture of the cerebral hemispheres and the cerebellum (as in sparrows or chickens), or the pineal may nest more deeply in the brain (as in rats and humans). Usually there is a pineal stalk reaching inward to the choroid plexus of the brain. In some species there is both a superficial pineal and a deep pineal. Investigators have claimed that the pineal gland does not exist as a discrete structure in owls, crocodiles, alligators, anteaters, sloths, dugongs, and armadillos. However, it is possible that these species have cells similar to those in the pineal but located elsewhere (e.g., the subcommissural region).

There are species of fish, amphibians, and reptiles (e.g., the lizard *Anolis carolinensis*) in which the pineal gland has an intriguing relationship to an eye-like structure in the top of the head. The so-called "third eye" (parietal eye, parapineal eye) can be visibly present as a spot (brow spot) on top of the head; the unpaired eye may be organized with a retina of photoreceptors and a lens; and the photoreceptor is connected to the pineal with a parietal nerve. The function of the third eye is one of the still unsolved great mysteries of comparative physiology. However, there is little question that the third eye is designed to detect light, because it has a photoreceptor-like anatomy.

But why do the redundant eyes exist in creatures that have two perfectly normal looking lateral eyes? One logical possibility put forward was that the third eye functions as a "radiation dosimeter"[3] which monitors the incident radiation (sunlight) for the purpose of thermoregulation in some cold blooded animals. A second idea is that third eyes function to permit their owners to detect overhead predators. A third idea is that the third eye functions to detect light for synchronizing circadian rhythms. A fourth idea is that it senses photoperiod for reproduction. And, lizard homing behavior was attributed to the parietal eye.[4] The third eye qualifies as an "extraretinal photoreceptor," but animals deprived surgically of their lateral eyes, pineal glands, and parietal eyes can still detect light.

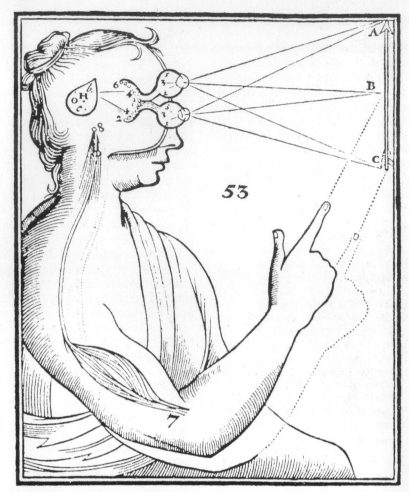

Figure 8.1 The figure illustrates pineal gland regulation according to Descartes. The seventeenth century engraving shows the regulation of the pineal gland (named for its pine cone shape, located more centrally than shown) by light perceived with the eyes. Reproduced, with permission. Crapo, L. Hormones: The Messengers of Life. W. H. Freeman Co.: New York; 1985; p. 80.

Embryologically, the pineal originates as an evagination from the roof of the diencephalon of the brain. Depending on the species, the pineal develops into (i) a strictly endocrine gland, (ii) a photoendocrine structure, (iii) a gland associated with a third eye, (iv) pineal cells are incorporated into brain regions, or (v) the pineal is absent.

Innervation of the pineal is by adrenergic sympathetic nerve endings whose cell bodies are located in the superior cervical ganglion. Parasympathetic axons run in a tract called the **nervi conarii**. There are also commissural fibers that access the pineal gland via the habenular and posterior commissures of the brain, peptidergic fibers which may release peptide hormones of the hypothalamus, neurons, nerve cell processes, and curious axon loops.

Arterial vessels to the pineal gland consist of 2–6 branches of posterior choroidal arteries that derive from the posterior cerebrals of the mesencephalon. The arteries branch in the capsule of the gland and then penetrate the gland. Venous drainage from the pineal is to the great cerebral vein and thence into the superior sagittal sinus which is close to the pineal. The rate of circulation is 4 ml/min/g which makes pineal blood flow second

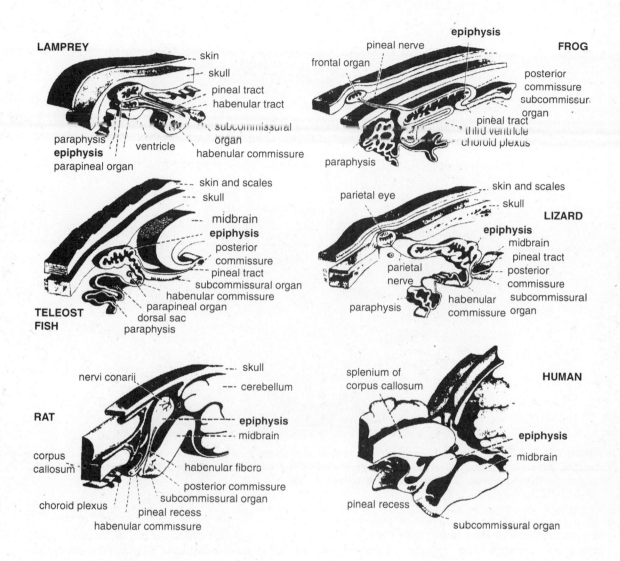

Figure 8.2 The diagrams show the comparative anatomy of the pineal gland and its associated organs for six vertebrates. In the diagrams, the main parts of the head surrounding the pineal gland (epiphysis) are arranged as follows: cerebrum left, cerebellum right, skull above, third ventricle below. Anterior is left, posterior is right. The posterior commissure, habenular commissure, the subcommissural organ, and the choroid plexus are found near the pineal stalk attachment point. Lampreys and teleost fish can have a parapineal organ and a paraphysis in the pineal region. Some frogs and lizards have a third eye, also called the parietal eye or parapineal eye, and a paraphysis in the pineal region. Unusual fibers from the habenular commissure loop through some pineals (shown for the rat). The pineals of some animals, for example birds, lie just beneath the skull, but the human pineal gland is in the center of the brain. Pineal innervation also includes the pineal tract (fish), pineal nerve (frog), parietal nerve (lizard), and nervi conarii (rat). Modified, with permission, from Wurtman, R.J.; Axelrod, J.; Kelly, D. The Pineal. New York and London: Academic Press; 1968; pp. 4–5.

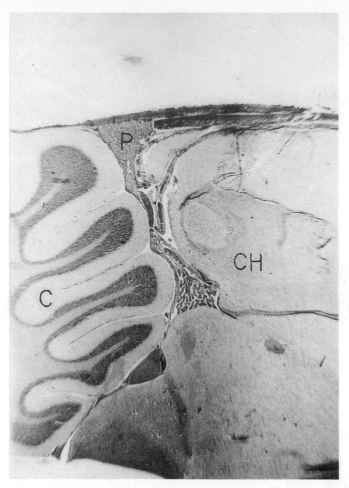

Figure 8.3 The figure shows a photograph of a section through the parts of the brain and the pineal of the house sparrow, *Passer domesticus*. P = pineal, C = cerebellum, CH = cerebral hemisphere. The long stalk of the gland ends at the choroid plexus. Photograph by the author.

only to the vascular flow through the kidney. The pineal is considered to be "outside" of the blood-brain barrier, so that the pineal responds to drugs that are injected systemically. The same drugs to which the pineal does respond may not affect brain cells because of the blood-brain barrier.

HISTOLOGY

A section through a whole pineal gland is shown in Figure 8.4. Pineal cells may be organized. The cells are laid out in layers that comprise rosettes or follicles surrounding a lumen. A number of cell types have been described. The cell

believed to be the endocrine cell of the pineal gland is called the **pinealocyte** (pineocytes, parenchymal cells, light and dark chief cells). Sensory pinealocytes of some species have anatomical characteristics of photoreceptor cells (lamellar whorls, cilia, synaptic ribbons, degenerated outer segments, cone-like outer segments). In other words, the cells resemble photoreceptor cells of the retina. A generalized description of a pinealocyte from "inside" to "outside" a follicle is: a residual lumen, an outer segment, a 9+0 cilium, an inner segment with two centrioles and mitochondria and microtubules, a Golgi region, a nucleus, a synaptic pedical with vesicle-crowned rodlets, and space with connective

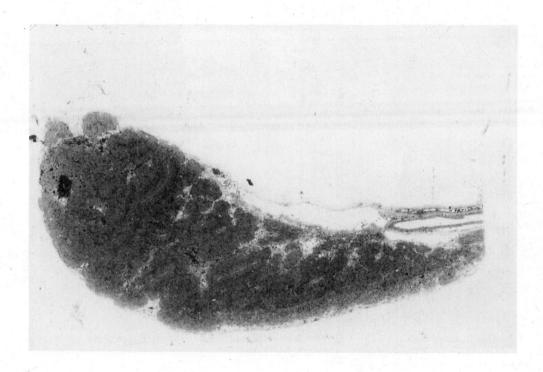

Figure 8.4 The photograph shows a section through the entire pineal gland of a three-week-old chick, *Gallus domesticus*. The top of the gland is near the skull (not shown). Photograph by M. Cioffi.

tissue. A second cell-type found in the pineal gland, stellate neuroglia, most likely are supportive cells. Neurons, nerve cell processes, and curious axon loops have been noted in pineal glands. The existence of these structures imply brain-pineal links. Pineal glands also possess connective tissue cells and striated muscle cells.

Weights of pineal glands range from 0.2 mg in the house mouse, *Mus musculus*, to 3500 mg in Weddell seals. Histological structure of the pineal gland varies with time of day, season of the year, reproductive state (gender, pregnancy, ovarian cycle stage, puberty, age), and latitude. The human pineal gland is pea sized.

HUMAN PINEAL ANATOMY

Human pineal glands are not considered to have the "photoreceptor-like" pinealocytes, and light-detecting ability is not proposed for the human pineal gland. However, the human pineal does have fascinating structures (Figure 8.5). The human pineal boasts "brain sand"—sand-grain sized, calcareous concretions, also called acervuli or corpora arenacea). Under close examination with a dissecting microscope, the concretions have a mulberry shape. They are chemically similar to tooth enamel.

Denervation of pineal glands reduces concretion formation in gerbils, so pinealogists view

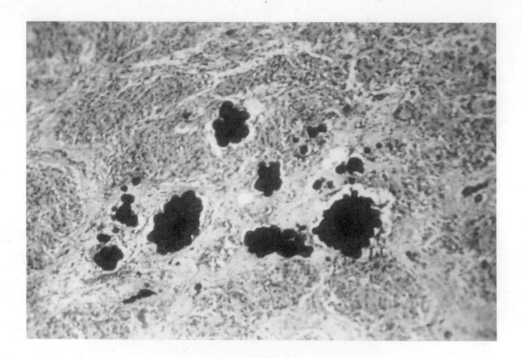

Figure 8.5 The figure shows a section through a human pineal gland. The dark structures are brain or pineal "sand." In three dimensions the sand grains are mulberry shaped. The photograph was made by S. Binkley from a transparency (source unknown).

concretions as indicative of pineal secretory activity.[5] Interestingly, the occurrence of the concretions in humans increases with age so that 3% of one-year olds, 7.1% of ten-year olds, and 33% of 18-year olds have concretions. Concretions are found in about 70% of humans during the fourth to seventh decades of life. The incidence of calcification is only half as much in American blacks as American whites and even smaller in Nigerian blacks. This topic deserves some re-examination with modern techniques which might link changes in concretions, secretory activity, and pineal function (e.g., lighting in the environment, diet).

BIOCHEMISTRY

The pineal hormone is named "melatonin" (MEL, M, MT). It is an indole molecule synthesized in the pineal gland from the indole serotonin.

Serotonin (5-hydroxytryptamine, 5-HT) in turn is synthesized from tryptophan. (Figure 8.6). The enzymes necessary for melatonin synthesis were found in the Harderian gland and in the retinas of some species,[6] and the retinal synthesis of melatonin can account for some circulating melatonin.[7] (The Harderian gland, also called Harder's gland, is a lacrimal gland located in the orbits of the eyes of vertebrates, especially those with a well-developed nictitating membrane. The gland is especially interesting because it may, as it does in the rat, contain porphyrins which fluoresce redly when the whole fresh gland is viewed with ultraviolet light.)

The discovery of rhythms in the enzyme that synthesizes melatonin stimulated investigation of rhythmic synthesis of hormones of other glands. In 1970, Klein and Weller[8] showed that an enzyme in the pineal gland (N-acetyltransferase, NAT, SNAT, serotonin N-acetyltransferase) that was responsible for melatonin synthesis, nightly soared

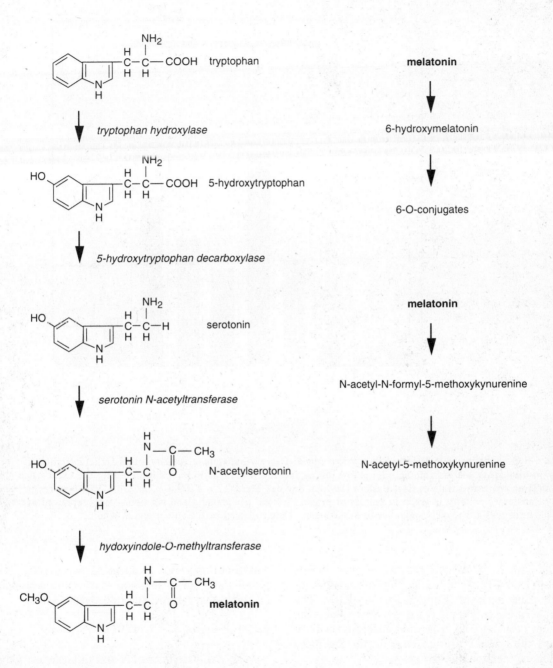

Figure 8.6 The pathway for melatonin synthesis is on the left. On the right are the conversion pathways for melatonin to conjugates in the liver and to kynurenine in the brain. Modified, with permission, Martin, C.R. Endocrine Physiology. New York: Oxford University Press; 1985; p. 853.

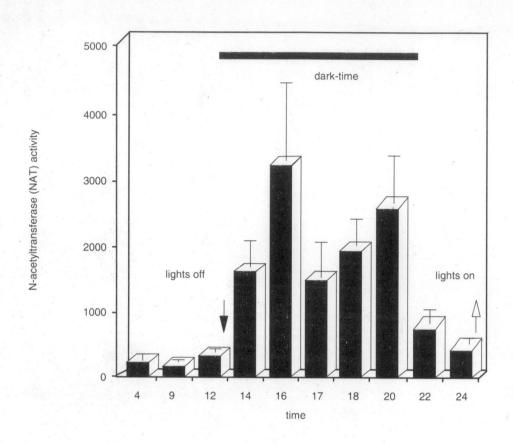

Figure 8.7 A daily cycle is found in sparrow pineal N-acetyltransferase activity. In LD12:12 (lights-off from noon to midnight), the enzyme activity is low during the day when it is light and high during the night when it is dark. Time represents time of day, Eastern Daylight Savings Time (12 = 1200 = noon; 24 = 2400 = midnight). N-acetyltransferase activity is given in pmoles of product formed per pineal gland per hour. Bars represent averages and the error tees are + one standard error of the mean. Data collected by the author and S. Klein.

in the dark to 30 times light-time activity in rats kept in LD14:10. The finding was extended to include other species (Figures 8.7 and 8.8). The rhythm in N-acetyltransferase activity explains the rhythm in melatonin; N-acetyltransferase has been called the "rate limiting" enzyme for the daily rhythm of melatonin synthesis.

Other substances synthesized by the pineal include arginine vasotocin (AVT), TRH, thyroid hormones, peptides, indoles, and ß-carbolines. These other products may also have rhythms (e.g., antidiuretic activity is highest in rat pineals in the

dark-time) and AVT peaks in August in rats. The pineal gland has large amounts of lipid (even lipid inclusions) and amines (taurine, cystathionine).

PHOTOPERIODIC CONTROL

Daily rhythms of N-acetyltransferase activity appear to have the major responsibility for generating the melatonin rhythm. The precursor, serotonin, is depressed at night when melatonin synthesis is high. The duration, phase, and amplitude of N-acetyltransferase activity is dependent upon the

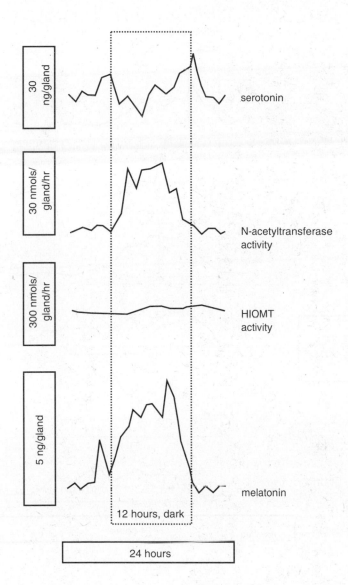

Figure 8.8 The graphs show the rhythms in four pineal biochemical parameters in chicks kept in an LD12:12 light-dark cycle. The 10-fold nocturnal peak in melatonin is believed to be derived from the 21-fold rhythm in pineal N-acetyltransferase activity which produces a mid-dark, 6-fold decrease in the substrate serotonin. Hydroxyindole-O-methyltransferase activity (HIOMT) exhibited a 1.3-fold change. The height of the rectangles on the y-axis are equal to the units inscribed within the rectangles. The chick pineal N-acetyltransferase rhythm was first published in Binkley, S.; MacBride, S.; Klein, D.; Ralph, C. Pineal enzymes: Regulation of avian melatonin synthesis. Science 181: 273–275; 1973; the serotonin data are from Brammer, M.; Binkley, S. Daily rhythms of serotonin and N-acetyltransferase in chicks. Comp. Biochem. Physiol. 63C: 305–307; 1979.

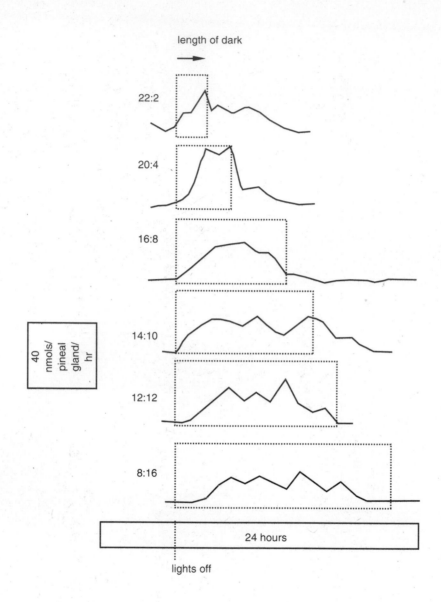

Figure 8.9 The graphs show the circadian rhythm of N-acetyltransferase activity in the pineal glands of chicks maintained in six different photoperiods from the day of hatching to three weeks of age. The legend on the left indicates the scale used for plotting N-acetyltransferase activity in nmol of enzyme activity per pineal gland per hour. The horizontal bar under the graphs indicates 24 hours. The dotted rectangles drawn over the graphs have vertical axes 0–40 nmol/pineal gland/hour enzyme activity, and horizontal axes show duration of the dark period (scotoperiod) in hours with respect to lights-off. The numbers to the left of the graphs are the hours of light:dark. The data are replotted from the first study to show the pineal amplitude and dark-time duration changes that are evoked by photoperiod. Binkley, S.; Stephens, J.; Riebman, J.; Reilly, K. Regulation of pineal rhythms in chickens: Photoperiod and dark-time sensitivity. General and Comparative Endocrinology 32: 411–416; 1977.

duration of the dark-time in a light-dark cycle (Figure 8.9).[9] Thus, melatonin synthesis is controlled by photoperiod.

The enzyme, HIOMT (hydroxyindole-O-methyltransferase) is sensitive to long-term changes in photoperiod. HIOMT displays dramatic seasonal changes in some species (such as the tortoise) and its activity is halved by 6–12 weeks of exposure to long days. The combined effect of the two enzymes is to provide a redundant system that reduces melatonin in long days.[10]

When a rhythm is synchronized to a light dark cycle, circadian biologists say that the rhythm is "entrained" to the light-dark cycle. When the timing of the light-dark cycle is changed (due to seasonal changing photoperiod, or, as occurs for humans in east-west travel), the timing of the cycle must be reset.

The time signals of N-acetyltransferase are conveyed to the rest of the brain and body by the hormone melatonin. The properties of the N-acetyltransferase rhythm are similar whether the organism is nocturnal (night-active: rat, hamster) or diurnal (day-active: chicken, sparrow, human). Melatonin is synthesized at night in vertebrate species.

NEURAL REGULATION

The pathways for regulation of pineal glands vary depending on species. However, there is one consistent, well established pathway for mammals including humans (Figure 8.10). Light is perceived by the retinas of the eyes. A special tract, the retinohypothalamic tract, which is separate from the optic nerve, connects the retina directly with the hypothalamus.[11] In the hypothalamus, the region that processes the light information is the suprachiasmatic nuclei (SCN). Here, scientists believe that information about light and dark entrain a circadian rhythm that is generated by the SCN acting as a biological clock. The rhythm information from the SCN is conveyed to the pineal gland via the sympathetic nervous system. The final neurons in the pathway originate in the superior cervical ganglia (SCG). Axons from the SCG travel the nervii conari to release norepinephrine (NE) at their endings in the pineal gland.

In the rat pineal gland, norepinephrine interacts with beta receptors[12] on pinealocyte cell membranes to stimulate cyclic AMP activity and

initiate a cascade of reactions. The cascade ends with the synthesis of N-acetyltransferase. The resulting increase in N-acetyltransferase activity increases the production of N-acetylserotonin from serotonin. HIOMT is highly active in the pineal gland and readily converts the N-acetylserotonin to melatonin. Melatonin, which is lipid soluble, is not stored in the pineal gland but is released into the blood stream when it is synthesized.

There is also the intriguing possibility that the pineal gland secretes hormones into cerebrospinal fluid (CSF). This is because there is an area of the third ventricle of the brain where the stalk of the pineal attaches that is called the pineal recess. Cells in the region offer the possibility for bidirectional transport of molecules.

Melatonin has been found in cerebrospinal fluid. So melatonin could directly target the brain and the spinal cord, not only via the bloodstream, but also via the fluids in the brain cavities. Binding studies with iodinated melatonin have pinpointed regions of the hypothalamus (pars tuberalis, median eminence, SCN) and the retina as a melatonin targets. Krause and Dubocovich list central nervous system, retina, and pituitary as targets for mammals.[13] The focus has been on mammalian targets in the head, but chromatophores and gonad cells may also be targets for melatonin in some species.

The pathway for light to influence the pineal may not be the same in all species because some species have extraretinal photoreceptors and/or pineal photoreceptors. Moreover, the pineals of some species (e.g., chickens or sparrows) are capable of both light sensitivity and generation of daily rhythms of N-acetyltransferase activity and melatonin synthesis when the glands are isolated in organ or superfusion cultures.[14]

SKIN COLOR

The role of the pineal in skin color is straightforward: when pineal glands were fed to tadpoles, their skin color lightened. The isolation of melatonin was based on lightening skin color.[15] Melatonin was named for its function in causing amphibian skin to become pale.[16] In view of our other information about how melatonin is regulated by light, the interpretation of the pineal role in lower vertebrate skin color is quite simple.

Melatonin, produced at night in the dark,

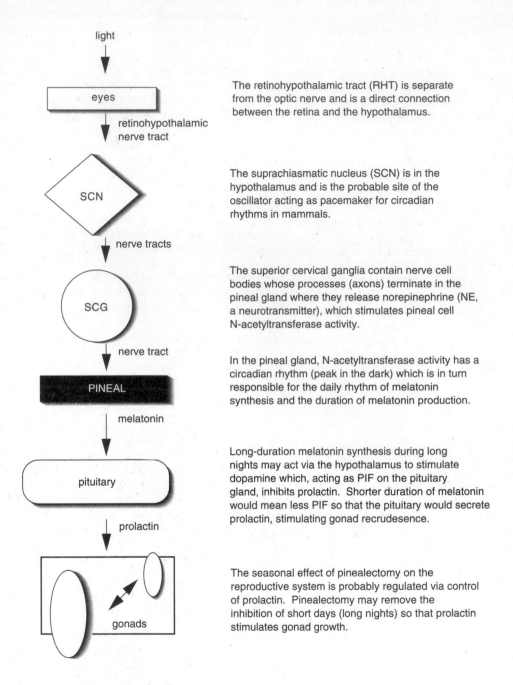

The retinohypothalamic tract (RHT) is separate from the optic nerve and is a direct connection between the retina and the hypothalamus.

The suprachiasmatic nucleus (SCN) is in the hypothalamus and is the probable site of the oscillator acting as pacemaker for circadian rhythms in mammals.

The superior cervical ganglia contain nerve cell bodies whose processes (axons) terminate in the pineal gland where they release norepinephrine (NE, a neurotransmitter), which stimulates pineal cell N-acetyltransferase activity.

In the pineal gland, N-acetyltransferase activity has a circadian rhythm (peak in the dark) which is in turn responsible for the daily rhythm of melatonin synthesis and the duration of melatonin production.

Long-duration melatonin synthesis during long nights may act via the hypothalamus to stimulate dopamine which, acting as PIF on the pituitary gland, inhibits prolactin. Shorter duration of melatonin would mean less PIF so that the pituitary would secrete prolactin, stimulating gonad recrudesence.

The seasonal effect of pinealectomy on the reproductive system is probably regulated via control of prolactin. Pinealectomy may remove the inhibition of short days (long nights) so that prolactin stimulates gonad growth.

Figure 8.10 The pineal gland is controlled by environmental light and in turn regulates seasonal breeding.

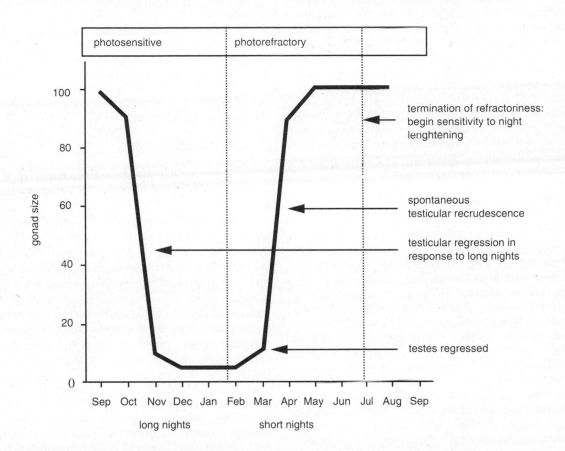

Figure 8.11 The annual progress of the reproductive system in a seasonal breeding animal, such as the hamster, is shown. Gonad size is represented as % on the left; descriptions refer to the testis on the right. The testes get smaller (regress) as the days shorten. The animals are reproductively quiescent. As the days lengthen, the testes enlarge and become functional (recrudesce) through the breeding season. In the absence of long days, the testes will still begin to enlarge which is called spontaneous recrudescence. However, early decline in testis size cannot be provoked by short days until the refractory period is completed. After Stetson, M.; Whitmyre, M. Physiology of the pineal and its hormone, melatonin, in annual reproduction in rodents. In Reiter, R., editor. The Pineal Gland. New York: Raven Press; 1984;.

is responsible for dark-time pallor. Like melatonin, dark-time pallor has a circadian rhythm that persists in constant dark in lizards and is damped by constant light. In constant light, melatonin is suppressed, and the color of the animals depends upon their background, and, presumably the hormone MSH.[17]

The targets of the melatonin include the melanophores themselves (since skins of some species turn pale if melatonin is added to the bathing medium), the hypothalamus, and the pituitary (inhibition of MSH). MSH inhibition could also be accomplished by decreasing the melatonin precursor, serotonin, which may be an MRF, by converting it to melatonin. The dark-time pallor of poikilotherms is not dependent upon the eyes; there is extra-retinal photoreception.

In higher vertebrates (weasel, Djungarian hamster), the change from white winter pelage can be delayed by implanting melatonin pellets.

Skin color responses were used as bioassays for melatonin before there was a radioimmunoassay. In one such assay, samples of melatonin standards over the range of 0.1 ng/ml to 2.5 ng/ml were prepared. Ten house-fly sized tadpoles were captured with an eyedropper, blotted gently, and transferred to a small beaker containing a test sample of melatonin standard or unknown. The tadpoles were kept under bright illumination for thirty minutes followed by determination of melanophore indices with visual inspection of the tadpoles with a dissecting microscope in a triangular area between the eye and mouth.[18]

REPRODUCTION

Seasonal reproduction is rigidly controlled by photoperiod (Figure 8.11). Organisms are able to distinguish long from short days (hamsters can discern as little as 15 minutes). In long-day breeders, such as hamsters, the long days of approaching spring stimulate growth (size, weight, cells) and function (sperm production, ovulations) of the gonads of both genders. Short days of approaching winter inhibit gonad function, the gonads actually become quiescent. In seasonal breeders, the animals cycle between reproductively active breeding and nonbreeding on an annual, or seasonal, basis. The rationale offered for seasonal breeding is that it ensures that the offspring are born at a time when conditions (temperature, food supply) are optimal for their growth and development.

The phenomena of reproductive response to photoperiod can be duplicated in the laboratory. In hamsters placed in short days (less than twelve hours of light per day, e.g., LD1:23) or blinded or placed in constant dark, regression of the testes takes about ten weeks; regression of the ovaries takes six to eight weeks. Removing the pineal gland abolishes the inhibition of reproduction that occurs in short days, the animals can reproduce all the time.[19]

This result supported the idea that the pineal gland was the source of an antigonadotrophic hormone. Melatonin is proposed to be that antigonadotrophic hormone. The idea is that on short days, N-acetylserotonin is synthesized by N-acetyltransferase throughout the long night and high HIOMT levels convert the N-acetylserotonin to melatonin so that melatonin is present for a long duration, resulting in inhibition of the reproductive system. Melatonin is believed to attain the inhibition by inhibiting prolactin which normally stimulates reproduction.

The whole process is very intriguing because, here, evolution has produced an exquisite system of natural birth control. Also, one wonders whether in organisms, such as humans, that reproduce throughout the year, this has been accomplished in part by suppressing the seasonal response to pineal hormones.

CIRCADIAN RHYTHMS

The pineal gland also functions in the regulation of circadian rhythms. Pinealectomizing house sparrows led to the momentous result that the animals lost their circadian rhythms of locomotor activity (Figure 8.12)[20] and body temperature.[21] It was also possible to suppress the locomotor rhythm with melatonin in the drinking water[22] or implanted in capsules constructed of Silastic tubing.[23] Rhythms were restored in pinealectomized recipient sparrows by implanting pineal glands from donor sparrows into the anterior chambers of the eyes.[24] So the pineal gland, like the hypothalamic SCN, contains a circadian oscillator (at least in some species). The evolutionary need to develop redundancy in circadian oscillators argues for their importance but seems unnecessary. Incredibly, the pineal glands of some species (chickens, sparrows, lizards) are capable of sustaining a circadian oscillation of N-acetyltransferase activity or of melatonin for several cycles when they are isolated in organ culture or grown in cell cultures (Figure 8.13).[25]

LIGHT AND DARK

The details of N-acetyltransferase activity regulation by light and dark have been studied by manipulating lighting schedules. In constant dark (DD), the rhythm of N-acetyltransferase activity persists, so that the rhythm is considered to be a true circadian rhythm (Figure 8.14). A circadian rhythm is a rhythm that continues with a period length near 24 hours, even in the absence of a 24-hour light-dark regimen. As a consequence of the rhythm in the enzyme, NAT, the melatonin rhythm is also a circadian rhythm.

Constant light (LL), on the other hand, abolishes or damps the rhythm in N-acetyltransferase activity. Amazingly, the abolition of the

24 hours

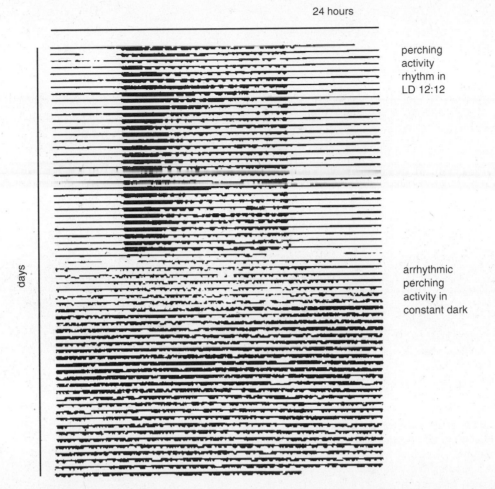

perching
activity
rhythm in
LD 12:12

arrhythmic
perching
activity in
constant dark

days

Figure 8.12 The raster graph of the rhythm of perch-hopping activity in the house sparrow shows the effect of pinealectomy. Each horizontal line displays 24 hours of data; the lines are arranged vertically in chronological order with the most recent data on the bottom. Pinealectomy abolished the circadian rhythm of perch-hopping which would normally have occurred in constant dark in the sparrow. Data collected by the author.

rhythm by constant light occurs even in blinded nonmammalian animals.[26] That is, N-acetyltransferase and the pineal gland can be controlled with extraretinal light perception.

Extending the photoperiod on a single day into the expected dark-time suppresses the normal rise in N-acetyltransferase activity. The enzyme rises when lights are finally turned out (L/D). The L/D transition thus provides the organism with a signal of when night begins. But the alternative experiment, turning the lights out early, does not provoke an immediate rise in N-acetyltransferase activity. Instead, the enzyme rises at the expected time of lights-out based on its previous cycles. Thus, a circadian rhythm governs when the pineal gland can begin to measure the length of a night.

Turning on the lights early during the dark-time causes an immediate suppression of N-acetyltransferase activity (halving time about 5 minutes), so that most of the activity is lost in fifteen minutes. This suppression of N-acetyltransferase activity by lights-on (D/L) provides the organism with a signal of when day begins.

Light and circadian clock regulation of N-acetyltransferase activity provides the organism with (i) a time standard (a circadian rhythm with

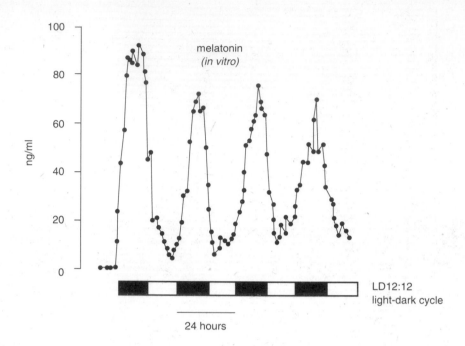

Figure 8.13 Daily cycle of melatonin secreted into the culture medium by a single pineal gland from a three-week-old chicken (*Gallus domesticus*). Courtesy Binkley and Tamarkin, 1980.

time settings derived from previous cycles), and (ii) means for detecting small changes (e.g., earlier lights-on) to reset the rhythm and to alter the rhythm in response to changing photoperiod.

INTRAOCULAR MELATONIN

When the enzymes for manufacture of melatonin were first discovered in the eye, pinealogists were relieved because ocular melatonin synthesis could explain the disappointing failure of pinealectomy to affect functions (e.g., reproduction) in experiments with some species.[27] Indeed, retinal melatonin does get into the circulation, at least in some species. Retinal N-acetyltransferase and melatonin respond to lighting just as in the pineal gland. In the retina, melatonin is synthesized in the dark, the rhythm persists in constant dark, the rhythm is damped by constant light, and there is a rapid plummet in response to lights-on at night.

However, it is also possible that retinal melatonin functions in the eye itself. Retinal melatonin may function in disk shedding, photoreceptor cell elongation, pigment migration, pigment aggregation, and ocular fluid regulation. Perfusion of isolated chick retinas with melatonin altered the membrane potentials and resistances of chick retinal pigment epithelium *in vitro* which means that the retinal cells themselves are melatonin targets.[28] There are daily rhythms of sensitivity to light in retinas[29] and it is possible that the hypothalamus and melatonin play roles in programming these rhythms.

In summary, it appears possible that the retina makes melatonin, responds to melatonin, and secretes melatonin to affect the brain via neural or endocrine routes.

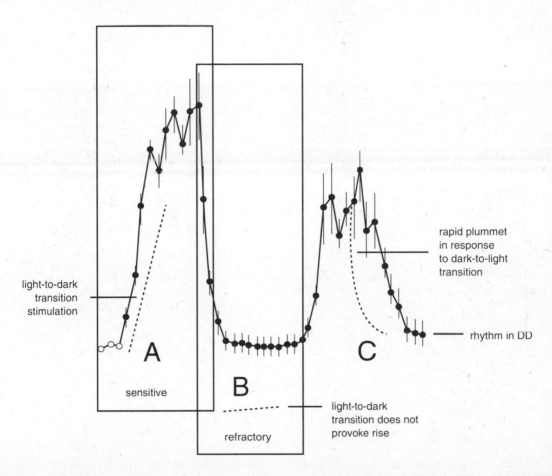

light-to-dark
transition
stimulation

rapid plummet
in response
to dark-to-light
transition

rhythm in DD

A

sensitive

B

refractory

C

light-to-dark
transition does not
provoke rise

Figure 8.14 The figure illustrates the author's model for the regulation of N-acetyltransferase activity by light and dark. The graph shows the first and second night peaks of the freerunning rhythm of N-acetyltransferase (NAT) in the chick pineal gland measured hourly in constant dark (points at one-hour intervals are mean ± SEM). Peak NAT activity is over 20 nmol/pineal/hour; nadir enzyme activity between the peaks is 2–3 nmol/pineal/hour. In the model, NAT rises during the expected dark-time (of the chicks' pretreatment LD12:12 light-dark cycle). (A) If the lights are turned off during the projected dark-time, NAT rises rapidly; the period in which the enzyme can rise is referred to as the "sensitive" phase of the rhythm. (B) However, if the lights are turned off during the projected light-time, NAT does not rise; the period during which the enzyme cannot be provoked is referred to as the "refractory" phase of the rhythm. (C) If the lights are turned on during the dark-time when the NAT is high, a "rapid plummet" occurs and the enzyme falls in 10–30 minutes. Binkley, S.; Geller, E. Pineal N-acetyltransferase in chickens: Rhythm persists in constant darkness. J. Comp. Physiol. 99: 67–70; 1975; Binkley, S.; MacBride, S.; Klein, D.; Ralph, C. Regulation of pineal rhythms in chickens: Refractory period and nonvisual light perception. Endocrinology 96: 848–853; 1975.

HUMAN PINEAL FUNCTION

People do have daily melatonin rhythms with peak synthesis in the dark time (Figure 8.15). Human melatonin is regulated by light and dark; seasonal alterations have been found.

One of the first notions about the function of the pineal gland was that it participated in the control of puberty. This was because in the final years of the nineteenth century, it was noticed that

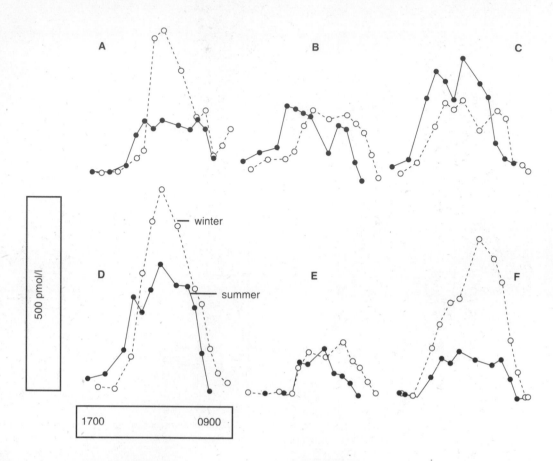

Figure 8.15 The graphs show melatonin rhythms in six human subjects for one night (1700 to 0900, 7 p.m. to 9 a.m., length of horizontal rectangle) in winter (open circles) compared to one night in summer (closed circles). The height of the vertical rectangle represents 500 pmol/l of melatonin in blood. The axes are the same for each of the six graphs. Modified, with permission. Illnerova, H.; Zvolsky, P.; Vanecek, J. The circadian rhythm in plasma melatonin concentration of the urbanized man: The effect of summer and winter time. Brain Research 328: 186–189; 1985; p. 187.

premature, or precocious, puberty was associated with pinealoma. The idea propounded back then was that the pineal gland inhibited reproduction in children. The number of cases of pineal tumors is small. They occur more often in young males and they are treated with surgery or radiotherapy. However, the idea that the pineal might function in controlling the time of onset in puberty never gained wide acceptance and was usually attributed to effects of the tumor pressing on other structures. Because the eyes make melatonin as well as the pineal gland, it is not sufficient to study melatonin

function with pinealectomy, and it is still possible that melatonin has a role in the control of the timing of human puberty. Moreover there are anecdotes about Eskimos and evidence that high and low latitude, where there are photoperiodic extremes, can affect menstruation and timing of births. These reproductive effects could be explained by melatonin, controlled by light, functioning in the regulation of human reproduction.

Because of the concretions, pineal glands are noticeable features on X-rays and CAT scans of human heads. In fact, calcified pineals serve as radiological markers. Displacement of the pineal from its normal central position is considered a radiological indicator of abnormalities in the brain.

Psychological depression may occur on a seasonal basis (usually in the form of winter depression). The syndrome has been called Seasonal Affective Disorder (SAD). SAD patients respond dramatically to treatments with bright light. While the light effects on depression seem clear, a possible role for the pineal has proved more elusive. Melatonin administration exacerbated the depression, but SAD patients had reduced dark-time melatonin.

The possibility of pineal function in human behavior has not eluded the imaginative pens of fiction writers. Dean R. Koontz writes about X-rays of one of his characters: "And there's been no shifting of the pineal gland, which you sometimes find in cases where the patient suffers from really vivid hallucinations."[30]

PINEAL OSCILLATION

It is interesting that Descartes connected light with the pineal gland:

> ...if we see some animal approach us, the light reflected from its body depicts two images of it, one in each of our eyes, and these two images form two others, by means of the optic nerves, in the interior surface of the brain which faces its cavities; then from there, by means of the animal spirits with which its cavities are filled, these images so radiate towards the little gland which is surrounded by these spirits...the two images which are in the brain form but one upon the gland....[31]

The pineal gland has much more remarkable abilities than were imagined by Descartes. Dark and light information that is perceived by the eyes is converted to a hormone signal, long nights cause lengthy melatonin production, and melatonin controls seasonal breeding by suppressing reproductive function. Some pineal glands actually detect light. And pineal glands are capable of oscillation even in the absence of the rest of the organism.

REFERENCES

1. Descartes, R. Les passions de l'ame (The Passions of the Soul). In Rene Descartes: Philosophical Works. Franklin Center, PA: The Franklin Library; 1981; p. 200.
2. Wurtman, R.; Axelrod, J.; Kelly, D.E. The Pineal. New York: Academic Press; 1968.
3. Eakin, R. The Third Eye. Berkeley: University of California Press; 1973.
4. Ellis-Quinn, B. A.; Simon, C.A. Lizard homing behavior: The role of the parietal eye during displacement and radio-tracking, and time compensated celestial orientation in the lizard Sceloporus jarrovi. Behav. Ecol. Sociobiol. 28: 397–407; 1991.
5. Reiter, R.; Johnson, L.; Steger, R.; Richardson, B.; Petterborg, L. Pineal biosynthetic activity and neuroendocrine physiology in the aging hamster and gerbil. Peptides 1: 69–77; 1980.
6. Binkley, S.; Hryshchyshyn, M.; Reilly, K. N-acetyltransferase activity responds to environmental lighting in the eye as well as in the pineal gland. Nature 281: 479–481; 1979.
7. Binkley, S. The Pineal: Endocrine and Nonendocrine Function. Englewood Cliffs, NJ: Prentice-Hall; 1988.
8. Klein, D.; Weller, J. Indole metabolism in the pineal gland: A circadian rhythm in N-acetyltranferase. Science 169: 1093–1095; 1970.
9. Binkley, S.; Stephens, J.; Riebman, J.; Reilly, K. Regulation of pineal rhythms in chickens: Photoperiod and dark-time sensitivity. Gen. Comp. Endocrinol 32: 411–416; 1977.
10. Vivien-Roels, B.; Arendt, J.; Bradke, J. Circadian and circannual fluctuations of pineal indoleamines (serotonin and melatonin) in *Testudo hermanni* Gmelin (Reptilia, Chelonia). Gen. Comp. Endocrinol 37: 197–210; 1979.
11. Moore, R.Y.; Klein, D. Visual pathways and the central neural control of a circadian rhythm in pineal serotonin N-acetyltransferase. Brain Research 71: 17–33; 1974.
12. Deguchi, T.; Axelrod, J. Control of circadian change of serotonin N-acetyltransferase activity in the pineal organ by the ß-adrenergic receptor. Proc. Nat. Acad. Sci. USA 69: 2547–2550; 1972.
13. Krause, D.N.; Dubocovich, M.L. Regulatory sites in the melatonin system of mammals. Trends in Neurosciences 13: 464–470; 1990.
14. Binkley, S.; Riebman, J.; Reilly, K.

Regulation of pineal rhythms in chickens: Inhibition of dark-time rise in N-acetyltransferase activity. Comparative Biochemistry and Physiology 59C: 165–171; 1978.

15. Lerner, A.; Case, J. Pigment cell regulatory factors. J. Invest. Derm. 32: 211–221; 1959.

16. McCord, C.; Allen, F. Evidences associating pineal gland function with alterations in pigmentation. J. Exp. Zool. 23: 207–224; 1917.

17. Binkley, S.; Reilly, K.; Hermida, V.; Mosher, K. Circadian rhythm of color change in *Anolis carolinensis*. Pineal Research Reviews 5: 133–151; 1987.

18. Ralph, C.; Lynch, H. A quantitative melatonin bioassay. General Comparative Endocrinology 15: 334–338; 1970.

19. Hoffman, R.; Reiter, R. Pineal gland: Influence on gonads of male hamsters. Science 148: 1609–1611; 1966.

20. Gaston, S.; Menaker, M. Pineal function: The biological clock in the sparrow? Science 160: 541–548; 1968.

21. Binkley, S.; Kluth, E.; Menaker, M. Pineal function in sparrows: Circadian rhythms and body temperature. Science 174: 311–314; 1971.

22. Binkley, S.; Mosher, K. Oral melatonin produces arrhythmia in sparrows. Experientia 41:1615–1617; 1985.

23. Turek, F.; McMillan, J.; Menaker, M. Melatonin: Effects on the circadian locomotor rhythm of sparrows. Science 194:1441–1443; 1976.

24. Zimmerman, N.; Menaker, M. Neural connections of sparrow pineal: Role in circadian control of activity, Science 190: 477–479; 1975.

25. Binkley S., Riebman, J.; Reilly, K. Regulation of pineal rhythms in chickens: Photoperiod and dark-time sensitivity. Science 202: 1198–1201; 1978.

26. Binkley, S.; MacBride, S.; Klein, D.; Ralph, C. Regulation of pineal rhythms in chickens: Refractory period and nonvisual light perception. Endocrinology 96: 848–853; 1975.

27. Binkley, S.; Hryshchyshyn, M.; Reilly, K. N-acetyltransferase activity responds to environmental lighting in the eye as well as in the pineal gland. Nature 281: 479–481; 1979.

28. Nao-i, N.; Nilsson, S.E.G.; Gallemore, R.P.; Steinberg, R.H. Effects of melatonin on the chick retinal pigment epithelium: Membrane potentials and light-evoked responses. Exp. Eye Res. 49: 573–589; 1989.

29. Bobbert, A.C.; van Wiechen, R.; Eggelmeijer, F. Imitations of the circadian changes in rabbit photic responses elicited by stimulation of the cervical sympathetic nerves and mediated by means of intraocular adrenergic alpha receptors. J. Interdiscipl. Cycle Res. 21: 273–288; 1990.

30. Koontz, D.R. The House of Thunder. New York: Berkley Books; 1992; page 189.

31. Descartes, R. Op. cit. p. 200.

SECTION III

AMINE AND PEPTIDE HORMONES FROM GLANDS IN OR NEAR THE GUT: THYROID, PARATHYROID, PANCREAS, AND GASTROINTESTINAL TRACT

This section covers a group of endocrine glands whose location is related to the alimentary canal. The glands make peptide and amine hormones that control metabolic rate, regulate sugars, maintain calcium levels, and aid in the digestion of food.

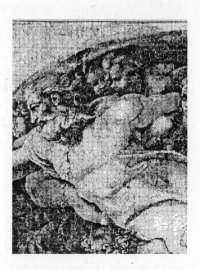

CHAPTER 9

T3 from the Thyroid, Immunology, and the Thymus

The hormones of the thyroid gland, thyroxine (T_4) and triiodothyroine (T_3), are iodinated forms of the amino acid tyrosine. The thyroid gland is distinguished by its ability to trap iodine. The thyroid hormones function to control basal metabolic rate—they stimulate oxygen consumption and they raise body temperature. Parafollicular, or C-cells, of the thyroid make the hormone calcitonin which, along with parathyroid hormone, regulates calcium. A second gland, the thymus gland, is found, like the thyroid gland, in the neck region. Thymus peptide hormones function in development and in immune responses.

HISTORY

The thyroid gland's location in the throat region by the voice box prompted the Greeks to suppose that the gland secreted a mucus to lubricate the larynx and pharynx. Or perhaps the function of the thyroid was conjectured to be aesthetic—it rounded the contours of the throat. A Roman poet and satirist, Juvenal, observed that the necks of women were swollen at puberty, during menstruation, and throughout pregnancy. The Romans used neck measurements as tests of premarital virginity. Another early idea that circulated at the time of Vesalius (1543) was that the purpose of the thyroid gland was to keep the throat warm.

The last hundred years have seen most of the advances in understanding the thyroid. In 1895 Magnus Levy found that oxygen consumption was raised by thyroid extract and Baumann discovered that the thyroid gland was the only structure in mammals that incorporated iodine.[1] Thyroxin was isolated by Kendall in 1915. TSH was demonstrated in 1929 by Loeb and Aron. TRH was isolated and synthesized in 1969.[2]

ANATOMY

In the human, the thyroid gland weighs 25–40 g (Figure 9.1). It is located in the neck and can be felt by palpation below the Adam's apple. The gland is wrapped around the trachea and the thyroid is divided into two lobes connected by a tissue bridge, the isthmus. The gland has a similar butterfly shape and neck location in the rat, but in some other species the thyroid tissue is in a single gland (e.g., snakes and turtles), is two separate glands (e.g., frogs and birds), or is not even organized into a gland (e.g., cyclostomes and teleosts).[3] The human thyroid gland is highly vascularized and its nerves regulate the blood supply. Parathyroid glands are closely associated with thyroid glands.

HISTOLOGY

The thyroid, like the mammary gland and the ovary, has follicular architecture. The basic structural unit of the thyroid gland is the **follicle** (Figure 9.2). The follicle is a ball made up of a one-cell-thick layer of epithelial cells enclosing a space that is filled with a viscous, homogeneous substance called **colloid**. The thyroid gland is usually a collection of follicles. A single follicle can be nearly a centimeter in diameter. The rat thyroid has 100,000 follicles.[4] Cells lying between the follicles are a different cell type and are called the parafollicular cells, or C cells.

The histology of the gland varies with thyroid activity. Follicle cells change from 0.02 to 0.1 mm in diameter[5] with changes in thyroid activity—follicles of rats with stimulated thyroids have thick, columnar, secretory epithelium and less colloid, while those from hypophysectomized rats have atrophic thyroids with low cuboidal follicle cells and large amounts of colloid.[6] A generality that increased colloid represents gland inactivity can be made. However, there are exceptions to this rule. Changes in thyroid function and cell sizes is an example of the way that "histometrics" can be used to understand the physiology of an endocrine gland.

EMBRYOLOGY

The follicles of the thyroid gland develop from alimentary tract progenitors and therefore from endoderm. The thyroid gland's development is described by Telford and Bridgman:

> The thyroid develops as a median endodermal downgrowth at the base of the tongue. In the adult, the telltale evidence of its origin is a prominent depression, the foramen cecum, at the back of the tongue. During embryonic development the thyroid descends inferiorly to its adult position in the lower neck.[7]

Iodinated amino acids are found in sponges, corals, protochordates, insects, molluscs, and polychaete worms. The wide distribution implies that iodinated amino acids appeared early in evolution. Iodinated amino acids have a wide distribution in invertebrates.

The C-cells of the thyroid (the source of the hormone thyrocalcitonin which functions in calcium regulation), however, have a neural crest origin.

SYNTHESIS, TRANSPORT, METABOLISM

The amino acid **tyrosine** is the precursor from which thyroid hormones are synthesized

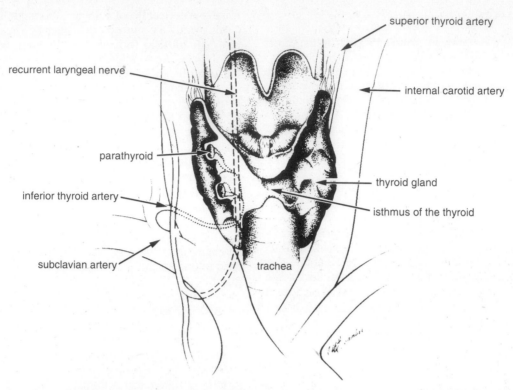

Figure 9.1 The figure shows the anatomy of the human thyroid from the ventral view; the four parathyroids are on the back of the gland. Modified, with permission. West, J. B. Physiological Basis of Medical Practice. Baltimore: Williams & Wilkins; 1991; p. 112.

(Figure 9.3). Tyrosine residues (123) are linked by peptide bonds in the glycoprotein **thyroglobulin**. Thyroglobulin has a molecular weight of 660,000. Thyroglobulin is synthesized with two subunits and 10% carbohydrate by the thyroid follicle cells. The thyroid follicle cells secrete the thyroglobulin by exocytosis into the colloidal interior of the follicles (Figures 9.4 and 9.5). In the cytoplasm, the thyroglobulin is found in granules where it is accompanied by an enzyme, thyroid peroxidase.

The thyroid gland actively transports iodide from the blood to the colloid. This feature of thyroid function is called the "iodide pump" or the **"iodide-trapping mechanism."** There are tissues other than the thyroid which possess the ability to concentrate iodide, and these include the mammary glands, salivary glands, gastric mucosa, placenta, ciliary body of the eye, and choroid plexus. The iodine budget—the amounts of iodine intake, use, and excretion—is shown in Table 9.1.

In the thyroid gland, iodide is oxidized to iodine and bound to tyrosine residues in the thyroglobulin. The reaction, called **iodination**, of a few of the tyrosines, takes place in seconds and is catalyzed by an enzyme, thyroid peroxidase, which is located at the cell-colloid interface. Iodinations at position three on tyrosine produce monoiodotyrosine (MIT) and again at position five produce diiodotyrosine (DIT). DIT and MIT are therefore examples of iodinated tyrosines. A pair of iodinated tyrosines is joined (oxidative condensation, the **coupling reaction**). If the pair is MIT and DIT, then T₃ (triiodothyronine) results; if the coupled pair is two DITs, then T₄ (thyroxine) results (Figure 9.6). Coupling liberates an alanine (amino acid) from one of the iodinated tyrosines. In the manufacture of T₃, whether the alanine is removed from the MIT or the DIT

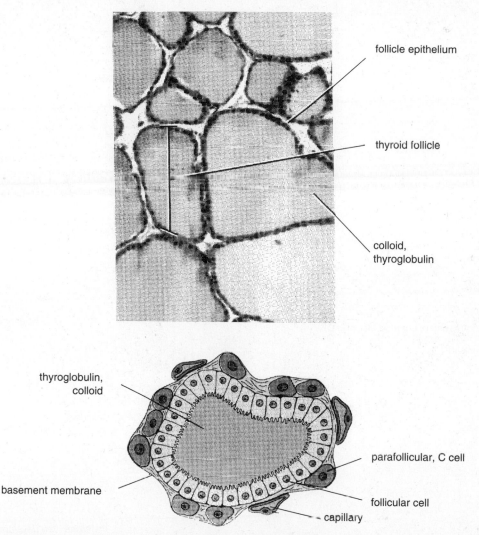

follicle epithelium

thyroid follicle

colloid, thyroglobulin

thyroglobulin, colloid

parafollicular, C cell

basement membrane

follicular cell

capillary

Figure 9.2 The figure shows thyroid histology (light microscopy, 230x) at the top and a diagrammatic representation of a thyroid follicle below. A thyroid follicle can be visualized as a sphere bound by a one-cell thick epithelium of follicle cells. The follicle is filled with colloidal thyroglobulin. Modified, with permission. Tortora, G.J.; Anagnostakos, N.P. Principles of Anatomy and Physiology, Sixth Edition. New York: Harper & Row, Pubs., 1990; p. 514.

determines whether T$_3$ or reverse T$_3$ (RT$_3$) is made. Scientists argue as to whether the coupling reaction takes place with the iodinated molecules attached to the thyroglobulin or whether they are disconnected from thyroglobulin during coupling. The coupling is catalyzed by coupling enzyme (thyroid peroxidase, TPO).

Secretion requires the liberation of the thyroid hormone from the thyroglobulin. Thyroid cells ingest colloid in globules by endocytosis. The ingestion leaves spaces (lacunae) in the colloid. Ingested colloid globules coalesce with lysozomes (phagolysosomes). The lysosomes contain enzymes, proteases and catheptases, which digest the thyroglobulin and thus set free T$_3$, T$_4$, DIT and MIT. T$_3$ and T$_4$ are secreted, probably by diffusion.

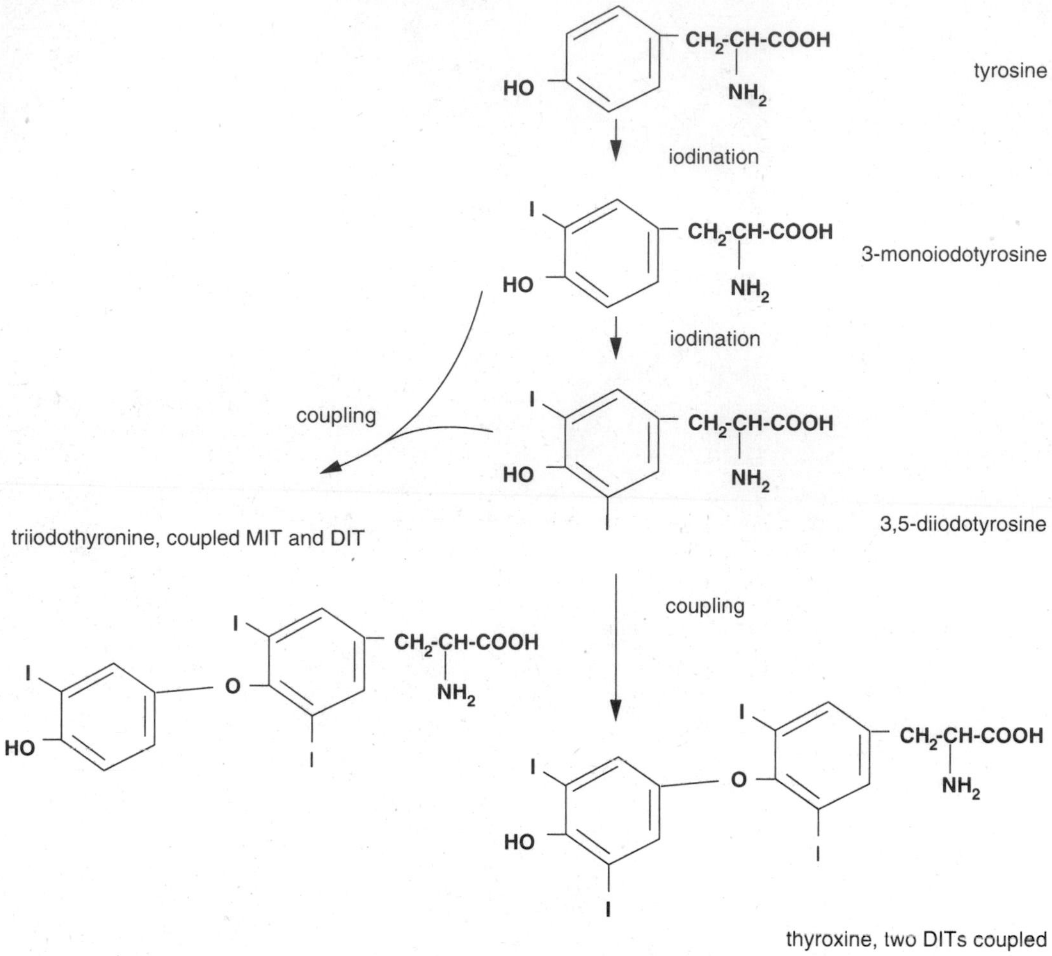

Figure 9.3 The pathway for the synthesis of thyroxine from tyrosine obtained in the diet is illustrated. MIT = monoiodotyrosine. DIT = diiodotyrosine. Two DITs are coupled to produce thyroxine (shown). When MIT and DIT are coupled, then triiodothyronine is made (not shown). Coupling and iodination details are still controversial. The amino acid alanine (not shown) is a biproduct of the coupling reaction.

In blood, plasma proteins transport over 99% of thyroxine. For example, thyroxine binding globulin (TBG)[8] transports 67% of T$_4$ and 46% of T$_3$; thyroxine-binding prealbumin (TBPA) transports 20% of T$_4$ and 1% of T$_3$; and albumin transports 13% of T$_4$ and 53% of T$_3$. The half-life of

thyroxine is 6–8 days, of T$_3$ is one day, and of RT$_3$ is 0.2 days. Thyroglobulin is also secreted but no function has been attributed to it once it has served its roles in the synthesis and storage of thyroid hormones in the thyroid gland.

Iodine and amino acids are conserved by

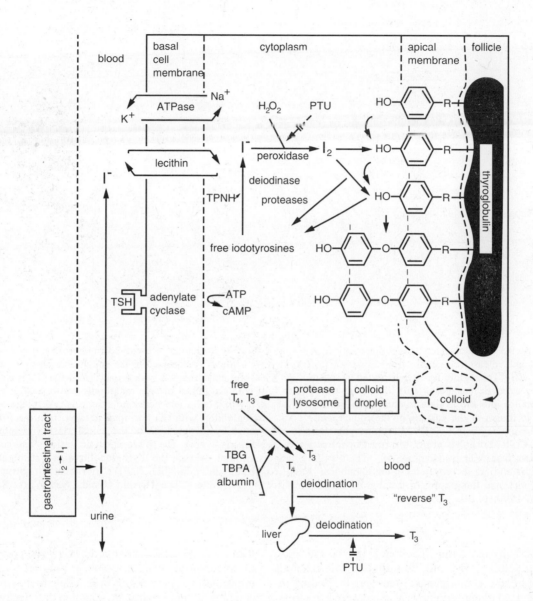

Figure 9.4 The diagram shows events of thyroid hormone synthesis and secretion by a thyroid follicle cell. TSH promotes thyroid function in many ways: blood flow, iodine trapping, peroxidase activity, iodination, coupling, phagolysosome activity, and TBG. Thyroid inhibitors act at sites of iodine trapping, peroxidase, coupling enzyme, and binding of hormones to TBG. Reproduced, with permission. Berkow, R., editor. The Merck Manual of Diagnosis and Therapy. Rahway, NJ: Merck Sharp & Dohme Research Laboratories; 1987; p. 1034.

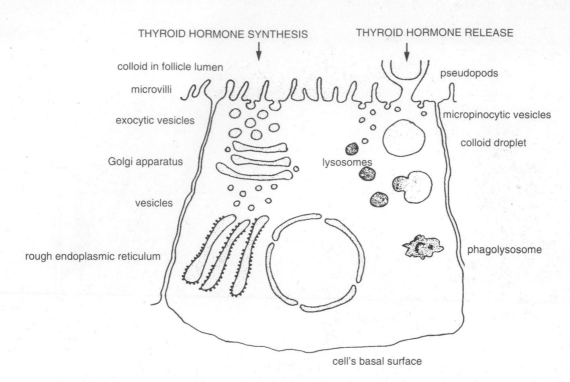

THYROID HORMONE SYNTHESIS   THYROID HORMONE RELEASE

colloid in follicle lumen   pseudopods

microvilli

exocytic vesicles   micropinocytic vesicles

                                                   colloid droplet

Golgi apparatus   lysosomes

vesicles

rough endoplasmic reticulum   phagolysosome

cell's basal surface

Figure 9.5 The diagram is a representation of the way the follicle lumen is involved in thyroid hormone synthesis and release (clockwise from lower left).   (i) Thyroglobulin is synthesized in the rough endoplasmic reticulum.   (ii) Thyroglobulin is transported to and through the Golgi apparatus via vesicles and from the Golgi apparatus by exocytic vesicles.   (iii) The exocytic vesicles fuse with the apical plasma membrane and release the thyroglobulin into the follicle lumen.   (iv) Iodination of the thyroglobulin and hormone synthesis take place in the follicle lumen at the surface of the follicle cell.   (v) Thyroglobulin with the hormone is taken into the follicle cell by endocytosis.   (vi) Micropinocytic vesicles are formed by invagination of the apical plasma membrane. (vii) Colloid droplets are also formed by retraction of pseudopods.   (viii) The micropinocytic vesicles and colloid droplets fuse with lysosomes.   (ix) The resulting phagolysosomes degrade the thyroglobulin with lysosomal hydrolases and (x) thereby release the hormones. Modified, with permission. Ekholm, R.; Bjorkman, U. Structural and functional integration of the thyroid Gland. In Greer, M.A., editor. The Thyroid Gland. New York: Raven Press; 1990; p. 39.

the body by recycling. The iodine in DIT and MIT is recycled. Thyroid deiodinase (microsomal iodotyrosine dehalogenase) recovers the iodine in the thyroid gland. Iodine is also recovered from the liver and other tissues. Although only a small amount of T$_3$ and RT$_3$ (4 mg each) are secreted by the thyroid gland, additional T$_3$ (27 µg) and RT$_3$ (36 µg) are formed from T$_4$ deiodination by 5'-deiodinase and 5-deiodinase in the liver, the kidney, and other tissues. The deiodinases further catalyze DIT production from T$_3$. T$_3$ and T$_4$ are conjugated to form glucuronides and sulfates in liver which are

then excreted in the feces via the bile. The presence of selenium as well as iodine in the diet may be important. Type I iodinase is a selenoenzyme, it contains selenocysteine. A selenium deficiency can contribute to hypothyroidism.[9]

Inhibition of the metabolism of thyroid hormones (e.g., their deiodination and conjugation with glucuronates and sulfates in the liver) can increase thyroid hormone levels. Hepatic enzyme inducers (drugs such as phenobarbitol and Dilantin, industrial compounds such as polyhalogenated biphenyls or PBB, and pesticides such as DDT)

Table 9.1 Values for Thyroid Parameters in Humans

Substance	Value
iodide (I-) in diet	500 µg/day
iodide trapped by thyroid	120 µg/day
iodide from thyroid	40 µg/day
iodide in thyroid hormones	80 µg/day
iodide in blood from liver	60 µg/day
iodide lost to feces via bile	20 µg/day
iodide lost in urine	480 µg/day
MIT in thyroid	23%
DIT in thyroid	35%
T$_4$ in thyroid	35%
T$_3$ in thyroid	7%
RT$_3$ in thyroid	traces
T$_4$ secretion by thyroid	80 µg/day (103 nmol)
T$_3$ secretion by thyroid	4 µg/day (7 nmol)
RT$_3$ secretion by thyroid	2 µg/day (3.5 nmol)
T$_4$ concentration in plasma	4–12 µg/dl (103 nmol/l)
T$_3$ concentration in plasma	0.15 µg/dl (2.3 nmol/l; 75–195 ng/dl)
protein-bound iodine in plasma	6.00 µg/dl
TBG capacity	15–25 µg T$_4$/dl
blood flow	4–6 ml/minute
TSH secretion rate	110 µg/day
TSH concentration in plasma	2 µg/ml (0.5–5.0 µU/ml)

Ganong, W. Review of Medical Physiology, Fourteenth Edition. Norwalk, CT: Appleton & Lange; 1989, pp. 267–274; Berkow, R. The Merck Manual, Sixteenth Edition, Vol. II. Rahway, NJ: Merck & Co.; 1992; p. 1430.

thus can have secondary effects on thyroid function.[10]

CALORIGENIC FUNCTION OF THE THYROID GLAND

The principal function of thyroid hormones is to stimulate oxygen consumption (Figure 9.7). Evolutionarily, the role of the gland in regulation of growth and development probably preceded its role in calorigenesis.

The idea of thyroid function in calorigenesis is attributed to Magnus Levy in 1890. Thyroid hormones raise basal metabolic rate (BMR; oxygen consumption determined at rest, at a comfortable temperature, and 12–14 hours after the last meal). Removing the thyroid drops the BMR to 40–50% of normal levels. The targets of thyroid hormones are metabolically active tissues such as liver, kidney, skeletal muscle, cardiac muscle, gastric mucosa, and diaphragm. Administration of thyroid hormones measurably increases oxygen consump-

monoiodothyronine

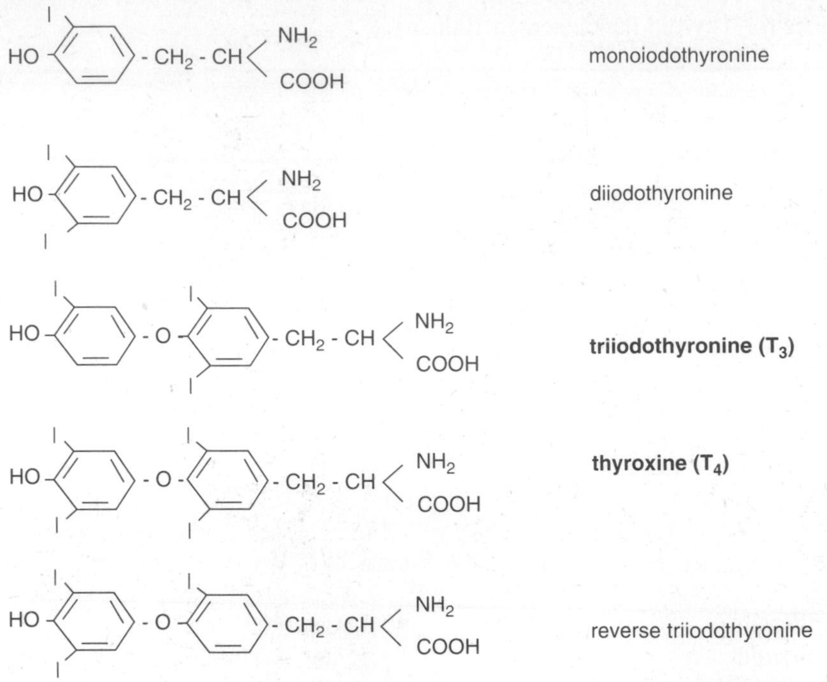

diiodothyronine

triiodothyronine (T$_3$)

thyroxine (T$_4$)

reverse triiodothyronine

Figure 9.6 Structures of thyroid hormones and related molecules are shown. Modified, with permission. Bjorkman, U.; Ekholm, R. Biochemistry of thyroid formation and secretion. In Greer, M.A. The Thyroid Gland. New York: Raven Press; 1990; p. 87.

tion after several hours, and, because of the long half-life of thyroxine, the effects may last as long as six days. Administration of thyroid hormones may even increase body temperature, and low morning body temperature may be an indication of low thyroid function. The size of the oxygen stimulation response to thyroid hormone depends upon existing status—the responses are greater if thyroid function and basal metabolic rate are low than if they are high.

The active thyroid hormone appears to be mainly T$_3$. Compared to T$_4$, T$_3$ has a shorter half-life, it acts more quickly, it is 3–5 times as potent, and it has greater binding to nuclear receptors. Apparently, T$_4$ is converted to T$_3$ and RT$_3$ by target tissues using 5'- and 5-deiodinases. According to Ganong the fourth iodine is not required for calorigenic action.[11]

There are some noteworthy exceptions, that is, tissues whose oxygen consumption is not stimulated by thyroid hormones. Brain, uterus, testes, spleen, lymph nodes, anterior pituitary, and the thyroid gland itself are all exempt from thyroid

hormone increases in oxygen consumption.

The ability of thyroid hormones to increase oxygen consumption is **calorigenesis** (heat producing ability). Various phrases have been used to describe this function of the thyroid gland: "It is a 'governor' of metabolism, or a 'thermostat', or it serves to 'fan the fires of life' or to 'regulate the rate of living.'"[12]

The sodium/potassium pump (Na$^+$/K$^+$ pump; Na,K-ATPase] functions continuously to generate gradients of sodium and potassium ions across membranes. It accounts for 20–45% of basal energy consumption, the thermogenic action, by cells.[13] T$_3$ increases the abundance of the mRNAs that encode the alpha and beta subunits of Na,K-ATPase. T$_3$ stimulates the biosynthesis of the ubiquitous plasma membrane-bound Na,K-ATPase. The activity of the enzyme is thereby increased by T$_3$.

Thyroid hormones are synergistic with somatotropin and epinephrine in calorigenesis. To reiterate, thyroid hormones achieve calorigenesis by

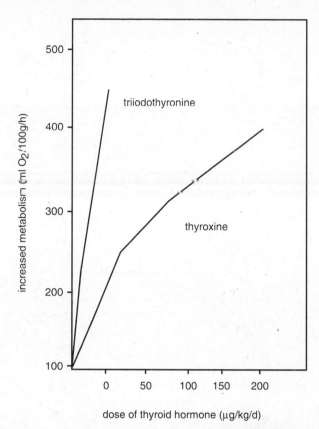

Figure 9.7 The graph shows the percentage changes in the basal metabolic rates of thyroidectomized rats injected with thyroid hormones. Note that the triiodothyronine is more effective at the same dose than the thyroxine. Redrawn. Barker, S.B. Peripheral actions of thyroid hormones. Federation Proceedings 21: 635; 1962.

increasing tissue energy production, increasing oxygen consumption, and by increasing the basal metabolic rate.

TEMPERATURE

A particularly interesting function of the thyroid gland is the role it plays in thermoregulation.[14]

Birds, mammals, and humans are homeotherms (they can maintain their body temperature in cold environments) whose thyroids are active the whole year. In cold winter conditions, thyroid activity and secretion increases compared to its activity in summer. Sudden exposure to cold increases thyroid hormone secretion, especially in animals and human babies.

However, some animals hibernate in winter (marmot, hedgehog, dormouse). Hibernating, they drop their internal body temperatures to a few degrees above ambient (outside, external) temperatures. The thyroid glands of hibernators cease activity during hibernation, but thyroid activity peaks in spring when the animals end their hibernation. Depriving hedgehogs of their thyroids did not prevent or induce hibernation, while thyroxine treatment did prevent hibernation in ground squirrels.[15]

Vertebrates that cannot maintain their body temperatures in cold environments are classified as poikilotherms. These animals warm themselves by behavioral thermoregulation. In *Anolis carolinenesis*, for example, the thyroid does not appear to function if the lizards live at 20–24 °C, but

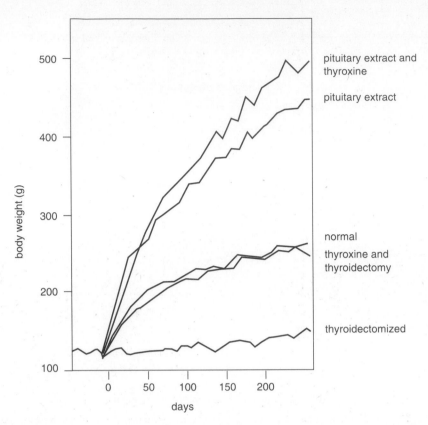

Figure 9.8 The graphs show the effects of various treatments on growth in normal and thyroidectomized female rats. The upper two graphs show the effects of pituitary extract and thyroxine on normal rats. The middle two graphs show normal growth and the effects of thyroxine replacement in thyroidectomized rats. The bottom graph shows the lack of growth in thyroidectomized rats which did not receive replacement therapy. Replacement therapy began on day zero. Redrawn. Evans, H.M.; Simpson, M.E.; Pencharz, R. Endocrinology 25: 275l; 1939.

does appear to affect oxygen consumption when the animals are at 30 °C.

GROWTH

Thyroid hormone causes protein anabolism in conjunction with stimulation of growth (Figure 9.8). Thyroid hormones cause elevation of urine nitrogen, potassium, and hexosamine excretion. And they cause catabolism of protein unless there is a compensatory increase in food intake. Thyroid hormones cause hyperglycemia by increasing the rate of absorption of carbohydrates from the intestinal tract. Thyroid hormones cause fat breakdown, decrease cholesterol by increasing formation of LDL receptors, and reduce weight unless there is a compensatory increase in the dietary intake. Starvation for six days decreases T₃ from 9 to 5 mg/dl, decreases T₄ from 180 to 140 ng/dl, and increases RT₃ from 2 to 5 mg/dl. The hormones return to normal levels four days after resumption of normal diets.[16]

Ganong discourages use of thyroid hormones as a quick fix for weight reduction: "use of thyroid to promote weight loss can be of value only if the patient pays the price of some nervousness and heat intolerance and curbs the appetite so that there is no compensatory increase in caloric intake."[17]

Untreated control tadpole

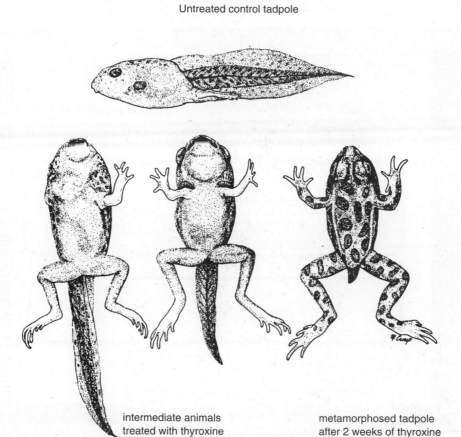

intermediate animals
treated with thyroxine

metamorphosed tadpole
after 2 weeks of thyroxine

Figure 9.9 The drawings are of responses to treatment with thyroxine in *Rana pipiens* tadpoles. The thyroxine was added to the bathing water in which the tadpoles were cultured. Modified, with permission. Turner, C.D.; Bagnara, J.T. Endocrinology, Sixth Edition. Philadelphia: Saunders; 1976; p. 210.

THYROID FUNCTION IN DEVELOPMENT

Remarkable effects of thyroid hormones are seen in development and growth. In particular, the thyroid functions in transitions required for juveniles to become adults. Thyroid hormones synergize with somatotropin in causing normal skeletal growth so that individuals who are hypothyroid during development fail to grow normally. Thyroxine has many diverse roles during development in mammals, such as a permissive action in

the ontogeny of digestion (e.g., jejunal sucrase in suckling rats[18]) and the transitions from the developmental to adult phase in salmon (the change from dependence on yolk to active feeding, smoltification, and adaptation to seawater).[19]

A dramatic example is found in the requirement of the thyroid gland for amphibian metamorphosis (Figure 9.9). Amphibian larvae, tadpoles, that are thyroidectomized do not metamorphose into adults (frogs and salamanders), but instead enlarge. Thyroid hormones produce

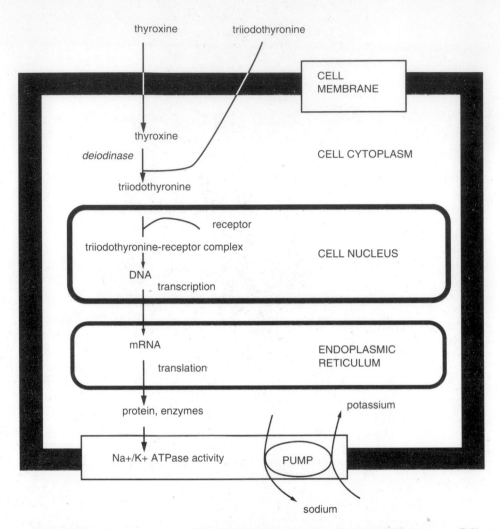

Figure 9.10 The diagram illustrates a simplified mechanism of action for thyroid hormones. Cell membranes are represented as black bars. Entering the cell, thyroxine is converted to triiodothyronine which binds to a nuclear receptor. The triiodothyronine-receptor complex causes DNA to produce new mRNAs which are translated to make new proteins. Here, the final result is shown as activation of ATPase (and/or the production of more "pumps") whose energy consumption in pumping sodium out of the cell is manifested as increased metabolic rate and calorigenesis, but other enzymes are also activated.

metamorphosis. The failure to metamorphose can also be found under natural conditions. The larval form persists and even becomes sexually mature. The word "neoteny" is used to describe this phenomena which is believed to involve thyroid hormone deficiency and lack of TSH production.

MECHANISM OF ACTION

The mechanism of action for thyroid hormones is similar to that for steroids in that the thyroid hormones enter the target organ cells and bind to receptors. T₄ is first converted to T₃ in the cytoplasm.

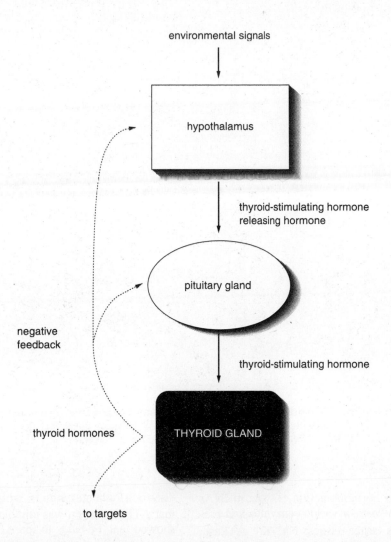

environmental signals

hypothalamus

thyroid-stimulating hormone
releasing hormone

pituitary gland

negative
feedback

thyroid-stimulating hormone

thyroid hormones

THYROID GLAND

to targets

Figure 9.11 Feedback regulation of the thyroid gland is illustrated. The thyroid hormones feed back negatively to control the hypothalamic production of TRH and the pituitary secretion of TSH. Sources vary as to whether the feedback of thyroid hormones on the hypothalamus exists, and thyroid hormone production is also controlled by a hypothalamic thermostat.

In the case of thyroid hormones, the receptors are located in the cell nuclei (Figure 9.10).

The high affinity and low capacity T$_3$ receptors are two species of nonhistone proteins with molecular weight about 50,500 which are similar in all species and tissues so far studied. The thyroid hormone receptor has strong peptide homology to the receptors for glucocorticoids, progesterone, estradiol, and v-erb A oncogene product.[20]

In the nucleus, a T$_3$-receptor complex is rapidly formed. The T$_3$-receptor complex binds to DNA. Specific genes are caused to express themselves and mRNAs are produced. There is a rapid response in liver mRNA-S14 to T$_3$, so mRNA-S14 has been used as a model target gene for the

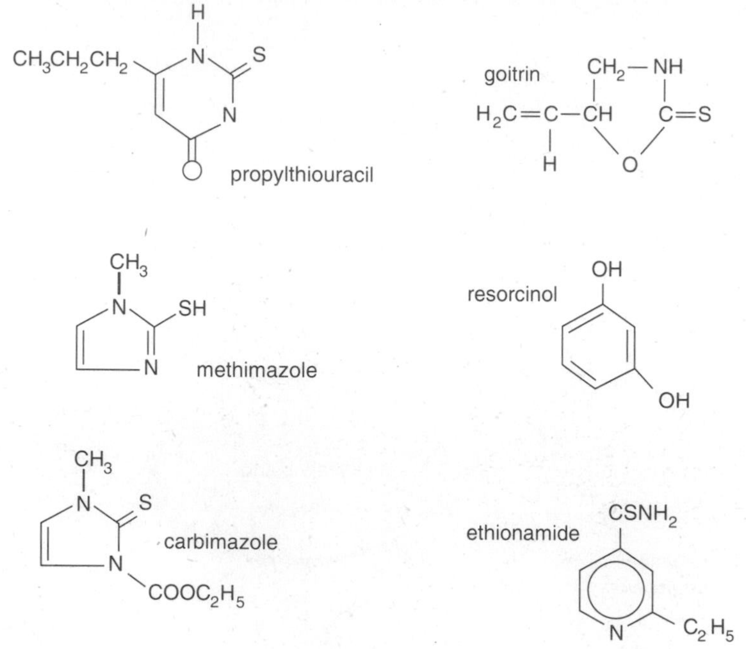

Figure 9.12 Structures of some thyroid inhibitors are shown. These inhibit iodination that is catalyzed by thyroid peroxidase. Modified, with permission. Cooper, D.S. Substances that affect thyroid function or thyroid hormone metabolism. In Greer, M.A. The Thyroid Gland. New York: Raven Press; 1990; p. 328.

study of thyroid hormone action.[21] The mRNAs increase the synthesis of various enzymes and proteins in various target tissues: Na^+-K^+ ATPase, hyaluronidase, malic dehydrogenase, mitochondrial α-glycerophosphate dehydrogenase, chromatin protein kinase, hepatic pyruvate carboxylase, α-lactalbumin, and carbamoyl phosphate synthetase.

The principal site of thyroid hormone action is believed to be the nucleus. But some investigators have challenged the idea of sole nuclear action of thyroid hormones and have proposed a mitochondrial alternative for the action of T₃. Investigators injected nanogram doses of T₃ into rats *in vivo*, killed them 30 minutes later, and found an activation of mitochondrial phosphorylation even when new protein synthesis was blocked. They supported this with an *in vitro* study of mitochondria freshly isolated from the livers of thyroidectomized rats. They incubated the mitochon-

dria for 15 minutes with or without T₃, and found that ATP formation was stimulated. Finally, they showed that T₃ binds to the ADP/ATP translocator, adenine nucleotide translocase. In the model for thyroid hormone action on mitochondria, the translocase serves as both hormone receptor and effector. The mitochondrial mechanism could provide for a rapid response (e.g., within 15–30 minutes) while the nuclear mechanism may provide for more sustained effects which are seen after a day or more.[22] Hadley writes: "For many years there was argument whether thyroid hormones mediated their effects through direct actions on mitochondria [and concludes that] indeed, another site of thyroid hormone action is the mitochondria."[23] On the other hand, Oppenheimer and his colleagues write that "there is no entirely convincing demonstrations to date that the binding of T₃ to extranuclear sites

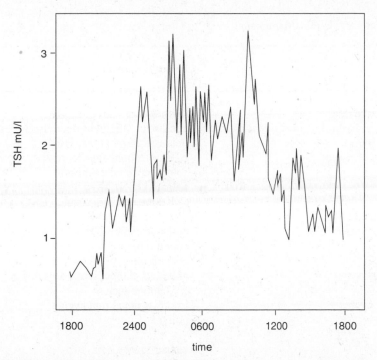

Figure 9.13 The graph shows the daily cycle of TSH in a single adult male subject who exhibited peak TSH from bedtime through noon. Redrawn, with permission. Brabant, G.; Prank, J.K.; Ranft, U.; Schuermeyer, T.; Wagner, T.O.F.; Hauser, H.; Kummer, B.; Feistner, H.; Hesch, R.D.; and von zur Muhlen, A. Physiological regulation of circadian and pulsatile thyrotropin secretion in normal man and woman. J. Clin. Endo. Metabol. 70: 403–409; 1990; page 405. Other investigators also measured the TSH cycle in human males and found peak TSH from 1900–0300.[24]

results in conventionally recognized hormonal actions."[25]

REGULATION

Regulation of thyroid hormone secretion is by a negative feedback system (Figure 9.11).

Heating and cooling of the blood directly affect the temperature of the hypothalamus. A hypothalamic "thermostat" is sensitive to the temperature changes and, in the case of cooling, stimulates thyrotropin-releasing hormone which in turn stimulates the thyroid gland to produce thyroid hormones. Thyroid hormones circulate to target tissues and feedback on the pituitary gland, and, possibly, the hypothalamus.

Thyrotropin-releasing hormone (TRH) is a hormone made from a precursor molecule (preproTRH with five TRH copies) in the medial paraventricular nuclei of the hypothalamus. TRH is the smallest hypothalamic peptide hormone having three amino acid residues: (pyro)glu-his-pro-NH₂. It appears that the heat production stimulated by thyroid hormones (thyroid hormone thermogenesis) is brought about by the detection of cold and subsequent increase in TRH. A symptom of hyperthyroidism is a 0.5°C increase in body temperature; and body temperature is lowered by about half a degree in hypothyroidism. TRH increases the activity of TSH by affecting its glycosylation. TRH also stimulates prolactin secretion. TRH secretion is inhibited by glucocorticoids.

Thyroid-stimulating hormone (TSH) is a glycoprotein with 211 amino acids and carbohydrate moieties (hexosamines, hexoses, sialic acid). It is chemically similar to LH and FSH; it has an alpha subunit identical to LH and FSH.[26] During TSH synthesis in the rough endoplasmic reticulum of anterior pituitary thyrotropes,[27] asparagine residues of the α and ß chains of amino acids attach to 14-

Table 9.2 Symptoms of Thyroid Malfunction

Hyperthyroidism	Hypothyroidism
thyroid hormones increased	thyroid hormones decreased
restless, hyperactive, irritable, short attention span, quick movements, tremor	apathetic, sluggish, decreased mentation, lethargy, depression, paranoia, fatigue
basal metabolic rate increased	basal metabolic rate decreased
insomnia	somnolence (sleepiness)
rapid heart rate	enlarged heart, slow heart rate
Q-Kd interval decreased in EKG	Q-Kd interval increased in EKG
blood pressure elevated	blood pressure low
body temperature elevated 0.5°C	body temperature low
appetite increased	appetite poor
diarrhea	constipation
skeletal muscle weakness	enlarged, flabby, weak muscles
heat intolerance	cold intolerance
irregular menstrual cycles	irregular menstrual cycles
goiter	goiter
exophthalmos	coarse, sparse hair
hung up reflex	sensitivity to light and sound increased
weight loss (despite increased feeding)	thickened tongue
sweating, warm moist palms	lower resistance to narcotics
	rise in plasma carotenes
	myxedema (puffy appearance, edema of face, eyelids)

In the upper part of the table, functions are paired for comparison between hyperthyroidism and hypothyroidism; in the lower part of the table, functions are not paired.

sugar units. The carbohydrate side chains are modified in the Golgi apparatus. Secretion of TSH is pulsatile and has a daily rhythm (rises in the evening to a midnight peak). The half-life of TSH is about 60 minutes. TSH is a 28,000 dalton protein in the family of pituitary hormones with LH and FSH and the placental hormone CG. It is synthesized in the pituitary thyrotropes and is stored there in secretory granules. TSH binds to and stimulates thyroid cells.[28]

In the absence of TSH, the thyroid gland atrophies. TSH stimulates thyroid follicle cell function at a number of points: blood flow to the thyroid, iodide trapping, synthesis of hormones, secretion of thyroglobulin into colloids, endocytosis of colloid, secretion of hormones and production of iodinated amines. Excess TSH causes the thyroid gland to enlarge—its weight increases and the cells hypertrophy because metabolism of phospholipids in the membrane is stimulated. TSH receptors in the thyroid cell membranes possess a ganglioside-glycoprotein which binds to TSH causing activation of adenyl cyclase. TSH secretion by the pituitary gland is inhibited by dopamine and somatostatin.

Thyroid hormones, mainly T$_3$, feed back (negative feedback) on the pituitary to inhibit TSH secretion. The possibility of feedback of thyroid hormones on the hypothalamus to inhibit TRH secretion is more controversial appearing in some models[29,30] but not others.[31]

There is a dietary influence on thermogen-

Table 9.3 Irradiation and Thyroid Lesions

Treated region	Dose (rads)	Goiter %	Cancer %
none	none	1–5	0.004
thymus	199	1.8	0.80
thymus	399	7.6	5.00
neck, chest	807	27.2	5.70
neck, chest	180–1500	26.2	6.80
fallout	<50	–	0.40
fallout	>50	–	6.70
fallout	175 γ, 700–1400ß	39.6	5.70
¹³¹I therapy	10,000	0.17	0.08

The table shows the incidence of nodular goiter and cancer after treatment of various areas of the body with irradiation given in the estimated dose to the thyroid gland. γ,ß refer to treatments with different types of radiation (column one fallout). The normal incidence of goiter depends upon age; it is less than 1% in young children but rising to 5% in persons over the age of 60 years. Greenspan, F. S.; Rapoport, B. Thyroid gland. In Greenspan, F.; Forsham, P., editors. Basic and Clinical Endocrinology, Second Edition. Norwalk, CT: Appleton & Lange; 1987; p. 193.

esis. Serum T₃ decreases during food deprivation and so does the resting metabolic rate. Serum T₃ increases during overeeding and so does the metabolic rate.[32]

THYROID SUBSTANCES

There are other substances to consider with the thyroid in addition to thyroid hormones, thyroid regulating hormones, thyroglobulin, and thyroid hormone-transporting molecules.

A number of substances, the **antithyroid substances**, inhibit thyroid gland function. The names of some of the antithyroid substances are anions (chlorate, perchlorate, pertechnetate, periodate, biodate, nitrate, thiocyanate), thiocarbamides (e.g., propylthiourea, PTU; and methimazole), thiocyanate (KSCN), thiouracil, sulfonamides, cobalt ions, allylthiourea, goitrin, and iodide (Figure 9.12). Some of these substances are found in food. Allylthiourea is a component of mustard, and progoitrin is found in rutabagas, cabbage, and turnips. Most of the antithyroid compounds block iodination or iodine trapping. By reducing thyroid hormones, the antithyroid substances remove the feedback inhibition of TSH so that TSH causes

thyroid enlargement (goiter). Inhibition of thyroid function by iodide (too much or too little is harmful) is called the Wolff-Chaikoff effect.

Other substances are related to disorders involving the thyroid gland. **Long-acting thyroid stimulator** (LATS; TSI = thyroid-stimulating immunoglobulin) is an immune globulin which is found in some hyperthyroid individuals. "Exophthalmos-producing substance" (EPS) is the name that was given to a substance from the pituitary gland that was thought to be distinct from TSH. It was believed to cause the "eye popping" characteristics of some thyroid disorders. However, now the explanation of exophthalmia based on animal studies is provocation of the Harderian glands by TSH digests.[33]

THYROID FUNCTION TESTS AND RHYTHMS

Thyroid hormones and TSH can be measured with RIA and these assays are used for clinical diagnoses. Response of plasma TSH to TRH injection, of thyroid hormones to TSH administration, and of TSH to T₃ treatment are tests used in evaluating thyroid system function.

Basal metabolic rate (BMR) can be measured by determining oxygen consumption with a spirometer and indicates hypothyroidism (reduced BMR) or hyperthyroidism (increased BMR). However, other factors (sex, age, size, height, weight, surface area, exercise, meals, environmental temperature, emotions, pregnancy, menstruation, or catecholamines) also influence BMR.

Another aspect of thyroid function involves its ability to utilize iodine. A radioisotope can be administered (NaI^{125}) and, 4–24 hours later, the thyroid's ability to acquire iodide can be assessed by scanning the neck region with a gamma scintillation counter to count the radioactivity (radioactive iodine uptake, RAIU); or alternatively, either a rectilinear or pinhole collimated gamma camera can be used to provide an image of iodine distribution in the thyroid. Protein-bound iodine (PBI) is a measurement of serum precipitatable iodine that was formerly used to indicate thyroid hormone levels (3.5–8 mg/100ml indicated 6–12 $\mu g/T_4$).

Daily cycles of thyroid hormones and TSH in serum of rats have light-time peaks and nadirs in the dark-time (Figure 9.13). TSH secretion is also pulsatile: there are 10–11 pulses of TSH per 24 hours with 50% of the pulses occurring at night (2000–0400).[34]

HYPOTHYROIDISM AND HYPERTHYROIDISM

The term euthyroidism is used to indicate conditions where the thyroid is functioning normally. Hypothyroidism refers to too little thyroid hormone production; it can be treated with thyroid hormone replacement therapy. Sometimes the therapy is simply referred to as treatment with "thyroid." Hyperthyroidism refers to too much thyroid hormone production. Hyperthyroidism can be treated with antithyroid drugs, partial thyroidectomy, and radioactive iodine. There is a multiplicity of causes for either of these conditions. Either of these abnormal conditions is accompanied by a characteristic set of symptoms (Table 9.2).

Myxedema is puffiness of the skin which results when there is a deficiency of thyroid hormone. The missing action of thyroid hormone is water retention and the accumulation of skin proteins which are combined with chondroitin sulfuric acid, with polysaccharides, and with hyaluronic acid. The skin has another symptom of hypothyroidism: carotene accumulates making the skin

yellow because thyroid hormones stimulate the liver to make vitamin A from carotene.

Thyroid hormones are necessary to prevent anemia. Without thyroid hormones, bone marrow decreases its metabolism and there is poor absorption of vitamin B_{12} from the intestine.

Reproduction is affected by thyroid hormones. Hypothyroid women have menstrual cycles that are irregular and lower fertility. Thyroid hormones may be necessary for normal LH release. Thyroid hormones also stimulate milk secretion and this effect is useful in increasing milk production in the dairy industry. Male reproduction also requires normal thyroid hormones. Hypothyroidism delays male reproductive development. For example, inhibition of the thyroid can be obtained experimentally by feeding mother rats thiouracil. The male offspring are hypothyroid (cretinic) and their testes at 40 days of age weigh only 112 mg whereas in normal controls they weigh 893 mg. Thyroid hormones can stimulate or impair the formation of spermatozoa.

The heart is a target of thyroid hormones. Thyroid hormones increase the number of ß-adrenergic receptors in the heart, and thereby thyroid hormones increase cardiac responsiveness to catecholamines. Because of the increase in receptors, thyroid hormones increase heart rate (tachycardia). Thyroid hormones also alter the myosin which could affect heart contractility and which may be correlated with changes in stroke volume. Hyperthyroidism is characterized by rapid heart rate, increased stroke volume, increased pulse pressure, and peripheral vasodilation. In hypothyroidism, the heart rate decreases, the amplitude of contraction is less, and the heart enlarges.

The effects of catecholamines are modulated by thyroid hormones. Thyroid hormones increase ß-adrenergic receptors. Thus, as just mentioned, a tissue, such as the heart, that responds to catecholamines using ß-receptors, has increased responses to epinephrine and norepinephrine in the presence of thyroid hormone. In turn, responses associated with excess thyroid hormone (cardiovascular, sweating, tremulousness, thyroid storms) may be ameliorated with ß-blockers such as propranolol.

The oxygen consumption of the brain is normal in hypothyroid and hyperthyroid individuals. Hypothyroidism causes serious mental retardation in infants where the absence of thyroid hormones causes abnormal synapse development and

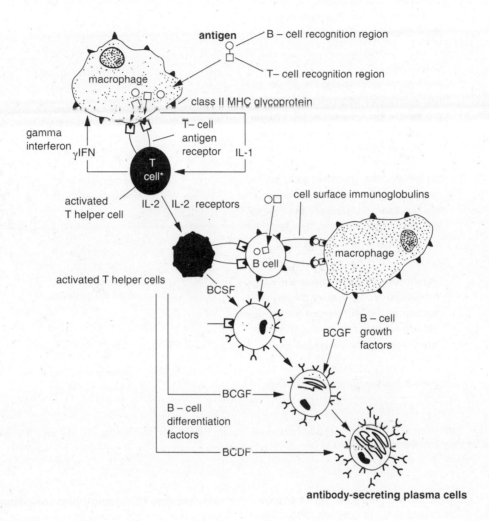

Figure 9.14 The model illustrates the way an antigen, via induction of B-cell differentiation by helper cells, causes secretion of antibodies. The macrophages (stippled) consume antigen (upper) and bind it to the surfaces of the class II MHC glycoprotein in their cell membranes. The antigen is recognized by the T-cells (black). The helper T-cells are activated by crosslinked antigen receptors and interleukin 1 (IL-1) from the macrophages. The activated helper T-cells make IL-2l, IL-2 receptors, and macrophage stimulatory gamma-interferon. Interaction with helper T-cells and macrophages activates B-cells via crosslinked cell surface immunoglobulins. Activated B-cells (unshaded) respond to B-cell growth and differentiation into plasma cells that secrete antibodies. Modified, with permission, Gilbert, S.F. Developmental Biology, Second Edition. Sunderland, MA: Sinauer Associates, Inc., Pubs.; 1988; p. 576.

CH₃COHN-
ser-asp-ala-ala-val-asp-thr-ser-glu-
ile-thr-thr-lys-asp-leu-lys-glu-lys-lys
glu-val-val-glu-glu-ala-glu-asn

thymosin a1
28 amino acids

CH₃CONH-
ser-asp-lys-pro-asp-met-ala-glu-ile-glu-
lys-phe-asp-lys-ser-lys-leu-lys-lys-thr-
glu-thr-gln-glu-lys-asn-pro-leu-pro-ser-
lys-glu-thr-ile-glu-gln-glu-lys-gln-ala-
gly-glu-ser-COOH

thymosin β4
43 amino acids

gly-gln-phe-leu-glu-asp-pro-ser-val-leu-
thr-lys-glu-lys-leu-lys-ser-glu-leu-val-
ala-asn-asn-val-thr-leu-pro-ala-gly-glu-
gln-arg-lys-asp-val-tyr-val-gln-leu-tyr-
leu-gln-*his*-leu-thr-ala-val-lys-arg

thymopoietin I
49 amino acids

ser-gln-phe-leu-glu-asp-pro-ser-val-leu-
thr-lys-glu-lys-leu-lys-ser-glu-leu-val-
ala-asn-asn-val-thr-leu-pro-ala-gly-glu-
gln-arg-lys-asp-val-tyr-val-gln-leu-tyr-
leu-gln-*thr*-leu-thr-ala-val-lys-arg

thymopoietin II
49 amino acids

gln-ala-lys-ser-gln-gly-gly-ser-asn

serum thymic factor
9 amino acids

Figure 9.15 The structures of some peptide hormones isolated from bovine thymus are shown. Thymopoietins I and II differ only by two amino acids.

defective myelination. Hypothyroidism is associated with slower mentation. In contrast, hyperthyroidism is associated with rapid mentation, irritability, restlessness, and shortened reaction time. At the spinal cord level, hypothyroidism also lengthens stretch reflex reaction times in adults (Achilles reflex, ankle jerk).

Skeletal muscle is a target of thyroid hormones. Hypothyroidism has muscular symptoms of stiffness, cramps, and muscle weakness. Hyperthyroidism also has symptoms of muscle weakness called thyrotoxic myopathy which may be due to changes in myosin and protein catabolism.

Electrolytes are affected by thyroid hor-

mones because of thyroid hormone-enhancing effects on the Na⁺/K⁺ pump. Hypothyroidism is associated with retention of sodium ions, chloride ions, and water. Thyroid hormones cause water loss.

HYPOTHYROID DISEASES

When severe hypothyroidism occurs in infants the disorder may be called **cretinism**. The disorder characterized by low T₄ and high TSH occurs in about 1/4000 newborns. The untreated syndrome includes mental retardation (because thyroid hormone is required for normal nervous system

Table 9.4 T- and B-lymphocyte distribution

	T-lymphocytes	B-lymphocytes
thymus	+++	rare
bone marrow	+	++++
circulating blood	+++	+
lymph nodes	+++	++
spleen	+++	++
thoracic duct	+++	+

The thymus is a source of lymphocytes and thymosin, a hormone that stimulates lymphocyte production and maturation. T-lymphocytes attain their immunocompetency in blood, lymph, or connective tissue and are responsible for cell-mediated immunity. T-lymphocytes cause B-lymphocytes to differentiate into cells that can synthesize antibodies. Modified, Telford, I.R.; Bridgman, C.F. Introduction to Functional Histology. New York: Harper & Row, Pubs.; 1990; p. 280.

development), short stature, puffy appearance, deafness, and muteness. Hypothyroidism in children can result from a variety of causes: failure of thyroid descent in development, thyroid antibodies from a mother with Hashimoto's thyroiditis, excess iodides, antithyroid drugs, or radioactive iodine, and pituitary deficiency.

When hypothyroidism occurs in adults it is called adult **myxedema** (Gull's disease). Sometimes the mental symptoms are so severe as to be called "myxedema madness." Vocalizations assume a characteristic nature: "The voice is husky and slow, the basis of the aphorism that 'myxedema is the one disease that can be diagnosed over the telephone.'"[35]

Hashimoto's thyroiditis is the most common cause of hypothyroidism. The disorder is thought to be an autoimmune disease. It is characterized by a chronic inflammation of the thyroid gland with infiltration of the gland by lymphocytes. The disease is treated with lifelong thyroid hormone replacement therapy (e.g., oral L-thyroxine, 150–200 µg/day).

GRAVE'S DISEASE

Hyperthyroidism (thyrotoxicosis) takes various forms. It can be caused by hyperactivity of the thyroid, by excess thyroid hormone ingestion, or may have a genetic component. One of the disorders, the most common, is called Grave's disease. It is characterized by thyrotoxicosis, goiter, exophthalmos, and thickening of the skin over the lower tibia. In Grave's disease TSI (thyroid-stimulating immunoglobulin) antibodies are are usually found. The effects on the appearance of the eyes (exophthalmos) is due to inflammation or autoimmune responses in the orbital muscles. Diseases of hyperthyroidism can involve an acute attack, a thyroid storm, which can be lethal. Usually the storm accompanies surgery, radioactive iodine treatment, or childbirth. Some of the characteristics of thyroid storm may be flushing, sweating, body temperature increases to 100–106 °F, rapid pulse, agitation, restlessness, delirium, coma, nausea, vomiting, diarrhea, and jaundice. A puzzle for the etiology of Grave's disease, which may be an autoimmune disease, was presented by its near simultaneous possible discovery in President George Bush, his wife Barbara, and their dog.

Hyperthyroidism was used by novelist Tom Robbins: "On the fifth morning, as the Indian summer sun popped up from behind the hills like a hyperthyroid Boy Scout, burning to do good deeds..."[36]

GOITER

"Goiter" is a word used to describe any enlargement of the thyroid gland. Often goiters are

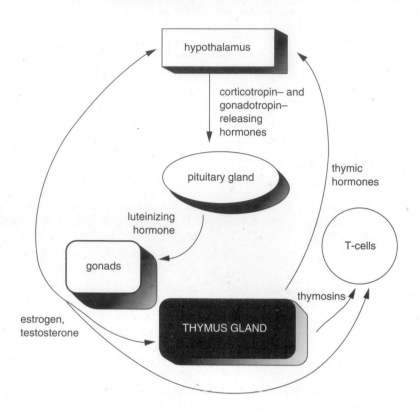

Figure 9.16 A regulation scheme for the thymus involves the gonads, nervous system, and pituitary gland. A more complicated model for endocrine and immunology system interactions also includes the adrenal and pineal glands. Growth hormone, prolactin, and action of the T-cells on the gonads are probably also involved.[37]

large enough to be seen externally. Goiter can occur with a number of causes (including Grave's disease). A particularly interesting form is called **endemic goiter**.[38] Endemic goiter is a regional disease. It is due to iodine deficiency in the diet. It is still found in the Himalayas, the Andes, Central Africa, and New Guinea. However, in other areas where the soils are deficient in iodine, fertilizers with iodide, "iodized salt," iodized animal feed, and food preservatives have prevented the disorder. The Chinese in 1600 B.C. knew that ashes of seaweed or burnt sponge was a remedy for a swollen neck. Adults require 150–300 μg/day of iodine in their diets if goiter is to be prevented. The mechanism causing endemic goiter is believed to be stimulation of thyroid growth by TSH attempting to respond to low thyroid hormone production.

Exposure to ionizing radiation (from radiation treatment or radioactive fallout) produces increases in nodular goiter and carcinoma (Table 9.3). This has led scientists to expect an increase in thyroid related changes in populations exposed to nuclear fallout from nuclear plant disasters such as that which occurred in Chernobyl.

THYMUS GLAND AND LYMPHOKINES

The thymus is a gland that is associated with development and the immune system (Figure 9.14).

In the young rat, the prominent thymus is found by gross dissection in the anterior neck and is about one centimeter in its largest dimension. The thymus atrophies in mammals and has virtually disappeared when the adult rat is dissected.

In humans, the thymus is a "well-developed, bilobed, greyish white body located in the superior part of the chest. It rests on the great vessels of the heart and extends into the root of the neck."[39] At birth the thymus is a large gland (12–15g), in puberty it reaches 40g, and its size then declines to less than 10g by age 50.

The immune system defends against foreign agents that invade the body; it has two components. The first component is the **humoral** defense system. The humoral defense system consists of antibodies which are plasma proteins in the gamma globulin fraction of blood proteins. The antibodies are used to defend against bacteria, viruses, and other foreign substances. The second component of the immune system is the **cellular** defense system. Cells named lymphocytes defend against some bacteria, viruses, fungi. In addition, the lymphocytes are involved in allergic reactions and reject foreign tissue. Lymphocytes are part of the white cell fraction which also includes neutrophils, eosinophils, basophils, monocytes, and macrophages.

Lymphocytes originate from white blood cells called leukocytes that are produced by the bone marrow during development (Table 9.4). Lymphocytes can be separated into subtypes using glycoprotein markers on their cell surfaces. Lymphocytes that are influenced by the thymus are called **T-lymphocytes** and they confer cellular immunity. Four subtypes of T-lymphocytes are killer cells (effector T-cells, cytotoxic T-cells, T$_8$-cells), memory T-cells, suppressor T-cells, and helper/inducer T-cells (T$_4$-cells). The killer cells attack foreign cells. The killer cells also act to inhibit tumor cell development so that they are of particular interest to cancer researchers. Moreover, the killer cells release substances called lymphokines which affect the activity of other white blood cells, called macrophages, which are essential for presentation of antigen to T-cells and B-cells. The helper/inducer T-cells regulate B-cell antibody production. The thymus is believed to confer competency on T-lymphocytes as they pass though the gland and are subjected to the thymus hormones and/or lymphocytes that reside in the thymus.

B-lymphocytes function to provide humoral immunity. They are apparently formed in mammals in bone marrow and maybe other locations. Most remain in the spleen and the fluid of the lymphatics. B-lymphocytes are formed in birds in the bursa of Fabricus which is located near the cloaca. Two subtypes of B-lymphocytes are memory B-cells and plasma cells.

Hormones of the thymus include thymosins, thymopoietin, serum thymus factor, and thymic humoral factor (Figure 9.15). Lymphocytes undergo a maturation process that appears to be regulated by chemical messengers. **Thymosin** is the name given to one of the collections of thymic polypeptides from thymus extracts which promote maturation of lymphocytes. Some names of thymosins are thymosin ß$_4$ and thymosin α$_1$. **Thymopoietin** is another group of thymus hormones including thymic factor, thymopoietin I (TPI), and thymopoietin II (TPII). Thymopoietin causes bone marrow cells to differentiate into T-lymphocytes. **Serum thymus factor** (STF) from thymus restores immunity to thymectomized mice. **Thymic humoral factor** (THF) similarly restores mouse immunity and the cellular host-versus-graft responses.

Ablation of the the thymus from neonatal animals, such as newborn mice, causes a wasting disease and a loss of lymphocytes. The wasting disease can be reversed with thymus implants. When the thymus does not develop in humans, the immune system deficiency is called DiGeorge's syndrome. The thymus enlarges in autoimmune disorders (myasthenia gravis) and sometimes in hyperthyroidism. Sudden Infant Death Syndrome (SIDS) was once though to be caused by suffocation due to enlargement of the thymus, but Martin discredits this idea by arguing that thymuses of normal and SIDS infants are within the same size range, that enlarged animal thymuses have not been observed to cause suffocation, and that enlarged thymuses are caused by adrenal cortex insufficiency.[40]

The thymus exhibits numerous physiological changes and has been linked to the function of most of the other endocrine glands. Its weight varies in response to hormones: androgens, estrogens, glucocorticoids, growth hormone, progesterone, prolactin, mineralocorticoids, and thyroid hormones. Thymus weight changes in correlation with physiological events: time of day, season, molting, metamorphosis, reproduction, and starvation. The thymus has also been implicated in the regulation of minerals: calcium, sodium, potassium, chloride. A hypothalamic-gonadal-thymic axis can be proposed (Figure 9.16).

The recent awareness of bi-directional interactions amongst the central nervous system, endocrine system, and immune system has created a new discipline for research called neuroimmunoendocrinology. This relatively new field is poised to take a fresh approach in answering some of biology's more intriguing questions, such as what is the underlying mechanism for sexual dimorphism in the immune response?[41]

REFERENCES

1. Ericson, L.E.; Fredrikson, G. Phylogeny and ontogeny of the thyroid gland. In Greer, M.A., editor. The Thyroid Gland. New York: Raven Press Ltd.; 1990; pp. 1–35.

2. Sawin, C.T. Defining thyroid hormone: Its nature and control. In McCann, S.M., editor. Endocrinology: People and Ideas. Bethesda, MD: American Physiological Society; 1988; pp. 149–199.

3. Eales, J.G.; Grau, G.E.; McNabb, F.M.A.; Specker, J.L. Introduction to the Symposium: Comparative Endocrinology of the Thyroid Gland. American Zoologist 28: 295–296; 1988.

4. Turner, C.D.; Bagnara, J.T. General Endocrinology, Sixth Edition. Philadelphia: W. B. Saunders Co.; 1976; p. 180.

5. Telford, I.R.; Bridgman, C.F. Introduction to Functional Histology. New York: Harper & Row; 1990; p. 457.

6. Turner, C.D.; Bagnara, J.T. Op. cit. p. 196.

7. Telford, I.R.; Bridgman, C.F. Op. cit. p. 457.

8. Bartalena, L. Recent achievements in studies on thyroid hormone-binding proteins. Endocrine Reviews 11: 47; 1990.

9. Berry, M. J.; Larsen, P. R. The role of selenium in thyroid hormone action. Endocrine Reviews 13: 207–219; 1992.

10. Curran, P.G.; DeGroot, L.J. The effect of hepatic enzyme-inducing drugs on thyroid hormones and the thyroid gland. Endocrine Reviews 12: 135–150; 1991.

11. Ganong, W. Review of Medical Physiology, Fourteenth Edition. Norwalk, CT: Appleton & Lange, Norwalk; 1989; p. 272.

12. Gorbman, A.; Dickhoff, W.; Vigna, S.; Clark, N.; Ralph, C. Comparative Endocrinology. New York: John Wiley & Sons; 1983; p. 260.

13. Ismail-Beigi, F.; Gick, G.C.; Edellman, I.S. Thyroid hormone regulation of Na,K-ATPase. In Lardy, H.; Stratman, F., editors. Hormones, Thermogenesis, and Obesity. New York: Elsevier Science Publishing Co., Inc.; 1989; pp. 269–278.

14. Lardy, H.; Stratman, F. Hormones, Thermogenesis, and Obesity. New York: Elsevier; 1989; 528 pages.

15. Gorbman, A.; Dickhoff, W.; Vigna, S.; Clark, N.; Ralph, C. Op. cit. p. 267.

16. Ganong, W. Op. cit. p. 271.

17. Ganong, W. Op. cit. p. 279.

18. Henning, S.J. Permissive role of thyroxine in the ontogeny of jejunal sucrase. Endocrinology 102: 9–15; 1978.

19. Specker, J.L. Preadapative role of thyroid hormones in larval and juvenile salmon: Growth, the gut, and evolutionary considerations. Amer. Zool. 28: 337–349; 1988.

20. Oppenheimer, J.H.; Schwartz, H.L.; Mariash, C.N.; Kinlaw, W.B.; Wong, N.C.W., Freake, H.C. Advances in our understanding of thyroid hormone action at the cellular level. Endocrine Reviews 8: 288–308; 1987.

21. Oppenheimer, J.H.; Freake, H.C.; Santos, A.; Perez-Castillo, A.; Schwartz, H.L.; Kinlaw, W.B.; Mariash, C.N.; and Strait, K. In Lardy, H.; Stratman, F., editors. Hormones, Thermogenesis, and Obesity. New York: Elsevier Science Publishing Co., Inc.; 1989; pp. 289–299.

22. Sterling, K. The mitochondrial pathway of thyroid hormone action. In Lardy, H.; Stratman, F., editors. Hormones, Thermogenesis, and Obesity. New York: Elsevier Science Publishing Co., Inc.; 1989; pp. 301–309.

23. Hadley, M. E. Endocrinology. New York: Prentice Hall; 1992; p. 348.

24. Chan, V.; Jones, A.; Liendo-Ch. P.; McNeilly, A.; Landon, J.; Besser, G.M. The relationship between circadian variations in circulating thyrotrophin, thyroid hormones, and prolactin. Clinical Endocrinology 9: 347–349; 1978.

25. Oppenheimer, J.H.; Schwartz, H.L.; Mariash, C.N.; Kinlaw, W.B.; Wong, N.C.W., Freake,

H.C. Op. cit. p. 294.

26. Magner, J. Thyroid-stimulating hormone: Structure and function. In Ekholm, R.; Kohn, L.D.; Wollman, S. H., editors. Control of the Thyroid Gland. New York: Plenum Publishing Corporation, 1989, pp. 27–103.

27. Magner, J.A. Thyroid-stimulating hormone: Biosynthesis, cell biology, and bioactivity. Endocrine Reviews 11: 354–385; 1990.

28. Magner, J. A. Ibid.

29. Dent, J.N. Hormonal interaction in amphibian metamorphosis. Amer. Zool. 28: 297–308; 1988.

30. Hadley, M. E. Op. cit. p. 343.

31. Greenspan, F.S.; Rapoport, M.B. Thyroid Gland. In Greenspan, F.S., editor. Basic and Clinical Endocrinology, Third Edition. Norwalk, CT: Appleton & Lange; 1991; p. 197.

32. Welle, S.L. Dietary effects on thermogenesis in man: Role of norepinephrine and triiodothyronine. In Lardy, H.; Stratman, F., editors. Hormones, Thermogenesis, and Obesity. Elsevier Science Publishing Co., Inc., 1989, pp. 279–288.

33. Martin, C.R. Endocrine Physiology. New York: Oxford University Press; 1985; p. 776.

34. Brabant, G.; Prank, K.; Ranft, U.; Schuermeyer, T.; Wagner, T.O.F.; Hauser, H.; Kummer, B.; Feistner, H.; Hesch, R.D.; von zur Muhlen, A. Physiological regulation of circadian and pulsatile thyrotropin secretion in normal man and woman. J. Clin. Endocrinol. Metab. 70: 403–409; 1990.

35. Ganong, W. Op. cit. p. 276.

36. Robbins, T. Even Cowgirls Get the Blues. New York: Bantam Books: 1976; p. 144.

37. Michael, S.D.; Chapman, J.C. The influence of the endocrine system on the immune system. Immunology and Allergy Clinics of North America 10: 215–233; 1990.

38. Gillie, R. B. Endemic Goiter. Scientific American 224 (6): 92–101; 1971.

39. Telford, I.R.; Bridgman, C.F. Op. cit, p. 277.

40. Martin, C.R. Op. cit. p. 882.

41. Michael, S.D.; Chapman, J.C. Ibid.

CHAPTER 10

Parathyroid Hormone and Calcitonin

Parathyroid hormone from the parathyroid glands raises blood calcium. Calcitonin is the hormone of the thyroid parafollicular cells which lowers blood calcium. Together with a derivative of vitamin D (1α,25-dihydroxycholecalciferol), parathyroid hormone and calcitonin act on bone, intestine, and kidney to control the exchange of calcium between these organs and the extracellular fluid. Parathyroid hormone also regulates phosphate which combines with calcium to form the hydroxyapatite salts which account for most bone mineral.

OSTEOTROPIC AND CALCIOTROPIC HORMONES

Plasma calcium (Ca^{2+}) is subject to exquisite, fine-tuned, regulation in a variety of circumstances. There is a three-fold control system for regulating calcium using (i) parathyroid hormone, (ii) calcitonin, and (iii) $1\alpha,25$-dihydroxycholecalciferol. These three hormones, the osteotropic or calciotropic hormones, regulate calcium by their actions on intestine, bone, and kidney functions.

Bone remodeling, its formation by osteoblasts and its resorption by osteoclasts, is a lifelong process. Bone can be thought of as a result of the reaction of calcium and phosphate to form calcium-phosphate. To maintain bone, the calcium and phosphate and calcium-phosphate are maintained in equilibrium. To deposit new bone, calcium phosphate compounds must precipitate out of solutions containing calcium and phosphate. If there is enough calcium and phosphate, the solution is saturated and calcium phosphate precipitates as hydroxyapatite. In organisms with internal living skeletons, plasma calcium is undersaturated with respect to itself; supersaturated with respect to calcium phosphate in bone.

ANATOMY OF THE PARATHYROID GLAND

The parathyroid glands were discovered by Owen in 1850 in the rhinoceros and described by Sandstrom in 1880 (Figure 10.1). The parathyroids are found in pairs (one or two pairs) in other vertebrate groups. Parathyroids are absent in most teleost fish and neotenous amphibians. The human has four parathyroid glands weighing 30–35 mg apiece (Figure 10.2). The rat has one pair of parathyroid glands. In most species, the parathyroid glands are closely associated with the thyroid and are even, as in humans, embedded in its surface. But in some species, the parathyroid glands are spatially separated from the thyroid gland. The parathyroids received their blood supply from the thyroid arteries.

The parathyroid glands develop from endoderm. In humans they develop from the third and fourth pharyngeal pouches. There are two kinds of cells in the parathyroid gland (Figure 10.3). Most of the cells are **chief cells** which are the cells responsible for secreting parathyroid hormone. The less numerous cells, the **oxyphil** cells, are named for their staining properties. Their function is not known but they may be degenerated chief cells.[1]

Only a few factors alter the appearance of the parathyroid cells. Interestingly, in humans, the oxyphil cells make their appearance near the time of puberty. There may be follicles in the parathyroid glands. In amphibians and reptiles there is seasonal variation in parathyroid gland cytology. For example, in the frog, *Rana pipiens*, the cells have whorls in the summer and exhibit reticular degeneration in the winter.[2,3]

HISTOLOGY OF THE THYROID PARAFOLLICULAR CELLS

Calcitonin is a hormone of the thyroid gland. The cells responsible for calcitonin synthesis in mammals are the thyroid parafollicular cells, or C-cells, or clear cells. The parafollicular cells also synthesize serotonin.

In some birds, reptiles, amphibians, and fish, cells that are the equivalent of the parafollicular cells are organized into separate glands called the ultimobranchial glands. Ultimobranchial glands, like the parathyroids and thyroid and thymus, arise embryologically from the pharynx. In mammals, the most posterior (fifth pair) branchial pouches give rise to ultimobranchial glands which develop into the thyroid parafollicular cells. In humans, the appearance of functional parafollicular cells coincides with the onset of calcification in the fetus.

CHEMISTRY

Parathyroid hormone (parathormone, parathyrin, PTH) is a polypeptide hormone secreted by the parathyroid chief cells. Parathyroid hormone has 84 amino acids and MW 9600 (Figure 10.4). It is synthesized from larger precursor molecules in the manner of peptide hormones (Figure 10.5). Preproparathyroid hormone (preproPTH) has 115 amino acids and is the initial product made from the genes. In the production of parathyroid hormone it is cleaved at five sites. The "pre" sequence is a 23 amino acid hydrophobic sequence which binds the polyribosome-precursor complex to the endoplasmic reticulum. The enzyme, clipase, removes the presequence. This leaves a 90 amino acid proparathyroid hormone (proPTH) with MW 12,000. In the Golgi apparatus, tryptic clipase cuts off a six residue sequence from proPTH to produce

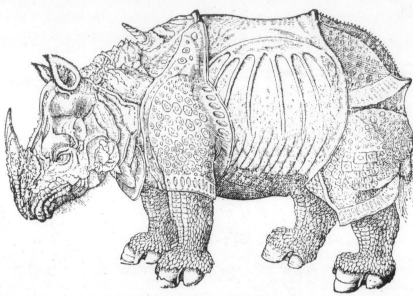

Figure 10.1 The parathyroid gland was discovered in the rhinoceros. The rendition of the rhinoceros is from Gesner's *Historiae Animalium* (1551–1587) which was translated into English by Topsell (1572–1638) as *The History of Four-Footed Beasts*. The drawing is not accurate; the position of the second horn is out of place. Reproduced, with permission. Moore, J.A. Understanding nature—Form and function. American Zoologist 28: 449–584; 1988.

parathyroid hormone which is secreted. Parathyroid hormone is cleaved into fragments in the chief cell secretory granules, chief cell cytoplasm, liver, and kidney. The mid and carboxy fragments are secreted by the chief cells; the amino fragment is recycled by the chief cell.

The PTH precursor molecules are not secreted under normal conditions, but pro-PTH has 3–50% of the activity of PTH. Pro-PTH is converted to PTH within 20 minutes after synthesis.[4] The 34 amino acids at the N-terminal of the PTH polypeptide (the amino fragment) have the biological activity. Bovine and porcine PTH differ from human PTH at eleven of the 84 amino acid residues.

Calcitonin is abbreviated CT.[5] Because of its thyroid gland origin in mammals, it has also been called thyrocalcitonin and abbreviated TC. Calcitonin has 32 amino acids, one disulfide bond, and MW 3000. Calcitonin is made and secreted in the parafollicular and ultimobranchial cells. Calcitonin levels are higher in human males than females and decrease with age. Calcitonin may come from other cells (extrathyroidal calcitonin) in addition to the parafollicular cells.

Vitamin D_3 (cholecalciferol) is a sterol (Figure 10.6). A derivative, **1α,25-dihydroxycholecalciferol** (1α,25 $(OH)_2$-D_3, calcitriol), can act like a hormone in the regulation of calcium. Some investigators do not discriminate between D_2 and D_3 (natural form), which differ by a double bond between C22 and C23, because in humans the metabolism and potency of both are similar, and these investigators refer to the active compound as 1,25 $(OH)_2$D.[6]

Vitamin D is synthesized in skin when ultraviolet light irradiates 7-dehydrocholesterol. Because of the requirement for light, vitamin D availability has seasonal and regional variations.

Vitamin D can also be obtained as a dietary supplement in the form of vitamin D_2 (ergocalciferol). Vitamin D_2 is made by irradiating ergosterol obtained from plants and adding the product to milk and dairy products as a food additive. Liver enzymes 25-hydroxylate vitamin D producing 25OH-D_3. Then, in the kidney, 25OH-D_3 is converted to the hormone form of vitamin D_3 by rate-limiting 1α-hydroxylation in the renal tubule mitochondria. 25OHD$_3$ has activity that

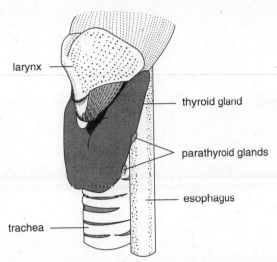

Figure 10.2 The internal gross anatomy of the human throat in three-quarters view shows two of the parathyroid glands along with the thyroid gland. Redrawn, with permission. Keeton, W. Biological Science, Third Edition. New York: Holt Rinehart and Winston; 1975; p. 368.

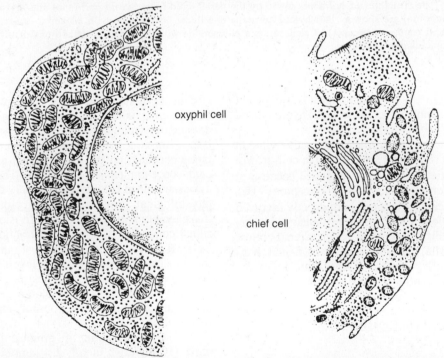

Figure 10.3 The figure shows sketches of two cell types of the parathyroid gland. The parathyroid gland is enclosed by a thin, fibrous capsule. The parathyroid parenchyma is divided into loose lobules by septa extending in from the capsule. Most cells are chief, or principal, cells that make parathyroid hormone. Chief cells are arranged in clumps or in cords and border on capillaries. Active chief cells have enlarged Golgi body, rER, small oval mitochondria, and 200–400 nm membrane-bound secretory granules near the cell membrane. The second cell type is the oxyphil or acidophil cell type which increase in number with age and appear in humans at the time of puberty. Oxyphil cells have smaller nuclei than chief cells and have an abundance of mitochondria with prominent cristae. Modified, with permission. Telford, I.R.; Bridgman, C.F. Introduction to Functional Histology. New York: Harper & Row, Pubs.; 1990; p. 461.

ser-val-ser-glu-ile-gln-leu-met-his-asn-
leu-gly-lys-his-leu-asn-ser-met-glu-arg-
val-glu-trp-leu-arg-lys-lys-leu-gln-asp-
val-his-asn-phe-val-ala-leu-gly-ala-pro-
leu-ala-pro-arg-asp-ala-gly-ser-gln-arg-
pro-arg-lys-lys-glu-asp-asn-val-leu-val-
glu-ser-his-glu-lys-ser-leu-gly-glu-ala-
asp-lys-ala-asp-val-asp-val-leu-thr-lys-
ala-lys-ser-gln

parathormone
84 amino acid residues

S-S

cys-gly-asn-leu-ser-thr-cys-met-leu-gly-
thr-tyr-thr-gln-asp-phe-asn-lys-phe-his-
thr-phe-pro-gln-thr-ala-ile-gly-val-gly-
ala-pro-NH_2

calcitonin
32 amino acid residues

Figure 10.4   The structures of hormones made by the parathyroid (parathyroid hormone) and thyroid parafollicular cells (calcitonin) are shown. Parathyroid hormone is a linear polypeptide with 84 amino acids (here arrayed in 10 amino acid residue sequences). Calcitonin is a polypeptide with 32 amino acids and one disulfide bond embracing amino acids one and seven.

may be biologically important, but it is less potent than the less abundant hormone, alpha hydroxylated vitamin D3 (Table 10.1).

A more general role for the active vitamin D derivative (dubbed 1,25(OH)2D) in cell growth and differentiation has been suggested because of the distribution of the 1,25(OH)2D receptor (VDL, vitamin D receptor) in tissues not directly involved in plasma calcium homeostasis (pituitary, pancreatic islet ß-cells, parathyroid gland, adrenal cortex, adrenal medulla, thyroid, ovary, testis, hematolymphopoietic cells, immune system, cardiac tissue, muscle, liver, central nervous system, skin, mammary gland, and placenta).[7,8]

BLOOD CALCIUM HOMEOSTASIS AND RHYTHMS

Blood calcium was viewed as being tightly regulated in a very narrow range, a concept referred to as "calcium homeostasis." **Homeostasis** is a term suggested by W.B. Cannon to describe "the various physiological arrangements which serve to restore the normal state, once it has been disturbed."[9] The concept of homeostasis plays a large

role in the understanding of calcium regulation. Homeostasis is achieved by mechanisms of endocrinology including set points and negative feedback. Hormones adjust calcium in order to maintain a constant internal environment as far as calcium concentrations are concerned. The idea is that a constant blood calcium is necessary for the many physiological processes (blood clotting, bone, transmembrane potentials, cell division, hormone signal conduction, stimulus contraction coupling, etc.). However compelling, the argument ignores the evidence that blood calcium levels are not constant: there are times of day, certain species, and physiological states in which blood calcium is well outside the narrow range supposedly maintained by homeostasis.

Blood calcium in humans is about 10 mg% (10 mg/dl, 5 meq/l, 2.5 mmol/l, 2,500,000 nmol/l).   A portion (46%) of the total blood calcium is bound to serum albumin. The remaining calcium, 54% is considered to be diffusible, and therefore available, in the form of ionized calcium (47% of total calcium is Ca^{2+}) or complexed with small molecules (bicarbonate, citrate, etc.).

The diffusible calcium, but not the bound calcium, is available and can be used for coagula-

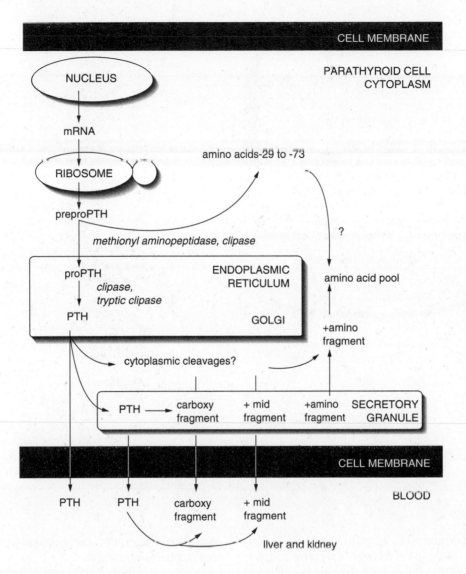

Figure 10.5 The diagram illustrates the synthesis and secretion of parathyroid hormone (amino acids 1–84) and its carboxy and mid fragments (amino acids 34–84) by a parathyroid chief cell. The amino fragment (amino acids 1–34) is recycled.

tion of blood, nerve activities, and muscle contraction. Blood calcium fluctuates with daily rhythms (Figure 10.7) that peak around 10 a.m. The changes are small (e.g., about 0.4 mg% for total blood calcium). PTH levels peaked at 0300–0600 in another study.[10]

Calcium acts in the mechanisms of action of some hormones. Calcium can act as a second messenger using calcium-binding proteins such as calmodulin. Hormones release calcium from the endoplasmic reticulum or increase transport of calcium into cells to increase intracellular calcium (extracellular calcium is 10^{-3}M; intracellular calcium is 10^{-7}M).

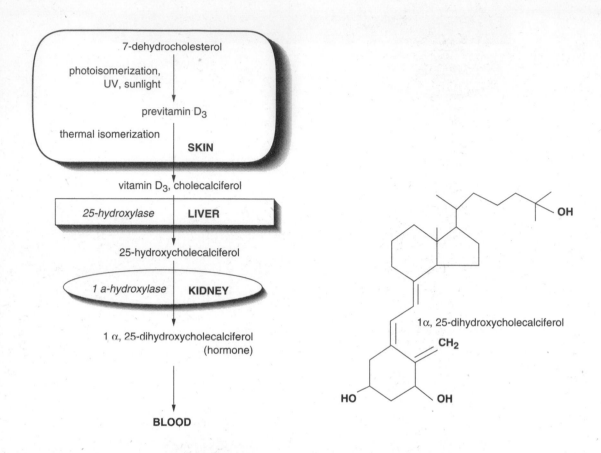

Figure 10.6 The diagram illustrates the synthesis of 1α,25-dihydroxycholecalciferol.

Calcium is supplied by the diet. Minimum daily **nutritional calcium** requirements in humans range from 360 mg in infants to 800 mg in children and adult women and 1200 mg in men.[11] It is absorbed from the gastrointestinal tract. Once in the body, calcium is transported in the fluids. Calcium absorption in food in the gastrointestinal tract requires both active transport and passive diffusion. The absorption process occurs at the brush border of the gastrointestinal cells and it involves an ATPase. Calcium absorption rates adapt to calcium intake levels; calcium absorption rates are higher when total calcium ingestion is reduced. Active transport and passive diffusion also function to transport inorganic phosphorus (P_i).

Phosphorus absorption rate is linearly proportional to phosphorus in the diet.

Much higher levels of blood calcium in species of animals which must meet a calcium challenge in the environment. For example, laying hens need high calcium to produce eggs and their blood calcium, particularly the bound calcium, is elevated as might be expected. Calcium metabolism was studied in pack rats (*Neotoma micropus*). The animals are abundant in southwest Texas where they feed upon and build large nests in the branching arms of the prickly pear cactus. However, the cactus (like spinach) has high levels of oxalate, a compound that chelates calcium making it physiologically unavailable. The pack

Table 10.1 Amounts of Hormones, Calcium, and Phosphorus

Parameter	Value
HORMONES	
parathyroid hormone blood	10–55 ng/l
parathyroid hormone half-life	2–4 minutes
calcitonin in human blood	0–28 pg/ml
$1\alpha,25(OH)_2D_3$ in human blood	30 pg/ml
25OHD$_3$ in human blood	30 ng/ml
CALCIUM	
total blood calcium in humans	8.8–10.4 mg%
ionized (or diffusible) blood calcium mammals	4.5 mg%
fish blood calcium	20 mg%
rooster blood calcium	10 mg%
laying hen (with estrogen) blood calcium	30–100 mg%
total adult calcium	1200–1400 grams
human cerebrospinal fluid calcium	5 mg%
free Ca^{2+} in interstitial fluid	1200 nmol/l
free Ca^{2+} in cytoplasm	100 nmol/l
hyperparathyroid mammal, blood calcium	>10 mg%
hypoparathyroid mammal, blood calcium	5–7 mg%
PHOSPHORUS	
adult human, total phosphate	500–800 grams
children, plasma phosphate	5–7 mg%
adult plasma phosphate	3.0–4.5 mg%
total plasma phosphorus	12 mg%

Ganong, W. Review of Medical Physiology, Fourteenth Edition. Norwalk, CT: Appleton & Lange; 1989; pp. 326–337; Arnaud, C.D.; Kolb, F.O. The calciotropic hormones and metabolic bone disease. In Greenspan, F.; Forsham, P. Basic and Clinical Endocrinology, Second Edition. Norwalk, CT: Appleton & Lange; 1987; pp. 202–271; Turner, D.C.; Bagnara, J.T. General Endocrinology, Sixth Edition. Philadelphia, PA: W. B. Saunders Co.; 1976; p. 233; Mallette, L.E.; Gagel, R.F. Parathyroid Hormone and Calcitonin. Primer on Metabolic Bone Diseases and Disorders of Mineral Metabolism, pp. 65–70; Berkow, R. The Merck Manual Sixteenth Edition. Rahway, NJ: Merck & Co. Inc.; 1992; p. 2584.

rats had high levels of blood calcium and possessed a huge cecum which may have been an adaptive response to the oxalate challenge. Possible sources of calcium for the rats were the abundant sea shells that littered the desert floor. Fish have high blood calcium levels but lack parathyroid glands.

Inside the body, calcium is distributed in the extracellular fluid and "stored" in large quantities, 99%, in **bone**. Bone turns over 100% of its calcium per year in children but only 18% per year in adults. The bone cells are the **osteocytes** (trapped in the bony matrix). The cells that form bone by secreting a protein collagen matrix are called **osteoblasts** (located near bony surfaces and interfacing with the vascular compartment); the calcium matrix subsequently calcifies. The cells that are responsible for resorption (reabsorption) of bone are the multinuclear **osteoclasts**.

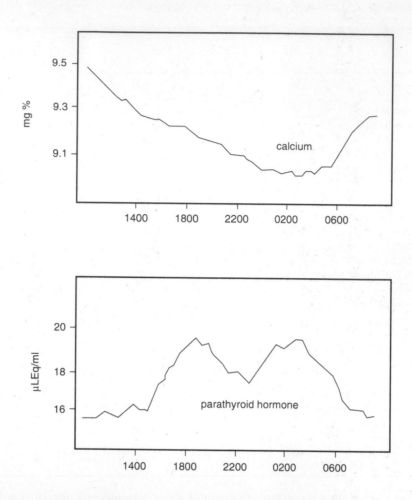

Figure 10.7 The graphs illustrate rhythms in human blood total calcium that peak in the morning and rhythms in parathyroid hormone which was high at night (1800–0800). Ionized calcium peaks around 0100 but has its nadir about 1700 (not shown); phosphate rose around 1700 and peaked at 0400 (not shown). In another study, the parathyroid hormone rhythm was quite different and peaked in the last part of the night (0300–0600). Redrawn, with permission. Markowitz, M.E.; Arnaud, S.; Rosen, J.F.; Thorpy, M.; Saximinarayan, S. Temporal interrelationships between the circadian rhythms of serum parathyroid hormone and calcium concentrations. J. Clin. Endocrin. Metab. 67: 1068–1073; 1988.

Calcium excretion is via the feces from the gastrointestinal tract and via the urine from the kidneys. The kidney proximal tubules and ascending Henle's loops and distal tubules reabsorb calcium, and thereby conserve, 98–99% of the calcium that filters in the glomerulus.

The calciotropic hormones, parathyroid hormone, calcitonin, and vitamin D regulate calcium balances in the gastrointestinal tract, bone, and kidneys.

PHOSPHORUS

Phosphorus is found in ATP and cyclic AMP and in other important biological molecules. But 85–95% of phosphorus is in the skeleton. In

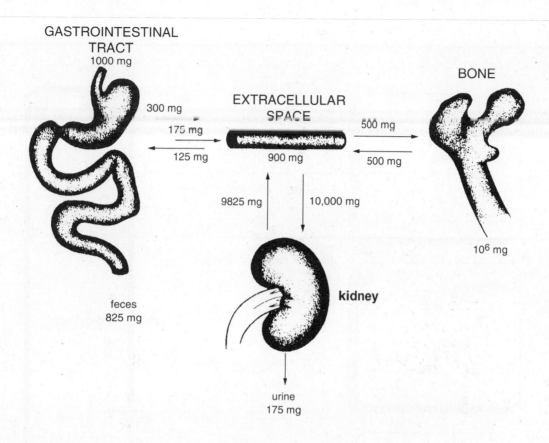

GASTROINTESTINAL
TRACT
1000 mg

EXTRACELLULAR
SPACE

BONE

300 mg

175 mg

125 mg

900 mg

500 mg

500 mg

9825 mg

10,000 mg

10^6 mg

kidney

feces
825 mg

urine
175 mg

Figure 10.8 The figure shows the calcium balance for a human subject on an average diet. Reproduced, with permission. West, J.B., editor. Physiological Basis of Medical Practice, Twelfth Edition. Baltimore: Williams & Wilkins; 1991; p. 834.

plasma, two-thirds of the phosphorus is in organic compounds. The other third of the phosphate is in inorganic compounds (designated Pi): 85% of the phosphorus is quite soluble phosphate, 15% is biphosphate which does not form calcium salt, and <1% is H_3PO_4 whose calcium salt is quite insoluble.

Calcium absorption from the gastrointestinal tract is decreased by compounds that bind calcium into salts or soaps (phosphate, oxalate, alkalis). Some plants (e.g., spinach) contain oxalates which might be detrimental to calcium acquisition. Urinary phosphate is decreased by parathyroidectomy. PTH injections increase urine phosphate (phosphaturia) by acting on the proximal convoluted tubule.

BONE

Bone is a target of parathyroid hormone. The osteoblasts are the likely target cells for parathyroid hormone. Parathyroid hormone in

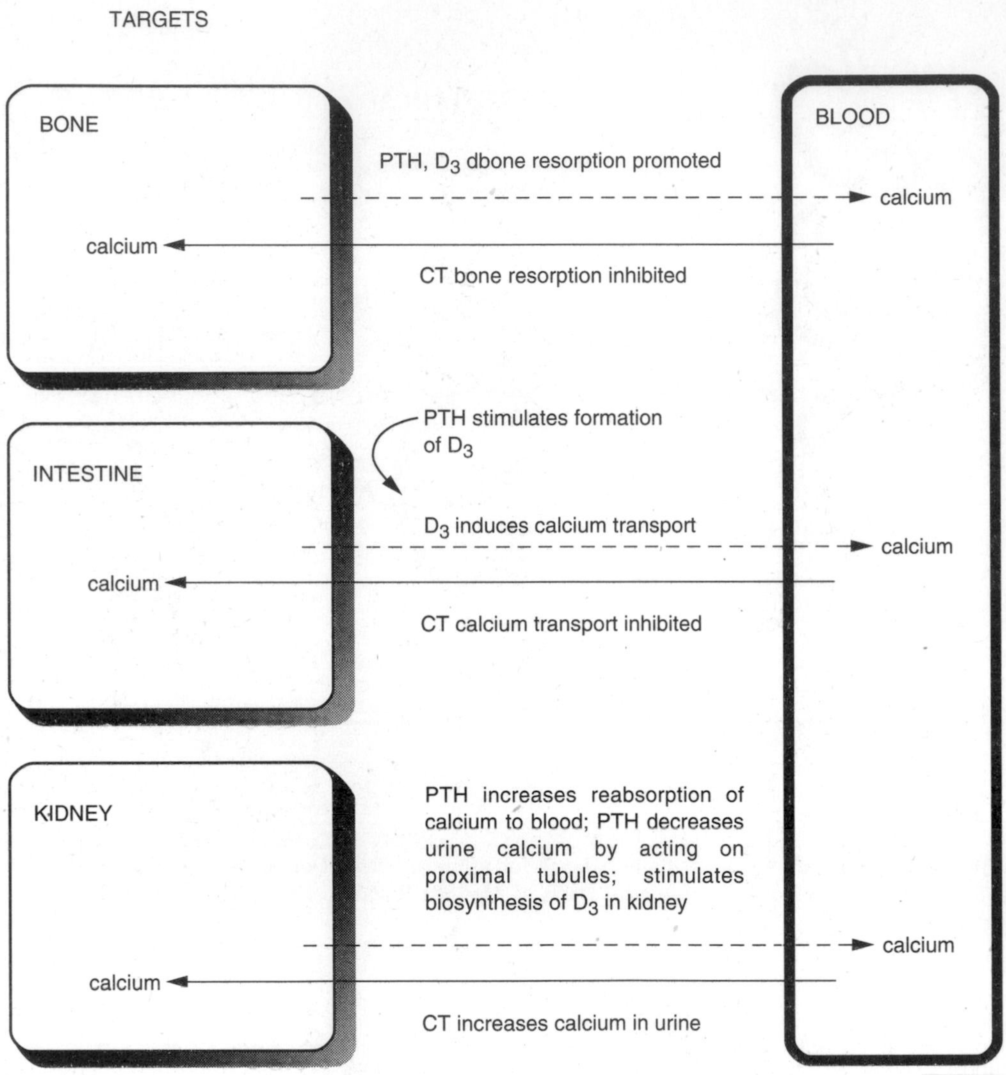

TARGETS

Figure 10.9 The diagram illustrates the influences of calcitropic hormones (parathyroid hormone and calcitonin) and vitamin D_3 on the calcium fluxes of the target organs (bone, kidney, intestine). Parathyroid hormone increases plasma calcium; calcitonin decreases plasma calcium.

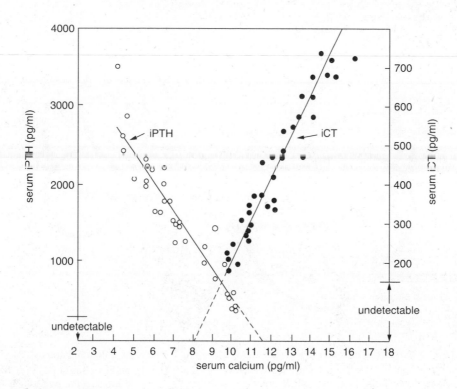

Figure 10.10 The graphs show the way that parathyroid hormone decreases and calcitonin increases with increasing serum calcium levels. iPTH = immunoreactive parathyroid hormone; iCT = immunoreactive calcitonin. With permission. Arnaud, C.D. et al. In Taylor, S., editor. Calcitonin: Proceedings of the Second International Symposium. Heinemann; 1969.

creases bone resorption, mobilizes Ca^{2+}, and thereby increases blood calcium.

Some investigators think that bone is also a target of calcitonin. Calcitonin inhibits bone resorption by inhibiting Ca^{2+} permeability of osteoclasts, preventing its return from the bone fluid compartment to the blood, but the role of calcitonin is less well established than that of parathyroid hormone. Low or high calcitonin has no adverse affects on bone and calcitonin has only short-term effects on blood calcium. Thus, investigators speculate that the role of calcitonin may be in meeting calcium challenges. For example, calcitonin could function in the development of the skeleton when bone turnover is high, or calcitonin may prevent hypercalcemia after a meal, or calcitonin could protect maternal bones from calcium loss during pregnancy or lactation.

GUT

Gastrointestinal acquisition of calcium and P_i from food is stimulated by $1\alpha,25$-dihydroxycholecalciferol (active hormonal form of vitamin D_3) when calcium is low. The mechanism of action of $1\alpha,25$-dihydroxycholecalciferol is the steroid type of mechanism of action. The mechanism involves a cytoplasmic receptor in intestinal epithelial cells, formation of a hormone-receptor complex that moves to the nucleus, and increased new mRNA which is translated to make new calcium-binding protein. The active transport mechanism becomes saturated when high calcium levels are in the diet, so that dietary calcium supplements

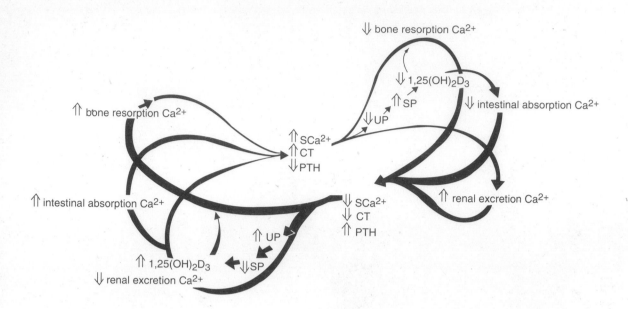

Figure 10.11 The diagram illustrates the maintenance of calcium levels, or calcium homeostasis. In the central region are blood levels of calcium (SCa^{2+}), parathyroid hormone (PTH), and calcitonin (CT). The loops relate the blood levels to three target organs: bone, intestine, and kidney. On the left are the events—increased bone resorption, increased intestinal absorption, and decreased renal excretion—that increase blood calcium concentration. On the right are the events—decreased bone resorption, decreased intestinal absorption, and increased renal excretion—that decrease blood calcium concentration. UP = urine phosphorus; SP = serum phosphorus. Modified, with permission. Arnaud, C.D. Calcium homeostasis: Regulatory elements and their integration. Federation Proceedings 37: 2557; 1978.

have limited value in increasing amounts of calcium that can be used by the body. Phosphates, oxalates, and alkalis that react with calcium prevent its absorption from the intestine, but high dietary protein increases calcium absorption. Parathyroid hormone stimulates formation of $1\alpha,25$-dihydroxycholecalciferol and thereby increases the absorption of calcium and phosphate from the gastrointestinal tract.

KIDNEY

Kidney function in calcium balance is regulated by hormones. Parathyroid hormone stimulates recovery of calcium from the lumen of the kidney tubules. Parathyroid hormone increases phosphate excretion by the renal tubules which stops serum phosphate from rising. Parathyroid hormone also stimulates the kidney mitochondrial enzyme, $25OHD_3$ 1α-hydroxylase, to promote formation of $1\alpha,25(OH_2)D_3$. Calcitonin acts on kidney to decrease the return of calcium and phosphate from the renal tubule. The kidney is a main target of vitamin D_3 where it increases phosphate and calcium reabsorption.

OTHER ACTIONS OF PARATHYROID HORMONE, CALCITONIN, AND VITAMIN D

The calciotropic hormones may have actions other than those in calcium regulation.

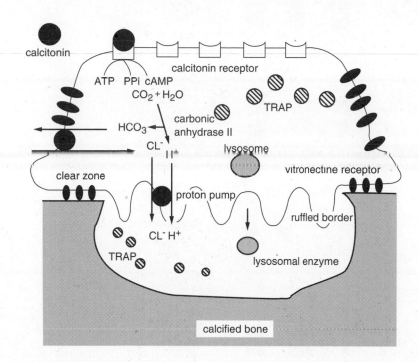

Figure 10.12 Osteoclasts, which have calcitonin receptors, are responsible for bone resorption which is accomplished by an acidic bone-resorbing area under a ruffled border. TRAP = tartrate-resistant acid phosphatase (a histochemical marker whose precise role is not known).   Modified, with permission. Suda, T.; Takahashi, N.; Martin, T.J. Modulation of osteoclast differentiation. Endocrine Reviews 13: 66–80; 1992.

Parathyroid hormone increases mitotic rates (mitogenic action) and has some vasodilator activity (vasodepressor action). Calcitonin may act as a satiety hormone and calcitonin injections may lower body weight.[12]

REGULATION AND MECHANISMS OF ACTION

Regulation of the hormones is straightforward and involves small serum calcium fluctuations (Figures 10.8, 10.9, 10.10, 10.11). Serum calcium is involved in negative feedback regulation of parathyroid hormone.[13] Increases in plasma calcium release calcitonin. Vitamin D formation is stimulated by parathyroid hormone.

Parathyroid hormone secretion is controlled by calcium acting directly on the glands—parathyroid hormone secretion is increased by hypocalcemia and decreased by hypercalcemia—parathyroid hormone secretion is inversely proportional to extracellular calcium concentration in the physiological range. This inverse relationship is paradoxical because increased intracellular calcium stimulates secretion; peak parathyroid hormone secretion occurs when intracellular calcium concentration is about 200 nM.[14]

The mechanism of action of parathyroid hormone on kidney and bones involves a membrane receptor and increased formation of cyclic AMP. Osteoclasts have calcitonin receptors (Figure 10.12). The model implies a role for calcitonin, mediated by cAMP, in lessening the acidity produced by the osteoclasts and thereby inhibiting bone resorption; calcitonin also inhibits bone resorption by reducing the number of osteoclasts.[15]

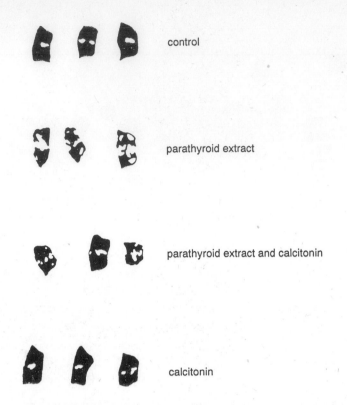

control

parathyroid extract

parathyroid extract and calcitonin

calcitonin

Figure 10.13 The figure illustrates alteration in bone by parathyroid extract and calcitonin. Bone (flat calvaria, cranium from young rats, represented here as three pieces per treatment) was cultured with control solutions, or with parathyroid gland extract (0.5 u/ml) and/or calcitonin (13 u/ml). Following culture the bone was stained. Bone resorption areas are white patches; unaffected bone is black. Parathyroid extract caused bone resorption; calcitonin inhibited the resorption caused by parathyroid extract. After Aliapoulios, M.A.; Goldhaber, P.; Munson, P. Thyrocalcitonin inhibition of bone reabsorption induced by PTH in tissue culture. Science 151: 330-331; 1966.

METHODS, ASSAYS, AND HETEROGENEITY OF PEPTIDE HORMONES

An interesting technique was used to study the functions of calcium-regulating hormones (sometimes called calciotropic hormones[16]). **Peritoneal lavage** was used to alter the levels of calcium in blood. In the procedure, a metal tube that penetrated the skin, muscles, and peritoneum was sewn into a rat's abdominal wall. The tube was threaded and closed externally with a screw-cap top. In an experiment, high or low calcium solutions were placed in the abdominal cavity through a catheter threaded into the metal tube. Thus the intestines and internal organs could be bathed in a solution and the blood calcium could be raised or lowered.

A bioassay was done with bone (Figure 10.13). In one bioassay, bone (e.g., from the cranium or calvaria of rats) could be cultured. Hormones (e.g., parathyroid gland extract, calcitonin) or control solutions were added to the culture medium. The effect on the bone was visualized by staining. However, bioassays were not sensitive enough to measure PTH in the blood. Ganong addresses this problem:

This obstacle has now been overcome by 2 novel approaches. One is a cytochemical bioassay that is based on the PTH-specific stimulation of glucose 6-phosphate dehydrogenase in guinea pig renal slices. This assay [measures] femtogram amounts of

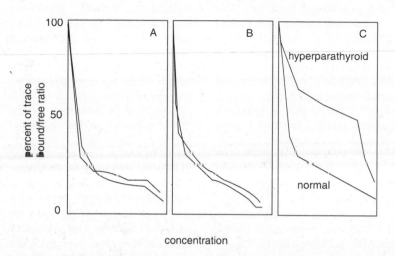

Figure 10.14 The graphs show the inhibition of binding of radioactively labelled bovine parathyroid hormone on three antisera (A,B,C) from a hyperparathyroid individual and by normal human parathyroid gland extract. The A and B antisera gave similar inhibitions for normal and hyperparathyroid samples as concentration increased (from left to right on the abscissa). But the C antiserum gave very different results for the two samples. The data are explained by hypothesizing that the A and B antisera recognized the same sites on both the normal and hyperparathyroid samples, but that the C antibody detected differences in the sites of the normal and hyperparathyroid samples implying that the peptides were different. After Yalow, R.S. Heterogeneity of peptide hormones. Recent Progress in Hormone Research 30: 596–632; 1974.

PTH . . . . The other assay...uses a non-hydrolyzable analog of guanosine triphosphate...to augment the sensitivity of adenylate cyclase to PTH in canine kidneys *in vitro* [and detects] as little as 10 pg/mL of intact PTH.[17]

Radioimmunoassays are used to measure parathyroid hormone and calcitonin. A problem for parathyroid hormone was inherent in the heterogeneity of peptide hormones. When different antisera were used to measure human parathyroid hormone, the different antisera did not give the same results (Figure 10.14). These differences were also proved with fractionation techniques for purification and sequencing hormones with physical and chemical systems. The differences in antisera findings are due to differences in the concentrations of the various forms of PTH and its fragments that are circulating in the blood.[18] Heterogeneity of peptide hormones also occurs for other peptide hormones (e.g., insulin, gastrin, corticotropin, and somato-tropin). Nevertheless, radioimmunoassays are still effective tools for measuring the concentrations of hormones.

DISEASES RELATED TO CALCIUM-REGULATING HORMONES

Hypoparathyroidism is the disorder of parathyroid hormone deficiency. Parathyroid hormone is essential for life. Parathyroidectomy can cause death within 6–10 hours. Neuromuscular hyperactivity, hypocalcemia, hyperphosphatemia, and low plasma parathyroid hormone are symptoms of hypoparathyroidism. Hypoparathyroidism can be idiopathic (no known cause), functional (after long-term magnesium deprivation from gastrointestinal failure to absorb magnesium), or resulting from surgical damage to or removal of the parathyroid glands. In hypoparathyroidism there is decreased bone resorption, renal phosphate excretion, and renal synthesis of $1\alpha,25\text{-}(OH_2)D_3$. Calcium excretion increases. The neuromuscular increase in excitability are a consequence of low calcium and alkalosis from reduced bicarbonate excretion. The neuromuscular effects can be dramatic: paresthesias (numbness and tingling in extremities), **low calcium tetany** (muscle spasms and contortion of hands, arms, and feet), hyperventilation, adrenergic symptoms (sweating, pallor, increased heart rate, anxiety from epinephrine), convulsions, Trousseau's sign of latent tetany (carpal spasm in the hand of a cuffed arm), Chvostek's sign (contraction of facial muscles in response to facial nerve tapping at the jaw), Parkinsonism, cataracts, prolongation of the cardiac Q-T interval, dental abnormalities, and intestinal malabsorption.

Hyperparathyroidism has several possible causes. The consequences of hyperparathyroidism include hypercalcemia, hypophosphatemia, bone demineralization, hypophosphaturia, kidney stone formation, excess parathyroid hormone secretion, and bone disease (osteitis fibrosa cystica). Hyperparathyroidism has also been called von Recklinghausen's disease for his description of the skeletal deformities in 1891. An array of symptoms includes weakness, anorexia, nausea, constipation, abdominal pain, intestinal obstruction, nocturia, polyuria, thirst, kidney stones, peptic ulcers, bone disease, confusion, depression, and psychosis.

Rickets (osteomalacia) results from any of several causes which include vitamin D deficiency and insufficient sunlight. In rickets, the normal bone mineralization and maturation does not occur in children or young animals.

Another disorder, **Paget's disease** (osteitis deformans), has excess osteoblasts and osteoclasts which result in isolated areas of very rapid bone remodelling. This leads to localized excessive bone loss resulting in fragile bones, especially the femur, skull, tibia, lumbosacral spine, and pelvis. It may be due to a slow virus. Paget's disease is found in about 4% of people in Germany and England after age 40, less in other regions, and rarely before age 40. Calcitonin is used in treating Paget's disease.

Still another disorder of calcium is hypercalciuria (>250–300 mg calcium in the urine per 24 hours) which can result in formation of calcium containing **kidney stones** if oxalate is present. Hypercalciuria can be due to hyperparathyroidism, high calcium ingestion (800–1400 mg/day), or high protein injections.

Osteoporosis is loss of bone quantity, or bone mass, which results in fragile bones which are easily broken. Arms, hips, and vertebrae are frequent fracture sites. Osteoporosis is common in postmenopausal women. Osteoporosis can result from genetic factors, nutritional deficiency, too little sunlight, hypogonadism (low estrogen), drugs, smoking, gastrointestinal or kidney disease, hyperparathyroidism, hyperthyroidism, immobilization, and excessive exercise or lack of exercise. Risk of osteoporosis is increased by Caucasian ancestry, northern European descent, small size, and female gender. Osteoporosis in postmenopausal women is associated with estrogen deficiency. Estrogen replacement therapy prevents bone loss in aging individuals. The estrogen may act by osteoblasts which have estrogen-binding sites. Estrogen replacement therapy is the main treatment for osteoporosis in women. Increased dietary calcium, moderate exercise, and even phototherapy (to increase vitamin D formation) have also been recommended for aging women in the hope of ameliorating osteoporosis. Older people with osteoporosis have reduced vitamin D and parathyroid hormone, so parathyroid hormone or calcitonin in combination with calcium supplements has been tried for treating osteoporosis with partial, but disappointing, success. Osteoporosis can also result from excess glucocorticoids as occurs in Cushing's disease. Disuse osteoporosis is another problem where bone resorption rate exceeds bone formation rate. On earth, disuse osteoporosis occurs in immobile patients. Disuse osteoporosis is a problem for space travel because of the reduction of gravity.

ANOTHER POINT OF VIEW

For the role of hormones in calcium regulation, as well as other areas of endocrinology, there are divergent points of view. While the preceding may be the view of 90% of endocrinologists, there are still some 10% mavericks who hold a different view, and a great many of us with specific questions.

After a lifetime of study of the hormones regulating calcium,[19,20] Talmage is convinced that "the basic role of PTH is to set and maintain within narrow limits the ionized calcium level of plasma."[21] He "doubts...the physiological role of calcitonin in controlling plasma calcium levels [and believes that it uses] phosphate in some manner to store calcium entering postprandially onto the surface of bone to provide a more balanced supply of this cation for bone metabolism."[22]

REFERENCES

1. Martin, C.R. Endocrine Physiology. New York: Oxford University Press; 1985; p. 464.

2. Cortelyou, J.R.; McWhinnie, D.J. Parathyroid glands in amphibians. Parathyroid structure and function in the amphibians, with emphasis on regulation of mineral ions in body fluids. Amer. Zool. 7: 843; 1967.

3. McWhinnie, D.J.; Cortelyou, J.R. Influence of parathyroid extract on blood and urine mineral levels in iguanid lizards. Gen. Comp. Endocrinology 11: 78; 1986.

4. Habener, J.F.; Kemper, J.F.; Rich, A.; Potts, J.T. Biosynthesis of parathyroid hormone. Recent Prog. Horm. Res. 33: 249–308; 1977.

5. Rasmussen, H.; Pechet, M.M. Calcitonin. Scientific American 223 (October): 42–50; 1970.

6. Bikle, D. D. Vitamin D, calcium, and epidermal differentiation. Endocrine Reviews 14: 3–19; 1993.

7. Walters, M.R. Newly identified actions of the vitamin D endocrine system. Endocrine Reviews 13: 719–764; 1992.

8. Bikle, D.D. Vitamin D: New Actions, new analogs, new therapeutic potential. Endocrine Reviews 13: 765–784; 1992.

9. Cannon, W.B. The Wisdom of the Body, New York: Norton; 1932.

10. Loque, F.C.; Fraser, W.D.; O'Reilly, St.J.; Beastall, G.H. The circadian rhythm of intact parathyroid hormone 1–84 and nephrogenous cyclic adenosine monophosphate in normal men. J. Clin. Endocrin. Metab. 121: R1–R3; 1989

11. Recommended Dietary Allowances, Ninth Edition, Food and Nutrition Board, National Research Council, National Academy of Sciences, 1980.

12. Freed, W.J.; Perlow, M.J.; Wyatt, R.J. Calcitonin: Inhibitory effect on eating. Science 206: 850–852; 1979.

13. Pocotte, S.L.; Ehrenstein, G.; Fitzpatrick, L.A. Regulation of parathyroid hormone secretion. Endocrine Reviews 12: 291–301; 1991.

14. Pocotte, S.L.; Ehrenstein, G.; Fitzpatrick, L. Ibid.

15. Suda, T.; Takahashi, N.; Martin, J.T. Modulation of osteoclast differentiation. Endocrine Reviews 13: 66–80; 1992.

16. Deftos, L.J.; Bayard, D.; Catherwood, M.D. Syndromes involving multiple endocrine glands. In Greenspan, F.; Forsham, P., Editors. Basic and Clinical Endocrinology, Second Edition. Norwalk, CT: Appleton & Lange; 1986; p. 202.

17. Deftos, L.J.; Bayard, D.; Catherwood, M.D. Ibid; p. 209.

18. Yalow, R. S. Heterogeneity of peptide hormones. Recent Progress in Hormone Research 30: 597–632; 1974.

19. Talmage, R.V.; Cooper, C.W. Physiology and mode of action of calcitonin. In DeGroot, L.J., editor. Endocrinology 2: 647; 1979.

20. Talmage, R.V. The influence of endogenous or exogenous calcitonin on daily urinary calcium excretion. Endocrinology 101: 1351–1357; 1977.

21. Talmage (Personal Communication).

22. Talmage, R.V. Comment on the physiological role of calcitonin. Bone and Mineral 16: 186; 1992.

CHAPTER 11

Insulin and Glucagon from the Pancreas

The pancreas secretes digestive enzymes and hormones that function in intermediary metabolism. Insulin is a hormone made in islets of cells in the pancreas. Insulin lowers blood sugar because it promotes the transport of glucose into most of the cells of the body. Deficiency of insulin is a characteristic of the disease diabetes mellitus. Glucagon, gastrin, somatostatin, and pancreatic polypeptide are other hormones of the pancreas.

PANCREAS

Pancreatic physiology is divided into exocrine and endocrine functions. The exocrine pancreas makes digestive enzymes. The hormones that the pancreas makes—insulin, glucagon, gastrin, somatostatin, pancreatic polypeptide—function in the regulation of intermediary metabolism (Figure 11.1). These functions make some anatomical sense because the pancreas is located adjacent to the small intestine in the abdomen. Simply put, sugar can be obtained from the digestion of foodstuffs (promoted by pancreatic enzymes) and by recovery from compounds in the body (e.g., glycogen).

Blood glucose is the major source of energy for the central nervous system, so brain function is particularly susceptible to abnormal swings in blood glucose levels. Indeed, 2-deoxyglucose, which is taken up like glucose but which is not metabolized, can be used to map regions of neuron activity in experimental animals or in living humans by PET scanning. The brain uses up its available glycogen and glucose in about two minutes if the blood supply is interrupted. The dogma—that insulin is not required for brain glucose utilization—has been challenged by evidence that insulin and its receptor are found in adult mammalian brain, that insulin may cross the blood brain barrier using a specialized transport system, and that alteration of food intake behavior by insulin.[1]

Diabetes, a disease involving the endocrine pancreas, is an important human disease because it affects large portions of the population. Because of this, there has been considerable research on diabetes, and this research has resulted in early prominence of insulin in biology and medicine that involve pancreatic function and the hormone insulin. Insulin was the first protein whose amino acid sequence was discovered (by Sanger, 1959 Nobel Prize), the first protein to be synthesized (by Katsoyannis and colleagues, 1963), and one of the first proteins whose three-dimensional structure was learned from X-ray crystallographic analysis (Dorothy Hodgkin, 1972). Insulin was used to develop the radioimmunoassay technique (Solomon Berson and Rosalyn Yalow). Insulin was one of the first human genes to be cloned (Bell and colleagues 1980), and it was the first commercial product of recombinant DNA (1979).[2,3]

Most endocrinology of the pancreas settles around the "islet organ" and the hormones insulin, glucagon, pancreatic polypeptide, and somatostatin. Epple and Brinn suggest that the islet organ should be interpreted in a larger way as one member of a group of endocrine organs and tissues that share a common ancestor identical with the open-type basal-granulated cells of the gastroderm of the hydra and the open cells in the digestive mucosa where the gastrointestinal contents provide stimuli (pH, amino acids) to which the cells respond with secretions.[4]

GROSS ANATOMY AND DEVELOPMENT

The pancreas is found nested in the greater curvature of the stomach and along the loops of the intestines in the region of the duodenum (Figure 11.2). Embryologically, the pancreas arises from endoderm from two duodenal diverticula which later fuse. So the origin of the pancreas is probably endoderm, but it has also been suggested that the endocrine portion develops from neural ectoderm. In the human, the pancreas is sometimes grossly described as having a "head," a "body," and a "tail."

EXOCRINE PANCREAS

The portion that produces digestive enzymes constitutes 97–98% of the weight of the pancreas and is the **exocrine pancreas**. The pancreas produces carboxypeptidase B, colipase, pancreatic lipase, cholesteryl ester hydrolase, pancreatic α-amylase, ribonuclease, deoxyribonuclease, phospholipase A_2, enteropeptidase, chymotrypsinogen, and aminopeptidases. The enzymes are secreted through the pancreatic duct into the duodenum of the alimentary canal in an alkaline pancreatic juice containing bicarbonate (HCO_3^-). The pancreatic enzymes act in the digestion of proteins, fats, triglycerides, cholesteryl esters, starches, nucleic acids, and phospholipids. The secretion of pancreatic juice is controlled by gastrointestinal hormones (secretin, cholecystokinin) and the transmitter, acetylcholine, from the vagus nerve.

Acinar cells comprise the exocrine pancreas that secretes pancreatic juice. The digestive enzymes are found in intracellular granules called the **zymogen granules**. The enzymes are secreted by exocytocis into pancreatic duct lumens which join to form a single duct (duct of Wirsung) which joins the bile duct forming the ampulla of Vater before opening into the duodenum.

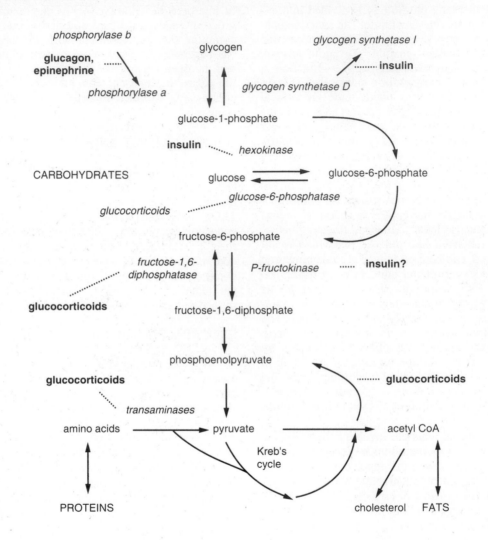

Figure 11.1 A simplified diagram of intermediary metabolism shows the points where hormones (glucocorticoids, insulin, glucagon, epinephrine) affect the activity of enzymes. Modified, with permission. Frieden, E.; Lipner, H. Biochemical Endocrinology of the Vertebrates. Englewood Cliffs, NJ: Prentice-Hall; 1971; p. 71.

ANATOMY OF THE ENDOCRINE PANCREAS

Islets of Langerhans (islet organs) make up the endocrine portion of the pancreas (Figure 11.3). The islet tissue accounts for two to three percent of the weight of the pancreas; islet tissue weighs only about one to two grams in adult humans. The islets secrete four peptide hormones—insulin, glucagon, somatostatin, and pancreatic polypeptide. In the human, the islets are egg

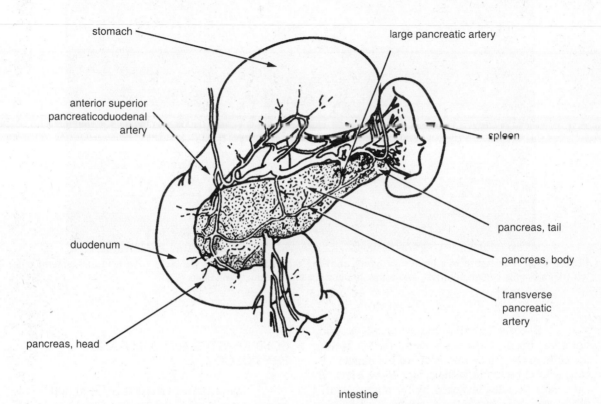

stomach

large pancreatic artery

anterior superior
pancreaticoduodenal
artery

spleen

duodenum

pancreas, tail

pancreas, body

transverse
pancreatic
artery

pancreas, head

intestine

Figure 11.2 The figures show a diagrammatic representation of the anatomical relationships of the pancreas (shaded) to the digestive tract (stomach, duodenum, intestine) and spleen. Modified, with permission. Hazelwood, R.L. The Endocrine Pancreas. Englewood Cliffs, NJ: Prentice-Hall; 1989; p. 11.

shaped; the islets measure about 76–175 micrometers; and there are one to two million islets. The islets have no duct but do have a rich blood supply and innervation.

The histology of the islets involves classification of the cell types. Ganong describes the problems with the cell type classifications:

> The cells in the islets can be divided into types on the basis of their staining properties and morphology. There are at least 4 distinct cell types in humans: A, B, D, and F cells. A, B, and D cells are also called α, ß, and

δ cells. However, this leads to confusion in view of the use of Greek letters to refer to other structures of the body, particularly adrenergic receptors.[5]

A-cells (α-cells) make the polypeptide hormone glucagon. A-cells are about 20% of the cells in human islets. The A-cells are usually found surrounding B-cells. The A-cells arise embryologically from one of the diverticula, the dorsal pancreatic bud. Within the A-cells, glucagon is contained in A-granules.

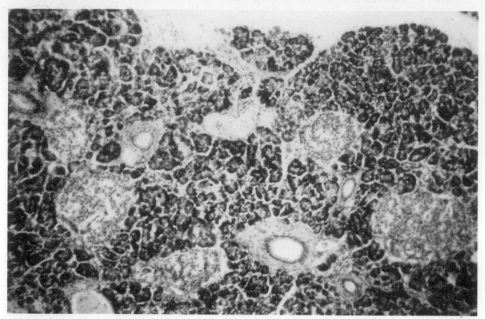

Figure 11.3 The figure is a photomicrograph showing the histology of the pancreas. An islet of Langerhans is left (A), a duct is center-right (B), and acinar tissue surrounds the ducts and islets (C).

B-cells (ß-cells) make the polypeptide hormone, insulin. B-cells account for 60–75% of the cells in the pancreatic islets of the human. B-cells tend to be found in the center of the islets. B-cells have vesicles enclosed by membranes called the B-granules. Inside the membrane is a halo, or relatively clear space. Inside the halo is a round or rectangular "packet" of insulin.

D-cells make somatostatin. D-cells are 3–5% of the islet mass. Somatostatin is also a hormone of the hypothalamus (it inhibits the release of somatotropin).

F-cells make pancreatic polypeptide. F-cells, less than 2% of islet mass, develop embryologically from the ventral pancreatic bud. F-cells are only found in the lobe of the pancreas that is in the posterior portion of the "head" of the pancreas. A partition of fascia sets off the posterior portion of the pancreatic head from the anterior portion. In this portion, the islets have mostly F-cells (80%) and some B-cells (11–20%), but only a few A-cells (0.5%).

The blood that carries secretions of the islets drains into the **portal vein** which drains blood from the intestine to the liver. In that regard, the endocrine circulation of the pancreas is unique. The arrangement is appropriate for the liver to be a major target of pancreatic hormones.

COMPARATIVE ANATOMY AND PHYSIOLOGY

Interspecies variation is found both in the pancreas itself and in the details of islet histology.[6]

For example, in cyclostomes the acinar cells have a diffuse distribution in the intestinal epithelium and the fishes lack A- or D-cells. In a second example, some species of teleost fish possess Brockmann corpuscles in which most of the islet tissue is located. Fishes, for example the anglerfish (*Lophius*), were of special use in the early efforts to isolate insulin because their islet tissue could be extracted without much contamination by the acinar tissue enzymes which destroy peptide hormones during extraction. Reptiles and birds have a greater proportion of A-cells than is found in humans or mammals in general. In birds the pancreas has four lobes and the islets are specialized so that there are A-cell islets and B-cell islets.

Invertebrates don't have a pancreas or glucagon, but insulin and glucagon-like activities and molecules have been located in echinoderms, crustaceans, tunicates, molluscs, insects (e.g., in royal jelly of bees[7]), and even in the bacterium *Escherichia coli*.[8]

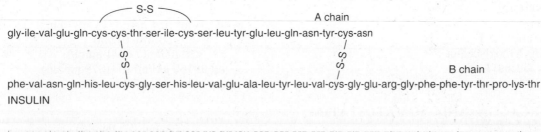

```
                    ┌──────── S-S ────────┐
                    │                     │                        A chain
gly-ile-val-glu-gln-cys-cys-thr-ser-ile-cys-ser-leu-tyr-glu-leu-gln-asn-tyr-cys-asn
                        \                                                        \
                         S-S                                                      S-S
                          \                                                        \
phe-val-asn-gln-his-leu-cys-gly-ser-his-leu-val-glu-ala-leu-tyr-leu-val-cys-gly-glu-arg-gly-phe-phe-tyr-thr-pro-lys-thr
INSULIN                                                                                           B chain
```

his-ser-gln-gly-thr-phe-thr-ser-asp-tyr-ser-lys-tyr-leu-asp-ser-arg-arg-ala-gln-asp-phe-val-gln-trp-leu-met-asn-thr
GLUCAGON

ala-gly-cys-lys-asn-phe-phe-trp-lys-thr-phe-thr-ser-cys
SOMATOSTATIN

Figure 11.4 The structures of hormones made by the pancreatic islets of Langerhans are shown. Somatostatin is also found in the central nervous system and intestine. Somatostatin may exist in both straight and cyclic forms.

CHEMISTRY OF INSULIN

The intracellular locations of insulin synthesis and secretion in the pancreatic B-cells are known and serve as a model for peptide hormone synthesis and secretion. In humans, the gene for insulin has two introns and three exons; the gene is on the short arm of chromosome eleven. Insulin is synthesized in the endoplasmic reticulum. RNA with 550 nucleotides is translated in the polysomes. Preproinsulin has a leader sequence or signal peptide of 23 amino acids which are removed as the preproinsulin enters the endoplasmic reticulum.

The remaining peptide is folded in the endoplasmic reticulum, and disulfide bonds are made to form **proinsulin**. Proinsulin contains insulin and a **connecting peptide**, or C-peptide, which has 31 amino acid residues. Proinsulin is then packed into its granules, or membrane-bound vesicles, in the Golgi apparatus. In the vesicles, connecting peptide is removed, possibly by an endopeptidase (converting enzyme, tissue kallikrein) whose distribution is similar to that of insulin. Using a process that involves microtubules, the granules move to the region of the cell membrane.

Secretion is by exocytocis. The membranes of the vesicles fuse with the cell membrane and empty their contents to the exterior of the cell. Insulin, connecting peptide (10% of insulin activity), and proinsulin (7–8% of insulin activity) are secreted. The hormones move across the B-cell basal lamina, and across the basal lamina and fenestrated endothelium of a nearby capillary to enter the blood.

Human insulin has 51 amino acids and molecular weight 5808 (Figure 11.4). The molecule has two chains and three disulfide bonds. The A-chain has 21 amino acids (not counting two cys involved in bonding to the B-chain), and the B-chain has 30 amino acids. Insulin was the first protein whose primary structure, that is, the amino acid sequence, was deciphered. The pioneering work by Sanger took place over the years from 1944 to 1955.

Insulin values (Table 11.1) may differ from measurement of insulin-like activity. One of the many bioassays for the measurement of insulin-like activity is to determine glucose uptake and gas exchange in fat tissue. However, anti-insulin antibodies only suppress 7% of this insulin-like activity. The suppressible insulin-like activity probably represents the contribution of pancreatic insulin.

Table 11.1 Hormones and Glucose in Human Blood

INSULIN

fasting	6–26 µU/ml (0.4 ng/ml, 43–187 pmol/l)
peak after meal	50–130 µU/ml
during hypoglycemia	<20 µU/ml (<144 pmol/l)
after glucose load	up to 150 µU/ml (0–1078 pmol/l)
secreted per day	40 U (287 nmol)

GLUCAGON AND SOMATOSTATIN

glucagon, fasting	75 pg/ml (25 pmol/l)
glucagon in portal vein	300–500 pg/ml
somatostatin	80 pg/ml

GLUCOSE

normal, fasting	60–110 mg%
normal, after glucose load, 500 mg/kg load	150 mg%
diabetic, fasting	150–200 mg%
diabetic, after glucose load, 500 mg/kg load	400–500 mg%
normal, fasting, elderly	80–150 mg%
diabetic coma	1000 mg%
insulin shock	30 mg%

To express glucose levels, mg/100 ml is sometimes referred to as mg%. Measurements after a glucose load were made at one hour after the load. The glucose level in diabetic may stay up 5 hours after the load. Blood glucose increases with aging so that 1 mg/dl is added per year for each year past age 60. Values are shown for humans, but for glucose values would be similar in rats. Compiled from data in Karam, J. H.; Salber, P. R.; and Forsham, P.H. Pancreatic hormones and diabetes mellitus. In Greenspan, F.; Forsham, P., editors. Basic and Clinical Endocrinology, Second Edition. Norwalk, CT: Appleton & Lange; 1987, pages 526–530; Ganong, W. Review of Medical Physiology, Fourteenth Edition. Norwalk, CT: Appleton & Lange; 1989; p. 280–300; Berkow, R. The Merck Manual Sixteenth Edition. Rahway, NJ: Merck Research Laboratories; 1992; p. 2585.

Because of that, the remaining insulin-like activity which is not affected by the anti-insulin antibodies has been called nonsuppressible insulin-like activity (NSILA). NSILA remains after the pancreas is removed so that it does not represent insulin. Five percent of NSILA is due to somatomedins (IGF-I and IGF-II) which have amino acid similarities to insulin. The remaining NSILA may be due to nonsuppressible insulin-like protein.

In the circulation, insulin's half-life is five minutes. Insulin is metabolized by most tissues, but 80% of insulin is degraded by liver and kidney. Insulin has a rhythm with the daily peak at about 7 p.m. (Figure 11.5). There are three insulin inactivating systems (insulinases) which inactivate insulin by breaking disulfide bonds (hepatic glutathione insulin transhydrogenase) or peptide bonds.

Species vary in the number of insulins secreted and in amino acids 8–10 on the A-chain and amino acid 30 on the B-chain. Insulin molecules are similar enough that insulin from one species has biological action in another, however, the insulin molecules are different enough to elicit immunological reactions. Pork insulin has only one amino acid that is different from humans (position 30 amino acid alanine instead of threonine) and elicits little immune response. Beef insulin produces antibodies in two months but the antibodies usually are not a clinical problem for most patients.

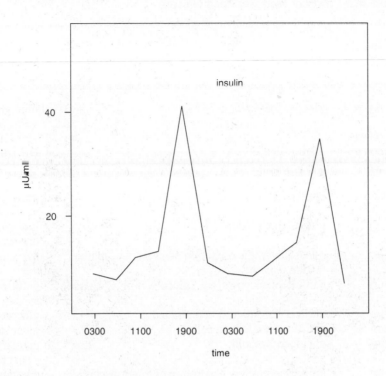

Figure 11.5 Two cycles of the daily rhythm in serum insulin concentration in humans are shown. The subjects ate a diet with 150 grams of protein/day. Insulin peaked at 1900 (7 p.m.) on that diet and also on diets with less protein. Redrawn, with permission. Fernstrom, J.D. The influence of circadian variations in plasma amino acid concentrations on monoamine synthesis in the brain. In Krieger, D.T. Endocrine Rhythms. New York: Raven Press; 1979; p. 95.

GLUCAGON, SOMATOSTATIN, AND PANCREATIC POLYPEPTIDE CHEMISTRY

Glucagon is synthesized in the A-cells. It is a polypeptide hormone, but it has only one chain of 29 amino acid residues and molecular weight 3485. The biological activity of glucagon is partly due to glucagon (30–40%) and partly due to the activity of its larger precursor molecule. Preproglucagon has 179 amino acids and contains glucagon, glycentin, and two other glucagon-like peptides; all the moieties have some glucagon activity. Half-life of glucagon is about 3–10 minutes. The kidneys and the liver remove glucagon from the circulation. The principal target of glucagon in mammals and birds is the liver which, in responding to glucagon, removes most of the glucagon from circulation.

Somatostatin has 14 amino acids, one disulfide bond, and molecular weight 1640. It was discovered and named in association with its ability to inhibit release of growth hormone from the anterior pituitary gland. It is synthesized in the pancreatic D-cells from a 28 amino acid precursor molecule, prosomatostatin. Its metabolism is rapid giving it a short half-life of less than two minutes.

Pancreatic polypeptide (PP) of the F-cells has 36 amino acids and molecular weight 4200. Pancreatic peptide secretion increases in response to a meal and the response is abolished by severing the vagus nerve.

TERMINOLOGY OF GLUCOSE METABOLISM

Pancreatic hormones function in intermediary metabolism to regulate sugar, or glucose. In

Table 11.2 Factors that Lower or Increase Blood Glucose

Hormone	Blood glucose	Glucose effect	Hormone regulation
insulin	down	glucose into cells	high glucose, nerves, secretin
somatostatin	down		via GH
somatomedins	down	insulin-like	GH stimulated
stress, exercise	down	use up sugar	
storage	down	produce glycogen	
excretion	down	eliminate sugar	glucose up, kidney threshold
glucagon	up	glucose out of liver	low glucose, low GI hormones stimulate
catecholamines	up	release liver glucose, counteract insulin, inhibit insulin release	nervous system, adrenal
glucocorticoids	up	stimulates enzymes, e.g., glucose-6-phosphatase	pituitary feedback system
GI hormones	up	indirect, food digestion promoted	glucose from food
GH	up	anti-insulin effect on cells	glucostat
ACTH, CRH	up	via glucocorticoids	pituitary feedback system
thyroid hormones	up	indirect, digestion, absorption of monosaccharides, increase insulin degradation	pituitary feedback system
angiotensin	up	indirect via epinephrine, insulin	blood pressure, blood glucose
food	up	stimulate hormones, add new sugar	
arginine (in food)	up	stimulate hormones, stimulate insulin release	

order to appreciate this function, an understanding of the terminology of glucose metabolism and the pathways for intermediary metabolism is needed.

A terminology (that can be confusing because of the similarity of the terms and diverse definitions) describes events in intermediary metabolism.

Glycolysis refers to the conversion of carbohydrates to pyruvic or lactic acid in tissues; it begins with hydrolysis of glycogen to form glucose (glycogenolysis);[9] alternatively, the term "glycolysis" has been used to refer to the formation of glucose or glucose 6-phosphate from glycogen.

Gluconeogenesis means the de novo synthesis of glucose from a large variety of substrates: amino acids, lactate, pyruvate, propionate, glycerol, galactose, and fructose. Glycogen is stored in muscle and liver.

Glycogenolysis is the word for the intracellular breakdown of glycogen to glucose.

Glycogenesis is the intracellular formation of glycogen from glucose.

A simplified representation of these terms is[10]

glycogenolysis = glycogen ➡ glucose
glycogenesis = glycogen ⬅ glucose
glycolysis = glucose ➡ lactate
gluconeogenesis = glucose ⬅ lactate

Hypoglycemia is low blood sugar, and **hyperglycemia** is high blood sugar. Pancreatic

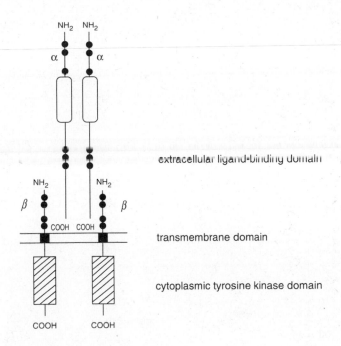

extracellular ligand-binding domain

transmembrane domain

cytoplasmic tyrosine kinase domain

Figure 11.6 The figure illustrates a model of the structure of the insulin receptor. The receptor has four peptide chains (two alpha- and two beta-chains). The beads represent single cysteine residues that may be involved in linking the alpha and beta subunits together with disulfide bonds. Ulrich, A.; Bell, J.R.; Chen, E.Y. et al. Human insulin receptor, and its relationship to the tyrosine kinase family of oncogenes. Nature 313: 756–761; 1987.

hormones are involved in the regulation of blood sugar, but many other hormones and factors, in addition to pancreatic hormones, affect blood sugar (Table 11.2).

FUNCTIONS OF INSULIN

Insulin has been called the "hormone of abundance" because it promotes the storage of carbohydrate, fat, and protein. As Ganong says: "There is an appealing parsimony to the concept that insulin has a single action that underlies all its diverse effects on metabolism."[11] This idea, that one mechanism is responsible for all insulin actions, is undoubtedly too simple, but the idea provides a basis for launching the discussion of insulin's varied activities–movement of small molecules into cells, activation of enzymes, inhibition of enzymes.

The mechanism involves the binding of insulin to insulin receptors which are located in the cell membrane. Insulin-sensitive cells (liver, muscle, fat) can bind an estimated 11,000 insulin molecules per cell. The **insulin receptor** has been characterized and cloned. The insulin receptor is a protein, 340,000 MW, found on the membranes of many different cells of the body, and has a half-life of 7 hours. The receptor has four glycoprotein subunits (two α subunits and two ß subunits) which are linked by disulfide bonds (Figure 11.6). When insulin binds to its receptor, it triggers autophosphorylation and phosphorylates other proteins to achieve the biological effect of insulin.

Cells have a mechanism for disposal of used insulin receptors (insulin-insulin receptor complexes). The insulin-receptor complexes gather in patches and are consumed by the cells (receptor-mediated endocytocis). Once inside the cells, the

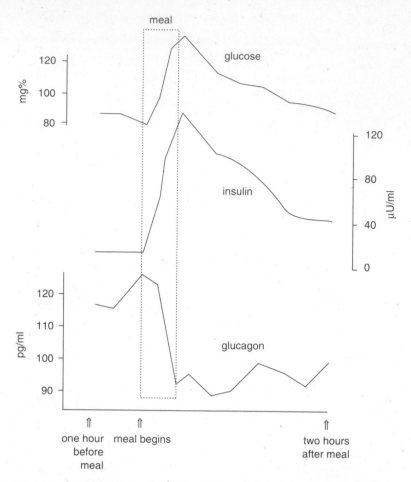

Figure 11.7 The graphs show the effects of a meal on glucose, insulin, and glucagon. Redrawn, with permission. After Muller, W.A.; Faloona, G.R.; Aguilar-Parada, E.; Under, R. Abnormal alpha cell function in diabetes. Response to carbohydrate and protein injection. New England Journal of Medicine 283: 109–115; 1970.

insulin-receptor complexes are broken down by lysosomes or recycled to plasma membrane. The insulin receptor is responsible for some of the regulation of insulin because the receptor numbers and affinity are changeable. The insulin receptors respond to insulin, other hormones, food, exercise, etc. Increasing insulin or starvation causes the receptor numbers to decrease which is termed "down regulation" of the receptors. Decreased insulin or adrenal hormone deficiency increases receptor affinity; excess glucocorticoid decreases receptor affinity.

Insulin is responsible for facilitating the movement of glucose into cells. Thus, insulin lowers blood sugar (hypoglycemic action). Excess insulin causes hypoglycemia. The process by which glucose enters cells is called facilitated diffusion. Insulin injections have a maximal effect on glucose transport in 30 minutes. Insulin causes insertion of more glucose carrier molecules, **glucose transporters**, into the cell membrane. The transporter is visualized as a large protein with twelve transmembrane regions. Insulin facilitates the movement of glucose into muscle cells, fat cells, leucocytes, fibroblasts, pituitary, mammary gland, aorta, pancreatic islet A-cells, and the crystalline lens of the eye.

Effects of a **meal** are straightforward. The

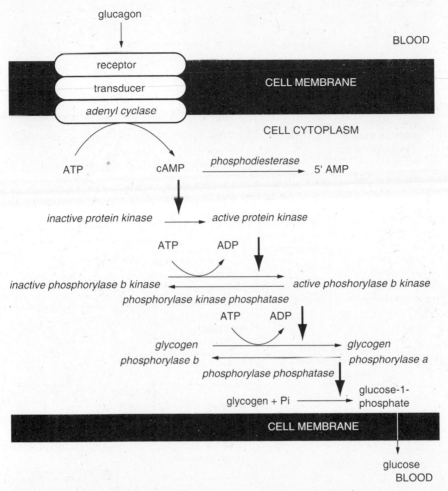

Figure 11.8 The diagram illustrates the classic mechanism of action of glucagon on a liver cell. There is a cyclic AMP mechanism and a cascade of reactions that are a consequence of the hormone, glucagon, on its target liver cell. Activations are represented by heavy arrows. Enzyme names are italicized.

meal provides nutrients, blood sugar increases to a peak in about an hour, and insulin imitates the glucose increase (Figure 11.7). **A glucose tolerance test** is a standardized "meal" given to a fasted individual to test the response of the pancreas. In the glucose tolerance test, the individual should eat at least 150–200g carbohydrate for three days before the test and then fast from midnight on the test day. Glucose (75g/300ml) is given to the subject and blood samples are tested for glucose at times 0, 30, 60, 90, and 120 minutes. In a normal test, plasma glucose rises from >115 mg% and returns in two hours to <140 mg%. An abnormal test, indicating diabetes mellitus, is a two-hour value >200 mg%.

A number of conditions can result in false positives: poor nutrition, inactivity, infection, emotional stress, diuretics, oral contraceptives, thyroxine, glucocorticoids, nicotinic acid, psychotropic drugs, and phenytoin.

The **liver** is a target of insulin. Because of the portal vein circulation, insulin arrives at the liver at 3–10 times the concentrations found in the peripheral circulation. Effects of insulin on the liver do not directly involve facilitation of glucose movement. Instead, insulin prevents glycogen breakdown and increases fat and protein synthesis. It does this by increasing glycogen synthesis, decreasing gluconeogenesis, and decreasing

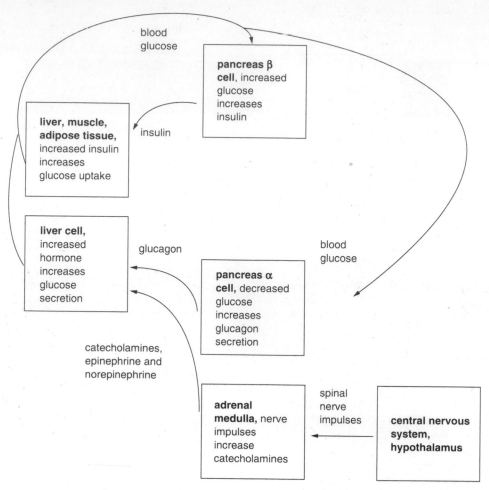

Figure 11.9 The figure illustrates some of the factors involved in the regulation of glucagon and insulin secretion in the pancreas by glucose.[12] Amino acids, fatty acids, and gastrointestinal hormones are also involved in the regulation.

ketogenesis.

Muscle is also a target of insulin. In muscle cells, insulin increases glucose admission, glycogen synthesis, amino acid uptake, protein synthesis, ketone uptake, and potassium uptake. Insulin decreases protein breakdown and decreases the release of amino acids derived from gluconeogenesis.

Fat, adipose tissue, is also a target of insulin. In fat cells, insulin increases glucose uptake, fatty acid synthesis, glycerol phosphate synthesis, triglyceride deposition, and increases potassium acquisition. Insulin activates lipoprotein lipase and inhibits hormone-sensitive lipase.

There are other tissues that are noteworthy because insulin does not facilitate glucose uptake. These tissues include the kidney tubules, erythrocytes, mucosa of the intestine, and the brain. All effects of insulin hypersecretion, besides hypoglycemia, are caused by the effects of low blood sugar on the nervous system. Normally glucose is the only energy source for the brain. Since the brain doesn't have much storage capacity, a constant supply of glucose is necessary for normal neural function.

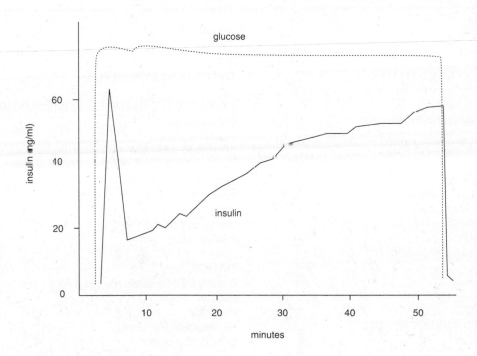

Figure 11.10 The graphs show the effect of glucose infusion on the plasma concentration of insulin in the rat pancreas. The level of glucose was almost 300 mg% during the infusion. After Grodsky, G.M. Further studies on the dynamic aspects of insulin release *in vivo* with evidence for a 2-compartmental storage system. Acta Dibetol. Lat. 6 [Suppl. 1], 554, 1969.

FUNCTIONS OF GLUCAGON

A high concentration of glucagon comes to the liver (300–500 pg/mL) compared to the amount of glucagon in the peripheral circulation (75 pg/ml). **Liver cells** are the principal targets of glucagon. Acting via a G_s protein which activates adenylate cyclase and raises cyclic AMP, glucagon promotes gluconeogenesis, glycogenolysis, lipolysis, and ketogenesis. The classic model for cyclic AMP is based on the action of glucagon on a liver cell (Figure 11.8). By activating phosphorylase, glucagon causes glycogen breakdown and release of glucose that increase blood glucose. Liver cells may have separate receptors that are stimulated by glucagon to activate lipase C,[13] increase cytoplasmic calcium, and thereby to stimulate glycogenolysis.

A meal has a dramatic effect on glucagon just as it does on insulin. However, glucagon levels drop after a meal. In some other situations the actions of glucagon and insulin are opposite to one another. For example, during physical exercise, glucagon increases and insulin declines. This increases glucose production by the liver. The opposing effects have led scientists to consider the insulin/glucagon ratio in regulation (high after glucose or a large carbohydrate meal; low after fasting or a low carbohydrate diet).

Glucagon has a **calorigenic action**. It increases the hepatic deamination of amino acids which produces heat. This is another action of gluconeogenesis. In the liver, then, glucagon causes proteolysis (protein breakdown). Fat is also a target of glucagon. Fat breakdown, lipolysis, is also stimulated by glucagon and leads to the

Table 11.3 Stimulation and Inhibition of Insulin and Glucagon Secretion[14]

Stimulators	Inhibitors
INSULIN SECRETION	**INSULIN SECRETION**
METABOLITES amino acids (arginine, leucine) glucose ß-keto acids (acetoacetate) mannose	METABOLITE-RELATED COMPOUNDS 2-deoxyglucose mannoheptulose potassium depletion
ENDOCRINE AGENTS ß-adrenergic agents cholecystokinin-pancreozymin (CCK) cyclic AMP gastrointestinal peptide (GIP) gastrin secretin glucagon	HORMONES epinephrine insulin norepinephrine somatostatin
NEUROTRANSMITTERS acetylcholine	DRUGS ß-adrenergic blockers (propranolol) alloxan diazoxide microtubule inhibitors thiazide diuretics
DRUGS chlorpropamide cyclic AMP agonists glipzide glyburide sulfonylureas theophylline tolbutamide	
GLUCAGON SECRETION	**GLUCAGON SECRETION**
amino acids (ala, cys, gly, ser, thr) hormones (cholecystokinin, cortisol, gastrin) exercise, infections ß-adrenergic stimulators theophylline, acetylcholine	glucose hormones (insulin, secretin, somatostatin) free fatty acids, ketones α-adrenergic stimulators phenytoin

production of free fatty acids which are converted to ketones (ketone bodies, ketogenesis) in the liver. Muscle glycogenolysis is not initiated by glucagon; there is a positive inotropic effect on the heart.

REGULATION OF THE PANCREAS

The major means for regulation of insulin is by **blood glucose feedback** on the pancreas B-cells (Figure 11.9). Perfusing the pancreas with blood containing >110 mg/dl glucose increases in

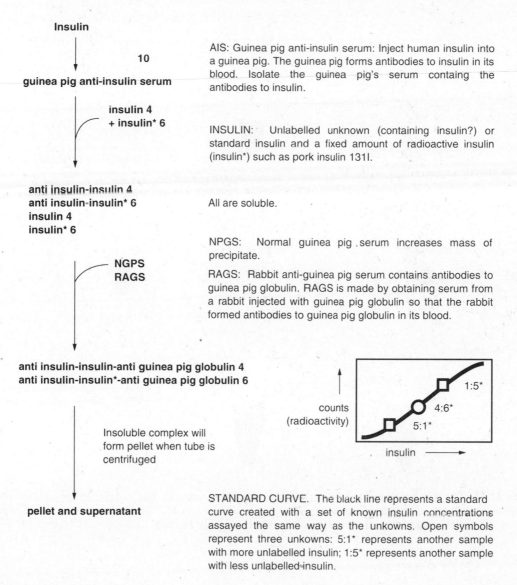

Insulin

10

guinea pig anti-insulin serum

AIS: Guinea pig anti-insulin serum: Inject human insulin into a guinea pig. The guinea pig forms antibodies to insulin in its blood. Isolate the guinea pig's serum containg the antibodies to insulin.

insulin 4
+ insulin* 6

INSULIN: Unlabelled unknown (containing insulin?) or standard insulin and a fixed amount of radioactive insulin (insulin*) such as pork insulin 131I.

anti insulin-insulin 4
anti insulin-insulin* 6
insulin 4
insulin* 6

All are soluble.

NGPS
RAGS

NPGS: Normal guinea pig serum increases mass of precipitate.

RAGS: Rabbit anti-guinea pig serum contains antibodies to guinea pig globulin. RAGS is made by obtaining serum from a rabbit injected with guinea pig globulin so that the rabbit formed antibodies to guinea pig globulin in its blood.

anti insulin-insulin-anti guinea pig globulin 4
anti insulin-insulin*-anti guinea pig globulin 6

counts
(radioactivity)

1:5*
4:6*
5:1*

insulin

Insoluble complex will form pellet when tube is centrifuged

pellet and supernatant

STANDARD CURVE. The black line represents a standard curve created with a set of known insulin concentrations assayed the same way as the unkowns. Open symbols represent three unkowns: 5:1* represents another sample with more unlabelled insulin; 1:5* represents another sample with less unlabelled insulin.

Figure 11.11 A radioimmunoassay for an unknown sample of insulin is described. The ratios (4:6) show how hypothetical antibody sites (10) would be occupied in one sample. The ratio is set up when the hormones are first added and is retained in the sample throughout the assay. The assay uses the double antibody method. Soeldner, J.; Slone, D. Critical variables in the radioimmunoassay of serum insulin using the double antibody technique. Diabetes 14: 771–779; 1965.

sulin secretion (Figure 11.10). Other factors also stimulate or inhibit insulin secretion (Table 11.3). The pancreatic islets are innervated by the right vagus nerve and stimulation of the right vagus triggers insulin secretion. Insulin secretion is also stimulated by glucagon and gastrointestinal hormones, by some amino acids from the diet or protein breakdown, and by ß-keto acids produced by fat breakdown. Catecholamines inhibit insulin secretion (α-adrenergic inhibition exceeds ß-adrenergic

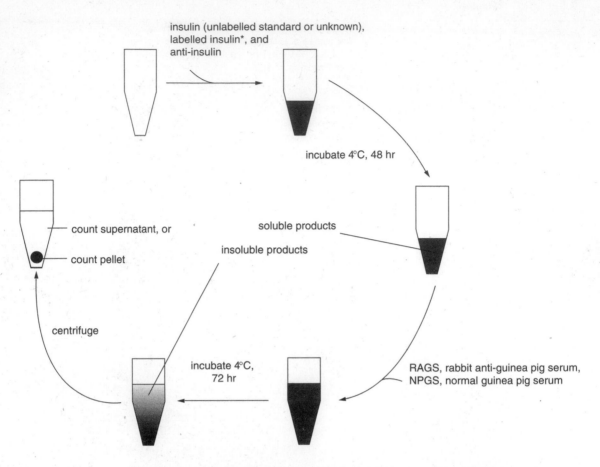

insulin (unlabelled standard or unknown),
labelled insulin*, and
anti-insulin

incubate 4°C, 48 hr

count supernatant, or

soluble products

insoluble products

count pellet

centrifuge

incubate 4°C,
72 hr

RAGS, rabbit anti-guinea pig serum,
NPGS, normal guinea pig serum

Figure 11.12 The diagram illustrates the sequence of steps for a test tube (one sample, either standard insulin or an unknown) in the insulin radioimmunoassay also shown in Figure 11.11. Soeldner, J.; Slone, D. Critical variables in the radioimmunoassay of serum insulin using the double antibody technique. Diabetes 14: 771–779; 1965.

stimulation).

Glucagon responds to blood glucose levels opposite to the manner of insulin. High blood glucose decreases glucagon secretion by the pancreatic A-cells. Signals via sympathetic innervation and the vagus nerve also increase glucagon via ß-receptors and cyclic AMP. Other glucagon stimulators include protein meals, amino acids, cholecystokinin, gastrin, cortisol, exercise, infections, theophylline, and acetylcholine. Inhibitors of glucagon include glucose, insulin, somatostatin, secretin, free fatty acids, ketones, phenytoin, and α-adrenergic agents.

INSULIN RADIOIMMUNOASSAY

Insulin is one of the many hormones that can be measured with radioimmunoassays. For their specificity, radioimmunoassays depend on differences and specificities of antibodies.

A radioimmunoassay measures a particular hormone or ligand (e.g., human insulin). **Antibodies** are produced ("grown") by injecting an animal with the hormone whose measurement is the desired goal (Figures 11.11, 11.12). In assaying insulin, for example, a guinea pig is

Table 11.4 Diabetes Mellitus

Juvenile-onset diabetes	Maturity-onset diabetes
OTHER NAMES	**OTHER NAMES**
type I diabetes	type II diabetes
insulin-dependent diabetes (IDDM)	non-insulin-dependent diabetes (NIDDM)
ketosis-prone diabetes	ketosis-resistant diabetes
CHARACTERISTICS	**CHARACTERISTICS**
less than 10% of diabetics	80–90% of diabetics
younger than 20 years at onset	over age 40 years at onset
abrupt onset	slow onset
decline in number of B-cells	normal beta cells
insulin deficiency	insulin normal or high
50% genetic concordance	100% genetic concordance
lower blood pH, diabetic ketoacidosis	insulin resistance
onsets more common in fall and winter	reduced number of insulin receptors
HD-DR3-HLA-DR4 histocompatibility antigens	obesity
polyuria (excess urination)	recurrent blurred vision
polydipsia (excess thirst)	vulvovaginitus or pruritus
polyphagia (excess eating with weight loss)	peripheral neuropathy
nocturnal enuresis	can be asymptomatic
THERAPY	**THERAPY**
hormone replacement with exogenous insulin	diet and weight reduction
	hypoglycemic agents (insulin, oral sulfonylureas, low-sugar diet)

injected with purified human insulin. The guinea pig's immune system recognizes the insulin as "foreign" and forms antibodies to the human insulin. The antibodies can be recovered from the guinea pig by obtaining blood by heart puncture. The blood is centrifuged to recover the serum fraction. The resulting serum with antibodies is the antiserum. Each molecule of antibody can have one or more binding sites for the hormone. In the case of insulin, the antiserum is called anti-insulin serum. Antibodies can be repeatedly harvested from the guinea pig. Goats and rabbits are other animals commonly used to raise antibodies.

To do an assay, a series of test tubes is set up. The series contains tubes with no insulin, tubes with **standard amounts** of insulin, and tubes with unknowns. Usually two or three replicates of each sample are assayed to improve accuracy. Sometimes the unknowns have to be diluted to bring them into the range that can be detected.

The assay requires **radioactive hormone** (radioactive ligand) which is obtained by reacting purified hormone with labelled hormone (e.g., radioactive iodine attached to the tyrosine residues in the hormone). For example, pork insulin can be radioactively iodinated with radioactive iodine (^{131}I). Fixed amounts of antiserum and radioactive hormone are added to each sample tube. The tube is permitted to react for a long time (e.g., two days) so that the reaction can go to completion. The tubes are refrigerated during reaction so that the protein components (hormone, antibody) will not break down. In the reaction, unlabelled standard or unknown hormone competes equally for antibody sites. The result is that the ratio of unla-

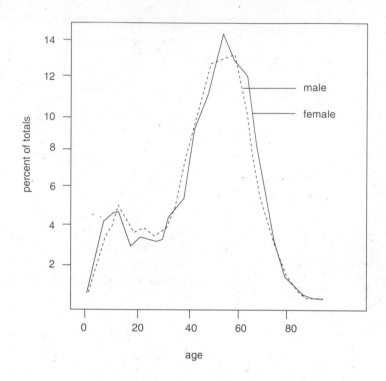

Figure 11.13 The graph shows the age of the onset of diabetes mellitus in humans. The graphs represent the frequency with which diabetes begins. There is a bimodal distribution with a peak around puberty and a second peak in the later years. Redrawn, Joslin, E.P.; Root, H.F.; Marble, A.; White, P. Treatment of Diabetes Mellitus, Tenth Edition. Philadelphia, PA: Lea & Febiger; 1959; p. 30.

belled to labelled hormone that binds is the same as the ratio of unlabelled to labelled hormone placed in the test tube. Samples differ in the amount of unknown hormone, so that the ratio is higher if there is more hormone and lower if there is less hormone.

It remains to separate the antibody-hormone complex from the free hormone. If the antibody-hormone complex is insoluble, the separation can be achieved by centrifugation. If the antibody-hormone complex is soluble, then a separate procedure must be done for a separation. Sometimes, as in the example shown for insulin, a second antibody is used in the separation. Once an insoluble antibody-hormone complex is obtained, centrifugation is used to separate the complex from unreacted hormone.

The radioactivity can be "counted" using a gamma counter. Either the supernatant or the pellet can be counted; but only one is counted routinely. If there is no hormone, most of the radioactivity will be in the pellet; if there is a very high amount of hormone, most of the radioactivity will be in the supernatant. Using the counts obtained for the standards, a standard curve is constructed for either the supernatant or the pellet (counts versus the amount of hormone). Unknowns are read by comparing their counts with the standard curve to obtain the value for the hormone.

Some advantages of radioimmunassays are that the assays have a high degree of specificity; radioimmunoassays are independent from bioassay variations; and radioimmunoassays can be used for large numbers of samples. Radioimmunoassays also do not require keeping a large animal colony; most reagents, including antibodies, can be pur-

Table 11.5 Alloxan Diabetes Experiment

Group	Preinjection glucose	Postinjection glucose	Postglucose load glucose
rats, buffer	131 ± 13	131 ± 12	168 ± 30
rats, alloxan	135 ± 90	297 ± 47	404 ± 49

The data in the table are mean ± one standard error of the mean for blood glucose in mg% (mg per 100 ml). In the experiment, normal human values were obtained in the afternoon; the values ranged from 49–165 mg% (N = 15). On the same day, blood glucose was determined in two groups of rats (preinjection, N = 10,22). The rats were then injected subcutaneously with either 0.8 ml buffer vehicle (N = 10) or alloxan dissolved in the vehicle (5 g alloxan/100 ml buffer; N = 21). One week later, blood glucose was again measured in the rats (postinjection values). Then, the rats were all injected with a glucose load (0.6 ml of 10% glucose, intraperitoneal). One hour later, blood glucose was again determined in the rat blood (postglucose). Alloxan increased both the baseline blood glucose and the response to a glucose load. Blood glucose was determined with the Statzyme Glucose (500 nm) method (Worthington®). Blood glucose measured in humans was 92 ± 15 mg%. The experiment was done at Temple University by a class of endocrinology students.

chased and stored in refrigerators or freezers.

One of the disadvantages of radioimmunoassays is that they do not necessarily detect biological activity. That is because the portion of the hormone that reacts with the antibody may not be the same as the portion of the hormone that is responsible for the biological action. Moreover, the insulin standard may not be the same as the endogenous or immunoactive hormone in the unknown (e.g., pork insulin standard, human insulin unknowns). Sometimes two different antibodies give different results for the same sample. This has been attributed to the "heterogeneity of peptide hormones."[15] Many, possibly all, peptide hormones exist in more than one form in the gland, extracts, and plasma, even in one individual. Another disadvantage of radioimmunoassays is that they involve handling radioactive materials. ELISAs eliminate this problem.

DIABETES

The disease of insufficient insulin action at the target tissue level is **diabetes mellitus**. The disease is of major importance. It is found in about 5% of the United States population. In the United States, diabetes mellitus is the third leading cause of death following cancer and heart disease.

Individuals have one chance in five of developing the disease and the risk doubles each decade of life for each 20% weight increase. The disease has serious complications: retinal scarring, kidney disease, 3.5 times increase in risk of cardiovascular death, male impotency, and loss of autonomic nerve function. Diabetics subdivide into separate clinical entities. Most diabetics have juvenile-onset diabetes or maturity-onset diabetes (Table 11.4, Figure 11.13), but there is also diabetes that is associated with other conditions (Cushing's syndrome, acromegaly, etc.)

Aretaius of Cappadocia is credited with naming the disease in 200 A.D. and describing it as a strange disease that consists of the flesh and bones running together into the urine. Hadley describes the origin of the name of the disease which the Romans thought was caused by the bite of the 'thirst adder.'

Diabetes mellitus was first described about 1500 B.C. in Egypt. Mellitus, the Latin word for honey, characterizes the high sugar content of the urine of diabetics. The word diabetes, derived from the Greek for siphon, refers to the copious excretion of water that characterizes the disease. For centuries the disease was known as

Table 11.6 Changes Following Binding of Insulin and Its Receptor and Activation of Tyrosine Kinase[16]

Intracellular change	Examples
increases in serine/threonine phosphorylation	acetyl-CoA carboxylase insulin receptor ribosomal protein S6
decreases in serine/threonine phosphorylation	glycogen synthase pyruvate dehydrogenase triacylglycerol lipase
translocation of proteins	glucose transporter IFG-II receptor insulin receptor
changes in transcription	PEPCK fructose 1,6-biphosphatase glucokinase pyruvate kinase

'the pissing evil' in England, an epi-
thet that appropriately characterizes
its most observable symptom.[17]

Minkowski and Mering are noteworthy for removing the pancreas from a dog in 1892 and observing that the dog's urine attracted flies. There are unsavory rumors, involving abuse of medical students, which tell that the urine of diabetics tasted sweet.

Juvenile-onset diabetes has been called the "poly" disease (polyphagia, polydipsia, and polyuria) for excess eating, drinking, and urinating symptoms. Although there is a genetic concordance of 50% implying a genetic predisposition to develop the disease, there is a belief that there is an environmental factor. Viruses have sometimes been suspected, but the likely causes of juvenile diabetes is autoimmunity. The individual forms antibodies against his own islet cells resulting in the loss of B-cells, decline in ability to produce insulin, and symptoms of insulin insufficiency. It has even been suggested that drinking cow's milk, which contains proteins with sequences similar to portions of insulin, might contribute to the development of the inappropriate immune re-

sponse. Therapy for juvenile-onset diabetes includes insulin replacement by injection or electromechanical pump. Human, pork, and beef insulins are used in the United States. Insulin is available in rapid acting (15–30 minutes), intermediate acting (1–3 hours), or long acting (4–8 hour) preparations.

Maturity-onset diabetes, on the other hand, has strong evidence for an inherited component. Maturity-onset diabetics do not lack insulin, instead they have reduced numbers of insulin receptors on their adipose cells. The hypothetical scenario is overeating leading to insulin secretion which causes down regulation of the receptors.

Experimental diabetes can be produced in the laboratory in vertebrates with a diabetogenic drug resembling dehydroascorbic acid named "alloxan." **Alloxan diabetes** can readily be produced in rats. Baseline levels of blood glucose and the response to a glucose load increase in rats after a single treatment with alloxan (Table 11.5). According to Turner and Bagnara:

> Three phases are generally observed
> after the administration of alloxan:
> transitory periods of hyperglycemia

Table 11.7 Fuel

Body fuel	Weight (g)	Calories	% Fuel
glycogen	225	900	0.5
protein	6,000	24,000	14.0
fat	15,000	141,000	85.0

The data are from Cahill, G. F. Starvation in man. New England Journal of Medicine 282: 668–675; 1970.

and hypoglycemia, followed by permanent hyperglycemia and other diabetic symptoms. Alloxan is thought to act directly and specifically on the B-cells, causing them to undergo degeneration and resorptions; the A-cells and the acinar tissue remain relatively unaffected.[18]

Coma can result from severe insulin deficiency (hyperglycemic coma, blood sugar of 1000 mg%). Or, coma can result from excessive use of agents, such as insulin, that lower blood sugar, or from too little food (hypoglycemic coma, blood sugar 30 mg%, **insulin shock**). Milder reactions to excess insulin in diabetic treatment are called insulin reactions. The symptoms of an insulin reaction are those of hypoglycemia, sometimes mistaken for drunkenness, and can be treated with candy or sugar.

Diabetes was associated with ovarian hyperandrogenism when a "diabetes of bearded women" was described.[19] **Insulin-induced hyperandrogenism** has since been divided into several syndromes.

HYPOGLYCEMIA

Hypoglycemia is low blood sugar (<50 mg%). The responses of men and women to fasting for three days differ; male fasting blood glucose levels rarely drop below 55 mg%; half of fasting females decrease levels to <50 mg%. Hypoglycemia is produced by excess insulin and the symptoms are mainly dependent upon the effects of inadequate energy supply for the brain.

Physiological countermeasures are taken by the body when blood glucose falls to 70 mg%. The countermeasures are secretion of hormones—glucagon, epinephrine, GH, ACTH, cortisol—which act to increase blood sugar.

Warning signs appear if the countermeasures fail to raise blood sugar. The warning signs begin when the blood sugar drops to 60 mg%. The warning signs are sweating, tremor, hunger, anxiety, palpitations. The warning signs are autonomic symptoms and they are attributed to the release of catecholamines and acetylcholine as countermeasures. Sometimes, however, blood sugar drops and without warning symptoms and this condition is called "hypoglycemia unawareness."[20] The phenomenon has been studied mainly in patients taking insulin.

Further symptoms of hypoglycemia (weakness, lethargy, blurred vision, confusion, dizziness) usually begin to appear when blood sugar drops to 50 mg% (2.8 mM). This set of symptoms, the neuroglycopenic symptoms, is a consequence of low blood sugar affecting brain function.

Reactive hypoglycemia is the response to a meal, specific nutrients, or drugs. The symptoms and signs are similar to responses to the hormone epinephrine: weakness, faintness, palpitation, tremulousness, diaphoresis, nervousness, and hunger. Reactive hypoglycemia follows an exogenous factor such as a drug (e.g., alcohol, salicylates, insulin, oral hypoglycemic agents, etc.), a carbohydrate meal, or a specific nutrient which inhibits hepatic glucose output (fructose, galactose, or leucine). Reactive hypoglycemia occurs 2–4

Table 11.8 Changes in Islet Cell Types in Human Babies and Adults

Hormone	F-cell rich areas % of cells	A-cell rich areas % of cells
INFANTS		
insulin	24	49
glucagon	2	17
somatostatin	16	33.5
pancreatic polypeptide	58	0.5
ADULTS		
insulin	16.5	77
glucagon	0.5	18
somatostatin	2	4.5
pancreatic polypeptide	81	0.5

Infants were 0–6 months old; adults were 29–80 years old. The data are from Orci, L.; Stefan, Y.; Lagae, F.M.; Perrelet, A. Instability of pancreatic endocrine cell populations throughout life. Lancet I: 615–616; 1979.

hours after a meal and is due to rapid glucose absorption from excess insulin secretion. The decrease in glucose overshoots on returning to normal after a meal-induced rise. In this disorder of "tense, conscientious people with symptoms of autonomic overactivity," the symptoms of hypoglycemia appear 3–4 hours after meals.[21]

Spontaneous hypoglycemia has another set of symptoms and signs: confusion, headache, palsy, ataxia, visual disturbances, and even personality changes. Spontaneous hypoglycemia includes metabolic processes that produce hypoglycemia in the fasting state (excess glucose utilization, exercise, fever, pregnancy, beta islet tumors or insulinoma, etc.). The dizziness and slurred speech symptoms of hypoglycemia can be mistaken for drunkenness. Low blood sugar stimulates epinephrine secretion which causes symptoms of sympathetic overactivity (nervousness, palpitations, tremor). The symptoms of hypoglycemia are usually worse in the morning because of the preceding night of fasting. The usual remedy is oral glucose (e.g., 2–3 teaspoons of granulated sugar in a glass of water or fruit juice). If the situation is not corrected with glucose, then convulsions and coma can ensue. Further prolongation of low sugar causes depression of the respiratory center of the brain followed by death.

INSULIN MECHANISM OF ACTION

Despite the great interest in insulin, the mechanism(s) of action of the hormone have been elusive and may include activation of tyrosine kinase, a novel second messenger, calcium ions, or effects on subcellular organelles (Table 11.6). In intact cells exposed to insulin, proteins (in glycogen particles, cytoplasms, microsomes, mitochondria, plasma membrane) change serine/threonine phosphorylation; in some increases, the effect is only obtained if another hormone first elevates cyclic AMP.[22]

INSULIN AND GLUCAGON, THE HORMONES OF FEASTING AND FASTING

Hazelwood views the opposing functions of glucagon and insulin in terms of fasting and feasting.[23] Insulin is an "anabolic islet hormone" which can be considered to function when food is plentiful and the organism is well fed ("feasting"). When food is plentiful, it is adaptive for the organisms to eat well and store food. Thus insulin can be viewed as acting to adapt the organism to a situation where food is plentiful and to promote storage of nutrients. Insulin's effects which would support use and storage of nutrients during feasting include

> ...the increase in glucose transport into cells, the uptake of amino acids (even in the absence of glucose, the stimulation of protein synthesis concomitant with an inhibition of protein catabolism, the inhibition of hormone-sensitive lipase in adipocytes, and the increase in membrane potential in adipose tissue and skeletal muscle.[24]

In contrast, glucagon can be viewed as a hormone that functions when the food supply is low ("fasting"). Glucagon participates in a "supply-demand" theory. Food deprivation (starvation, temporary denial during the first few postpartum hours, delayed delivery during nightly sleep episodes, stress from bone fracture or surgery) causes the release of glucagon which marshalls carbohydrate and amino acids into the blood stream so that glucose is available for metabolism and for repairs.

> From a nutrient-fuel standpoint, glucagon is a catabolic hormone which in many ways counteracts the action of insulin on the same tissue . . . . glucagon should be viewed as a retrieval hormone [that acts] on nutrient depots to release previously stored forms of energy substrate . . . which were deposited earlier at times of metabolic surplus.[25]

One of the most dramatic effects of insulin is on fat. As can be seen from Table 11.7, when it comes to fuel storage, fat is responsible for 85% of stored fuel. Hazelwood points out that insulin has both rapid and slow effects on fat: "Translocation of glucose into adipocytes represents one of insulin's fastest effects (seconds), while that of activating lipogenic enzymes and repressing sensitive lipases are temporally slower (minutes to hours)."[26]

The proportion of pancreatic islet cells of various types changes throughout life (Table 11.8). The percentage of islet cells that produce insulin increases between infancy and adulthood; the percentage of cells that produce glucagon remains rela-

tively constant. Obesity is a frequent concomitant of maturity-onset. Moreover, maturity-onset diabetes can usually be treated effectively with diet and weight reduction.

An interesting phenomenon has been observed with regard to **fat atrophy**. It is common for the subcutaneous fat to atrophy at the insulin injection site. But, paradoxically, insulin promotes fat deposition. Gorman hypothesized[27] that the fat atrophy might be due to small amounts of fat-mobilizing glucagon (up to 0.5%) that were present in commercial insulins. This leads to the interesting speculation that there might be a means of making use of hormone injections or implants to selectively reduce fat deposits.

A "neuroendocrine dysregulaton hypothesis" accounts for some individual variation in regional fat distribution. Stressful stimuli (social, behavioral, biological) initiate chronic neuroendocrine dysregulations. A state of chronic hypothalamic arousal results over time in a more pronounced android profile of fat deposition (higher amounts of abdominal fat in males or a propensity to develop android fat distribution phenotype in females).[28]

REFERENCES

1. Schwartz, M. W.; Figlewicz, D.P.; Baskin, D.G.; Woods, S.C.; Porte, D. Insulin in the brain: A hormonal regulator of energy balance. Endocrine Reviews 13: 387–414; 1993.

2. Tepperman, J. A view of the history of biology from an islet of Langerhans. In McCann, S. M., editor. Endocrinology: People and Ideas. Bethesda, MD: American Physiological Society; 1988; 285–333.

3. Ashcroft, F.M.; Ashcroft, S.J.H., editors. Insulin: Molecular Biology to Pathology. New York: Oxford University Press; 1992; 421 pages.

4. Epple, A.; Brinn, J.E. The Comparative Physiology of the Pancreatic Islets. New York: Springer Verlag; 1987; 223 pages.

5. Ganong, W. Review of Medical Physiology, Fourteenth Edition. Norwalk, CT: Appleton & Lange; 1989, p. 280.

6. Epple, A.; Brinn, J.E.; Ibid.

7. O'Connor, K.J.; Baxter, D. The demonstration of insulin-like material in the honey bee, *Apis mellifera*. Comp. Biochem. Physiol. 81B: 755–760;

1985.

8. LeRoith, D.; Hendricks, S.A.; Lesniak, M.A.; et al. Insulin in brain and other extrapancreatic tissues of vertebrates and nonvertebrates. Adv. Metabol. Disorders 10: 303–340; 1983.

9. Hoerr, N.L.; Osol, A. Blakiston's New Gould Medical Dictionary. New York: The Blakiston Division, McGraw-Hill Book Co.; 1956; 1463.

10. Devlin, T. M. Textbook of Biochemistry with Clinical Correlations. New York: John Wiley & Sones; 1982; p. 326.

11 . Ganong, W.; Op.cit.; p. 290.

12. Frieden, E.; Lipner, H. Biochemical Endocrinology of the Vertebrates. Englewood Cliffs, NJ: Prentice Hall; 1971; p. 7.

13. Ganong, W.; Op.cit.; p. 294.

14. Ganong, W.; Op.cit.; p. 292,295.

15. Yalow, R. S. Heterogeneity of peptide hormones. Recent Progress in Hormone Research 30: 597–632; 1974.

16. Denton, R.M.; Tavare, J.M. Mechanisms whereby insulin may regulate intracellular events. In Ashcroft, F.M.; Ashcroft, S.J.H., editors. Insulin: Molecular Biology to Pathology. New York: Oxford University Press; 1992; 421 pages.

17. Epple, A.; Brinn, J.E.; Op. cit.; pages 247–248.

18. Turner, C.D.; Bagnara, J.T. General Endocrinology, Sixth Edition. Philadelphia, PA: W. B. Saunders Co.; 1976, p. 278.

19. Poretsky, L. On the paradox of insulin-induced hyperandrogenism in insulin-resistant states. Endocrine Reviews 12: 3–13; 1991.

20. Gerich, J.E.; Mokan, M.; Veneman, T.; Korytkowski, M.; Mitrakou, A. Hypoglycemia unawareness. Endocrine Reviews 12: 356–370; 1991.

21. Ganong, W.; Op.cit.; p. 299.

22. Denton, R.M.; Tavare, J.M.; Op. cit.; 421 pages.

23. Hazelwood, R.L. The Endocrine Pancreas. Englewood Cliffs, NJ: Prentice-Hall; 1989, p. 126–146.

24. Hazelwood, R.L.; Ibid.; p. 126.

25. Hazelwood, R.L.; Ibid.; p. 137.

26. Hazelwood, R.L.; Ibid.; p. 132.

27. Gorman, C.K. Diabetes mellitus. In Ezrin, C.; Godden, J.O.; Volpe, R.; Wilson, R. Systematic Endocrinology. New York: Harper & Row, Pubs.; 1973, p. 336–337.

28. Bouchard, C.; Despres, J.; Mauriege, P. Genetic and nongenetic determinants of regional fat distribution. Endocrine Reviews 14: 72–93; 1993.

CHAPTER 12

Gastrointestinal Hormones

The gastrointestinal tract in the transport, digestion, and absorption of food. Hormones (mainly gastrin, secretin, cholecystokinin, and gastric inhibitory peptide) open and close sphincters, contract muscles, and cause digestive secretions in response to nutrients. The autonomic nervous system, the enteric nervous system of the intestinal walls, and hormones work together to regulate and fine tune gastrointestinal function. The gastrointestinal hormones are made in cells scattered through the gastrointestinal tract, but some are also made in the pancreas and neurons. In addition to the peptides discussed in this chapter, there are hormones from other glands that also have roles to play in the metabolism and use of nutrients, such as insulin, somatotropin, prolactin, and glucocorticoids.

HISTORICAL PERSPECTIVE: SECRETIN

Secretin played an important role in the development of the field of endocrinology.[1] As put by Turner and Bagnara:

> The real science of endocrinology was probably born through the experiments of Bayliss and Starling (1902-1905). Their work showed the existence and manner of action, at the level of the whole organism, of the hormone *secretin*. This secretion is released from cells of the duodenal mucosa when acidified food enters from the stomach; it is conveyed by the circulation to the pancreas, where it stimulates the rapid discharge of pancreatic juice through the pancreatic duct. Although it had been recognized before this time that a variety of endocrine glands exert influences on the body, this discovery was epoch-making because it proved unequivocally for the first time that chemical integration could occur without assistance from the nervous system. It clearly confirmed the idea that special glands elaborate chemical agents, which are freed into the blood and exert regulatory effects upon distant target organs and tissues."[2]

Starling is even given credit for coining the word "hormone." The word is derived from a Greek word, *hormaein*, variously translated as to excite, to arouse, to set into motion, or to bring into play. According to Douglas Wright, Starling was the first to use the word "hormone" to refer to chemical messengers–adrenalin, thyroid extract, secretin, gastrin, female sex hormones, hormones of pancreatic diabetes–in the Croonian Lectures which he delivered to the college of Physicians of June 20, 1905.[3] But Bayliss apparently noted that the word "hormone" was proposed by Mr. W. B. Hardy, and Needham says that "hormone" was suggested by W.T. Vesey. Added to this confusion, there apparently was some early scientific dispute over the word "hormone" because chemical messengers are responsible for inhibition as well as excitation. In any case, the work of Bayliss and Starling, two Canadian physiologists, is the cornerstone of the field of endocrinology. Hadley considers their first experiment critical, and dubs it the *experimentum*

cruces.[4]

GASTROTINTESTINAL ENDOCRINE SYSTEM

Secretin and the other gastrointestinal hormones do not fit comfortably into the classical definition of an endocrine system since they are not synthesized and secreted by discrete endocrine glands. Instead, most gastrointestinal hormones are produced by cells that are scattered in regions of the gastric or intestinal mucosa.

Deveney and Way specify criteria for gastrointestinal hormones: "(1) postprandial [after a meal] release, as demonstrated by measuring a rise in blood levels; and (2) elicitation of physiologic response of target organ by infusing exogenous hormone at a rate that reproduced postprandial blood levels."[5] These criteria are met by four hormones: gastrin, secretin, cholecystokinin, and gastric inhibitory polypeptide. The gastrointestinal hormones are synthesized by large portions of the gastrointestinal tract (Figure 12.1).

Other peptides may be potential gut hormones because of (i) potential function as gastrointestinal hormones, (ii) localization in gastrointestinal tract, or (iii) structural or functional similarities to the four gastrointestinal hormones. The list of gut peptides is extensive; in addition to the four hormones, it includes calcitonin gene-related peptide, dynorphin, enteroglucagon (nonpancreatic-type glucagons in the gut), met-enkephalin, leu-enkephalin, galanin, gastrin-relasing peptide, motilin, neuromedin B, neuromedin K (neurokinin B), neuromedin U, neuropeptide Y, neurotensin, peptide histidine isoleucine, peptide histidine methionine, pancreastatin, peptide YY, substance K (neurokinin A), substance P, somatostatin, valosin, and vasoactive intestinal peptide.[6]

GASTROINTESTINAL TRACT

To appreciate the functions of hormones in the regulation of digestion, there must first be a minimal understanding of the anatomy of the digestive system, the timing of food passage through the tract, and the physiology of digestion (Figure 12.2).

Food enters the **mouth** where it is mechanically broken into smaller parts by chewing. The chewed food descends the **esophagus** to the **stomach**. The length of the mouth, esophagus, and stomach average 65 centimeters in humans.

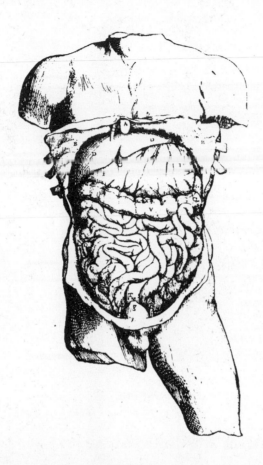

Figure 12.1 The artwork shows the human gastrointestinal tract in its portrayal of the human visceral organs. The drawing is from Vesalius book of woodcuts, *De Humani Corporis Fabrica*, and was probably done hundreds of years ago by students in Titian's studio. Reproduced, with permission, from Moore, J.A. Understanding nature—Form and functions. American Zoologist 28: 449–584; 1988.

From the stomach, the chyme (a thick slush of partly digested food) passes through the pyloric sphincter into the 25-cm-long **duodenum** which is the first part of the small intestine. The bolus passes through the 260-cm-long **small intestine.** The upper 40% of the intestine is called the jejunum; the lower 60% is called the ileum). From there, the bolus enters the **large intestine** (the large bowel, or colon, is 110 cm long), and, finally, is excreted as feces via the **rectum** which ends externally as the **anus.** Gastrointestinal hormones are involved in organizing some of the events of digestion (Figure 12.3).

DIGESTION

Digestion is accomplished by mastication (chewing), enzymes, acid (hydrochloric acid in the stomach), diluents, lubricants, emulsifying salts, and colonic bacteria. Enzymes in the mouth include starch-digesting salivary α-amylase (ptyalin) secreted by the salivary glands. In the stomach, pepsins are released from precursors (pepsinogens) from the mucosa by hydrochloric acid, and there is a gelatinase. In the duodenum, pancreatic enzymes work on breaking down protein

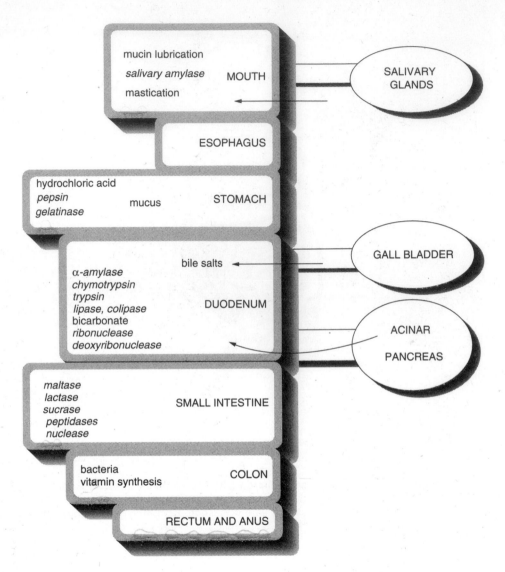

Figure 12.2 The figure shows the locations of some of the enzymes and other factors involved in the process of digestion. Enzymes are italicized.

(chymotrypsin, trypsin, elastase, carboxypeptidases A and B), starch (α-amylase), fats (lipase, phospholipase, esterase) and nucleic acid (ribonuclease, deoxyribonuclease). The gallbladder secretes bile salts into the duodenum; the bile salts emulsify fats. The small intestine mucosa secretes peptidases which break down protein, oligosacchari-dases which break down sugars (maltose, α-limit dextrins, lactose, sucrose), and nucleases which break down nucleic acid. Components of a test meal reach the colon in 4–9 hours and may remain in the rectum up to 72 hours. Bacteria, mainly in the colon, also participate—they synthesize vitamins and function in cholesterol metabolism.

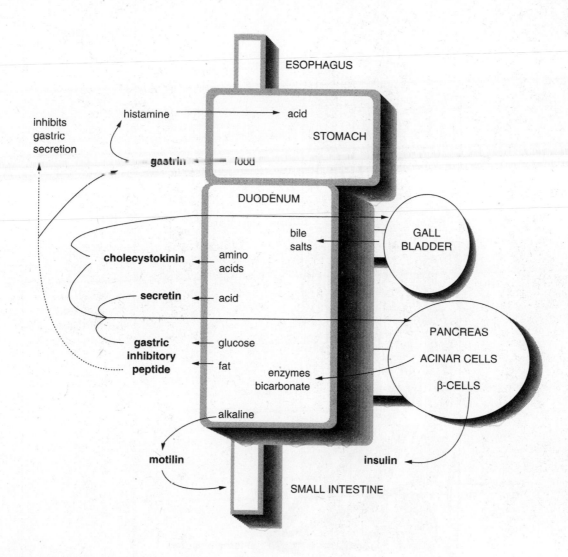

Figure 12.3 The figure represents some of the ways in which nutrients act on the mucosa to stimulate some of the gastrointestinal hormones (bold type).   Nutrients in the lumen of the gastrointestinal tract stimulate the secretion of the gastrointestinal hormones. The gastrointestinal hormones act on targets (stomach, gall bladder, pancreas) and cause them to secrete digestive acid, enzymes, and bile salts that participate in the digestion of the food.

GASTROINTESTINAL ENDOCRINE CELLS

The gastrointestinal tract (posterior pharynx to anus) has four layers: serosa or adventitia (outer), muscularis externa, submucosa, and mucosa (inner, adjacent to lumen).[7] Except for the esophagus, the gastrointestinal tract is lined with the **mucosa**. The mucosa is folded (plicae circularis) and has 0.5–1.5 mm long villi which project into the intestine and increase its surface area. Between the

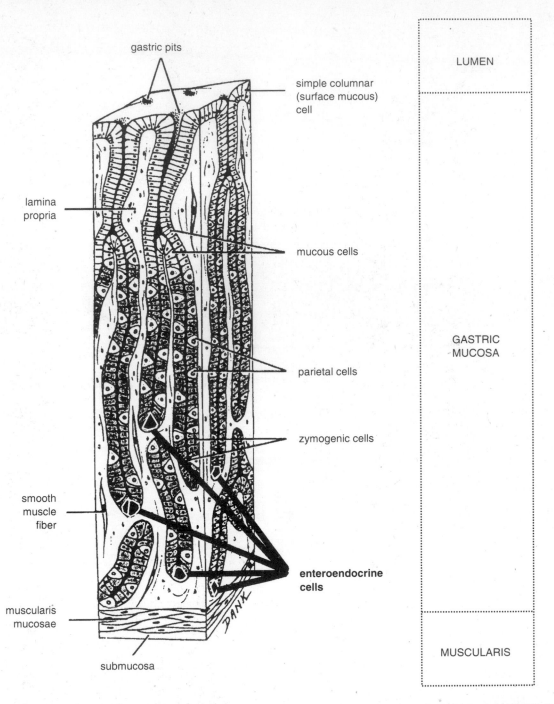

gastric pits

simple columnar
(surface mucous)
cell

lamina
propria

mucous cells

parietal cells

zymogenic cells

smooth
muscle
fiber

**enteroendocrine
cells**

muscularis
mucosae

submucosa

LUMEN

GASTRIC
MUCOSA

MUSCULARIS

Figure 12.4 The figure is a diagrammatic representation of the histology of the gastric mucosa showing the location of the enteroendocrine cells. Modified, with permission. Tortora, G.J.; Anagnostakos, N.P. Principles of Anatomy and Physiology, Sixth Edition. New York: Harper & Row, Pubs.; 1990; p. 747.

Table 12.1. Map of Gastrointestinal Peptide Locations

Cell type	Stomach fundus	Stomach antrum	Intestine duodenum	Intestine jejunum	Intestine ileum	Colon
G		+gastrin	gastrin	gastrin		
A		+glucagon	glucagon	glucagon		
S			+secretin	+secretin	secretin	
I			+CCK	+CCK	CCK	
K			+GIP	+GIP	GIP	
EC_2			+motilin	+motilin	+motilin	
D_1	VIP	VIP	VIP	VIP	+VIP	+VIP
EC_1	substance P	substance P	substance P	substance P	substance P	substance P
	glicentin	glicentin	glicentin	glicentin	+glicentin	+glicentin
D	+somatostatin	+somatostatin	somatostatin	somatostatin	somatostatin	somatostatin
K	+GIP	+GIP	GIP	GIP	GIP	GIP
N				neurotensin	+neurotensin	
	enkephalins	enkephalins	enkephalins			
			peptide YY	peptide YY	peptide YY	

Gastrin-secreting cells are divided into Ga cells in the antrum and GI cells in the intestine; + means higher concentration. Some of the hormones—glucagon, somatostatin, VIP, substance P, gastrin, bombesin, and pancreatic polypeptide—are also hormones of the pancreas. Other hormones—VIP, substance P, motilin, CCK, gastrin, neurotensin, bombesin—are also peptides of the nervous system. P-cells make bombesin; D_2F cells are the source of pancreatic polypeptide. Ganong, W. Review of Medical Physiology, Fourteenth Edition. Norwalk, CT: Appleton & Lange; 1989, p. 411; and Said, S.I. Peptides common to the nervous system and the gastrointestinal tract. Frontiers of Neuroendocrinology 6: 293–331; 1980.

villi bases, there are the intestinal glands (crypts of Lieberkuhn) 0.3–0.5 mm deep where the **enteroendocrine cells** are found. The enteroendocrine cells of the intestinal mucosa are the sources of the hormones (Figure 12.4).

The osmiophilic, basigranular yellow, or acidophil cells of the gastrointestinal mucosa were ascribed an endocrine function by Masson in 1914. The endocrine cells constitute the dispersed endocrine system (DES) and are some of Fuyrter's "specialized clear cells" which react to silver salts (argentaffin, argyrophil). They are enterochromaffin cells. The cells later became part of the APUD (amine precursor uptake and decarboxylation) concept, but the gut and pancreas endocrine cells, though they handle amines and produce peptides, probably do not originate from neural crest cells as do many of the other APUD cells. The cells were also called "paraneurons" by Fujita. The distribution of the cells that are intermingled nonendocrine cells varies along the gastrointestinal tract, and certain regions (e.g., gastric antrum) have more of them.[8]

Efforts to classify the cell types by the hormone they secrete have been made (Table 12.1).[9] Investigators have listed over fifteen cell types with some cells secreting more than one product. Some surfaces of endocrine cells have cell membranes at the gastrointestinal lumen. The lumenal membranes provide an opportunity for the cells to respond to metabolites from food in the lumen as the metabolites arrive at the cells' locations.

gastic inhibitory peptide 42 amino acids	glucagon 29 amino acids	secretin 27 amino acids	vasoactive intestinal peptide 28 amino acids	cholecystokinin 33 amino acids	cholecystokinin 39 amino acids	gastrin 34 amino acids
tyr	**his**	**his**	**his**		tyr	
ala	**ser**	**ser**	**ser**		ile	
glu	gln	asp	asp		gln	
gly	**gly**	**gly**	ala		gln	
thr	**thr**	**thr**	val		ala	
phe	**phe**	**phe**	**phe**		arg	(pyro)-glu
ile	**thr**	**thr**	**thr**	**lys**	**lys**	leu
ser	**ser**	**ser**	asp	**ala**	**ala**	gly
asp	**asp**	glu	asn	**pro**	**pro**	**pro**
tyr	**tyr**	leu	**tyr**	**ser**	**ser**	gln
ser	**ser**	**ser**	thr	**gly**	**gly**	**gly**
ile	lys	**arg**	**arg**	**arg**	**arg**	pro
ala	tyr	leu	**leu**	val	met	pro
met	leu	**arg**	**arg**	**ser**	**ser**	his
asp	**asp**	glu	lys	met	ile	leu
lys	ser	gly	gln	ile	**val**	**val**
ile	arg	ala	met	**lys**	**lys**	ala
his	**arg**	**arg**	ala	**asn**	**asn**	asp
gln	ala	leu	val	**leu**	**leu**	pro
gln	**gln**	**gln**	lys	**gln**	**gln**	ser
asp	**asp**	arg	lys	ser	asn	lys
phe	**phe**	leu	tyr	**leu**	**leu**	lys
val	**val**	leu	**leu**	**asp**	**asp**	gln
asn	**gln**	**gln**	asn	**pro**	**pro**	gly
trp	**trp**	gly	ser	**ser**	**ser**	pro
leu	**leu**	**leu**	ile	**his**	**his**	trp
leu	met	val-NH$_2$	**leu**	**arg**	**arg**	leu
ala	asn		asn-NH$_2$	**ile**	**ile**	glu
glu	thr			**ser**	**ser**	glu
lys				**asp**	**asp**	glu
gly				**arg**	**arg**	glu
lys				**asp**	**asp**	glu
lys				tyr	tys	ala
asn				**met**	**met**	tys
asp				**gly**	**gly**	**gly**
trp				**trp**	**trp**	**trp**
lys				**met**	**met**	**met**
his				**asp**	**asp**	**asp**
asn				**phe-NH$_2$**	**phe-NH$_2$**	**phe-NH$_2$**
ile						
thr						
gln						

Figure 12.5 The amino acid sequences for the gastrointestinal peptides in the secretin and gastrin families are shown. In cholecystokinin and gastrin, tys = sulfated tyrosine. Bold face amino acid residues indicate common features of the secretin (left four) and gastrin (right three) families of polypeptide hormones.

CHEMICAL GROUPS OF THE GASTROINTESTINAL HORMONES

The gastrointestinal hormones are peptides and polypeptides (Figures 12.5 and 12.6). There are three groups of peptide and polypeptide gastrointestinal hormones based on structural relationships. The cholecystokinin-gastrin family contains cholecystokinins (CCKs), gastrin, cerulein, and phyllocerulein. The secretin family is composed of

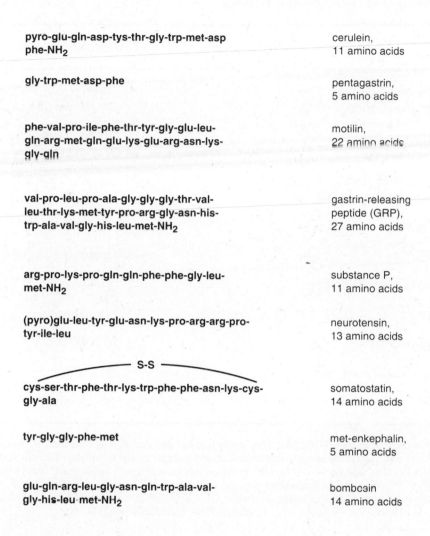

pyro-glu-gln-asp-tys-thr-gly-trp-met-asp phe-NH$_2$ — cerulein, 11 amino acids

gly-trp-met-asp-phe — pentagastrin, 5 amino acids

phe-val-pro-ile-phe-thr-tyr-gly-glu-leu-gln-arg-met-gln-glu-lys-glu-arg-asn-lys-gly-gln — motilin, 22 amino acids

val-pro-leu-pro-ala-gly-gly-gly-thr-val-leu-thr-lys-met-tyr-pro-arg-gly-asn-his-trp-ala-val-gly-his-leu-met-NH$_2$ — gastrin-releasing peptide (GRP), 27 amino acids

arg-pro-lys-pro-gln-gln-phe-phe-gly-leu-met-NH$_2$ — substance P, 11 amino acids

(pyro)glu-leu-tyr-glu-asn-lys-pro-arg-arg-pro-tyr-ile-leu — neurotensin, 13 amino acids

S-S
cys-ser-thr-phe-thr-lys-trp-phe-phe-asn-lys-cys-gly-ala — somatostatin, 14 amino acids

tyr-gly-gly-phe-met — met-enkephalin, 5 amino acids

glu-gln-arg-leu-gly-asn-gln-trp-ala-val-gly-his-leu-met-NH$_2$ — bombesin 14 amino acids

Figure 12.6 The amino acid sequences for the gastrointestinal peptides that are not in the gastrin and secretin families are shown.

glucagon, secretin, vasoactive intestinal peptide (VIP), and glycentin. There are other peptides and polypeptides involved in gastrointestinal function: motilin, substance P, gastrin-releasing peptide, and somatostatin. Some of the gastrointestinal hormones are synthesized in the pancreas and salivary glands while the rest are synthesized by the mucosa. The locations of hormones along the tract can be mapped, and their concentrations in blood can be measured (Table 12.2).

The actions of gastrointestinal peptides are variously considered to be endocrine (acting as hormones transported in the blood), neurocrine (acting as neurotransmitters or neuromodulators), or paracrine (transported by extracellular fluid to adjacent surrounding cells). Because of these diverse

Table 12.2 Amounts of Gastrointestinal Hormones

Substance	Concentration in blood
cholecystokinin, blood, fasting	0–20 pmol/l
cholecystokinin, blood, postprandial	20–100 pmol/l
gastrin, serum	10–50 pmol/l
gastrin, serum, postprandial	20–40 pmol/l increases
gastrointestinal peptide, basal levels, blood	250 pg/ml (50 pmol/l)
gastrointestinal peptide, postprandial, serum	1000 pg/ml
secretin, fasting, serum	1–5 pmol/l
motilin, blood	4–350 pmol/l (median 60)
vasoactive intestinal peptide, fasting	<7 pmol/l
substance P, serum	40–300 pg/ml
peptide YY, postprandial	200–300 pg/ml
pancreatic polypeptide, fasting, blood	50–200 pg/ml
glucagon, blood	50–150 pg/ml

Hormones were assayed with RIA. Gastrin is most easily assayed and therefore is well studied. Existence of multiple forms of CCK and gastrin complicate measurements and interpretations of levels. Secretin is difficult to measure with RIA because it has no tyrosine residues which can be iodinated. Substance P is only found in disease states. Deveney, C.W., Way, L.W. Regulatory peptides of the gut. In Greenspan, F.; Forsham, P., editors. Basic and Clinical Endocrinology, Second Edition. Norwalk, CT: Appleton & Lange; 1987; pp. 501–522; Norman, A.W.; Litwack, G. Hormones. Orlando, FL: Academic Press Inc.; 1987, pp. 758–760.

roles, Deveney and Way suggest referring to the group as "regulatory peptides."[10]

CHOLECYSTOKININ

Cholecystokinin (CCK) is a polypeptide hormone in the "gastrin family" of gastrointestinal peptides. Cholecystokinin is also called cholecystokinin-pancreozymin (CCK-PZ) because pancreozymin was formerly thought to be a separate hormone. Cholecystokinin shares three amino acids with gastrin and also an N-terminal sequence of five amino acids which are also called pentagastrin.

Cholecystokinin also has amino acid sequences similar to those in a decapeptide named **caerulein**.[11] Caerulein has 10 amino acids and comes from frog skin (Australian *Hyla caerulea*). It shares seven amino acids with gastrin which may account for the fact that it has properties of gastrin and cholecystokinin.

Cholecystokinin is present in nerve endings (where it may function as a neurotransmitter), and it is localized in the mucosa I cells of the small intestine found in the duodenum, jejunum, and ileum (from which it is secreted into the blood as a hormone).

Cholecystokinin is synthesized, as are other polypeptide hormones, from a large precursor. There are a number of cholecystokinin fragments that are designated by a number representing their numbers of amino acids. CCK39, CCK58 (a larger form of cholecystokinin), CCK33, CCK12, CCK8, CCK4, and pentagastrin are all synthesized as fragments of prepro-CCK. Cholecystokinin is found in the cerebral cortex of the brain (CCK8, CCK58), in the upper small intestine mucosal I cells (CCK8, CCK12, CCK58), in ileum and colon and nerves (CCK4), and in blood (CCK8, CCK33, CCK58). Forms of CCK share eight amino acids at the carboxy-terminal which also compose CCK8. The octapeptide is responsible for the biological activity and has high potency. Activity varies among CCK fragments; for example, CCK8 is has up to six times the activity of CCK 33. Sulfation is necessary for biological activity. CCK is described variously as possessing a sulfated tyrosine (tys or tyr-HSO_3) on the seventh amino acid from the N-terminal[12] or on position seven from the C-terminal.[13] The half-life of CCK is 2.5–7 minutes.

Cholecystokinin has several targets based on uptake—lung, spleen, intestine, stomach, liver, kidney—and several known functions. Its established functions are stimulation of gall bladder contraction and secretion of pancreatic juice, but there are many other actions having to do with digestive function that have been proposed.

Cholecystokinin functions to facilitate physical and chemical activities of the digestive tract. (i) CCK contracts the lower esophageal sphincter by stimulating contraction of smooth muscle. (ii) Cholecystokinin stimulates contraction of the antrum stomach. (iii) Cholecystokinin and secretin may act together to contract the pyloric sphincter which keeps the duodenal contents from backing up (refluxing) into the stomach. (iv) Cholecystokinin causes gall bladder contraction. (v) CCK, with secretin, stimulates the pancreas to secrete alkaline pancreatic juice and (vi) CCK, with gastrin, stimulates the pancreas to secrete glucagon by activating a phospholipase C. (vii) Cholecystokinin stimulates motility in the intestine. (viii) Cholecystokinin may stimulate colon contractility. Deveney and Way suggest that CCK "acts as a neurotransmitter to stimulate postganglionic inhibitory neurons...and acts directly on

smooth muscle."[14]

Cholecystokinin was named for its function in stimulating gall bladder contraction after a meal, or **postprandial gall bladder contraction**. Agents that stimulate the gall bladder are called cholagogues. When food enters the mouth, the sphincter of Oddi around the opening from the bile duct into the duodenum relaxes. The sphincter opening permits bile to be expelled from the gall bladder when cholecystokinin stimulates gall bladder contraction in response to digestive products entrance into the duodenum from the stomach.

Cholecystokinin functions in stimulating the secretion of other hormones. Cholecystokinin and gastrin stimulate secretion of glucagon and augments amino acid stimulation of insulin secretion. Cholecystokinin also stimulates pancreatic insulin release, pancreatic polypeptide release, and calcitonin release.

Cholecystokinin stimulates secretions that are important to digestion. Cholecystokinin causes secretion of pancreatic juice. Cholecystokinin, together with secretin, increases pancreatic juice concentration of bicarbonate which increases juice alkalinity. Cholecystokinin also stimulates secretion of hepatic bile and Brunner's glands of the duodenum. Cholecystokinin stimulates growth of pancreatic acinar cells via a mechanism of action involving phospholipase C activation.

Regulation of cholecystokinin secretion in the digestive system is by a positive feedback loop involving the digestive products in the lumen of the intestine. It was an early discovery that introduction of fat into the small intestine caused the gall bladder to contract. Presence of digestive products in the lumen of the duodenum stimulate the intestinal mucosa to secrete cholecystokinin. The digestive products are (i) amino acids such as tryptophan and phenylalanine from a protein meal, (ii) fatty acids that have more than 9 carbons, (iii) acids, and (iv) calcium. Cholecystokinin concentration in blood rises in ten minutes after a meal and stays up for two hours. The cholecystokinin, in turn, stimulates gall bladder contraction and production of pancreatic juice so that the fats and proteins are further digested. When the digested products exit the upper intestine, cholecystokinin secretion stops.

Longer chain fatty acids (up to 18 carbons) increase CCK and the amount of CCK produced depends on the length of intestine exposed to stimulating agents. Bile acids in the intestine reduce the effectiveness of digestive products as stimuli which may provide an additional means of shutting off CCK secretion.

Cholecystokinin may play roles in the regulation of eating and in gall bladder disease. A role in feeding behavior seems likely. Satiety induction in humans and some other species is a consequence of CCK and requires vagal innervation. For example, injecting rats, humans, or monkeys with cholecystokinin produces satiety as measured by feeding reduction, between-meal interval is lengthened in rats injected with CCK.[15,16] Calcitonin may act synergistically with cholecystokinin to induce satiety.[17] A role for CCK has been proposed in eating disorders such as **anorexia nervosa.** Deveney and Way discuss the possibility that cholecystokinin functions in obesity:

> ...[CCK8] inhibits appetite in mammals when infused into the cerebral ventricles. This polypeptide....is found in higher concentrations in the central nervous system than in plasma. Deficiencies in levels of CCK8 and of its central nervous system receptors have been postulated to exist in genetic animal models of obesity.[18]

Thus, a simple but appealing hypothesis would be that excess CCK is responsible for diminished eating because it produces satiety (in anorexia nervosa) and that deficient CCK is responsible for excess eating because it fails to produce satiety (in obesity). Where does CCK act? Hadley suggests a tentative hypothesis:

> CCK released by the gastrointestinal tract or afferent vagal neurons is stimulatory to noradrenergic neurons of the [ventral medial hypothalamus satiety center] which, through the release of norepinephrine, are inhibitory to the lateral hypothalamic feeding centers."[19]

It is also interesting that 40 percent of anorexics have elevated serum cholesterol which could be caused by excess CCK (anorexic cholesterol 400–600 mg/dl; normal cholesterol <260 mg/dl). This possibility exists because cholecystokinin plays a role in cholesterol regulation since cholesterol is excreted in the bile. Formation of one kind of **gallstones** (cholelithiasis) can be due to excess cholesterol which has low solubility in bile and formation of gallstones has been associated with low-calorie diets.

CCK is also found in brain regions. For example, frontal cortex of the cat has 36.8 pmol/g and hippocampus has 42.7 pmol/g.[20]

GASTRIN

Gastrin is synthesized in G-cells that are found in the mucosa of the antral, or lower, portion of the stomach. The G-cells are amine precursor uptake and decarboxylation (APUD) cells, which means that they share an origin from neural crest with other types of endocrine cells. The G-cells have characteristic histology: the cells have a narrow apex with microvilli projecting into the lumen of the stomach. The other end of the cells is broader, making them "flask" shaped. The broad region of the G-cells has granules that contain gastrin. There are additional cells that produce gastrin called the TG-cells. The TG-cells are found scattered throughout the small intestine and stomach. Gastrin is also a putative neurotransmitter or neural hormone found in the hypothalamus (G17, G34) and medulla oblongata of the brain. In fetuses, the pancreas secretes gastrin. Gastrin's functions are endocrine and neurocrine.

The gastrins are synthesized from a large precursor molecule called preprogastrin. Forms of gastrin include G14, G17, G34, G-45, and C-terminal gastrin tetrapeptide. Forms that are sulfated at amino acid six and forms that are not sulfated circulate. Some forms are amidated at the C-terminal phenylalanine. Gastrin shares a five-amino acid carboxy terminal sequence with cholecystokinin. G17 is the principal form and has 6–10 times the potency of the tetrapeptide. In serum G34 is the main form; the form secreted by antral G-cells is G17; the form made by duodenal cells is G34; G17 and G34 are found in the brain. The half-lives of G14, G17, and G34 are short, ranging is 2–15 minutes. The kidneys are responsible for metabolism of gastrin and excretion of gastrin breakdown products.

A main function of gastrin is stimulation of gastric acid secretion in the stomach. In this role, gastrin causes the parietal cells of the stomach to secrete an acid-rich juice (pH = 2, high H^+).

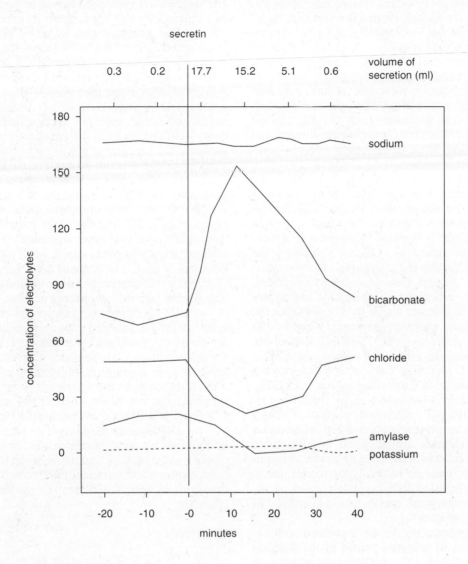

Figure 12.7 The illustration shows effects of secretin (12.5 units/kg IV) at time zero on the volume of secretions (top bar) and the concentration of bicarbonate and other electrolytes in the gastrointestinal tract (graphs). Concentrations of electrolytes are in meq/l; concentration of amylase is U/ml. Modified, with permission. After Janowitz, H.D. Pancreatic secretion. Physiol. Physicians (November) 2: 11; 1964.

Gastrin releases histamine from cells near the parietal cells and the histamine in turn causes the parietal cells to secrete hydrochloric acid. Gastrin also promotes the stomach to secrete pepsin. The pepsins (pepsinogens) are enzymes of the stomach that break peptide bonds that are next to aromatic amino acids. A second main function is stimulation of the growth of the gastric mucosa. A third function of gastrin is stimulation of physical changes in the gastrointestinal tract. Gastrin stimulates gastric motility. The muscles that close the opening from the stomach to the esophagus contract in response to gastrin. Gastrin relaxes the pyloric sphincter and stimulates the pancreas to secrete enzymes and bicarbonate and water. Gastrin increases intestinal motility. A fourth function of gastrin is stimulation of the secretion of other hormones. After a protein meal, gastrin causes glucagon and insulin secretion. Gastrin may also stimulate somatotropin. A fifth function of gastrin is stimulation of gastrointestinal growth. Gastrin stimulates gall bladder contraction and pancreas enzyme secretion, but it is less potent than cholecystokinin in these actions.

Gastrin is regulated by nerves, nutrients, and hormones. The innervation is by the vagus nerves. The neurotransmitter for the vagal stimulation of gastrin is probably gastrin-releasing peptide (GRP). Gastrin is secreted in response to a meal reaching the stomach. Gastrin stimulates the sphincter of the lower esophagus so that the opening closes. Protein derived nutrients—peptides, amino acids (especially phenylalanine and tryptophan)—in the stomach signal the G-cells to release gastrin. Gastrin concentrations are elevated by 30–60 minutes after a meal. Stomach distention, blood calcium, and circulating epinephrine also increase gastrin secretion. Gastrin causes an increase in stomach acid, but the acid feeds back and inhibits gastrin secretion. Gastrin secretion is inhibited by secretin, VIP, GIP, calcitonin, somatostatin, and glucagon. Gastrin levels are reduced in starvation or when nutrients are supplied intravenously. Gastrin secretion is stimulated by electrical stimulation of the vagus nerve, by hypoglycemia due to insulin, by injected 2-deoxyglucose, and by atropine. Removing the antrum results in atrophy of pancreas and mucosa.

Duodenal ulcers are associated with excess secretion of acid and pepsin by the stomach into the duodenum. The parietal cells of afflicted individuals have larger acid-secreting responses to histamine and gastrin. However, the number of gastrin-secreting cells and serum G17 and serum G34 are normal. The response to a meal is larger than normal and lasts for a longer time.

GASTRIC INHIBITORY POLYPEPTIDE

Gastric inhibitory polypeptide (GIP) is found in duodenal and jejunal and ileal mucosa. GIP is most abundant in the jejunum. Its function is endocrine. Gastric inhibitory polypeptide has 43 amino acids and is related structurally to secretin.

GIP is probably synthesized from a larger precursor molecule. GIP's half-life is about 20 minutes.

The pancreas is a target of GIP. GIP stimulates insulin secretion by increasing beta cell cyclic AMP. Ganong considers GIP to be the "gut factor" that regulates insulin's response to a meal.[21] GIP is also called glucose-dependent insulinotropic peptide because of its function in stimulating insulin secretion. Why glucose-dependent? GIP potentiates the insulin-releasing response of the pancreas to glucose injection, but the same amount of glucose evokes greater insulin release when the glucose is administered orally. Increasing GIP without glucose does not stimulate insulin release. Regulation of gastric inhibitory polypeptide is like that for other gastrointestinal hormones in that it involves nutrients. Gastric inhibitory polypeptide rises after a meal, peaks about 60 minutes later, and remains high for 3 hours. Glucose in the intestinal lumen stimulates GIP. The glucose response takes about an hour.

GIP is the active principle in enterogastrone which was believed to be responsible for the inhibition of gastric acid secretion in response to fat consumption. Triglycerides derived from fat breakdown in the intestinal lumen stimulate GIP. The fat response takes longer than the glucose response, about two hours. Again, the fat-induced GIP increase does not stimulate insulin secretion.

GIP inhibits the release of gastrin and it inhibits gastric acid secretion (for which it is named), and stimulates ileal mucosal electrolyte and fluid secretion and intestinal juice secretions from the duodenal glands of Brunner near the pyloric sphincter.

SECRETIN

In the gastrointestinal tract, secretin is produced in the duodenum and the jejunum. Secretin's function is endocrine, but secretin is nonetheless found in various parts of the brain: olfactory bulb, brain stem, cerebral cortex, hypothalamus, septum, hippocampus, and thalamus.

Secretin's structure shares a 14 amino acid sequence with glucagon; and secretin has structural similarities to glicentin, vasoactive intestinal peptide, and GIP. Secretin has 27 amino acids and a 3–7.5 minute half-life.

The cellular targets are the pancreatic and biliary tract duct cells. Using a cyclic AMP as a second messenger, secretin causes the pancreas to produce a watery, alkaline juice (Figure 12.7). In a clinical test used to evaluate human pancreatic function, 0.25 µg of secretin per kg body weight causes >2ml/kg flow over 80 minutes. The pancreatic juice is alkaline because of the high concentration of bicarbonate (HCO_3^-). In the same clinical test, normal bicarbonate concentration is >90 meq/l. So secretin's main function is, via promoting secretion of alkaline juice, to counteract, or neutralize, the acidity of the chyme that leaves the stomach. It is logical then, that secretin is secreted in response to lumen acid coming into contact with intestinal mucosa cells. There is a pH threshold for secretion of secretin. Secretin is secreted when lumen pH falls below 4.5. Secretin may also be stimulated by response to protein digestion products and bile salts, but it is not directly regulated by the vagus nerve. When the intestinal contents are neutralized, secretin secretion stops because the acidic signal is no longer present. Secretin decreases gastric acid secretion, stimulates bile secretion, and increases insulin secretion. Secretin may also cause contraction of the pyloric sphincter.

MOTILIN

Motilin is found in cells in mucosa of various parts of the intestine and stomach (duodenum, jejunum, antrum, fundus), neurohypophysis, cerebellum, and cerebral cortex. Its function is endocrine. Motilin has 22 amino acids. Motilin contracts smooth muscle mainly of the duodenum, but also to a lesser degree in the gall bladder, ileum, and colon. Smooth muscle in stomach and small intestine has characteristic electrical activity called "interdigestive migrating myoelectric complex."[22,23] The electrical response is subdivided into four phases of which two phases, which coincide with a peristaltic wave and motilin increases, recur in fasting dogs at 90–120 minute intervals. Following the origination of the myoelectric activity in the duodenum, the wave propagates slowly down the intestine so that it reaches the distal ileum in 60–80 minutes; thus it appears that motilin may function in the movement of food during between meal cyclic peristalsis. Motilin also stimulates gall bladder contraction and gastric acid secretion. The stimulus for motilin release may be alkalinity in the intestine lumen because motilin was discovered by the observation that increasing the alkalinity in the dog duodenum causes contractions in the stomach.

GLICENTIN

Glicentin is also called "glucagon-like immunoreactivity" (abbreviated GLI), "glucagon-like immunoreactive factor," "enteroglucagon," "enterogluconoid," and "proglucagon."

Molecules with GLI activity were suggested as present in gastrointestinal mucosa and pancreas A-cells. A component with GLI activity is a 100 amino acid peptide with MW 11000, so glycentin is larger than the 29 amino acid glucagon, but it has some glucagon activity. Because of this, glycentin is included in the secretin family of peptides. The ileum and colon have the greatest levels of glicentin, and it has been found in cells that look like pancreatic A-cells.

Glicentin may have neurocrine, paracrine, and endocrine function. Food, including carbohydrates, is hypothesized to release glycentin. Glycentin may release insulin, increase liver glucose, promote intestinal motility, and foster growth of the mucosa.

The term "gut glucagon" has been equated with total GLI, glucagon plus enteroglucagon.

VASOACTIVE INTESTINAL PEPTIDE

Vasoactive intestinal peptide (VIP) is found in the gastrointestinal tract, postganglionic cholinergic neurons, hypophysial portal blood, hypothalamus, cerebral cortex, retina, vasomotor nerves, pancreas D-cells, and the intestinal D-cells—indeed the entire intestinal tract from the esophagus to the colon. Based on structure, VIP is classified in the secretin family of polypeptides. VIP has 28 amino acid residues and is synthesized from prepro-VIP (also a precursor for another blood polypeptide, human PHM-27 or porcine intestinal peptide, PHI-27).[24,25] In blood, VIP has a 1–3 minute half-life. The name of the hormone derives from apparent circulatory function and the hormone's isolation from intestine.

Some functions of VIP appear to be neurocrine and paracrine, rather than endocrine, and include vasodilation of peripheral vessels, smooth muscle relaxation, inhibition of gastric acid secretion, potentiation of acetylcholine, stimulation of lipolysis, stimulation of glycogenolysis, stimulation of insulin secretion, stimulation of small intestine secretion of electrolytes, retinal neurotransmitter, and sphincter relaxation.

VIP does not increase in blood after meals. However, VIP may act as a cotransmitter for neural signals to cause salivary gland vasodilation which results in saliva secretion. Salivation is a "reflex" that can be conditioned. The salivation reflex was used by Pavlov in his experiments: dogs salivated in response to a bell that had previously been associated with the presentation of meat.[26] It would be interesting to know if VIP functions as a conditioned hormone reflex in the Pavlovian response.

SUBSTANCE P

Substance P has historical importance because it was the first peptide that was found in nervous tissue of both gut and brain. It is also found in the retina, and it has 11 amino acids. It is found in the blood in disease states so that it is possible that its functions are limited to paracrine and neurocrine roles, perhaps as a neurotransmitter. In the human brain substance P was particularly located in the caudate nucleus (85 units/g), hypothalamus (102 units/g), thalamus (12 units/g), and substantia nigra (699 units/g).[27]

Substance P has actions of a neurotransmitter and some actions on endocrine events. It stimulates prolactin secretion, growth hormone secretion, gut smooth muscle contraction, increases intestinal motility, pancreatic acinar secretions, salivary gland secretions, gall bladder contraction, vasodilation, and histamine release from Mast cells. Substance P may not enter the blood from the gastrointestinal tract.

The axon reflex is a local neural mechanism by which nerve endings control circulation. Substance P release from nerve endings results in increased capillary permeability and vasodilation.[28]

GASTRIN-RELEASING PEPTIDE

Gastrin-releasing peptide, abbreviated GRP, has 21 amino acids of which ten are shared with amphibian bombesin. Gastrin-releasing peptide can be found in the endings of the axons of the vagus nerve which terminate at the G-cells. Gastrin-releasing peptide is the putative neurotransmitter by which the vagus nerve stimulates the G-cells to produce gastrin. Bombesin has 14 amino acids and is found in frog skin. Bombesin-like immunoreactivity (BLI) is found in nerves of the gut and in the mucosa endocrine cells of the stomach antrum and the duodenum.

NEUROTENSIN

Neurotensin has 13 amino acids and is found in nerve cells and gut N-cells of the ileum. Neurotensin decreases gastric acid secretion, decreases gut peristalsis, contracts smooth muscle, causes hypoglycemia, causes hypotension, causes vasodilation, inhibits gastrin-stimulated acid secretion, and retards release of chyme from the stomach. It may act on mast cells causing the release of histamine.

PEPTIDE YY

Peptide YY, abbreviated PYY, is named for the fact that tyrosine (abbreviation Y) amino acid residues are located at both the carboxy and amino terminals of the 36 amino acid chain that makes up the polypeptide. Its structure bears similarities to pancreatic polypeptide. Peptide YY is found in the colon and ileum. Peptide YY inhibits secretion of pancreatic enzyme and bicarbonate.

PANCREATIC POLYPEPTIDE

Pancreatic polypeptide, abbreviated PP, has 36 amino acids. Pancreatic polypeptide comes from pancreatic islets in which the F-cells that secrete PP are located at the islet periphery near the acinar tissue.

Secretion of PP is stimulated by meals that contain meat or fish (i.e. a protein meal), exercise, fasting, and acute hypoglycemia and inhibited by glucose and somatostatin. The vagus nerve probably regulates pancreatic polypeptide secretion.

Pancreatic polypeptide inhibits pancreatic secretion of protein and bicarbonate, relaxes the gall bladder, decreases bile secretion, and slows the absorption of food.

Hadley suggests that somatostatin-containing D-cells and pancreatic polypeptide-containing F-cells regulate the secretory activity of each other by a paracrine mechanism.[29]

ENKEPHALINS AND ENDORPHINS

Enkephalins are among the gastrointestinal peptides that are also neuropeptides that may function as neurotransmitters. Enkephalins are found in nerves, stomach, duodenum, and gall bladder. The enkephalins are five amino acid residue fragments of the **endorphins** that are synthesized from pro-opiomelanocortin. The enkephalins are particularly interesting because they mimic opiate actions and they bind to opiate receptors which are found in both gut and in the substantia gelatinosa of the brain. In the gastrointestinal tract there are two enkephalins, leu-enkephalin and met-enkephalin. The precursor molecule for enkephalins, ß-**endorphin**, also has interesting actions. ß-Endorphin has 30 amino acids and it is synthesized from a still larger precursor, ß-lipotropin which has 91 amino acids. Collectively, endorphin and enkephalin belong with the eighteen opioid peptides that are also sometimes referred to generically as the endorphins. The word "endorphin" means "the morphine within." Thus, the opioid peptides are viewed as internal opiates.

The effects of enkephalins on the gastrointestinal tract on gut are constipation, initial contractions of gut regions (stomach, duodenum, jejunum), later distension and lack of tone of gut regions, colon contraction without peristalsis, and anal sphincter contraction. Opiate peptides also inhibit pancreatic bicarbonate secretion and inhibit pancreatic protein secretion. Enkephalins also inhibit release of substance P.

SOMATOSTATIN

Somatostatin (SS) is found not only in the hypothalamus, but in the mucosal endocrine cells in the antrum of the stomach and in the pancreatic islet D-cells. There are two forms with activity, a somatostatin 14 and a somatostatin 28 (prosomatostatin). Somatostatin is synthesized from the carboxy end of a preprosomatostatin that has 116 amino acid residues. Somatostatin is stimulated by gastrointestinal hormones, glucose, arginine, and tolbutamide. Its half-life is three minutes.

Somatostatin inhibits secretion of pancreatic hormones (insulin, glucagon, pancreatic polypeptide) and pituitary somatotropin. Somatostatin lengthens the time for gastric emptying. It decreases gastric acid, gastrin, pancreatic enzymes, splanchnic circulation, and xylose absorption. An analogue of somatostatin, octreotide, reduces kidney hyperfiltration and hypertrophy in insulin-dependent diabetes.[30] Individuals with somatostatin-secreting tumors have slow gastric emptying, decreased secretion of gastric acid, gallstones, and diabetic symptoms (hyperglycemia). CCK, arginine, leucine, and glucose stimulate somatostatin secretion by the pancreas and the gastrointestinal tract.

OTHER GASTROINTESTINAL PEPTIDES

Some other peptides have putative gastrointestinal function: **bulbogastrone** inhibits gastric acid secretion; **urogastrone** inhibits gastric acid secretion (epidermal growth factor, 53 amino acids); **chymodenin** stimulates pancreatic chymotrypsin (MW5000); and **villikinin** stimulates movement of the villi.

Glucagon, a hormone of the pancreas, is also made in stomach and duodenum A-cells (it is also the A-cells in pancreatic islets that secrete glucagon). Glucagon release is stimulated by amino acids, CCK, catecholamines, gastrin, GIP, glucocorticoids, and by autonomic nerves.

ENTERIC NERVOUS SYSTEM

Gastrointestinal regulation involves more than the gastrointestinal hormones. The gastrointestinal tract is innervated by interconnected plexuses of nerve cells. The myenteric nerve plexus, also called "Auerbach's plexus," and the submucous plexus, also called "Meissner's plexus," are located between the outer longitudinal muscle layer, the inner circular muscle layer, and the mucosa. Most of the cell bodies of the enteric neurons are found in the two plexuses.[31] Mucosal receptors respond to stretch and chemicals, and send information via processes to the nerve cell bodies in the plexuses. The whole system of a million receptor cells and interneurones and plexuses is a third portion of the autonomic nervous system called the "enteric nervous system." Neurochemicals in the enteric nervous system include the peptides (CCK, VIP, substance P, somatostatin, neurotensin, enkephalins, GRP, angiotensin II) and biogenic amines (serotonin, acetylcholine, norepinephrine).

GI HORMONES AND EATING DISORDERS

By sending information back to the nervous system directly or indirectly, the GI hormones may send signals about satiety. It would make a logical sequence: low blood nutrients $\Rightarrow$ brain (hunger) ⇒ feeding behavior ⇒ food in gastrointestinal tract ⇒ gut hormones secreted into blood ⇒ brain (satiety) ⇒ stop feeding behavior.

The possibility has been suggested that the GI hormones play a causative role in eating disorders. This idea was espoused by Anne H. Rosenfeld:

> Researchers...have preliminary evidence that bulimia may stem, in part from a biological abnormality—and may yield to a biological treatment. The culprit....is cholecystokinin (CCK), a hormone found in the intestines, blood plasma and brain. Animal studies have shown that CCK affects food satiety; injections of the hormone reduce the amount of food animals will eat. It's thought that CCK sets off a chain of neural messages to the hypothalamus...The message: I'm full now; turn off the munchies.[32]

If this idea is correct, there are possibilities for altering feeding behavior by altering the gut hormones which could lead to solutions for all sorts of weight and eating disorders.

REFERENCES

1. Bayliss, W.M.; Starling, E.H. The mechanism of pancreatic secretion. Journal of Physiology 28: 325–353; 1902.

2. Turner, C.D.; Bagnara, J.T. Endocrinology, Sixth Edition. Philadelphia, PA: W.B. Saunders; 1976, p. 13–14.

3. Starling, E.H. The chemical correlations of functions of the body. Lancet 11: 339–341; 1905.

4. Hadley , M. E. Endocrinology, Sixth Edition. Englewood Cliffs, NJ: Prentice Hall; 1988; p. 2.

5. Deveney, C. W.; Way, L. W. Regulatory peptides of the gut. In Greenspan, F.; Forsham, P., editors. Basic and Clinical Endocrinology, Second Edition. Norwalk, CT: Appleton & Lange; 1987; page 501.

6. Makhlouf, G.M., volume editor. The Gastrointestinal System, Volume II. In Schultz, S.G., Section editor. Handbook of Physiology. Bethesda, MD: American Physiological Society; 1989; p. 1–722.

7. Telford, I.R.; Bridgman, C.F. Introduction to Functional Histology. New York: Harper & Row; 1990; p. 348.

8. Polak, J. M. Endocrine Cells of the Gut. In Makhlouf, G.M., volume editor. The Gastrointestinal System, Volume II. In Schutz, S.G., Section editor. Handbook of Physiology. Bethesda, MD: American Physiological Society; 1989; p. 79–96.

9. Said, S.I. Peptides common to the nervous system and the gastrointestinal tract. Frontiers in Neuroendocrinology 6: 293–331; 1980.

10. Deveney, C. W.; Way, L. W.; Op. cit.; p. 501.

11. Bertaccini, G.; Decarlo, G.; Endean, R.; Erspamer, V.; Impicciatore, M. The action of caerulein on pancreatic secretion of the dog and biliary secretion of the dog and the rat. Brit. J. Pharmacol. 37: 185; 1969.

12 . Ganong, W. Review of Medical Physiology, Fourteenth Edition. Norwalk, CT: Appleton & Lange; 1989; p. 410.

13. Deveney, C. W.; Way, L. W.; Op. cit.; p. 507.

14. Deveney, C. W.; Way, L. W.; Op. cit.; p. 508.

15. Mueller, K.; Hsiao, S. Current status of cholecystokinin as a short-term satiety hormone. Neurosci. Behav. Rev. 2: 79–87; 1978.

16. Myers, R. D.; McCaleb, M.L. Feeding: satiety signal from intestine triggers brain's noradrenergic mechanism. Science 209: 1035–1037; 1981.

17. Pietrowsky, R.; Preuss, S.; Born, J.; Pauschinger, P.; Fehm, H.L. Effects of cholecystokinin and calcitonin on evoked brain potentials and satiety in man. Physiology & Behavior 46: 513–519; 1989.

18. Deveney, C. W.; Way, L. W.; Op. cit.; p. 620.

19. Hadley , M. E.; Op. cit.; p. 512.

20. Wang, J.-Y.; Yaksh, T.L.; Go, V.L.W. In vivo studies on the basal and evoked release of cholecystokinin and vasoactive intestinal peptide in rat and cat spinal cord. Brain Res. 242: 279–290; 1982.

21 . Ganong, W.; Op. cit.; p. 393.

22. Chey, W.; Lee, K.Y. Motilin. Clin. Gastroenterol. 9: 645; 1980.

23. Poitros, P., et al. Motilin-independent ectopic fronts of the interdigestive myoelectric complex in dogs. Am. J. Physiol. 239: 215; 1980.

24. Ganong, p. 412.

25. Takemoto, K.; Mutt, V. Isolation and characterization of the intestinal peptide porcine PHI (PHI-27), A new member of the glucagon secretin family. Proc. Natl. Acad. Sci. USA 78: 6603–6607; 1981.

26. Pavlov, I.P. Conditioned Reflexes. Oxford University Press; 1928.

27. Ganong, W.; Op cit.; p. 219.

28. Ganong, W.; Op. cit.; p. 506.

29. Hadley, M.; Op. cit.; p. 288.

30. Serri, O.; Beauregard, H.; Brazeau, P.; Abribat, T.; Lambert, J.; Harris, A.; Vachon, Luc. Somatotatin analogue, octreotide, reduces increased glomerular filtration rate and kidney size in insulin-dependent diabetes. JAMA 265: 888–892; 1991.

31. Costa, M.; Furness, J.B. Structure and neurochemical organization of the enteric nervous system. In Makhlouf, G.M., editor. The Gastrointestinal System, Volume II. In Schultz, S. G., Section editor. Handbook of Physiology. Bethesda, MD: American Physiological Society; 1989; p. 97–109.

32. Rosenfeld, Anne H. New treatment for bulimia. Psychology Today; March; 1989.

SECTION IV

STEROID, AMINE, AND PEPTIDE HORMONES RELATED TO THE GONADS AND ADRENALS

This section deals with the group of glands that make steroid hormones—adrenal glands and gonads. The section includes the peptide and amine hormones from these glands and other glands that are involved in the regulation and function of the adrenals and gonads. The adrenals and gonads function in water balance, responses to stress, growth, development, and reproduction.

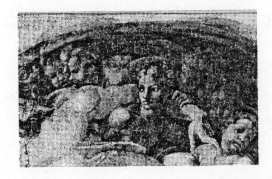

CHAPTER 13

Steroid Hormones

This chapter covers general principles for steroids. Steroids include the hormones of the adrenal cortex, testes, ovaries, and placenta. Subcategories of steroids from the adrenal cortex are the glucocorticoids and mineralocorticoids. The testes and adrenal cortex make androgens. The ovaries make estrogen and progestogens. The steroid hormones act via intracellular receptors.

STEROIDS

Today the word "steroids" makes most people think of muscles and their development (Figure 13.1). But steroids have a much broader role in endocrinology in keeping with their diverse sources and structures.

Steroids have in common a "cyclopentanoperhydrohenanthrene nucleus" which is a structure consisting of four attached rings (Figures 13.2 and 13.3). Steroids differ from one another by the number and location of double bonds in the rings and by the side chains attached to the rings. There is a standard method for describing steroid structures. The four rings are designated by letters (A, B, C, D). The carbon atoms at the vertices of the rings and in the side chains are designated by numbers. Systematic chemical names of steroids are derived from the numbering system. So progesterone (common, or trivial, name) also has a less used systematic chemical name (pregn-4-ene-3,20-dione) in which the numbers indicate vertices where double bonds appear and groups are attached. Steroids are grouped either by structure or function.

The steroids can be grouped based on structure. Most of the steroids with 19 carbon atoms and with a keto (=0) or hydroxyl (–OH) group attached at position 17 are called 17-ketosteroids or **C_{19} steroids**. The steroids that have 21 carbons and a two-carbon side chain at position 17 are the **C_{21} steroids**. If they also have a hydroxyl group at position 17, they are 17-hydroxycorticoids or **17-hydroxycorticosteroids** (17-OHCS).

The steroids can also be grouped by function. In vertebrates, steroids are synthesized mainly by the adrenal cortex, testes, ovaries, and placenta. The steroids have been divided into five groups: **androgens, estrogens, progestogens, mineralocorticoids**, and **glucocorticoids** (Table 13.1). There are other steroids that do not fit into these five groups. Related compounds include cholesterol, ergosterol, and bile acids. There are also steroids in invertebrates (such as ecdysone, the insect moulting hormone) and there are synthetic steroids.

The structural components of individual steroids confer their biological activity. Corticoid activity accompanies C4 double valence, C3 and C20, and ketone groups. Sodium retention is linked to the C21 hydroxyl group. Action on carbohydrates is associated with ketone oxygen or hydroxyl groups at C17 and C11. Electrolytes and water are altered by steroids with no oxygen at C11 and an aldehyde (-CHO) at C18. The A-ring is unsaturated (3 double bonds) in estrogens. C17 ketone groups are on steroids that are excreted.

SYNTHESIS

Vertebrates manufacture steroids from cholesterol (Figure 13.4) using enzymes. The biosynthesis of steroids is sometimes referred to as steroidogenesis. Typical amounts of adrenocortical steroid hormones in human adults are in Table 13.2. Relative potencies of some steroids in various bioassays are in Table 13.3.

Steroid-producing tissues practice conservation in their use of enzymes. The use of the enzymes in steroid production is efficient, because the organisms can make more steroids than the number of enzymes they possess. With only five enzymes (17-α-hydroxylase, 17 desmolase, 3ß-hydroxysteroid dehydrogenase (3BDI), 21ß-hydroxylase (21BHL), and 11ß hydroxylase (11BHL), ten steroid products can be made from cholesterol (Figures 13.5 and 13.6, Table 13.4). Moreover, several routes exist for the synthesis of some steroids.

COMPARTMENTALIZATION

Steroid synthesis involves several parts of the adrenocortical cell as envisioned for aldosterone as a specific example (Figure 13.7). Cholesterol can be synthesized from acetate, but most comes from plasma lipoproteins or low density lipid (LDL) in the blood. Specific LDL receptors assist adrenocortical cells in taking up cholesterol from the circulation. The cholesterol undergoes esterification. Esterified cholesterol is stored in intracellular lipid droplets. Free cholesterol is formed by cholesterol ester hydrolase in the lipid droplets. A sterol carrier protein transports cholesterol to the mitochondria.

The cholesterol is converted into pregnenolone in the mitochondria. The enzyme involved in the conversion is variously referred to as pregnenolone synthetase, cholesterol desmolase, side-chain cleavage enzyme, P450scc, or cholesterol 20,22-hydroxylase:20,22-desmolase complex.

The pregnenolone then moves to the smooth endoplasmic reticulum (SER) where 3BDI converts it to progesterone. The progesterone is

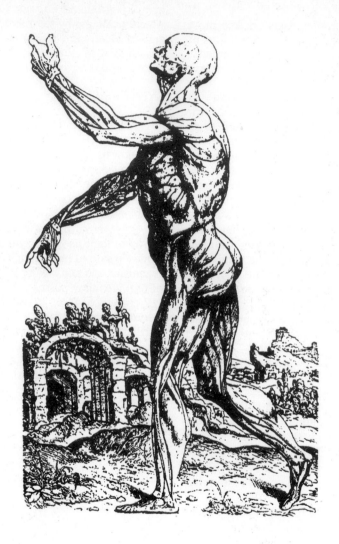

Figure 13.1 The muscles are one of the many systems of the body that are affected by steroids. The illustration shows a rendering of the human muscular system by Vesalius in *De Humani Corporis Fabrica*. Reproduced, with permission. Moore, J.A. Understanding nature—form and function. American Zoologist 28: 449–584; 1988.

the substrate for 21BHL whose product is 11-deoxycorticosterone. Smooth endoplasmic reticulum is abundant and well-developed in steroid secreting cells.

The 11-deoxycorticosterone travels back to the mitochondria where 11BHL converts it to corticosterone. The enzymes, 18-hydroxylase and 18-

dehydrogenase, make further conversions to produce aldosterone. The specialization of the zona glomerulosa occurs at these steps; the zone glomerulosa makes aldosterone but does not make glucocorticoids or reproductive steroids.

In the mitochondria, some of the enzymes (21BHL, 11BHL, cholesterol desmolase, 17α-

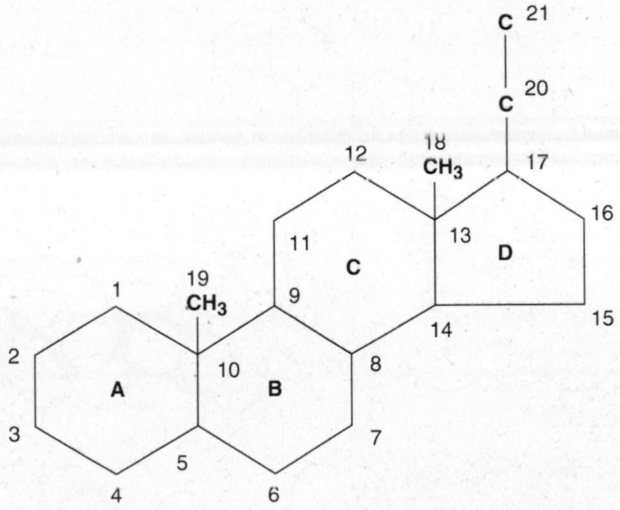

Structure of the cyclopentanoperhydrohenanthrene nucleus showing the alphabet designation of the rings and the numerical designation of the carbon atoms that appear in the vertices (C not shown) and side chains (C shown)

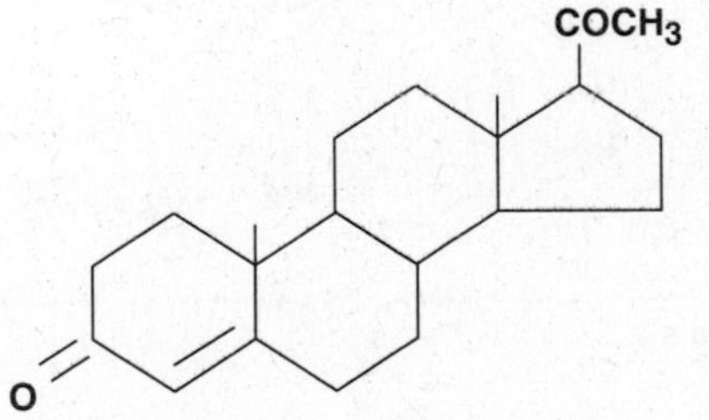

Structure of progesterone, a C21 steroid

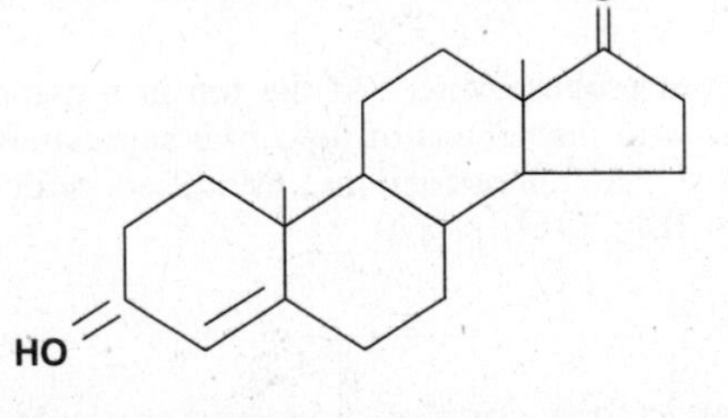

Structure of dehydroepiandrosterone, a C19 steroid, DHEA

Figure 13.2 The chemical structures of steroids are shown.

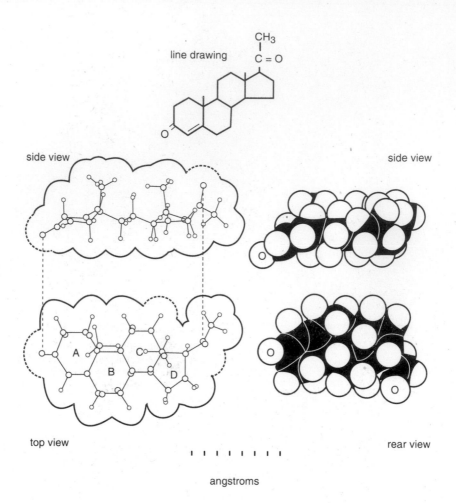

line drawing

side view   side view

top view   rear view

angstroms

Figure 13.3 The diagram shows representations of the steroid progesterone. At the top is a two-dimensional line drawing. The two diagrams on the left show "stick" views with the centers of the atoms represented. The two diagrams on the right represent two views of three-dimensional "ball" constructions. Modified, with permission. Reithel, F.J. Concepts in Biochemistry. New York: McGraw-Hill; 1967; p. 270.

hydroxylase) are classified as P450 enzymes, or cytochromes.

Similar compartmentalization occurs in the synthesis of cortisol. In cortisol synthesis, the 11-deoxycorticosterone made from pregnenolone moves back to the mitochondria for 11 hydroxyla-

tion to form corticosterone and cortisol.

ENZYME TRACKING

Variation occurs in the profile of steroids produced. The variation is achieved by "enzyme

Table 13.1 Groups of Steroids

Group	Specific example
androgens	testosterone
estrogens	17-ß-estradiol
progestogens	progesterone
glucocorticoids	cortisol
mineralocorticoids	aldosterone

tracking," that is, the array of enzymes present and their relative activities determine which steroids will be made from cholesterol and the amounts that will be produced. Enzyme tracking can be demonstrated in tissue specialization, chemical blockers, and genetic deficiencies of steroid biosynthesis.

TISSUE SPECIALIZATION

The zona glomerulosa specializes in the production of the mineralocorticoid aldosterone. The zona glomerulosa has the enzymes required to convert cholesterol to corticosterone, but, in addition, it has the enzymes 18-hydroxylase and 18-dehydrogenase which form aldosterone from corticosterone. Similarly the zona fasciculata and zona reticularis, with 17α-hydroxylase and 17-desmolase, specialize in production of glucocorticoids and adrenal androgens; but they do not make aldosterone because the cells lack 18-hydroxylase and 18-dehydrogenase. The adrenal cortex normally secretes mineralocorticoids (deoxycorticosterone, aldosterone), glucocorticoids (cortisol, corticosterone), and adrenal androgens (dehydroepiandrosterone, and androstenedione).

CHEMICAL BLOCKERS

The idea of enzyme tracking applies to chemical blockers. Some examples follow.

Metapyrone blocks 11BHL. A metapyrone test is used clinically to produce a temporary cortisol deficiency so that pituitary ACTH feedback response can be assessed by measuring an increase in 11-deoxycortisol secretion.

Amphenone, a derivative of DDT, blocks all steroid secretion by blocking 11BHL, 17α-hydroxylase, and 21ß-hydroxylase.

DDD (dichlorodiphenyldichlorethane) and o,p' DDD kill cells of the zona glomerulosa and zona reticularis.

Aminoglutethimide may block hydroxylations. Concern about these compounds relates to pesticides.

Cyanoketone blocks 3BDI.

SU-9055 blocks 17- and 18-hydroxylation.

Heparin, a drug that is commonly used to prevent blood clotting, blocks 18-hydroxylation thereby affecting aldosterone production; this blockage is probably indirect since Heparin should remain extracellular.

Triparanol inhibits synthesis of cholesterol.

The chemical blockers can be used as treatments to alter steroid profiles that result from disorders of the adrenal cortex. Chemical blockers are also useful for clinical or research testing of adrenal function.

CONGENITAL ENZYME DEFICIENCIES

Enzyme tracks are altered by enzyme deficiencies. In endocrinology, the concept of enzyme tracking is most clearly illustrated with congenital deficiencies in adrenal enzymes. Deficiency in the activity of an enzyme should result in accumulation of a precursor, a shortage of the products of that particular enzyme, and a decrease in the steroids that

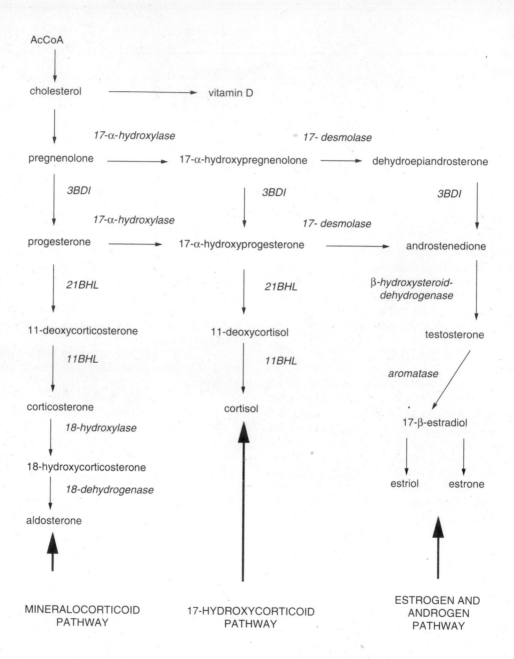

Figure 13.4 The diagram shows the biosynthetic pathways for steroids. Enzyme names and abbreviations are italicized; Acetyl-CoA (acetyl coenzyme A) is the only nonsteroid shown in plain type. 3BDI = 3-ß-hydroxysteroid dehydrogenase; 21 BHL = 21ß-hydroxylase; 11BHL = 11ß-hydroxylase. The pituitary hormone ACTH (corticotropin) stimulates conversion of cholesterol to pregnenolone.

Table 13.2 Steroid Amounts

Steroid	Average amount secreted (milligrams/24h)	Average plasma concentration free and bound (micrograms/dl)
cortisol	20	13.9
corticosterone	3	0.4
aldosterone	0.15	0.006
deoxycorticosterone	0.20	0.006
dehydroepiandrosterone	10 (females)	45.0
	15 (males)	

After W. Ganong. Review of Medical Physiology, Thirteenth Edition. Norwalk, CT: Appleton & Lange; 1987; p. 298.

are made from the products of that particular enzyme. A congenital deficiency creates a biochemical "dam" (Figure 13.8). The well documented maladies are disorders of inborn metabolism and consist of some physiological failure based on the inability to synthesize an enzyme. In these disorders, products of the deficient enzyme are usually low, but substrates usually accumulate.

Congenital hypoaldosteronism is a consequence of a deficiency in 18-hydroxysteroid dehydrogenase.

In another example, a deficiency of 11ß-hydroxylase (11BHL) leads to a deficiency not only of mineralocorticoids, but also of cortisol and mild virilization—the hypertensive form of congenital virilizing adrenal hyperplasia.

A deficiency of 21-hydroxylase (21BHL) produces the salt-losing form of congenital virilizing adrenal hyperplasia which is accompanied by the most virilization.

Congenital 17α-hydroxylase deficiency results in feminization and hypertension.

Deficient 3ß-hydroxysteroid dehydrogenase (3BDI) causes a third kind of congenital adrenal hyperplasia.

Inability to convert cholesterol to pregnenolone (failure of cholesterol desmolase) has a global effect so that steroids can't be produced and the disease, congenital lipoid adrenal hyperplasia, is fatal.

STEROID SECRETION AND RHYTHMS

Because of their lipid solubility, steroids pass easily through cell membranes so that when they are synthesized they can immediately be secreted and are not stored. Therefore, the rate of secretion parallels the rate of synthesis.

The rate of steroid synthesis is dependent upon the rate-limiting enzymes in the pathway for steroid biosynthesis. The step in synthesis, from cholesterol to pregnenolone (mitochondrial hydroxylations and side-chain cleavage), may be rate limiting. The stimulation of cyclic AMP (by ACTH in the adrenal cortex, or by pituitary gonadotropins in the gonads) affects the activity of the enzyme complex that synthesizes pregnenolone from cholesterol. Calcium is required for the ACTH stimulation of cyclic AMP.

The steroids are replete with well-defined rhythms. There is a daily cycle in a hormone that stimulates steroid synthesis, corticotropin, or

Table 13.3 Steroid Relative Activities

Steroid	Relative biological activity			

ESTROGENS

	MOUSE	RAT		
estrone	1.00	1.0		
ß-estradiol	10.00	10.0		
α-estradiol	0.08	0.1		
estriol	0.40	0.2		
stilbesterol	5.00	5. 0		

ANDROGENS

	CAPON			
testosterone	67			
androsterone	10			
dehydroepiandrosterone	4			
androstenedione	10			
17-methyltestosterone	83			
17-ethynyltestosterone	110			

GLUCOCORTICOIDS AND MINERALOCORTICOIDS	LIFE	SODIUM	LIVER GLYCOGEN TEST	ANTI-INFLAM-MATORY TEST
cortisol	1.00	1.0	1.00	1.00
cortisone	1.00	0.7	0.70	<0.60
11-deoxycorticosterone	4.00	10.0	<0.01	<0.01
corticosterone	0.75	1.6	0.30	0.30
aldosterone	80.00	300.0	0.30	0
prednisolone	2.00	1.0	4.00	3.00
methylfluorocortisol	–	1000.0	10.00	10.0

Mouse or rat test: The minimum dose necessary to produce nucleated epithelial or cornified cells in vaginal smears of ovariectomized rats or mice (0.2 micrograms subcutaneously injected is effective for mice). **Capon test:** The data are given in IU/mg. One IU stimulates capon comb growth equivalent to 100 micrograms of crystalline androsterone. 48–72-hour-old cockerels are injected with androgen, combs are removed and weighed on the eighth day. **Life maintenance test:** Survival of adrenalectomized rats on salt and water diet; life maintenance dose of cortisol is 2 mg/100 g body weight per day. **Sodium retention test:** Na^+ and K^+ excretion of adrenalectomized rats after controlled water intake. **Liver glycogen test:** Amount of liver glycogen 1 hour after a series of glucocorticoid injections in adrenalectomized, fasting mice or rats. An effective dose of cortisol is 100 micrograms/100 g. **Anti-inflamatory test:** Reduction of the size of a granuloma (fibrotic deposit) produced by a cotton ball in the wound on an adrenalectomized rat after treatment with adrenal steroids. Methylfluorocortisol is 2-alpha-methyl-9-alpha-fluorocortisol. Modified, with permission. Frieden, E.; Lipner, H. Biochemical Endocrinology of the Vertebrates. Englewood Cliffs, NJ: Prentice-Hall; 1971, pp. 84, 85, 88.

ACTH (Figure 13.9).

In the mechanisms by which ACTH causes increased steroidogenesis, a steroid activator polypeptide (SAP) has been suggested as having a role in influencing the intramitochondrial cholesterol access to its cytochrome $P-450_{scc}$ substrate

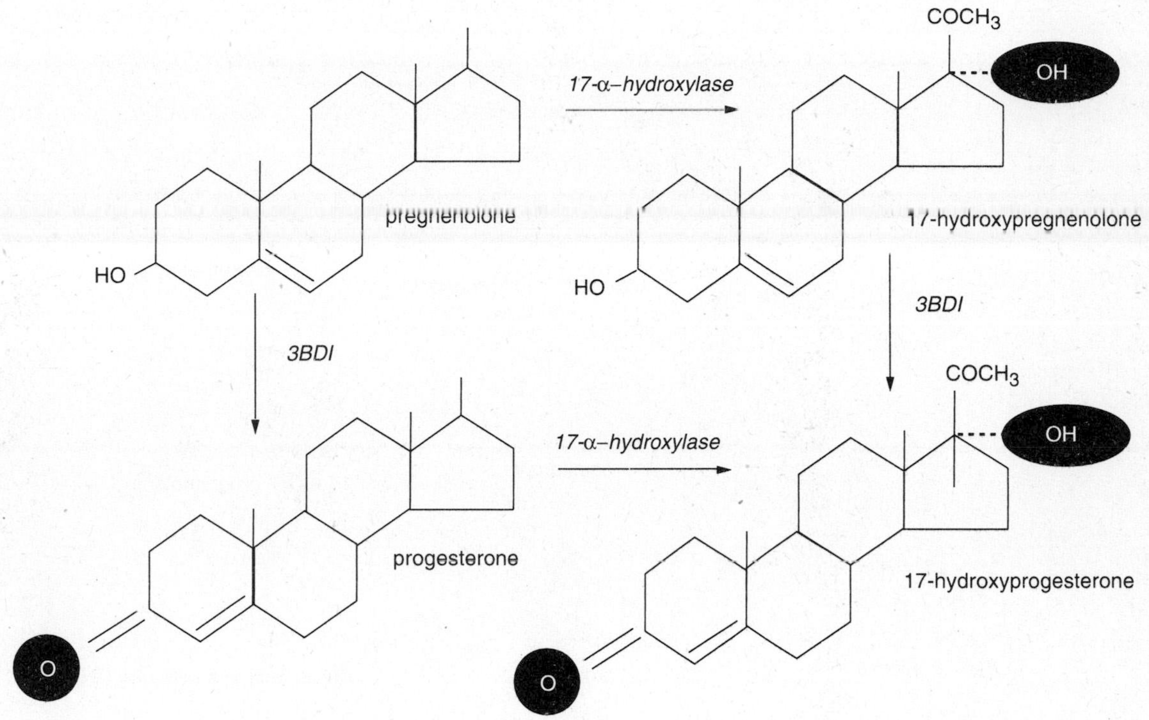

Figure 13.5 The figure illustrates "conservation" of enzymes. The chemical change in the product appears on a black background. Using one substrate (pregnenolone) and two enzymes (3BDI and 17α-hydroxylase), three products (17-hydroxypregnenolone, progesterone, and17-hydroxyprogesterone) are made.

binding site. SAP has a daily rhythm—activity is 0.10 pmol/mg protein at 0800 and rises over ten-fold to 1.36 pmol/kg protein at 1800 h in rats.[1]

The activity of cholesterol 7α-hydroxylase has a daily cycle in rat liver. Male rats had 10.25 pmol/min/mg protein of cholesterol 7α-hydroxylase activity at 9 a.m. (midlight of lights-on 3 a.m. to 3 p.m.) and three times more, 33.43 pmol/min/mg protein of cholesterol 7α-hydroxylase activity at 9 a.m. (middark of a reversed cycle, lights-on 3 p.m. to 3 a.m.).[2]

Particularly well known is the rhythm that occurs in plasma 11-OHCS.[3] The rhythms are characterized by a rise in hormones that occurs late in sleep and early in the morning. Steroid secretion is also episodic; that is, there are spikes of hormone that appear at short intervals.

STEROID-BINDING GLOBULINS

Steroids travel in the bloodstream, for the most part, bound to specialized transport proteins and to blood proteins such as albumin (Table 13.5). The reasons for this association are a source of speculations. (i) It is possible that the formation of complexes is to suppress biological activity dur-

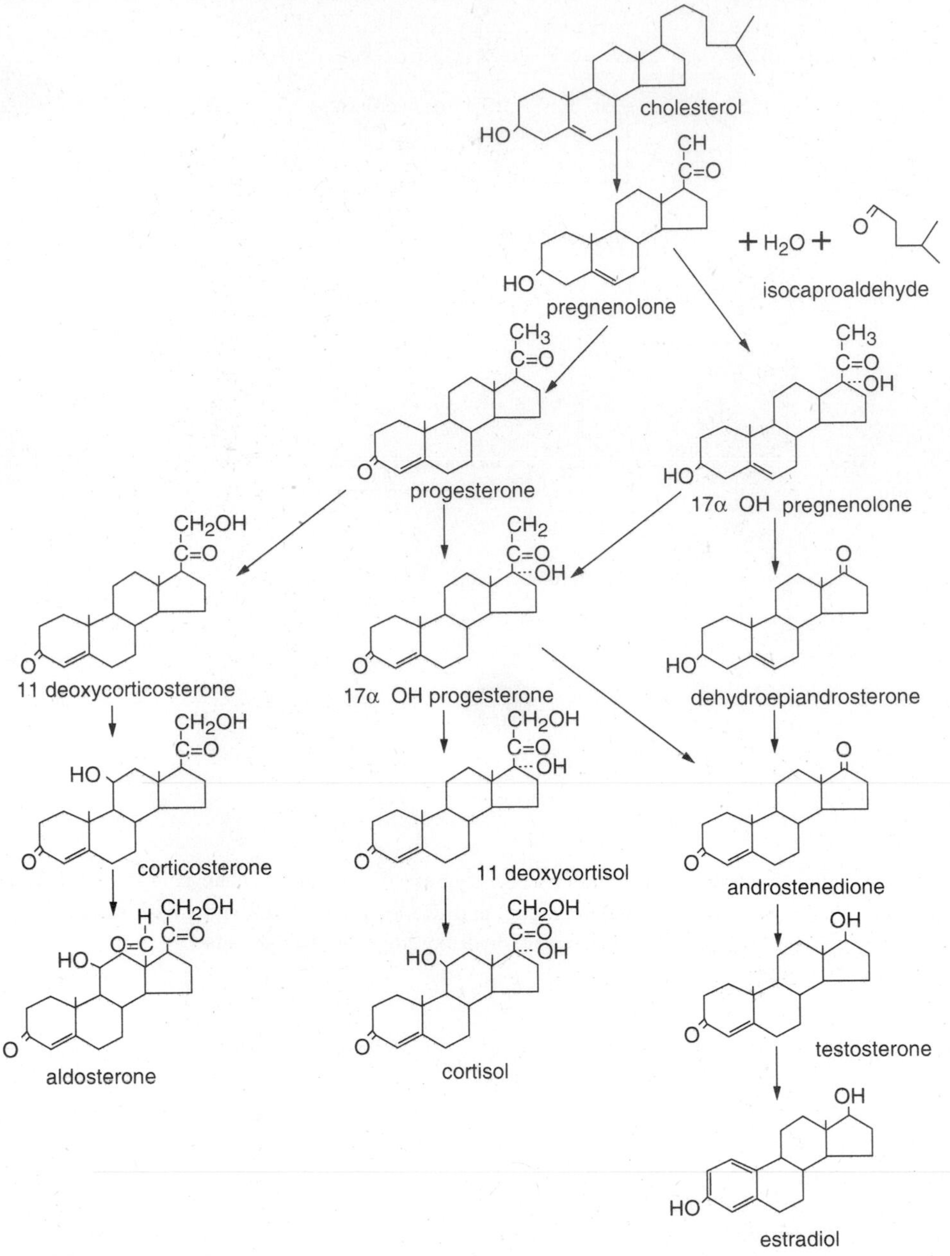

Figure 13.6 Steroid biosynthesis is shown for the adrenal gland (left mineralocorticoid pathway, center glucocorticoid pathway, right estrogen and androgen pathway). Redrawn, with permission. West, J.B., editor. Best & Taylor's Physiological Basis of Medical Practice, 12th Edition. Baltimore: Williams & Wilkins; 1991; p. 823.

Table 13.4 Enzymes of Corticoid Synthesis

Enzyme	Substrates	Products
cholesterol 20,22-hydroxylase: 20,22-desmolase complex	cholesterol	pregnenolone
3BDI = 3-ß-hydroxysteroid dehydrogenase	pregnenolone 17-α-hydroxypregnenolone dehydroepiandrosterone	progesterone 17-α-hydroxyprogesterone androstenedione
21BHL = 21-ß-hydroxylase	progesterone 17-α-hydroxyprogesterone	11-deoxycorticosterone 11-deoxycortisol
11BHL = 11 ß-hydroxylase	11-deoxycorticosterone	corticosterone
17-α-hydroxylase	pregnenolone progesterone	17-α-hydroxypregnenolone 17-α-hydroxyprogesterone
17 desmolase	17-α-hydroxypregnenolone 17-α-hydroxyprogesterone	dehydroepiandrosterone androstenedione
sulfokinase	dehydroepiandrosterone	dehydroepiandrosterone sulfate
18-hydroxylase	corticosterone	18-hydroxycorticosterone
18-dehydrogenase	18-hydroxycorticosterone	aldosterone

The adrenal gland is divided into histological zones (zona). The enzymes listed here are found in the zona fasiculata and zona reticularis of the adrenal cortex except for the 18-hydroxylase and 18-dehydrogenase which are found in the zona glomerulosa. 3BDI is also called 3-ß-hydroxysteroid dehydrogenase: Δ-5-oxosteroid isomerase complex. 17-Desmolase is also called 17,20-lyase and 17,20-desmolase.

ing transport; the bound steroids seem to be physiologically inert. (ii) Another possibility is that the steroids, being hydrophobic, attach to proteins for transport in order to become soluble in the plasma. (iii) A logical idea is that the steroid transport molecules are involved in the recognition of the steroids by target sites. (iv) Or perhaps, bound hormone provides a reservoir of hormone so that a supply of free hormone can be quickly made available. (v) It is further possible that the purpose of transporting proteins is to protect the steroids from chemical degradation and thereby to extend the steroid hormones' half-lives.

The alpha globulin, a blood protein that binds to cortisol, is named **corticosteroid-binding globulin** (CBG), or transcortin. CBG is a plasma glycoprotein with 383 amino acids and a polypeptide molecular weight of 42,646 (Figure 13.10).[4] The liver synthesizes CBG. Concentration of CBG in sera ranges from 3.4×10^{-7} M in the rabbit to 11.3×10^{-7} M in the rat. CBG and steroid hormones form complexes held together with covalent bonds which dissociate easily. CBG has a high affinity for cortisol: the cortisol binding capacity for CBG in plasma is about 25 μg/dl. Another way of saying this is that binding sites for cortisol on CBG saturate at plasma cortisol > 20 μg/dl. Steroids do compete with each other for

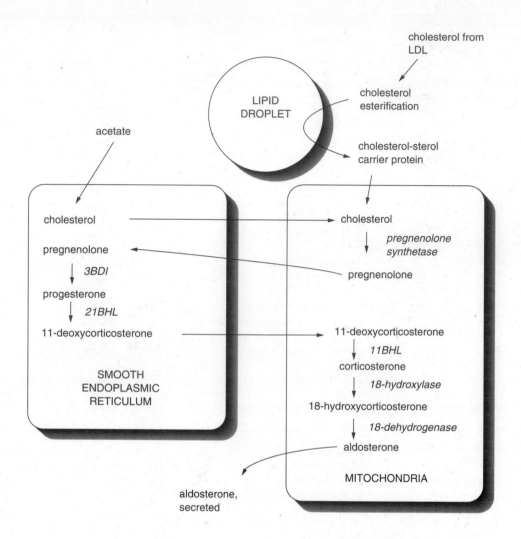

Figure 13.7 The figure shows "compartmentalization" in the cells that synthesize aldosterone. Synthesis of the steroids involves several organelles of the cell: lipid droplets, endoplasmic reticulum, and mitochondria. Cholesterol is either taken up from plasma LDL or synthesized in the cell from acetate; cholesterol ester hydrolase frees cholesterol from its esterified form in the lipid droplets; aldosterone is secreted by the cells.

binding sites on CBG and SHBG (sex hormone binding globulin). For example, progesterone may bind to 25% of CBG sites in late pregnancy and prednisolone, a synthetic steroid, has a high affinity for CBG.

Changes in CBG concentrations alter the availability of cortisol (increased CBH, more cortisol bound). Factors that increase CBG are estrogen (pregnancy, oral contraceptives, estrogen therapy), hyperthyroidism, diabetes, genetics, and blood disorders; factors that decrease CBG are myeloma, nephrosis, cirrhosis, hypothyroidism, and protein deficiency. Deficiency in CBG can be inherited. CBG binds less corticosterone than cortisol; the difference in binding seems to correlate with different half-lives; corticosterone's half-life is less than cortisol's half-life. The amount of cortisol bound to CBG is greater at 4°C (99% bound) and less at body temperature, 37°C (90%).

Still another blood protein, a beta globulin, transports testosterone and estradiol. It is variously called **sex hormone binding-globulin** (SHBG), sex steroid-binding globulin, and gonadal steroid-binding globulin (GBG). SHBG is different from the androgen-binding protein from Sertoli cells. Instead, SHBG, like CBG, is synthesized by the liver. Estrogen, thyroid hormone, hyperthyroidism, and cirrhosis increase SHBG; androgens, growth hormone, hypothyroidism, acromegaly, and obesity decrease SHBG. In the blood, 97% testosterone is bound to protein.

Albumin (human serum albumin, molecular weight about 69,000) has considerable capacity for binding cortisol and also for synthetic glucocorticoids (e.g., dexamethasone); but its affinity for cortisol is lower than that of CBG. Albumin also binds androstenedione, DHEA (dehydroepiandrosterone), and DHEA sulfate.

In contrast to testosterone and cortisol, more than 50% of aldosterone circulates free, unbound, in the plasma. The greater amount of free aldosterone may explain why aldosterone has a shorter half-life (30 minutes) than cortisol (about 80 minutes).

STEROID RECEPTORS

As mentioned in the earlier discussion of receptors, steroid hormones find their receptors in the cell cytoplasm. This is in contrast to the receptors for amine and protein hormones which reside in the cell membrane.

Hormone receptors were suspected to exist in target cells almost a hundred years ago. Early evidence for steroid receptors was the finding of "estrogen-binding proteins" in the mammalian uterus. The term "receptors" (R), as it applies to steroids, is now used to designate the "intracellular high-affinity steroid hormone-binding proteins."

Baulie and Mester[5] summarized the arguments for steroid receptors: (i) There is good correlation between the biological effect and its affinity for the receptor. (ii) Agonist and antagonist actions of modified steroid hormone structures can be explained by interactions with receptors. (iii) Biological effects correlate with receptor alterations: changes in the physicochemical properties of receptors (transformation) and changes in receptor distribution in subcellular fractions of target cell homogenates (translocation). (iv) Receptors are present in targets (levels vary from 10^3 to 10^4 molecules per cell). (v) Steroid hormone receptors show preferential binding to specific DNA sequences.

Simply put, the steroid hormone enters a cell. In the cytoplasm the steroid hormone (steroidal ligand) binds with a receptor (cognate receptor) which is specific for the hormone. The receptor-hormone complex migrates to the nucleus. The hormone-receptor complex has a "DNA binding domain" which has cysteine-rich regions involved in folding the peptide into loops stabilized by zinc, the steroid receptor zinc finger regions (Figure 13.11). Sequences of DNA in the target gene act as steroid response elements (SRE).[6] The zinc fingers interact with the hormone response elements. "The receptor regulates gene transcription presumably by interacting with the transcription machinery at the target promoter."[7] The consequence of this interaction is that messenger RNA is made from the DNA. The messenger RNA is used by the target cell to make new protein. The responses are specific to the target—estrogen causes the uterus to make more uterine protein.

STEROID METABOLISM AND EXCRETION

Generally, the steroids are hydrophobic, they are generally oil soluble but have little solubility in water. In order to excrete steroids, they must be converted to some water soluble form. Steroids are metabolized by the liver to more water soluble derivatives. Liver enzymes include Δ-4-reductase (hydrogenation at 4–5 double bonds), dehydrogenases (hydrogenation at 3-, α-, or 3-ß-keto groups), sulfatase (sulfonation), and ß-glucuronidase (adds a sugar). (Parenthetically, these inactivations are not the only peripheral conversions of steroids. The liver also converts cortisol to cortisone; and testosterone is metabolized to more active 5-α-dihydrotestosterone by enzymes in the target tissues.)

The steroids appear in urine as 17-ketosteroids that have less activity than their parent compounds. The 17-ketosteroids can be measured

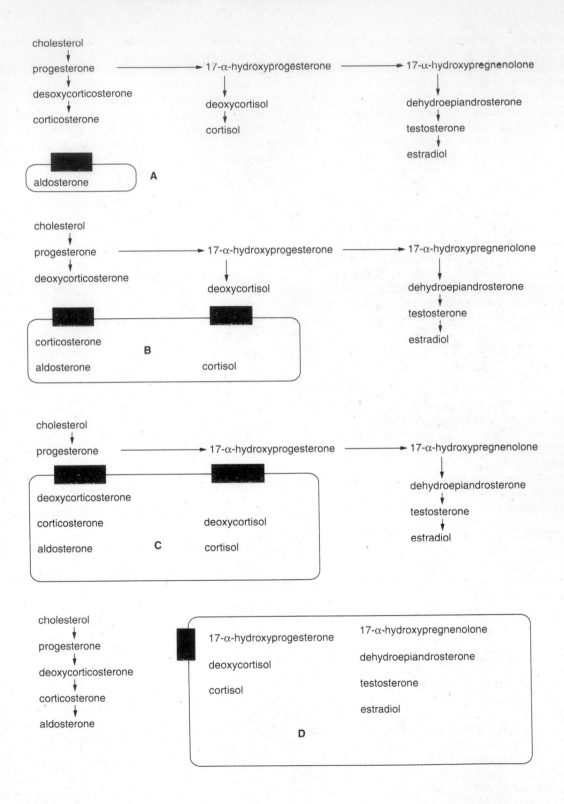

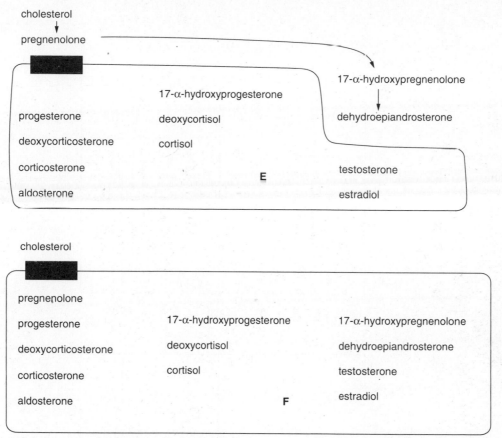

cholesterol

pregnenolone

17-α-hydroxypregnenolone

17-α-hydroxyprogesterone

progesterone   deoxycortisol   dehydroepiandrosterone

deoxycorticosterone   cortisol

corticosterone   testosterone

aldosterone   E   estradiol

cholesterol

pregnenolone

progesterone   17-α-hydroxyprogesterone   17-α-hydroxypregnenolone

deoxycorticosterone   deoxycortisol   dehydroepiandrosterone

corticosterone   cortisol   testosterone

aldosterone   F   estradiol

Figure 13.8 The effects of different enzyme deficiencies on the profile of steroids that are produced is illustrated. Enzyme presence is indicated by arrows; absence by black boxes. The names of the steroids that are missing or produced only in small amounts are encircled. **A = 18-hydroxysteroid dehydrogenase deficiency.** Afflicted individuals have sodium depletion, potassium retention, dehydration, hypotension, and increased plasma renin activity. Secretion of 18-hydroxycorticosterone occurs in Ulick's syndrome. **B = 11-ß-hydroxylase (11BHL) deficiency.** Symptoms are low plasma cortisol, renin activity, and aldosterone; low urine tetrahydrocortisol and tetrahydrocortisone; high plasma 11-deoxycortisol, deoxycorticosterone, ACTH, MSH; high urine tetrahydro derivatives of 11-deoxycortisol and deoxycorticosterone and 11-deoxy-17-ketosteroids. 11-ß-hydroxylase is found only in the adrenal cortex. Virilization and hypertension are symptoms of the deficiency so 11BHL is called the hypertensive form of congenital virilizing adrenal hyperplasia. **C = 21-hydroxylase deficiency.** The production of glucocorticoids and mineralocorticoids is impaired. There is low blood cortisol, high ACTH, high 17-α-hydroxyprogesterone, excess DHEA (which increases urine 17-ketosteroids). The salt-losing form of congenital virilizing adrenal hyperplasia is the most common form. **D = 17-α-hydroxylase deficiency.** The production of glucocorticoids, androgens, and estrogens is blocked. In the blood there is low cortisol, estrogen, and testosterone; and in the blood there is elevated ACTH, deoxycorticosteroids, deoxycorticosterone, corticosterone, and gonadotropins. Urine has high 17-OHS and 17-ketosteroids. Clinical symptoms in females include hypertension and sexual infantilism. Affected male fetuses do not secrete androgen which leads to failure to develop male external genitalia. **E = 3-ß-hydroxysteroid dehydrogenase deficiency.** All the steroids that are synthesized from progesterone are reduced. Blood has low cortisol and aldosterone. There are ambiguous neonatal genitalia, failure of the males to develop normal external genitalia, and partial masculinization of the external genitalia of females. **F = failure of the conversion of cholesterol to pregnenolone.** Blood and urine have low steroids; circulating ACTH is high. Infant survival rates are low, there are enlarged adrenal glands with excess cholesterol, and males have female external genitalia. Congenital (lipoid) adrenal hyperplasia is fatal. Redrawn, with permission. Williams, R. Textbook of Endocrinology. W. B. Philadelphia, PA: W. B. Saunders; 1987.

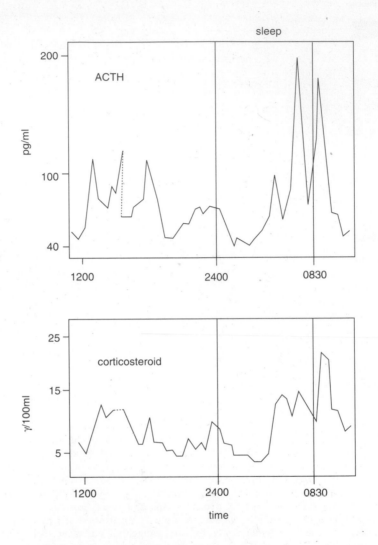

Figure 13.9 The graphs show daily rhythms in human male plasma corticotropin (ACTH) and corticosteroid (11-OHCS). The hormones were measured in samples taken every thirty minutes over a period of twenty-four hours. Redrawn, with permission. Krieger, D.; Allen, W.; Rizzo, F.; Krieger, H.P. Characterization of the normal pattern of plasma corticosteroid levels. J. Clin. Endocrinol. Metab. 32: 266–284; 1971.

with the Zimmerman reaction. In this test, the dried residue urine is heated with 1,3-dinitrobenzene at alkaline pH. A purple color is a positive reaction. The results of the test reflect daily secretion rates. 17-ketosteroids in males measured with this test are 8–30 mg/day; in females, 5–20 mg/day; and increase 3-fold at puberty.

By now, a student of endocrinology would expect to find hormones in blood and hormones, or their by-products, in urine. Interestingly, steroids can also be measured in saliva where the levels of most steroids reflect the unbound and biologically

Table 13.5 Steroid Distribution in Plasma

	Total plasma concentration nmol/l	Free %	SHBG %	CBG %	Albumin %
estradiol	0.29	1.81	37.3	<0.1	60.8
estrone	0.23	3.58	16.3	<0.1	80.1
progesterone	0.65	2.36	0.63	17.7	79.3
testosterone	1.3	1.36	66.0	2.26	30.4
dihydrotestosterone	0.65	0.47	78.4	0.12	21.0
androstenedione	5.4	7.54	6.63	1.37	84.5
cortisol	400	3.77	0.18	89.7	6.33

The values (%) show the percentages of the total plasma concentration that exists free or bound (to SHBG = sex hormone-binding globulin, CBG = corticosteroid binding globulin, or serum albumin). The values are for women during the early follicular phase of their menstrual cycles. In the luteal phase, the distributions are the same but total estradiol rises to 0.72 nmol/l and progesterone rises to 38 nmol/l. Dunn, J.F.; Rodbard, D. Transport of steroid hormones: Binding of 21 endogenous steroids to both testosterone-binding globulin and corticosteroid-binding globulin in human plasma. Journal of Clinical Endocrinology and Metabolism 53: 58–68; 1981; p. 61.

active concentrations found in plasma.[8] Steroid presence in saliva makes possible noninvasive testing.

CHOLESTEROL

Cholesterol is mainly important in this chapter as a precursor for the synthesis of steroid hormones.

But there has been a great deal of interest in the possible health hazards of dietary cholesterol (North Americans eat 0.4–2 g/day; but in other parts of the world people eat <0.2 g/day).[9] Thus, a little more discussion of cholesterol may be of interest.

Animals, but not plants, can synthesize cholesterol in all their cells. Acetyl-coenzyme A (Acetyl-CoA) is the precursor of cholesterol. HMG-CoA reductase is an enzyme that forms mevalonic acid which is an intermediate between acetyl-CoA and cholesterol. In the testes, luteiniz-

ing hormone increases cyclic AMP which activates protein kinase A and increases conversion of cholesteryl esters to cholesterol and conversion of cholesterol to pregnenolone. Most cholesterol synthesized in the liver is incorporated into very low density lipoproteins (VLDL). Cholesterol is an essential molecule in cell membranes of animals. Cholesterol absorption from the intestine involves its incorporation into intestinal chylomicrons whose remnants carry cholesterol to the liver. There are nonabsorbable plant sterols from soybeans that reduce cholesterol absorption.

The cholesterol circulates in the blood as cholesterol and as cholesteryl esters in lipoprotein complexes (bound to chylomicron remnants or albumin). The blood contains lipoproteins including chylomicrons, chylomicron remnants, very low density lipoproteins (VLDL), low density lipoproteins (LDL), and high density lipoproteins (HDL); the blood lipoproteins function in trans-

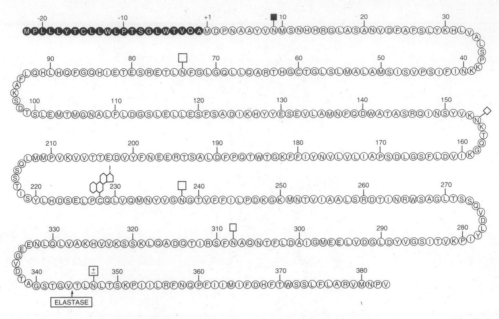

Figure 13.10 The figure shows the proposed primary structure of human corticosteroid binding globulin (CBG). Amino acids are represented by single letters. The shaded circles represent the signal peptide. Sites of N-glycosylation are squares; there is a cleavage site at elastase which releases bound glucocorticoid; and near 230 there is a cysteine (C) which may interact with 6-bromo progesterone. Reproduced, with permission. Hammond, G.L. Molecular properties of corticosteroid binding globulin and the sex-steroid binding proteins. Endocrine Reviews 11: 65–79; 1990.

portation of ingested exogenous lipids, triglycerides, and cholesterol. An LDL receptor that is a very large mosaic protein has been described. Levels of serum cholesterol below 260 mg/dl are considered to be medically desirable.

> The optimum serum cholesterol for a middle-aged American man is probably 200 mg/dL, or less. Hypercholesterolemia is defined as a value above the 95th percentile for the population, which in Americans ranges from 210 mg/dL in individuals <20 yr old, to >280 in individuals >60 yr old. However, these limits are clearly excessive because of the known cardiovascular risk of cholesterol values at these levels, and a convenient rule of thumb is than any level of serum cholesterol >180 mg/dL plus the person's age should be considered abnormal. . . . In women, values are slightly higher [by 10 mg/dL] after the reproductive years . . . . Mean values are lower among children before age 10 [125-195 mg/dL].[10]

Cholesterol is provided to the tissues for their cell membranes and steroid synthesis by LDL. 93% of cholesterol is in the cells; only 7% of cholesterol is in the circulation (but it is this fraction that is important to atherosclerosis).[11] Cells esterify cholesterol and store the esters in lipid droplets. An enzyme, cholesterol ester hydrolase, catalyzes the formation of free cholesterol.

Cholesterol, in turn, serves as the precursor of both steroid hormones and bile acids. Cholesterol 7α-hydroxylase is the first enzyme in the pathway for metabolism of cholesterol to bile acids. It is also the rate-limiting enzyme.[12] As mentioned, the activity of the enzyme has a daily rhythm in LD12:12 with low activity in the light-time and high activity in the dark-time. The distri-

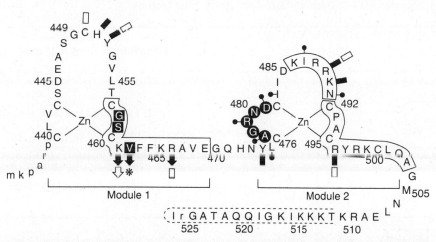

Figure 13.11 The diagram shows the zinc coordination scheme for the rat GR DNA binding domain. Numbers are based on the full-length receptor; rectangles show locations of phosphate backbone contacts; solid arrows show where there is contact with bases; solid dots show amino acids involved in dimer interface interactions; black boxed letters indicate residues that confer specificity in mutagenesis experiments; black circled letters show the residues that confer half-site spacing requirements; solid lines enclose alpha helical regions; dashed lines enclose a disordered section at the C terminus. Some amino acid designations are derived from vector sequence of the overexpression plasmid. Reprinted, with permission. Luisi, B.F.; Xu, W.X.; Otwinowski, Z.; Freedman, L.P.; Yamamoto, K.R.; Sigler, P.B. Crystallographic analysis of the interaction of the glucocorticoid receptor with DNA. Nature 352: 497–505; 1991. ©MacMillan Magazines.

bution of the activity of the enzyme varies among tissues (Table 13.6). Cholesterol is excreted by the liver in bile; in the bile it is present in free form and as bile acids. Obstruction of the bile duct consequently raises cholesterol.

A number of endocrine factors affect the amounts of cholesterol that are produced. Cholesterol partially inhibits its own synthesis by reducing the activity of one of the enzymes (HMG-CoA reductase). Cholesterol is decreased by thyroid hormones and estrogen. ACTH stimulates the formation of steroids by increasing the conversion of cholesterol to pregnenolone, thereby reducing the cholesterol pool.

Diet and liver interact to regulate the amount of cholesterol. Cholesterol can be absorbed from bile acids and from food in the intestines (mainly from egg yolks and animal fat). Diets high in cholesterol decrease liver biosynthesis of cholesterol. Low cholesterol diets increase hepatic synthesis, but diets low in cholesterol usually reduce blood cholesterol. Kane and Malloy comment on the value of diet in managing cholesterol:

Restriction of dietary cholesterol to less than 200 mg/d in normal individuals usually results in a decrease of 10–15% in serum cholesterol . . . . Although much attention has been devoted to the possible role of fiber in the development of coronary heart disease and levels of triglyceride and cholesterol in serum, there is little evidence that plasma lipids can be significantly affected by intake of most forms of fiber . . . . Several other nutrients have been studied in relation to atherosclerotic heart disease, including calcium, magnesium, trace elements, vitamins D, E, and C, and pyridoxine. The results of these studies are generally equivocal, and the observed effects on serum lipids are small. Caffeine and sucrose have negligible effects on serum lipids, and their statistical relationship to coronary heart disease is generally unimpressive when data are corrected for cigarette smoking.[13]

Table 13.6 Cholesterol 17-α-hydroxylase Activity in Microsomes

Tissue	Cholesterol 17-α-hydroxylase activity
liver	171.0 pmol/min/mg tissue
kidney	12.4 pmol/min/mg tissue
heart	18.9 pmol/min/mg tissue
lung	46.3 pmol/min/mg tissue

Chiang, J.Y.; Miller, W.F.; Lin, G. Regulation of cholesterol 17-α-hydroxylase in the liver. J. Biol. Chem. 265: 3889–3897; 1990.

Although the idea prevails that associates high cholesterol with obesity, 40% of people with anorexia nervosa have high serum LDL and cholesterol levels (400–600 mg/dl).[14]

Cholesterol has received great attention because of atheroschlerosis. In atherosclerosis, or hardening of the arteries, blood vessels become rigid because of lesions containing foam cells and cholesterol. Serious illness (myocardial infarction and strokes) have atherosclerosis as part of their etiology. Atherosclerosis in turn has been associated with high circulating cholesterol. A high LDL/HDL ratio is associated with disease; smoking, obesity, and sedentary lifestyle are associated with low HDL. Mutations in the LDL receptor produce familial hypercholesterolemia. A low LDL/HDL ratio decreases the incidence of serious illness; HDL is higher in women, and HDL is increased by exercise and alcoholic drinks. Atherosclerosis is a special problem in diabetes where cholesterol in the blood is also high.

Gallstones also have to do with cholesterol. The presence of gallstones is called cholelithiasis and is found in 5% of men and 20% of women aged 50–65 in the USA. In the USA and Europe, 85% of the gallstones are "cholesterol stones." The stones form when the bile fluid doesn't move, or when the bile is supersaturated with cholesterol, or due to "nucleation factors," possibly gall bladder mucus glycoproteins, which cause the stones to crystalize.

STEROID SUBDIVISIONS

Cholesterol has been made into a villain in the etiology of some diseases. But, getting back on track, cholesterol, as a precursor for steroid hormones, is essential for the endocrine glands that make steroid hormones. The steroids that are made primarily by the adrenal gland have been subdivided into glucocorticoids and mineralocorticoids. The androgens are the steroid hormones associated mainly with the testes. The estrogens and progestogens are the steroid hormones mainly association with female reproduction (ovaries, pregnancy, lactation). The steroid hormones function in the regulation of salt, glucose, and reproduction. The study of these steroid hormones comprises a large portion of the subject of endocrinology.

REFERENCES

1. Mertz, L.M.; Pedersen, R.C. The kinetics of steroidogenesis activator polypeptide in the rat adrenal cortex. J. Biol. Chem. 264: 15274–15279; 1989.
2. Chiang, J.Y.; Miller, W.F.; Lin, G. Regulation of 7α-hydroxylase in the liver. J. Biol. Chem. 265: 3889–3897; 1990.
3. Krieger, D.; Allen, W.; Rizzo, F.; Krieger,

H.P. Characterization of the normal temporal pattern of plasma corticosteroid levels. J. Clin. Endocrinology Metabolism 32: 266; 1971.

4. Hammond, G. L. Molecular properties of corticosteroid binding globulin and the sex-steroid binding proteins. Endocrine Reviews 11: 65–79; 1990.

5. Baulieu, E.; Mester, J. Steroid Hormone Receptors, Chapter 3. In DeGroot, L. J., editor. Endocrinology. Philadelphia, PA: W. B. Saunders Co.; 1989; p. 16.

6. Freedman, L.P. Anatomy of the steroid receptor zinc finger region. Endocrine Reviews 13: 129–145; 1992.

7. Bagchi, M.K.; Tsai, M.; O'Malley, B.W.; Tsai, S. Analysis of the mechanism of steroid hormone receptor-dependent gene activation in cell-free systems. Endocrine Reviews 13: 525–535; 1992.

8. Wilson, D.W.; Falker, R.F.; Read, G.F.; Griffiths, K. Potential value of salivary steroids in chronoepidemiological and endocrine-related studies. In: Chronobiology: Its Role in Clinical Medicine, General Biology, and Agriculture, Part A, Wiley-Liss, Inc.: New York; 1990; pp. 119–130.

9. Kane, J.P.; Malloy, M.H. Disorders of lipoprotein metabolism. In Greenspan, F.S., editor. Basic and Clinical Endocrinology, Third Edition. Norwalk, CT: Appleton & Lange; 1993; p. 670.

10. Berkow, R., editor. The Merck Manual, Fifteenth Edition. Rahway, NJ: Merck Sharp & Dohme Research Laboratories; 1987; p. 1003.

11. Ganong, W. Review of Medical Physiology, 14th edition. Norwalk, CT: Appleton & Lange; p. 258.

12. Chiang, J.Y.; Miller, W.F.; Lin, G.; Op. cit.

13. Kane, J.P.; Malloy, M.H. Disorders of lipoprotein metabolism. In Greenspan, F.S., Forsham, P.H., editors. Basic and Clinical Endocrinology, Second Edition. Los Altos, CA: Lange Medical Publications; 1986; p. 610.

14. Kane, J.P.; Malloy, M.H.; Ibid.; p. 605.

CHAPTER 14

Glucocorticoids and the Adrenal Cortex

The adrenal gland of mammals has two parts, an outer cortex and a central medulla. The cortex of the adrenal gland makes the corticosteroid hormones. Some of the hormones regulate glucose metabolism and are therefore classified as glucocorticoids. These hormones are the subject of this chapter. Other corticosteroids, especially aldosterone, regulate salt and water balance and are therefore classified as mineralocorticoids. The adrenal medulla, in contrast to the steroid-secreting cortex, makes catecholamine hormones. Glucocorticoids control glucose in concert with other hormones (insulin, glucagon, growth hormone, epinephrine, etc.).

ADRENAL GLAND ANATOMY

Each vertebrate individual has two adrenal glands. Each of the paired adrenal glands is really two glands, the adrenal cortex and the adrenal medulla (Figures 14.1 and 14.2). Adrenal glands in human adults together weigh 8–10g.[1] The adrenal glands of humans and other mammals ride atop the kidneys (Figure 14.3). Early erroneous speculations about its function included the ideas that it was a prop for the stomach, that it pressed on the kidneys to squeeze out the urine, and that it stored "black bile" humors. Adrenal glands of other vertebrates are also associated with the kidneys; however, there is variation in the anatomical arrangement. The distinct outer-cortex and inner-medulla arrangement is only found in mammals. In contrast to mammals, the frogs have elongated red-brown kidneys and the adrenal glands run along them as a bright yellow stripe.

The adrenal cortex and medulla can be compared (Table 14.1). The adrenal medulla occupies the center part of each adrenal gland where it accounts for 22% of the weight of the gland. The remaining 78% of the weight of the gland is adrenal cortex and the adrenal gland's surrounding capsule. The medulla is not steroidogenic, but instead makes amine hormones. The cortex is the portion of the adrenal gland that makes steroid hormones, the corticoids. The layers are so different that they can be distinguished with the naked eye. If an adrenal, for example, of a rat, is sliced in half, the inner medulla is deep red and the outer cortex is light tan.

ADRENAL GLAND HISTOLOGY

The histology of the mammalian adrenal cortex is characterized by zonation. The adrenal gland is enclosed in a fibrous capsule. The cortex has been subdivided into three layers: zona glomerulosa, zona fasciculata, zona reticularis. The cells that comprise the adrenal cortex are collectively referred to as **foam cells**. All three layers make corticosterone, but otherwise, the layers are specialized as regards their main hormone products. The cells have large amounts of smooth endoplasmic reticulum that is associated with their production of steroid hormones. The structure of cortical steroid-secreting cells is similar to that of other steroid-secreting cells in the body.

The **zona glomerulosa** (15% of adrenal weight) is the outer layer of the adrenal cortex. It specializes in production of the steroid hormone aldosterone (Figure 14.4). It is deficient in 17-α-hydroxylase activity, so it cannot produce cortisol or androgens. Its whorls of cells have less lipid than the cells of the other zones. The zona glomerulosa is not regulated by ACTH. The zona glomerulosa also forms new cortical cells and is responsible for the regenerating ability of the adrenal cortex.

The **zona fasciculata** (50% of adrenal weight) is the central, and widest, layer of the adrenal cortex. They have sometimes been called "clear cells" because they contain more lipid. The cells are loosely organized into columns extending from the zona reticularis to the zona glomerulosa. The zona fasciculata secretes cortisol and androgens. The zona fasciculata atrophies in the absence of ACTH and hypertrophies in response to excess ACTH. ACTH also causes depletion of lipid from the clear cells making them look more like cells of the zona reticularis.

The **zona reticularis** (10% of adrenal weight) is the innermost layer of the adrenal cortex; it surrounds the medulla. The interlaced network of "compact cells" have little lipid but do contain granules that stain lipofuscin-positive. The zona reticularis secretes cortisol and androgens, atrophies in the absence of ACTH, and hypertrophies in response to excess ACTH.

There is a vigorous blood supply. In cats, the blood flow through the adrenal is 4.9–7.0 ml per minute per gram. The blood supply for the adrenal glands arises from branchlets of the renal and phrenic arteries and the aorta. Blood flows through cortical sinusoids to the medulla from a plexus in the capsule. At the corticomedullary junction, there is a subcapsular plexus from which venules extend through the medulla. Venous drainage is by a single adrenal vein (also called the medullary vein). The blood exits via the renal vein to the inferior vena cava.

Factors that affect size of the adrenal glands are gender, domestication, and salt supply. Sexual dimorphism in the size of the adrenal glands can be seen in humans and rats (where females have larger adrenal glands) and hamsters (where males have larger adrenal glands). Wild rats have larger adrenal glands with more lipid, more aldehyde, more ketone groups, and a richer blood supply than laboratory rats. Rabbits and kangaroos have low

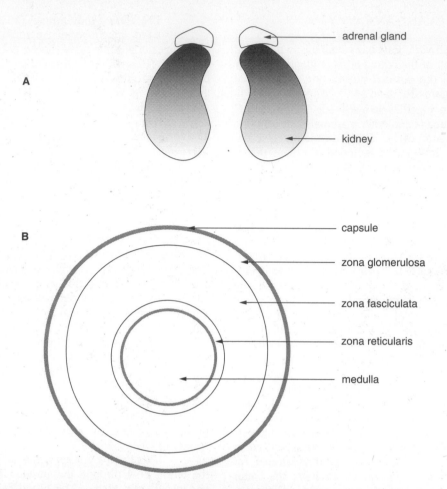

Figure 14.1 Diagrammatic anatomy of the mammalian adrenal gland is shown. (A) Location of adrenal glands and kidneys. (B) Layers of the adrenal glands. The three "zonas" make up the adrenal cortex.

salt diets and an enlarged zona glomerulosa; but, paradoxically, marine birds that have high salt diets have big adrenal glands as well.

FUNCTIONS OF THE GLUCOCORTICOIDS

The adrenal glands of humans make 40–50 steroids, but only a few of them are secreted in biologically interesting amounts: aldosterone, cortisol, corticosterone, dehydroepiandrosterone, androstenedione, deoxycorticosterone, aldosterone. Of these, the steroids made by the zona fasciculata and the zona reticularis that affect sugar metabolism are glucocorticoids. Cortisol is the main glucocorticoid secreted in humans, monkeys, sheep, and cats

(Table 14.2). Rats, mice, and birds secrete mainly corticosterone. Dogs secrete corticosterone and cortisol equally. A well-known effect of glucocorticoids is to raise blood sugar.

Glucocorticoids derive their name from the synthesis of glucose and glycogen. The glucocorticoids affect "intermediary metabolism" by alteration of the activity of enzymes in the pathways (Figure 14.5). Glucocorticoids increase **gluconeogenesis** in liver cells by stimulating phosphoenolpyruvate carboxykinase and glucose 6-phosphatase. They also increase liver glycogen formation by stimulating glycogen synthetase activity. At the same time, glucocorticoids

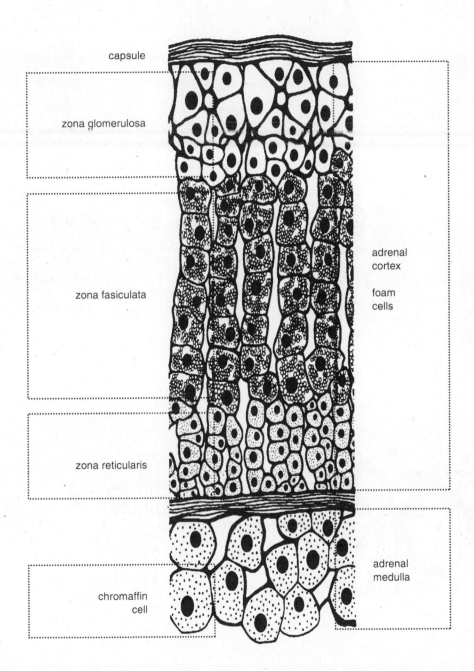

Figure 14.2 The diagram represents the cellular structure of the adrenal gland. Modified, with permission.
Norris, D.O. Vertebrate Endocrinology. Philadelphia, PA: Lea & Febiger; 1980; p. 303; and Gorbman, A.; Bern,
H. A Textbook of Comparative Endocrinology. New York: John Wiley and Sons; 1962; p. 310.

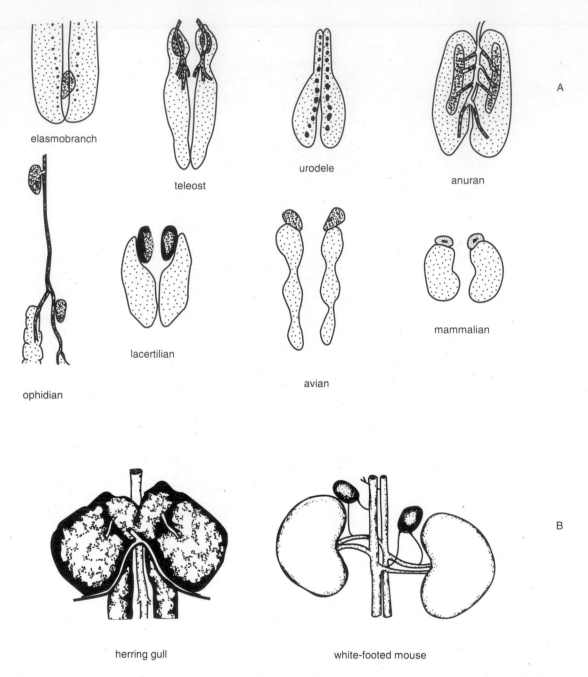

elasmobranch

teleost

urodele

anuran

A

ophidian

lacertilian

avian

mammalian

B

herring gull

white-footed mouse

Figure 14.3 The figure illustrates the comparative anatomy of the adrenal glands and kidneys in a variety of vertebrates. (A) For the upper eight organisms, chromaffin tissue is black, adrenals are dense stipple, and kidneys are light stipple. Modified, with permission. Gorbman, A.; Bern, H.A. A Textbook of Comparative Endocrinology. New York: John Wiley & Sons; 1962; p. 299. (B) The lower two diagrams, obtained from a different source, show the arteries and veins for two additional species. Hartman, F.A.; Brownell, K.A. The Adrenal Gland. Philadelphia, PA: Lea and Febiger; 1949; p. 27, 31.

Table 14.1 Comparison of Adrenal Cortex and Medulla

Parameter	Cortex	Medulla
% of gland	78%	22%
hormones	steroids	amines
embryonic origin	mesoderm	neural crest
innervation	nearly none	medulla consists of modified postganglionic cells (sympathetic division, autonomic nervous system)
regeneration	yes	no
essential for life	yes	no
cell characteristics	lipid droplets	amine granules

increase the availability of substrates derived from proteins (glucocorticoids reduce peripheral amino acid uptake and reduce peripheral protein synthesis) and fats (glucocorticoids increase lipolysis). So the glucocorticoids direct intermediary metabolism to substrates (amino acids and fatty acids) that can be used to increase sugar. Glucocorticoids further increase blood glucose by inhibiting glucose uptake by muscle and fat tissues. So, as far as metabolic effects are concerned, glucocorticoids act principally on liver, muscle, and fat. The effects of glucocorticoids are brought into play during fasting. The enzymes of intermediary metabolism are also regulated by other hormones (e.g., epinephrine from the adrenal medulla; glucagon and insulin from the pancreas).

Glucocorticoids are well known for their **anti-inflammatory** action. Inflammation is characterized by redness of the skin, swelling, and pain. The reaction is complex involving over fifty factors, but glucocorticoids suppress every known aspect. Martin says, "Attempts have been made to form a unifying hypothesis [for steroid influences on macrophages, lymphocytes, fibroblasts, neutrophils, mast cells, capillary endothelium, basement membranes, cell proliferation, antibody pro-

duction, mediator release] but no satisfactory one has been found."[2] The ability to suppress the inflammation response makes glucocorticoids useful in the treatment of any condition that involves inflammation: infection, rheumatoid arthritis, allergies, transplant rejection, and asthma. However, the use of glucocorticoids has side effects, symptoms similar to those of a disease of excess cortisol production, Cushing's disease. So while glucocorticoids do not cure inflammations, they assist in the response to injury by suppressing the harmful consequences of the defense system. For example, in poison ivy, the itchy rash, which is the problem, is suppressed by glucocorticoids, but prevention or cure of poison ivy requires removal of the the ivy's oleoresin, urushiol, which causes the reaction in the first place.

Glucocorticoids inhibit prostaglandins by causing synthesis of a polypeptide, macrocortin.[3] The macrocortin inhibits cell membrane phospholipase needed for the release of precursors of prostaglandin synthetase.

The glucocorticoids have effects on the lymphatic system and upon the cells that circulate in the blood. The glucocorticoids mobilize blood

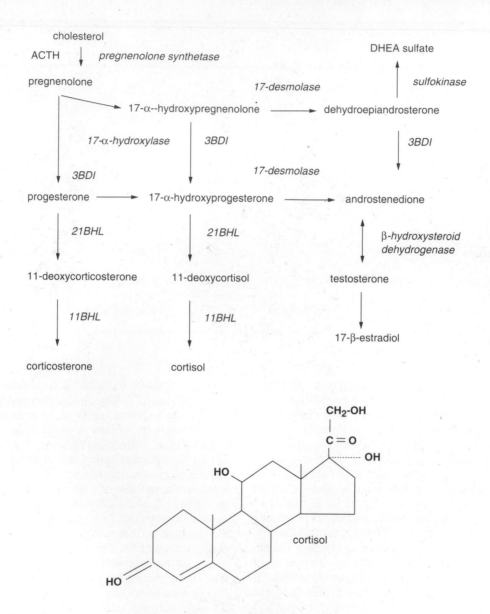

Figure 14.4 The figure illustrates the biosynthesis of steroids from cholesterol in the zona fasiculata (Zf) and zona glomerulosa (Zg) of the adrenal cortex. Enzymes are in italic and the structure of cortisol is shown, and the hormones that are secreted are in boldface.

cells. The glucocorticoids increase the function and movement of leukocytes. Particularly, glucocorticoids increase the number of circulating polymorphonuclear (PMN) leucocytes by releasing them from the bone marrow into the blood. The glucocorticoids stimulate the migration of inflammatory cells (PMNs, monocytes, lymphocytes) to injury locations.

Table 14.2 Amounts of Corticoids in Humans[4]

Parameter	Hormone	Amount
secretion	cortisol	25 mg/day
	corticosterone	5 mg/day
	aldosterone	0.25 mg/day
excretion	17-ketosteroids, male	8–30 mg/day
	17-ketosteroids, female	5–20 mg/day
blood	cortisol	5–25 µg/100ml
	corticosterone	1–1.5 µg/100ml
	aldosterone	0.004–0.008 µg/100ml

The skin, bone, and intestines are targets of glucocorticoids. Excessive glucocorticoids cause the skin to become thin, form stripes, and bruise easily. This is because the glucocorticoids inhibit fibroblasts and lead to loss of collagen and connective tissue. Bone formation is inhibited by excess glucocorticoids. Glucocorticoids decrease calcium absorption by the intestine. Overall, excessive glucocorticoids increase calcium loss in the urine together with decreased absorption from the intestine thereby producing a negative calcium balance. Serum calcium levels are maintained, but the bone loses calcium.

Glucocorticoids promote growth and development, unless they are in excess, and then they inhibit growth in children. The glucocorticoids act on the heart and blood vessels to maintain vascular tone and increase cardiac output. In excess, glucocorticoids produce hypertension.

Glucocorticoids influence electrolyte and water balance. They cause sodium and water retention, hypokalemia (low serum potassium), hypertension (high blood pressure), and increased glomerular filtration rate. Some of these effects may be due to stimulation of mineralocorticoid receptors.

The brain responds to excess glucocorticoids with initial euphoria. Irritability, emotional lability, depression, overt psychoses, increased appetite, decreased libido, insomnia, and decreased REM sleep are among the psychological effects of long-term glucocorticoid treatment. Glucocorticoid deficit is also accompanied by behavioral effects: irritability, apathy, depression, negativity, reclusivity, reduced appetite, and increased sensitivity to tastes and smells.

The liver metabolizes cortisol to cortisone (Figure 14.6). It also inactivates cortisol and other glucocorticoids by conjugation with glucuronic acid. Cortisone does have activity which makes it useful clinically, but very little endogenously produced cortisone reaches potential target cells. Cortisol metabolites are excreted in the urine and feces. Surgery, stress, and liver disease decrease metabolism of glucocorticoids and thus may raise plasma cortisol.

STRESS

Selye proposed a **General Adaptation Syndrome** involving the adrenal glands on a global scale. A representation of stress responses appears in Figure 14.7; however, it seems likely that the adrenal cortex is involved in the short term as well as the long term because ACTH secretion rises quickly in response to stress; Martin says TSH is inhibited by stress and that the response is mediated by somatostatin.[5] He proposed that the

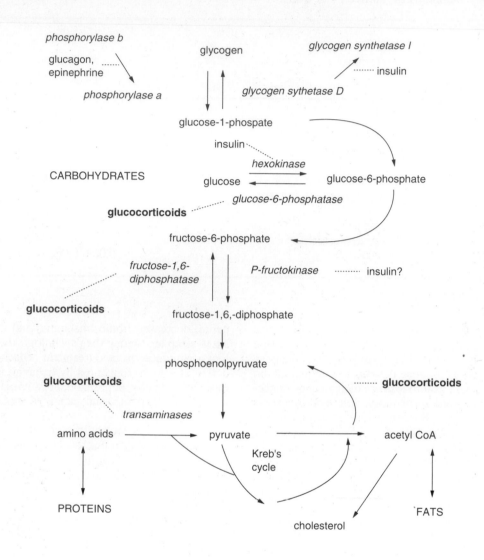

Figure 14.5 A simplified diagram of intermediary metabolism shows the points where hormones (glucocorticoids, insulin, glucagon, epinephrine) affect the activity of key enzymes. Modified, with permission. Frieden, E.; Lipner, H. Biochemical Endocrinology of the Vertebrates. Englewood Cliffs, NJ: Prentice-Hall; 1971; p. 71.

response of an organism to nonspecific stress involved steroid suppression of inflammatory reactions while, at the same time, permitting infection to spread. He called the resulting diseases the Adaptation Diseases. The Adaptation Diseases included nervous and emotional disturbances, high blood pressure, gastric and duodenal ulcers, rheumatic diseases, allergies, and diseases of the heart and kidneys. Stress was viewed broadly as the rate of all the wear and tear caused by life. Selye coined the terms, "glucocorticoid" and "mineralocorticoid."

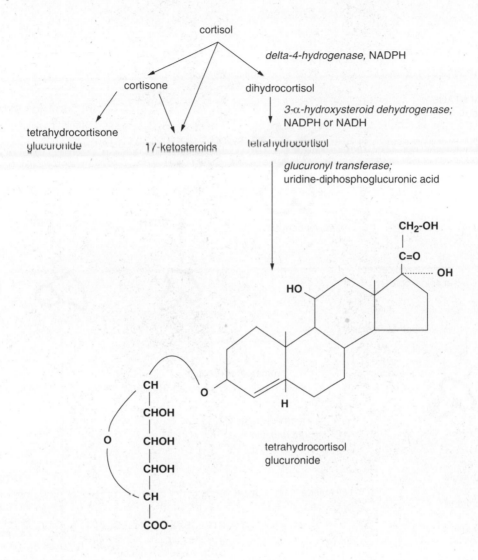

Figure 14.6 Metabolism of cortisol in the liver to form cortisone and glucuronides. The structure of tetrahydrocortisol glucuronide is shown.

Stress (any of a variety of noxious stimuli, Selye's "stressors") increase ACTH secretion with subsequent glucocorticoid increases. This response is essential for life. Hypophysectomized or adrenalectomized animals cannot survive stressful stimuli (such as cold exposure). Replacement glucocorticoids prolong survival in the operated animals.

In the context of biology and medicine, the word "stress" should be used cautiously. Ganong gives a clear clinical definition of stress: "The word is a short, emotionally charged word for something that otherwise takes many words to say, and it is a convenient term to use as long as it is understood that...it denotes only those stimuli that have been proved to increase ACTH secretion in

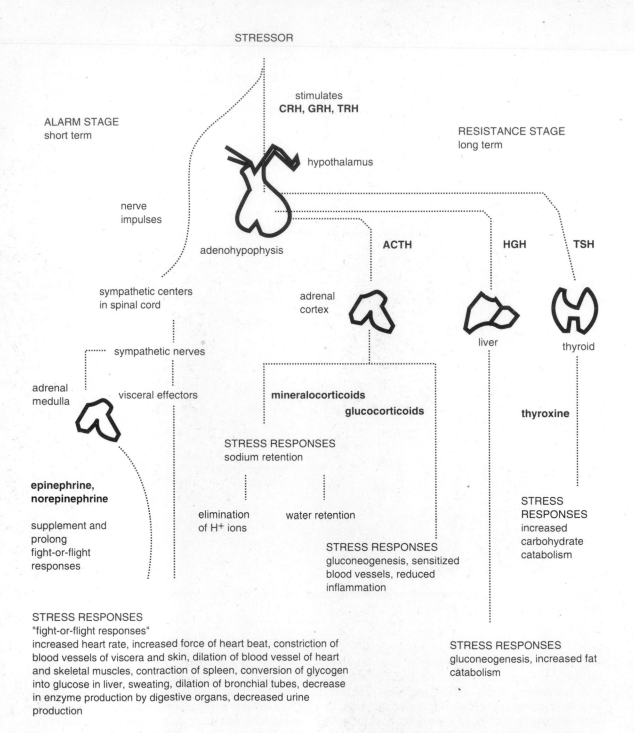

STRESSOR

stimulates
CRH, GRH, TRH

ALARM STAGE
short term

RESISTANCE STAGE
long term

hypothalamus

nerve
impulses

adenohypophysis

ACTH   **HGH**   **TSH**

sympathetic centers
in spinal cord

adrenal
cortex

liver   thyroid

sympathetic nerves

adrenal
medulla

visceral effectors

mineralocorticoids

glucocorticoids

thyroxine

STRESS RESPONSES
sodium retention

**epinephrine,
norepinephrine**

supplement and
prolong
fight-or-flight
responses

elimination
of H+ ions

water retention

STRESS
RESPONSES
increased
carbohydrate
catabolism

STRESS RESPONSES
gluconeogenesis, sensitized
blood vessels, reduced
inflammation

STRESS RESPONSES
"fight-or-flight responses"
increased heart rate, increased force of heart beat, constriction of
blood vessels of viscera and skin, dilation of blood vessel of heart
and skeletal muscles, contraction of spleen, conversion of glycogen
into glucose in liver, sweating, dilation of bronchial tubes, decrease
in enzyme production by digestive organs, decreased urine
production

STRESS RESPONSES
gluconeogenesis, increased fat
catabolism

Figure 14.7 The diagram shows the responses to stressors during the General Adaptation Syndrome. Names of hormones are italicized. Tortora, G. J.; Anagnostakos, N. P. Principles of Anatomy and Physiology, Sixth Edition. New York: Harper & Row; 1990; p. 535.

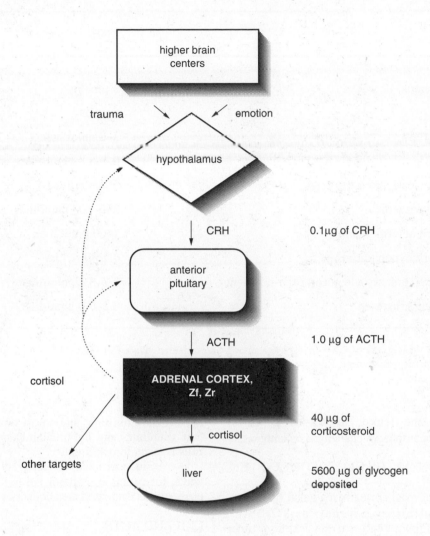

Figure 14.8 The figure illustrates the regulation of glucocorticoids by ACTH. The regulation scheme involves the hypothalamo-pituitary-adrenal axis, negative feedback by cortisol (left), and amplification (56,000x, right). Data for amplification are from Brown, J.; Barker, S. Basic Endocrinology, Second Edition. Philadelphia, PA: F. A. Davis Co.; 1966; p. 138.

normal animals and humans."[6]

    Long-term, or chronic, stress can be obtained for study by infecting rats with a mycobacterial Freund's type adjuvant which induces inflammatory joint disease. The consequence of the experimental treatment was associated with increased

morning ACTH and corticosterone levels and loss of the diurnal rhythms of ACTH and corticosterone.[7] Moreover, the glucocorticoids have been implicated in the function of the immune system. For example, they inhibit production of IL-1 which is a monokine (of the family of

Table 14.3 Corticotropin-Releasing Hormone

Location	CRH
fetal hypothalamus, 12 weeks	2 pmol/g
urine	5 µg/day
lumbar spinal fluid	3–8 nmol/liter
plasma, normal subjects 0800–1000 h	0.4–8.8 pmol/liter
plasma, women, early third trimester	55 pmol/liter
plasma, women at term	250–300 pmol/liter
plasma, women at term, twins	1460 pmol/liter
plasma, primary hypopituitarism	4.2 pmol/liter
plasma, untreated primary adrenocortical insufficiency	3.2–8.2 pmol/liter
plasma, Cushing's disease	0.2–0.6 pmol/liter

Orth points out that reports of CRH levels vary among investigators. Data from Orth, D. Corticotropin-releasing hormone in humans. Endocrine Reviews 13: 164–191; 1992.

interleukins, the leukocyte-derived peptides) produced by macrophages challenged by antigens.[8]

REGULATION OF THE GLUCOCORTICOIDS

The adrenal cortex is regulated by the **hypothalamo-pituitary-adrenal axis** (HPA).[9] This system (Figure 14.8) is a classical third order endocrinological negative feedback system involving a releasing hormone (CRH), a pituitary hormone (ACTH), and glucocorticoid hormones (cortisol). The brain processes signals from sensory pathways such as pain, trauma, or emotion. The signal for the circadian rhythm originates in nuclei of the hypothalamus: the suprachiasmatic nuclei (SCN).

Regulation of the adrenal cortex illustrates an advantage of hierarchical organization: **amplification**. For every 0.1 microgram of CRH, 5600 micrograms of glycogen are deposited in the liver. The overall amplification is 56,000 times! Even more impressive amplification can be calcu-

lated if the miniscule amount of neurotransmitter that stimulates the hypothalamic neurosecretory cells is taken into account.

Glucocorticoids are also regulated in other ways; for example, cortisol is raised as a consequence of its decreased metabolism by liver.

CRH AND ACTH

Corticotropin-releasing hormone (CRH) is a hormone made in the hypothalamus. Human CRH has molecular weight 4758.[10] The hormone triggers release of ACTH from the pituitary gland. Vasopressin can also release ACTH, but this may be a nonspecific or pharmacological effect. It is found in the hypothalamus in the supraoptic nucleus, paraventricular nucleus, and arcuate nucleus. In humans, CRH is found in fetal hypothalamus; it increases with age; and women have more than men in their hypothalami (Table 14.3). CRH is also found in other brain regions, cerebrospinal fluid, placenta, amniotic fluid, and various tumors. In

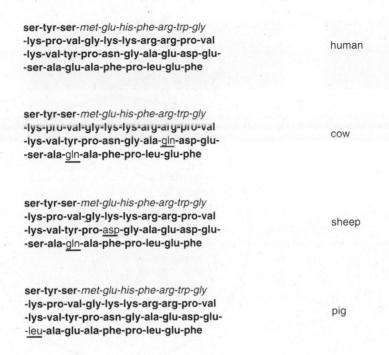

ser-tyr-ser-*met-glu-his-phe-arg-trp-gly*
-lys-pro-val-gly-lys-lys-arg-arg-pro-val
-lys-val-tyr-pro-asn-gly-ala-glu-asp-glu-
-ser-ala-glu-ala-phe-pro-leu-glu-phe   human

ser-tyr-ser-*met-glu-his-phe-arg-trp-gly*
-lys-pro-val-gly-lys-lys-arg-arg-pro-val
-lys-val-tyr-pro-asn-gly-ala-<u>gln</u>**-asp-glu-**
-ser-ala-<u>gln</u>**-ala-phe-pro-leu-glu-phe**   cow

ser-tyr-ser-*met-glu-his-phe-arg-trp-gly*
-lys-pro-val-gly-lys-lys-arg-arg-pro-val
-lys-val-tyr-pro-<u>asp</u>**-gly-ala-glu-asp-glu-**
-ser-ala-<u>gln</u>**-ala-phe-pro-leu-glu-phe**   sheep

ser-tyr-ser-*met-glu-his-phe-arg-trp-gly*
-lys-pro-val-gly-lys-lys-arg-arg-pro-val
-lys-val-tyr-pro-asn-gly-ala-glu-asp-glu-
-<u>leu</u>**-ala-glu-ala-phe-pro-leu-glu-phe**   pig

Figure 14.9 The sequence of 39 amino acids of corticotropin is shown for four species. ACTH is one of the melanotropins and has a seven-amino acid residue sequence that is also found in MSH, the "common heptapeptide," amino acids 4–10 (italics). Variations between amino acids among the species are underlined. ACTH is synthesized from POMC (pro-opiomelanocortin) along with melanotropins and lipotropin. Redrawn, with permission. Ganong, W. Review of Medical Physiology, Fourteenth Edition. Norwalk, CT: Appleton & Lange; 1989; p. 317.

blood there is a CRH-binding protein. CRH receptors are found in the pituitary on the corticotrophs. They are also found in the adrenal medulla, erythrocyte and immunocyte cell membranes, so CRH is thought to act in catecholamine secretion and T-cell function as well as in regulation of pituitary ACTH release.

Corticotropin, ACTH, is synthesized, like the melanotropins, from pro-opiomelanocortin. The structures of ACTH exhibit interspecies variation (Figure 14.9). The mechanism of action of ACTH involves a cAMP second messenger (Figure 14.10). The ACTH arrives at the target cells of the zona fasciculata and zona reticularis of the adrenal cortex. The target cell membranes contain receptor

proteins that interact with the ACTH. The receptors are coupled to the adenyl cyclase by a nucleotide regulatory protein (G_S). Stimulated adenyl cyclase increases cyclic AMP. Cyclic AMP activates protein kinase which in turn phosphorylates cholesterol ester hydrolase. The enzyme, cholesterol ester hydrolase, frees cholesterol from cholesterol esters in the lipid droplets. Cholesterol is converted to cortisol at the smooth endoplasmic reticulum. Cortisol is predominantly secreted in humans; some corticosterone is also secreted.

Long-term ACTH stimulation has still further effects on adrenal cortex cells. It increases the mitochondrial enzymes (P450s, cytochromes) involved in steroid formation.

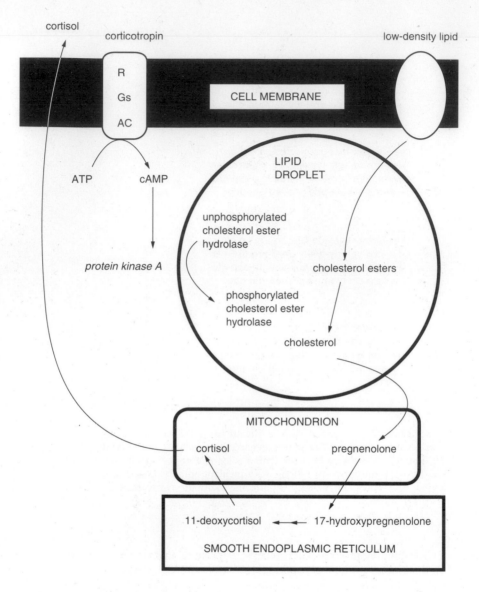

Figure 14.10 The diagram shows the mechanism of action of ACTH. ACTH acts on cells that secrete cortisol in the zona fasciculata and the zona reticularis.

MECHANISM OF ACTION OF GLUCOCORTICOIDS

Glucocorticoids are like other steroids. They achieve their actions by binding to receptor sites (GR, glucocorticoid receptors, which have been partially purified from rat liver) inside target cells. The receptor-hormone interacts with a DNA bound glucocorticoid response element (GRE) using the steroid receptor zinc finger region. The DNA is transcribed to make new mRNA. The mRNA in turn is responsible for making new enzymes that carry out glucocorticoid actions.[11]

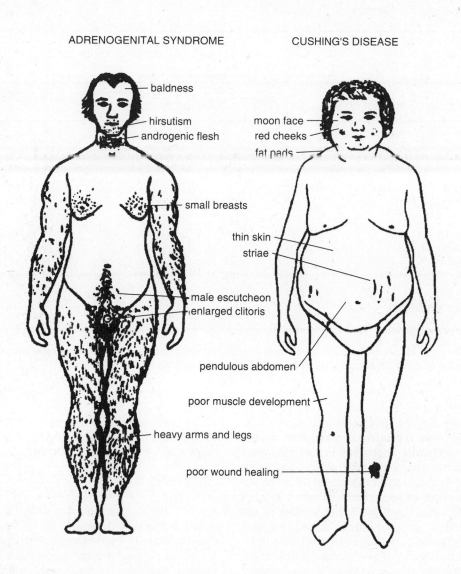

Figure 14.11 The sketches of two women show characteristics of disorders related to the adrenal gland: adrenogenital syndrome (left) and Cushing's disease (right). Adrenogenital syndrome has characteristics due to excess androgen such as hirsutism (hairiness) and male escutcheon (pubic hair pattern). Cushing's disease results from excess cortisol; the disease is characterized by easy bruising and striae (stripes). Modified, with permission. Forsham, R.P.; DiRaimondo, V. Traumatic Medicine and Surgery for the Attorney. Stoneham: MA; Butterworth; 1960.

ADRENAL ANDROGENS AND ESTROGENS

The adrenal gland also secretes androgens. The principal secreted adrenal androgen is DHEA (DEA, dehydroepiandrosterone). Most of it, 99%, is secreted in sulfate conjugated form. In plasma, DHEA in adult humans of both genders is 175–300 μg/dl and about 20 mg are secreted in 24 hours.

Table 14.4 Relative Potency of Corticoids[12,13]

	% of Cortisol Activity	
	Glucocorticoid	Mineralocorticoid
cortisol	100	100
cortisone	70	100
aldosterone	30	300000
corticosterone	30	1500
deoxycorticosterone	20	100
dexamethasone	2500	0
9-α-fluorocortisol	1000	12500
prednisolone	400	80
triaminolone	300	–
prednisone	400	70
6-α-methylprednisolone	500	50

The upper five steroids are natural; the lower three steroids are synthetic. The unit, % of cortisol activity, is used to show relative activity as compared to cortisol (set arbitrarily at 100).

Usually they do not produce virilization (masculinization) and the adrenal androgens cannot replace the testicular androgens in castrated men. However, under some conditions, adrenal androgens are secreted in excess and can then have masculinizing consequences (accentuated virilization in adult males, precocious development of secondary sex characteristics in prepuberal boys, pseudohermaproditism and adrenogenital syndrome in females). It has been suggested that DHEA might have an important role in retarding aging, preventing weight gain, and reducing cancer.

The pituitary gland stimulates adrenal androgen secretion with ACTH and, possibly, another hormone, but not with gonadotropin. The putative additional stimulating hormone, pituitary adrenal androgen-stimulating hormone (AASH), may be responsible for adrenarche. Adrenarche is an increase in adrenal androgens which occurs at 8–10 years of age. Peak DHEA in both sexes occurs in the early twenties with a gradual decline to prepuberal levels by about age fifty.

The adrenal gland also secretes estrogen. Normally too little estrogen is secreted for feminization to occur, but sometimes there is excess estrogen secretion by estrogen-secreting adrenal tumors which is sufficient for feminization.

ADDISON'S DISEASE

Hyposecretion of adrenal hormones is called **Addison's disease**. The symptoms of the disease include pigmentation increases, muscle weakness, hypoglycemia, gastrointestinal disturbances, low body temperature, kidney failure, weight loss, amenorrhea, cessation of growth, poor appetite, low plasma sodium, low blood pressure (hypotension), low metabolic rate, EEG abnormalities, and heart problems (small heart size, decreased cardiac work). In Addison's disease, ACTH levels increase. Presumably, low circulating cortisol means that cortisol does not feed back and inhibit the pituitary so that the pituitary secretes ACTH. ACTH in normal subjects is 0.5 mU/ml, but in Addison's disease the ACTH rises to 15 mU/ml. The skin darkening symptoms (tanning, black freckles, pigmentation of scars, dark palm creases, darkening nipple areolas, pigmentation at pressure points, gum pigmentation, bluish-black discolorations of mucous membranes) are attributed to the melanotropic action of ACTH and/or to MSH secretion. Causes of the disease include autoimmunity, tuberculosis, and cancer. If the entire adrenal glands are destroyed, the disease is fatal, but most people retain some adrenal tissue and do well in nonstressful situations. The disease is treated successfully with hormone (hydrocortisone and fluorocortisone) replacement therapy. Symptoms of Addison's disease can be produced experimentally in animals by adrenalectomy.

Stress can cause an acute attack called an **adrenal crisis** (Addisonian crisis) in which symptoms are headache, lassitude, confusion, restlessness, vomiting, pain in the abdominal or legs or lower back, and circulatory collapse. Other symptoms include fever, dehydration, and hypoglycemia. Untreated, an adrenal crisis leads to unconsciousness and death. An adrenal crisis can be caused by trauma, operations, infection, and by hot weather (causing salt loss through sweating).

CUSHING'S SYNDROME

Excess glucocorticoid secretion results in **Cushing's syndrome** (Figure 14.11). The visible symptoms may include moon-face (moon facies), trunk obesity, buffalo hump, purple abdominal stripes (striae), slender fingers and toes. Less visible symptoms include hypertension, osteoporosis, protein depletion, psychiatric abnormalities, muscle wasting, thin skin, susceptibility to bruising, kidney stones, menstrual irregularities, balding, and diabetes mellitus. Plasma cortisol normally peaks to 10–25 µg/100 ml between 6 a.m. and 8 a.m., but in Cushing's syndrome, high levels of plasma cortisol are present throughout the day and night. The rhythm of cortisol is lost and the 24-hour production is increased. The disease is treated with adrenalectomy or pituitary irradiation. After removing the adrenal, the pituitary sometimes secretes increasing amounts of ACTH and MSH which produces hyperpigmentation (Nelson's syndrome).[14] Some of the symptoms of Cushing's syndrome appear as side effects of steroid hormone treatments.

ADRENOGENITAL SYNDROME

Adrenogenital syndrome (adrenal virilism) is a consequence of hypersecretion of adrenal androgen. The syndrome is named for masculinization effects (pseudopuberty or female pseudohermaphroditism). Symptoms in an adult woman would include hirsutism (hairiness), baldness, androgenic flush, small breasts, heavy arms and legs, muscularization, male escutcheon, acne, deepened voice, amenorrhea, uterine atrophy, increased libido, and enlarged clitoris. Causes are congenital enzyme deficiencies in steroid production or tumors. Treatment is by adrenalectomy.

Congenital defects in steroid synthesis also produce a variety of adrenal related symptoms in addition to adrenogenital syndromes.

SYNTHETIC GLUCOCORTICOIDS

Synthetic steroids that are more potent than natural glucocorticoids have been produced by chemists and are available for clinical use (Table 14.4). Some of their names are 9-α-flurocortisol, prednisolone, and dexamethasone. The latter two have long half-lives and dexamethasone has a high affinity for glucocorticoid receptors. Extension of half-life and high affinity may explain the high potency. The steroids are useful in treatment of inflammation.

FETAL ADRENAL GLAND

The adrenal glands arise embryologically from coelomic mesoderm in the embryo's genital ridge. Human fetuses, but not other mammals, have an extensive cortex, the fetal adrenal cortex; 80% of the fetal cortex rapidly degenerates after birth. Adrenal cortical synthesis of steroids agrees with the generalization that glands that originate embryologically from mesoderm make steroid hormones.

The adrenal gland function is prominent in development:

> In most mammalian species, products of the fetal adrenal gland appear to play an important role in regulating maturation of various organ systems in the fetus, providing the fetus homeostatic mechanisms to respond to stress, and initiating and/or participating in the cascade of events culminating in the birth of a newborn. Thus, cortisol, presumably of fetal origin, is one of the chemical messengers involved in the stimuli to

lung maturation, deposition of glycogen in the liver, and induction of several enzymes in the fetal brain, retina, pancreas, and gastrointestinal tract that normally are associated with late intrauterine life.[15]

The fetal adrenal cortex makes sulfate conjugates of androgens; in turn the placenta converts the androgens to estrogens. The adrenal may play a role in parturition of some species, but maybe not primates, because removing the sheep fetal adrenal prevents lambing, and cortisol or ACTH infusion into sheep induces premature birth.[16]

REFERENCES

1. Tyrrell, J.B.; Aron, D.C.; Forsham, P.H. Glucocorticoids and adrenal androgens. In Greenspan, F.S., editor. Basic and Clinical Endocrinology, Third Edition. Norwalk, CT: Appleton & Lange; p. 323.

2. Martin, C. Endocrine Physiology. New York: Oxford University Press; p. 228.

3. Norman, A.; Litwack, G. Hormones. New York: Academic Press; 1987; p. 439.

4. Hawker, R. Notebook of Medical Physiology: Endocrinology. New York: Churchill Livingstone; 1978, page 49.

5. Martin, C; Op. cit.; p. 768.

6. Ganong, W. Review of Medical Physiology, Fourteenth Edition. Norwalk, CT: Appleton & Lange; 1989; p. 314.

7. Sarlis, N.J.; Chowdrey, H.S.; Stephanou, A.; Lightman, S. Chronic activation of the hypothalamo-pituitary-adrenal axis and loss of circadian rhythm during adjuvant-induced arthritis in the rat. Endocrinology 130: 1775–1779; 1992.

8. Bateman, A.; Singh, A.; Kral, T.; Solomon, S. The immune-hypothalamic-pituitary-adrenal axis. Endocrine Reviews 10: 92–112; 1989.

9. Jacobson, L.; Sapolsky, R. The role of the hippocampus in feedback regulation of the hypothalamic-pituitary-adrenocortical axis. Endocrine Reviews 12: 118; 1991.

10. Orth, D.N. Corticotropin-releasing hormone in humans. Endocrine Reviews 13: 164–191; 1992.

11. Freedman, L.P. Anatomy of the steroid receptor zinc finger region. Endocrine Reviews 13: 129–145; 1992.

12. Ganong, W.; Op. cit.; p. 308.

13. Liddle, G.W. The adrenals. In Williams, R., editor. Textbook of Endocrinology. W. B. Saunders: Philadelphia; 1987; page 259.

14. Berkow, R., editor. The Merck Manual, Fifteenth Edition. Rahway, NJ: Merck Sharp & Dohme Research Laboratories; 1987; p. 1275.

15. Pepe, G.J.; Albrecht, E.D. Regulation of the primate fetal adrenal cortex. Endocrine Reviews 11: 151–176; 1990.

16. Liggins, G.C.; Fairclough, R.J.; Grimes, S.A.; Kendall, J.Z.; Knox, B.S. The mechanism of initiation of parturition in the ewe. Recent Prog. Horm. Res. 29: 111; 1973.

CHAPTER 15

Aldosterone and Adrenals, Angiotensin and Kidneys

Mineralocorticoids are steroids, mainly the steroid aldosterone, from the adrenal cortex that regulate water and electrolytes. The complex multi-factor system for regulation of water and electrolytes also controls blood pressure. Aldosterone is not the only hormone involved; the regulation of water balance also includes angiotensin II made from a liver precursor molecule, atrial natriuretic peptide from the heart, antidiuretic hormone from the hypothalamus, and other factors.

ALDOSTERONE, ANGIOTENSIN, ATRIAL NATRIURETIC PEPTIDE, CATECHOL- AMINES, ANTIDIURETIC HORMONE

The regulation of body water and electrolyte content is complex, requiring control of thirst, concentrations of ions in the blood, urine formation, and blood pressure. A number of hormones are involved in the control of water and electrolytes: antidiuretic hormone (vasopressin) from the hypothalamus, catecholamines from the adrenal medulla, aldosterone from the adrenal cortex, angiotensin which is formed in the blood with the aid of an enzyme (renin) from the kidney, and atrial natriuretic peptide from the heart. Water consumption, total body water, plasma volume, rate of urine formation, and blood pressure are all involved in the regulation of body water and electrolyte content.

BIOCHEMISTRY OF ALDOSTERONE

The mineralocorticoids are the steroid hormones named for their role in electrolyte regulation. Aldosterone is the principal mineralocorticoid having the highest activity. Aldosterone has 3000 times the mineralocorticoid potency of cortisol, cortisone, and deoxycorticosterone, and it has 200 times the mineralocorticoid potency of corticosterone. Even so, the synthetic acetate of deoxycorticosterone (DOCA, desoxycorticosterone acetate) is used clinically because it is inexpensive.

Aldosterone is a steroid synthesized from cholesterol in the zona glomerulosa of the adrenal cortex (Figure 15.1). The structure of aldosterone is distinct among steroids because it has an aldehyde group (-CHO) at position C13.

In the blood, aldosterone has a half-life of 20 minutes. It is transported free and binds only marginally to carrier proteins. Normal plasma aldosterone in humans is only 0.006 µg/dl, which is a low concentration compared to some of the other steroids (e.g., cortisol 5–25 µg/dl). Peak aldosterone occurs at 0600 hours and nadir aldosterone occurs at 2100 hours (Figure 15.2).

Aldosterone is metabolized by liver and kidneys. Liver and kidney can convert aldosterone to an 18-glucuronide, and liver also forms a tetrahydroglucuronide. Of the aldosterone that is secreted from the adrenal gland, only 1% is excreted in free form in the urine, 5% is excreted as the glucuronide, and 40% is excreted as the tetrahydroglucuronide.

FUNCTIONS OF ALDOSTERONE

The function of aldosterone is to increase the **sodium reabsorption** from the various fluids in which it is lost: urine, gastric juice, saliva, and sweat. Aldosterone accomplishes this by exchanging hydrogen ion (H^+) and potassium (K^+) ions for sodium (Na^+) ions. Because of this ion exchange in sodium reabsorption, aldosterone also causes potassium excretion and lower urine pH. The sodium is retained in the extracellular fluid (ECF). The principal targets of aldosterone are the distal tubule and collecting duct epithelia in the kidney. Muscle and brain cells are also targets where aldosterone reduces the sodium and raises the potassium. Gut, skin, nasal salt glands, and salivary glands are also targets.

The mechanism of action of aldosterone is similar to other steroidal mechanisms of action. Aldosterone binds to mineralocorticoid receptors in the target cell. The hormone-receptor complex provokes transcription of RNA from DNA. The mRNA participates in translation for new proteins to be synthesized. The exact action of the proteins to achieve sodium retention is not known. There are several hypotheses, some of which involve the substrate for ATP, the synthesis of sodium-potassium ATPase, and the permeability of the cell to sodium (Figure 15.3).

The hormones that affect water balance affect blood pressure. One attempt to show the interactions of the hormones, sodium, and blood pressure is represented in Figure 15.4.

The kidneys participate in salt and water balance. But they are not the only organs involved in all vertebrates. The nasal salt glands (e.g., of marine birds and reptiles) and the cloaca (e.g., of amphibians) also participate in the control of electrolytes and water. Moreover, water is lost through the skin during perspiration and through the lungs during respiration.

Removing the adrenal results in loss of sodium ions in the urine and a concomitant rise in plasma potassium ions because potassium is retained (Table 15.1). Salt and water are lost. The plasma volume is reduced. Hypotension and failure of the circulation ensue, leading to fatal shock. These dire consequences can be partially prevented simply by increasing the dietary salt.

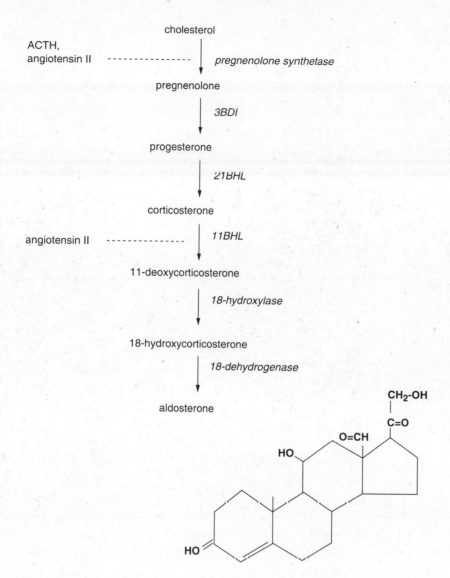

Figure 15.1 The figure illustrates the biosynthesis of aldosterone from cholesterol in the zona glomerulosa and the structure of aldosterone. Angiotensin II stimulates formation of pregnenolone and 11-deoxycorticosterone.

REGULATION OF ALDOSTERONE

Aldosterone is stimulated by surgery, anxiety, bleeding, and physical trauma (which also increase glucocorticoids). However, it is also stimulated by electrolyte intake (high potassium, low sodium). Factors that increase blood pressure (standing, constriction of the vena cava) also in-crease aldosterone. Aldosterone is also stimulated by hormones and electrolytes that circulate through the adrenal gland (angiotensin II, rise in plasma potassium, drop in plasma sodium, ACTH).

Angiotensin II has an important role in the regulation of aldosterone. Angiotensin II stimulates formation of aldosterone at two steps in its

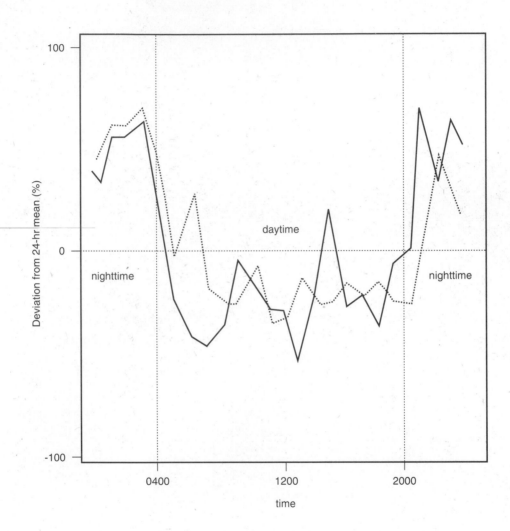

Figure 15.2 The graphs show the daily rhythm of human plasma aldosterone. The graphs are from two separate studies in which there were 4 or 6 subjects for each data point. The data are plotted as a percentage deviation from the mean. Average aldosterone in one study was 119 pg/ml and in the other study was 470 pg/ml. Data for the two graphs were obtained from Breuer, H.; Kaulhausen, H.; Muhlbauer, W.; Fritzsche, G.; Vetter, H. Circadian rhythm of the renin-angiotensin-aldosterone system in Chronobiological Aspects of Endocrinology Symp. Med. Hoechstg, Verlag, F. K. Schattauer, Stuttgart; 1974; pp. 101–109; Vagnucci, A.H.; McDonald, R.H.; Drash, A.L.; Wong, A.K.C. Intradiem changes of plasma aldosterone, cortisol, corticosterone, and growth hormone in sodium restriction. J.Clin. Endocrinol. Metab. 38: 761–776; 1974. In yet another study by Stern of older men in 1987, nadir aldosterone was near 40 pg/ml at 2100 and peak aldosterone was near 140 pg/ml at 0600.

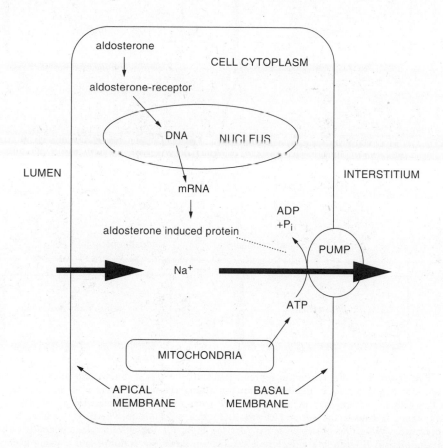

Figure 15.3 The mechanism of action for aldosterone on kidney is hypothesized as involving the Na+ pump. Modified, with permission. Ganong, W. Review of Medical Physiology, Fourteenth Edition. Norwalk, CT: Appleton & Lange; 1989; p. 595.

synthesis.

ACTH elevates both aldosterone and corticosterone, but the effects are transient. Even prolonging ACTH for several days cannot keep aldosterone levels up.

ANGIOTENSIN

Angiotensin II is the active chemical messenger of the peripheral renin-angiotensin system (RAS). Most of the RAS components have since been found in the kidney, arterial wall, heart, pituitary gland, adrenal gland, gonads, and brain. The peripheral RAS functions to control fluid homeostasis and regulate blood pressure. The peripheral RAS finds receptors in kidney (sodium retention), adrenal (aldosterone release), and vascular smooth muscle (vasoconstriction). Central RAS functions are cardiovascular, fluid homeostasis, and pituitary hormone release.[1]

BIOCHEMISTRY OF ANGIOTENSIN

Angiotensin II is an octapeptide whose amino acids come from a precursor molecule that is synthesized in the liver (Figure 15.5). The precursor is a glycoprotein called angiotensinogen (also called renin substrate, preangiotensin, angiotensin

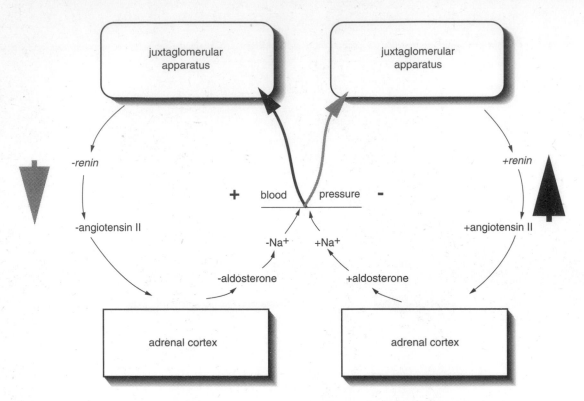

Figure 15.4 The figure is a diagrammatic representation of the means by which aldosterone and angiotensin regulate sodium and blood pressure (decreases, down-pointing arrow, -, on the left; and increases, up-pointing arrow, +, on the right). A decrease in blood pressure causes the juxtaglomerular apparatus to secrete renin. Increased angiotensin II causes the adrenal cortex to secrete aldosterone which, by causing sodium retention, raises blood pressure. When the blood pressure goes too high, the juxtaglomerular apparatus stops renin secretion, reducing angiotensin II, stopping aldosterone production, lowering sodium, and causing a decrease in blood pressure. [2]

precursor, hypertensinogen). The precursor is found circulating in the α2 globulin fraction of plasma proteins. It has 453 amino acid residues. The N-terminal of angiotensinogen consists of 13 amino acids which are cleaved to yield angiotensins.

    Renin is an enzyme, an acid (aspartyl) protease, with 340 amino acid residues. It is secreted into the blood from the kidneys. Renin is synthesized from prorenin (383 amino acid residues) which in turn comes from a preprorenin with 406 amino acid residues. Renin is a glycoprotein with a molecular weight of 37,325 in humans. Renin is the rate-limiting enzyme in the RAS system.

    In the blood, renin cleaves three amino acid residues from angiotensinogen to produce a de-

capeptide, angiotensin I (AI). Angiotensin I (AI) is physiologically inactive. Still in the blood, but primarily as angiotensin I passes through the endothelial cells of the lung, **angiotensin converting enzyme** (ACE, dipeptidyl-carboxypeptidase, angiotensin convertase, kinikinase II) splits off two more amino acids to produce **angiotensin II** (AII, ANG II, hypertensin, angiotonin). Angiotensin II is the most active form of the hormone. Angiotensin II has a short half-life (one to two minutes in humans).

    Angiotensinases in the red blood cells degrade angiotensin I or II into fragments. An aminopeptidase cleaves the asp residue from the N-terminal of AII to produce angiotensin III. Angiotensin III and angiotensin-(1-7) have some

Table 15.1 Adrenal Diseases and Electrolytes

Disease	Plasma Electrolytes (meq/l)			
	Sodium Na^+	Potassium K^+	Chloride Cl^-	Bicarbonate, HCO_3^-
normal	142	4.5	105	25
adrenal insufficiency	120	6.7	85	25
hyperaldosteronism	145	2.4	96	41

After data in Ganong, W. Review of Medical Physiology, Fourteenth Edition. Norwalk, CT: Appleton & Lange; 1989; p. 321.

biological activity but less than angiotensin II.

AMOUNTS AND RHYTHMS OF ANGIOTENSIN

In supine subjects consuming normal sodium, angiotensin II concentration is 25 pg/ml. Plasma renin is measured by its ability to produce angiotensin I from angiotensinogen. Plasma renin activity is 1 ng angiotensin/ml/hr.

There is a diurnal rhythm in plasma renin activity (PRA); plasma renin activity rises about 0900 and decreases about 2100. Plasma renin activity is higher in hypertensive subjects. Furthermore, angiotensin-converting enzyme is higher in smokers, which invites the speculations that angiotensin alterations are associated with high blood pressure or heart disease.

ANATOMY OF THE KIDNEY

The **juxtaglomerular cells** (JG cells) and lacis cells in the kidney produce renin (Figure 15.6). The cells are located by the juncture of the afferent arterioles with the glomeruli. (The relationship of the glomerulus to the kidney tubules was shown previously in Figure 5.6). At the start of the distal convoluted tubule, which lies near the arterioles of the glomerulus, the tubule is thickened and the thickened area is called the **macula densa**. The macula densa, the lacis cells, and the juxtaglomerular cells are collectively referred to as the

juxtaglomerular apparatus (JGA). The kidney is equipped with many JGAs. Each human kidney has about 1.3 million nephrons, each nephron has a juxtaglomerular apparatus.

There are mesangial cells (stellate cells also called Polkissen cells from the German pole cushions), whose processes penetrate the basal lamina and the endothelium between capillary loops of the glomerulus inside Bowman's capsule. The contractile mesangial cells may function to change the glomerular filtration rate by supporting and contracting the walls of the adjacent arterioles,[3] or they may be macrophages.[4] The cells contract and relax in response to various circulating factors.

FUNCTIONS OF ANGIOTENSIN II

Angiotensin has a number of functions.

(i) Angiotensin raises blood pressure. It is a vasopressor that increases both systolic and diastolic blood pressure by constricting the arterioles. It is 4–5 times as potent as norepinephrine as a vasoconstrictor. There are angiotensin receptors in the smooth muscles of the blood vessels. Drugs, such as Losartan, that are angiotensin receptor (AT_1) antagonists, act as antihypertensive agents.

(ii) Angiotensin stimulates zona glomerulosa cell production of aldosterone secretion.

(iii) Angiotensin causes increased water intake, a dipsogenic effect. Angiotensin causes drinking by its action on two circumventricular organs

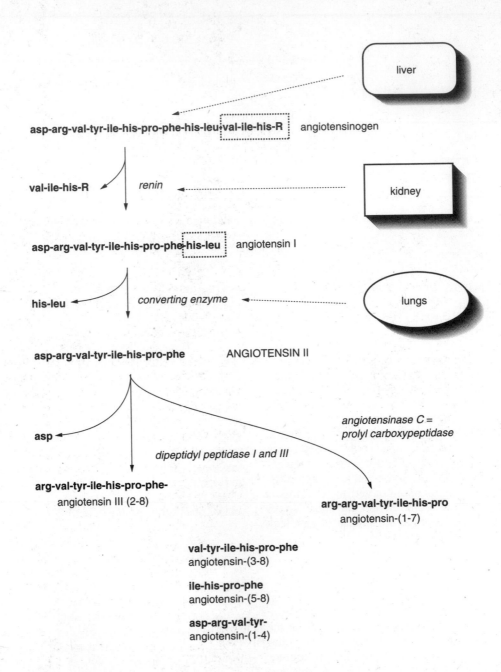

Figure 15.5 The figure illustrates the biosynthesis of angiotensin II, which occurs in the blood, and the catabolism of angiotensin II into fragments. Names of enzymes are italicized. In angiotensinogen, R represents the rest of the molecule. Angiotensin II is the most active, angiotensin III and angiotensin-(1-7) have some activity, and the smaller fragments are inactive.

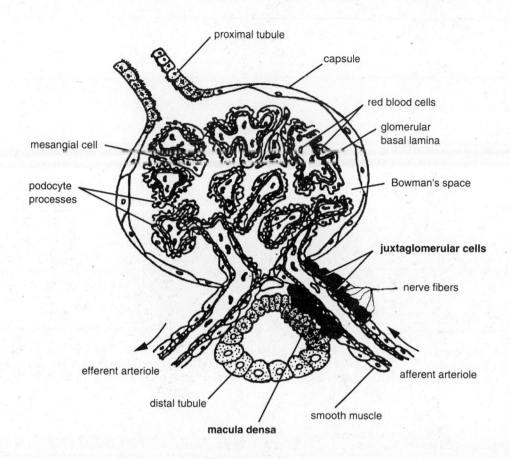

Figure 15.6 The figure is a diagrammatic representation of a glomerulus of a nephron in kidney which illustrates a juxtaglomerular apparatus (JGA). The juxtaglomerular apparatus consists of the macula densa, which are lacis cells at the junction of the arterioles which contain renin, and the juxtaglomerular cells (JG cells) which secrete renin. Modified, with permission. Wyngaarden, J.B.; Smith, L.N. Jr., editors. Cecil Textbook of Medicine, Philadelphia, PA: W. B. Saunders, 1988.

of the brain. These small organs (e.g., area postrema, organum vasculosum of the lateral terminalis) are outside the blood brain barrier. Injections of renin increased salt appetite in rats.

(iv) Angiotensin stimulates secretion of vasopressin, oxytocin, ACTH, prolactin, GH, TRH, and ß-endorphin by action on the four circumventricular organs of the brain.

(v) There are actions of angiotensin involving catecholamines, glucose, ACTH, uterine contractions, and fertility.

(vi) The kidneys respond to angiotensin.

Angiotensin reduces glomerular filtration rate by contracting mesangial cells (Table 15.2).

Targets of angiotensin II thus include the adrenal cortex, the brain, and the kidneys. Receptors complex with angiotensin and activate phospholipase C to increase calcium in the cytosol (Figure 15.7). The receptors have been subcategorized into AT_1 and AT_2 receptors based on differences in agonist and antagonist potency and affinity and sensitivity to disulfide-reducing agents. Receptors are found in kidney, blood vessel smooth muscle, adrenal cortex, zona glomerulosa, lung,

Table 15.2 Factors Which Alter Mesangial Cell Responses

Relaxation	Contraction
atrial natriuretic peptide	angiotensin II
dopamine	vasopressin
prostaglandin E_2	norepinephrine
cyclic AMP	platelet-activating factor
	platelet-derived growth factor
	thromboxane A_2
	prostaglandin F_2
	leukotrienes C, D
	histamine

Relaxation of mesangial cells reduces the glomerular filtration rate in the kidneys. The table shows the factors, including angiotensin II, which alter mesangial cells and thereby affect the glomerular filtration rate. Schlondorff, D. The glomerular mesangial cell: An expanding role for a specialized pericyte. FASEB J 1: 272; 1987.

liver, and brain (Figure 15.8).

REGULATION OF RENIN AND ANGIOTENSIN

Angiotensin formation depends on its enzymes. Renin can be artificially inhibited with drugs that inhibit prostaglandin synthesis (indomethacin), beta blockers (propranolol), and a peptide (pepstatin). Angiotensin-converting enzyme inhibitors (captopril) block angiotensin formation. Competitive inhibitors for angiotensin action with its receptors, such as saralasin, reduce angiotensin activity.

Renin is increased by bleeding, hypotension, diuretics, standing, dehydration, cardiac failure, cirrhosis, psychological stimuli, sodium depletion, constriction of renal artery, and constriction of the aorta. There may be many regulating factors: (i) JG cells secrete renin when pressure falls. JG cells are baroreceptors and apparently respond to stretching. (ii) The macula densa responds by se-creting renin when the rate of chloride or sodium transport is increased. (iii) Prostacyclin, a prostaglandin, causes JG cells to secrete renin. (iv) Plasma K+ level increases produce renin decreases. (v) Angiotensin II inhibits renin secretion (feedback). (vi) Vasopressin inhibits renin secretion. (vii) Catecholamines (from sympathetic nerve endings or the circulation) increase renin secretion via beta receptors.

ATRIAL NATRIURETIC PEPTIDE FROM THE HEART

Cantin and Genest wrote about the discovery of atrial natriuretic peptide:

"...it has been discovered that the heart is something more than a pump. It is also an endocrine gland. It secretes a powerful peptide hormone called atrial natriuretic factor (ANF). The hormone has an important role in

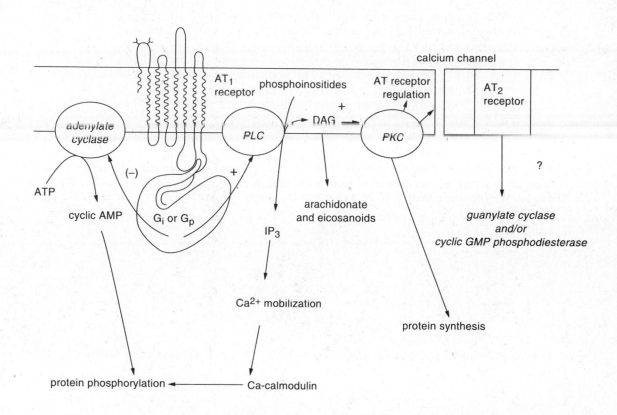

Figure 15.7 The figure illustrates a scheme proposed for the mechanism of action of angiotensin. Redrawn, with permission. Saavedra, J. M. Brain and pituitary angiotensin. Endocrine Reviews 13: 333; 1992.

the regulation of blood pressure and blood volume and in the excretion of water, sodium and potassium. It exerts its effects widely: on the blood vessels themselves, on the kidneys and the adrenal glands and on a large number of regulatory regions in the brain."[5]

Atrial natriuretic peptide (ANP, atrial natriuretic factor, ANF, atrial natriuretic hormone) has actions that are opposite to the actions of angiotensin. The cardiocytes, or heart muscle cells, have granules that have characteristics of the granules of hormone-secreting endocrine cells. The granules cluster near the nucleus of atrial cardiocytes of a normal rat, and the number increases if the rat is fed a sodium-deficient diet for 30 days.[6,7]   The granules are believed to contain ANP. ANP concentration in blood in the coronary sinus which drains the heart is 2–8 times the levels in peripheral blood.

ANP is a peptide with 28 amino acids and a disulfide bond (Figure 15.9). ANP is synthesized in atrial muscle cells of the heart. ANP is synthesized in the usual manner of peptides from a larger molecule, a 125-amino acid precursor called pro-ANP (pro-ANF). Injected extracts of heart atria cause natriuresis and diuresis. The peptide is se-

```
MALNSSAEDGIKRIQDDCPKAGRHSYIFVMIPTLYSIIFVVGIFGNSLVV–
IVIYFYMKLKTVASVFLLNLALADLCFLLTLPLWAVYTAMEYRWPFGNHL–
CKIASASYVFNLYASVFLLTCLSIDRYLAIVHPMKSRLRRTMLVAKVTCI–
IIWLMAGLASPAVIHRNVYFIENITNITVCAFHYESRNSTLPIGLGLTKN–
ILGFLFPFLIILTSYTLIWKALKKAYEIQKNKPRNDDIFRIIMAIVLFFF–
FSWVPHQIFTFLDVLIQLGVIHDCKISDIVDTAMPITICIAYFNNCLNPL–
FYGFLGKKFKKYFLQLLKYIPPKAKSHSSLSTKMSTLSYRPSDNMSSSAK–
KPASCFEVE
```

Figure 15.8 A representation of the AT$_1$ receptor of the rat. The receptor has 359 amino acid residues which are represented by single letters, instead of by three letters each, because of the large size of the molecule. Bernstein, K.E.; Alexander, W. Molecular analysis of the angiotensin II receptor. Endocrine Reviews 13: 384; 1992.

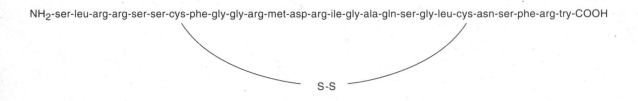

NH$_2$-ser-leu-arg-arg-ser-ser-cys-phe-gly-gly-arg-met-asp-arg-ile-gly-ala-gln-ser-gly-leu-cys-asn-ser-phe-arg-try-COOH

S-S

Figure 15.9 The structure of human atrial natriuretic peptide is shown. The peptide is synthesized as amino acid residues 99-126 from a larger precursor molecule. Cartin, M.; Genest, J. The heart as an endocrine gland. Scientific American 254: 76–81; 1986.

creted by the heart's atrial muscle cells that respond to increased sodium chloride intake and extracellular fluid expansion. The peptide is probably secreted by atrial muscle cells in direct response to stretching. Natriuretic agents inhibit reabsorption of cations, especially sodium, from the urine.

An interesting effect is that ANP secretion increases, and aldosterone and renin decrease, during immersion in water up to the neck. Immersion in-

creases central venous and atrial blood pressure. Immobilization stress increases the blood ANP five- to twenty-fold in rats.

ANP inhibits aldosterone production, inhibits renin release, inhibits vasopressin secretion and action on kidney, and relaxes blood vessels in opposition to angiotensin II. The consequence of ANP secretion is expansion of water volume and reduction of sodium retention.

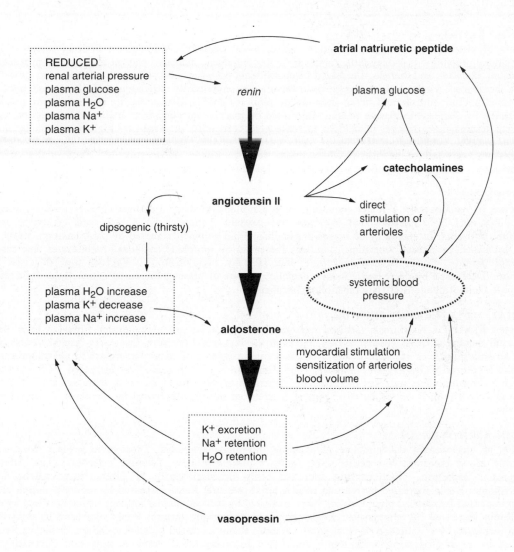

Figure 15.10 The figure is a diagrammatic representation of the hormones (bold) that control water, salt, and blood pressure. Arrows in this diagram represent interactions, not necessarily stimulation.

ANP probably has a daily rhythm though early reports on the subject have generated controversy. In one report, ANP had a daily cycle with amplitude of 19.4 pg/ml and with the time of the daily peak values estimated in the early morning, at 0400 hours, in ten normal men and women (16–76 years old). In the same report, the rhythms in blood pressure and heart rate had 5–7 fold rhythms with peak values in the afternoon (1500–1700).[8]

It is believed that ANP release is stimulated by stretching the atrial muscle cells. ANP becomes depleted during hypertension. Infused into hypertensive animals (1 µg/h) it lowers blood pressure to normal levels after the second

Table 15.3 Interacting Hormones that Affect Water Balance

ALDOSTERONE
Effects of aldosterone. Sodium retention (urine, sweat, saliva, gastric juice); Sodium retention in the ECF; Sodium retention in kidney distal tubule and collecting ducts; Increased percent filtered sodium reabsorbed; Potassium excretion and diuresis; Decreased percent filtered potassium reabsorbed; Water retention; Lower creatinine clearance. **Factors that change aldosterone.** Stimulated by angiotensin II; Increased potassium; Decreased sodium muscle and brain; Increase by pituitary ACTH; Stimulated by rise in plasma potassium; Stimulated by decrease in plasma sodium; Decreased by plasma water increase; Increased by surgery, anxiety, physical trauma, hemorrhage—these also increase glucocorticoids; Increased by high potassium intake, low sodium intake, constriction of inferior vena cava in thorax, standing, secondary hyperaldosteronism (congestive heart failure, nephrosis)—these things do not increase glucocorticoids. **Factors that decrease aldosterone.** Decreased by plasma water increase; Decreased by immersion in water.

VASOPRESSIN
Affected by vasopressin. Water retention; Increase blood pressure (mammals); Increased by increased osmolality of ECF. **Factors that increase vasopressin.** Increased by increased effective osmotic pressure of plasma; Increased by decreased extracellular fluid volume; Increased by pain, emotion, stress, exercise; Increased by nausea, vomiting, standing; Increased by morphine, nicotine, barbiturates; Increased by chloropropamide, clofibrate, carbamazepine; Increased by angiotensin II. **Factors that decrease vasopressin.** Decreased by decreased effective osmotic pressure of plasma; Increased extracellular fluid volume; Alcohol; Opiate antagonists (butorphanol, oxilorphan).

ATRIAL NATRIURETIC PEPTIDE
Affected by ANP. Natriuresis (sodium excretion) due to increase in glomerular filtration rate; Relaxes glomeruli mesangial cells; Tubular sodium excretion; Lowers blood pressure; Decreases responsiveness of vascular smooth muscle to vasoconstrictors; Decreases responsiveness of zona glomerulosa to aldosterone stimuli; Inhibits secretion of vasopressin. **Factors that stimulate ANP.** Increased by increased ECF volume due to high sodium or saline infusion; Increased by immersion in water up to the neck; Increases slightly on rising to standing position; Released by atrial muscle if stretched in vitro; Increased by increases in central venous pressure.

RENIN-ANGIOTENSIN II
Effects of angiotensin II. Stimulate aldosterone; Stimulate arterioles; Dipsogenic (causes thirst); Raise systemic blood pressure; Vasoconstriction; Increase plasma glucose; Increase catecholamines; Stimulates vasopressin secretion. **Factors that increase renin or angiotensin II.** Renin increased by drop in ECF volume; Renin increased by reduced renal arterial pressure; Renin increased by reduced plasma glucose; Renin increased by reduced plasma water; Renin increased by reduced plasma sodium; Renin increased by diuretics; Renin increased by hypotension; Renin increased by upright posture; Renin increased by dehydration; Renin increased by constriction of renal artery or aorta; Renin increased by cardiac failure, cirrhosis; Renin increased by psychological stimuli; Renin stimulated by sympathetic nerve activity and circulating catecholamines; Renin stimulated by prostaglandins (especially prostacyclin). **Factors that decrease renin or angiotensin II.** Renin inhibited by increased pressure which increases stretch of the JG cells; Renin inhibited by angiotensin II; Renin inhibited by vasopressin; Renin inhibited by increased chloride or sodium ion reabsorption across macula densa; Renin reduced by increased plasma potassium (secondary to potassium effects on sodium and chloride); Renin inhibited by inhibitors of prostaglandin synthesis (indomethacin); Renin inhibited by propranolol; Renin-to-angiotensin conversion inhibited by pepstatin; Angiotensin-converting enzyme (ACE) inhibitors (captopril, saralasin).

GLUCOCORTICOIDS
Repair inability to excrete a water load; Raise glomerular filtration rate.

CATECHOLAMINES
Raise systemic blood pressure.

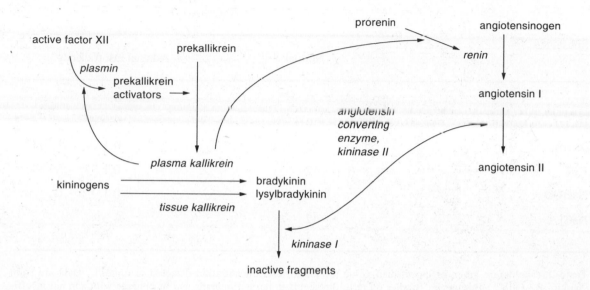

Figure 15.11 A representation of the role of kinins (bradykinin synthesized in plasma; lysylbradykinin synthesized in kidney, sweat glands, pancreas, intestine, and salivary glands),which are vasodilating peptides, in the renin-angiotensin system. Redrawn, with permission, Ganong, W. Review of Medical Physiology. Norwalk, CT: Appleton & Lange; 1989; p. 505.

day. There are also changes in ANP that correlate with the progress of congestive heart failure in animals. The properties of ANP hold promise for treatment of vascular difficulties, and it is important that it is physiologically active in humans.[9]

REGULATION OF WATER BALANCE

Angiotensin, aldosterone, and antidiuretic hormone all interact in complex ways to regulate water balance and electrolytes. In turn, water balance affects blood pressure. Blood pressure regulation involves other factors (catecholamines and atrial natriuretic peptide). Some of these complex interactions are indicated in the scheme for regulation of water balance (Figure 15.10, Table 15.3). Not shown, but also affecting water balance in some species, is the hormone prolactin.

COMPARATIVE ENDOCRINOLOGY

The mineralocorticoids have the same general function in water and electrolyte balance in the various vertebrate classes. However, in some species, the mineralocorticoid function is carried out by glucocorticoid steroids.

Perhaps the most interesting aspect of the comparative endocrinology of salt and water balance is the adaptive variation to differing challenges due to salt and water in the environment that has brought about the evolution of unique targets. In order to meet their particular challenges, some species have target organs other than the kidneys— toad skin, fish gills, avian nasal salt glands—that are involved in salt and water balance.

In birds, the nasal salt glands are located in the circular orbits above the eyes. Marine birds drink hypertonic saline. In order to dispose of the excess salt, the birds secrete a salty solution from

Table 15.4. Adrenal and Taste Thresholds

Substance	Threshold	
	Normal	Adrenal insufficiency
urea	90	0.8
HCl	0.3	0.006
sucrose	12	0.1
KCl	12	0.1
NaHCO3	12	0.1
NaCL	12	0.3

Taste thresholds are given as the median value for the lowest concentration detected in mmol/l. Data are from Henkin, R.; Gill, J.; Bartter, F. Studies on taste thresholds in normal humans and in patients with adrenal insufficiency: The role of the adrenal cortical steroids and serum sodium concentration. J. Clin. Invest. 42: 727; 1963.

their nasal salt glands which trickles down the bill. The adrenal glands have a corresponding increase in size; adrenalectomy abolishes nasal salt gland secretion; corticosterone restores nasal salt gland secretion. Nasal salt glands are also present in desert and marine reptiles. The marine iguana surprises a visitor by ejaculating a stream of salt from its nasal salt gland, so that it appears to be spitting, which the visitor should not take personally because the iguana is just eliminating salt in this manner.

KININS

Kinins are polypeptide hormones that come from plasma protein precursor molecules. Kallikreins are enzymes that release kinins. A renal kallikrein releases renin from its precursor, prorenin. In turn, angiotensin I-converting enzyme is the same as kininase II which inactivates bradykinin. Bradykinin, like renin, is released from affinity and sensivitity to disulfide-reducing agents. Receptors are found in kidney, blood vessel smooth muscle, adrenal cortex, zona glomerulosa, lung, liver, and brain (Figure 15.11).

DISEASES OF MINERALOCORTICOIDS AND RENIN

Aldosterone is reduced in enyzme deficiencies. For example, aldosterone is reduced due to deficient 18-hydroxysteroid dehydrogenase, and hypoaldosteronism is associated with congenital adrenal hyperplasia (except for a simple virilizing form of 21-hydroxylase deficiency in which aldosterone is increased).[10] There are diseases involving hypersecretion and hyposecretion of mineralocorticoids besides those due to congenital steroid-synthesizing enzyme deficiencies

Aldosteronism, hypersecretion of aldosterone, is associated with expected effects on electrolytes and water: sodium retention, potassium depletion, alkalosis, expanded extracellular fluid volume, increased body sodium, resistance to antidiuretic hormone, and suppressed renin. A plethora of symptoms are associated with potassium depletion: hypertension, fatigue, weakness, loss of stamina, transient paralysis, tetany, weakness, nocturia, increased thirst, polyuria, headache, and paresthesias. Aldosteronism can be primary (Conn's syndrome[11]) with adenoma, due to diuretic therapy, or adrenal carcinoma. Treatments include adrenalectomy or treatment with spironolactone. Spironolactone is an aldosterone antagonist that binds to mineralocorticoid receptors of the distal renal tubule.

Aldosteronism can be secondary to diseases in which increased renin is secreted (rare renin-secreting tumors) or in edematous disorders (cardiac failure, cirrhosis, nephrotic syndrome). These diseases usually have associated hypertension. Use of estrogen therapy or oral contraceptives can increase plasma angiotensinogen and renin activity, but hypokalemia is rarely associated with this type of aldosteronism.

An interesting possible consequence of adrenal hormone deficiency is salt appetite or salt craving. In some studies, adrenalectomized rats permitted choices between salty and unsalty water have been observed to increase their salt preference after adrenalectomy. Human ability to taste salt and other substances, as measured by thresholds for detection, is increased in individuals with adrenal insufficiency (Table 15.4).[12]

Hypertension, high blood pressure, has numerous causes. Increased activity of any vasoconstrictors can cause hypertension. Either high or low renin or normal renin activity can be found in people with high blood pressure, and renin correlates with dietary sodium content. Renin and angiotensin are probably important factors in most kinds of hypertension. Saralasin blocks angiotensin II receptors, and oral captropril inhibits converting enzyme, and both drugs have lowered blood pressure in some hypertensive patients.

REFERENCES

1. Saavedra, J.M. Brain and pituitary angiotensin. Endocrine Reviews 13: 329–380; 1992.

2. Goss, R. J. The Physiology of Growth. New York: Academic Press; 1978.

3. Ganong, W. Review of Medical Physiology, Fourteenth Edition. Norwalk, CT: Appleton & Lange; 1989; p. 595.

4. Telford, I.R.; Brighman, C. F. Introduction to Functional Histology. New York: Harper & Row, Pubs.; 1990; p. 414.

5. Cantin, M.; Genest, J. The heart as an endocrine gland. Scientific American 254: 76–81; 1986; p. 76.

6. Cantin, M.; Genest, J.; Ibid.

7. Cantin, M., Genest, J. The heart and the atrial natriuretic factor. Endocrine Reviews 6: 107–127; 1985.

8. Portaluppi, F.; Montanari, L.; Bagni, B.; Uberti, E.; Trasforini, G.; Margutti, A. Circadian rhythms of atrial natriuretic peptide, blood pressure, and heart rate in normal subjects. Cardiology 76: 428–432; 1989.

9. Richards, A.M.; McDonald, D.; Fitzpatrick, M.A.; Nicholls, M.G.; Espiner, E.A.; Ikram, H.; Jans, S.; Grant, S.; Yandle, T. Atrial natriuretic hormone has biological effects in man at physiological plasma concentrations. J. Clin. Endocrinol. Metab. 67: 114–139; 1988.

10. Yanase, T.; Simpson, E.R.; Waterman, M. 17 alpha-hydroxylase/17,20-lyase deficiency: From clinical investigation to molecular definition. Endocrine Reviews 12: 91–108; 1991.

11. Conn, J. Primary aldosteronism: a new clinical entity. J. Lab. Clin. Med. 45: 3–17; 1955.

12. Richter, C.P. Increased salt appetite in adrenalectomized rats. Amer. J. Physiol. 115: 155–161; 1936.

CHAPTER 16

Catecholamines and Adrenal Medulla

Epinephrine and norepinephrine are the hormones of the adrenal medulla. But catecholamines are also secreted at some nerve endings. So the adrenal medulla is considered to be part of the sympathetic nervous system. The hormones stimulate the heart. The adrenal medulla functions together with the adrenal cortex and the sympathetic nervous system in marshalling responses to physiological emergencies.

ADRENAL MEDULLA ANATOMY

In mammals, the adrenal medulla occupies the center of the adrenal gland. The endocrine tissue of the adrenal medulla is called **chromaffin** tissue (or chromaffin cells) because of its staining properties. In other vertebrates, however, the chromaffin tissue is also associated with the adrenal and the kidney (Figure 16.1). In addition, there are other organs in mammals and other vertebrates that have chromaffin tissue: paraganglia (located near sympathetic ganglia), carotid glands (near common carotid arteries), Organs of Zuckerkandl (by the inferior mesenteric artery), liver, heart, kidney, gonads, etc. The wide distribution of chromaffin cells accounts for the fact that the adrenal medulla is not essential for life. Chromaffin cells are found in amphibian skin glands, and invertebrates also have chromaffin cells. For example, chromaffin cells are found in the mantles of molluscs and in the nervous systems of leeches.

Histologically, chromaffin cells are characterized by their possession of chromaffin granules which contain catecholamines and adenine nucleotides. The classic Hillarp and Falck histochemical technique is to expose freeze-dried tissue to paraformaldehyde. The catecholamines and indoleamines undergo the Pictet-Spengler reaction to form fluorescent products. Viewed with a fluorescent microscope using purple excitation lighting (410 nanometers), catecholamines emit yellow light (480 nanometers), and serotonin fluoresces at a higher wavelength (520 nanometers). Use of a blue filter makes the catecholamines appear green and the serotonin appear yellow.

Chromogranin A (CgA) is the major soluble protein (49 kilodaltons) in the adrenal medulla chromaffin cells. Chromogranin A is also found in the electron-dense core secretory granules of a variety of endocrine and neuroendocrine cells, but it is not found in exocrine cells. Thus, although its function is not known, it serves as a marker of endocrine cells and tumors. It can be detected with immunohistology in cells and with immunoassay in serum.[1] Higher chromogranin A compared to substances in synaptic vesicles is common in Alzheimer's disease.[2]

Release of endogenous morphine and codeine by chromaffin cells has been suggested because the adrenomedullary equivalent and plasma of the American eel contain endogenous morphine and codeine. The opiates are found in similar concentrations in rat adrenal and human plasma.[3]

CATECHOLAMINE BIOCHEMISTRY

The catecholamines are named for their characteristic single "catechol" ring structure (Figure 16.2). The catecholamines (CAs) are **dopamine** (DA), **norepinephrine** (NE, noradrenalin), and **epinephrine** (E, adrenalin). The catecholamines are synthesized from amino acid precursors, phenylalanine and tyrosine (Figure 16.3). Epinephrine was the first hormone to be isolated and chemically identified by Abel in 1904.

The precursor of catecholamines is an essential amino acid, **phenylalanine**. That means that it must be obtained from the diet. Another precursor of the catecholamines, **tyrosine**, is also an amino acid. But it is not essential because most people can synthesize tyrosine from phenylalanine. The enzyme that catalyzes the reaction, phenylalanine hydroxylase, is found in liver and nerve. Deficiency of the enzyme is a genetic recessive defect in 1/200 humans. When it occurs in the newborn, the disease is named **phenylketonuria** (phenylpyruvic oligophrenia). However, the defect is detected routinely at birth and treated with a diet low in phenylalanine.

The rate-limiting step in catecholamine biosynthesis is the conversion of tyrosine to **DOPA** (dopa, L-dopa, dihydroxyphenylalanine, dioxyphenylalanine). So tyrosine hydroxylase is the rate-limiting enzyme for catecholamine production. The enzyme is found in cytoplasm. Tetrahydrobiotin is the cofactor for tyrosine hydroxylase; dihydrobiotin is a by-product of the reaction. The activity of tyrosine hydroxylase is induced by ACTH and enhanced by adrenal nerve stimulation. Dopamine, epinephrine, norepinephrine, and iodinated tyrosines block tyrosine hydroxylase activity (product feedback inhibition, end-product inhibition).

DOPA is an interesting molecule. It crosses the blood-brain barrier and is used to treat **Parkinson's disease**. Dopaminergic neurons project from the substantia nigra to the striatum. The motor dysfunction associated with Parkinson's disease results from degeneration of the nigrostriatal system.

Dopamine may also be involved in the pathology of schizophrenia because schizophrenics

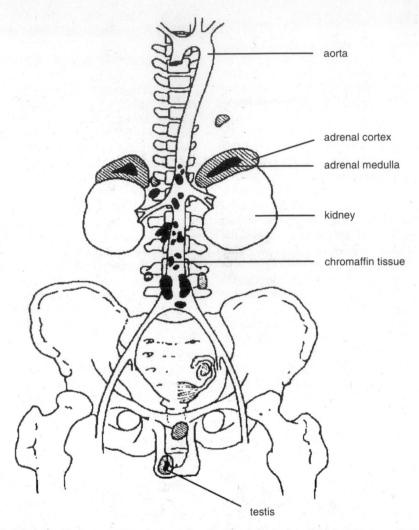

Figure 16.1 The diagram illustrates the anatomy of the human torso showing the location of the adrenal glands atop the kidneys. Black represents chromaffin tissue, found in the adrenal medulla, in the testis, and elsewhere in this diagram. Modified, with permission. Bethune, J.E. The Adrenal Cortex: A Scope Monograph. Kalamazoo, MI: Upjohn Co.; 1974; p. 11.

have increased numbers of dopamine receptors, dopamine stimulators (amphetamine) produce psychoses like schizophrenia, and phenothiazine tranquilizers that block dopamine relieve symptoms of schizophrenia.

DOPA is converted to dopamine by DOPA decarboxylase (aromatic L-amino acid decarboxylase) in the cell cytoplasm. The adrenal enzyme is inhibited by alpha methyl dopa and alpha methyl tyrosine. The reaction uses vitamin B_6

(pyridoxine) and produces carbon dioxide as a byproduct.

Dopamine is converted to **norepinephrine** inside granulated vesicles. The enzyme for the reaction, dopamine beta hydroxylase, is in chromaffin granules. The enzyme contains copper, and the enzyme is inhibited by disulfuram. Oxygen and ascorbic acid are needed for the reaction.

Norepinephrine is converted to

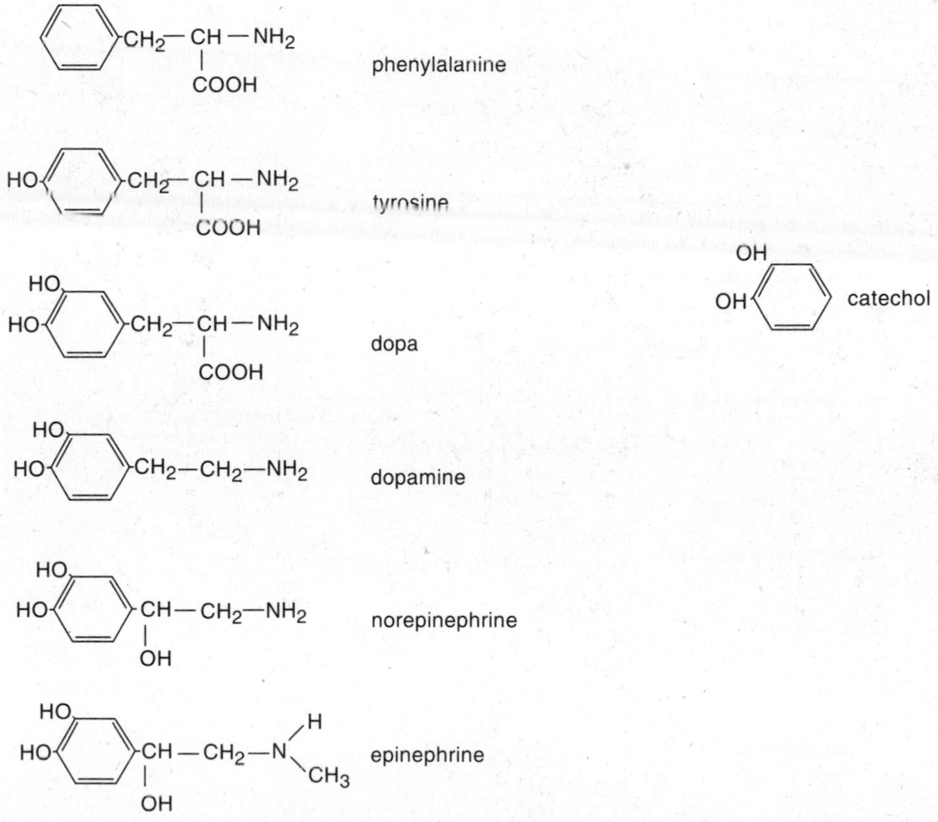

Figure 16.2 The structures of catechol, catecholamines (dopamine, norepinephrine, epinephrine), amino acid precursors of catecholamines (phenylalanine, tyrosine) and dopa are shown. Modified, with permission. Lightman, S. Adrenal Medulla. In James, V., ed. The Adrenal Gland. New York: Raven Press; 1979.

epinephrine by the enzyme PNMT (phenylethanolamine-N-methyltransferase). S-adenosylmethionine (SAM) acts as the methyl donor. S-adenosylhomocysteine (SAH) is a produce of the reaction. The enzyme, PNMT, is found in some neurons and cells of the adrenal medulla. It appears that the sequence involves the exit of norepinephrine from vesicles, conversion to epinephrine in the cytoplasm, and restorage in other vesicles. The result is that the chromaffin granules contain either epinephrine or norepinephrine. PNMT is characteristic of forms that have epinephrine. The activity of the enzyme PNMT is stimulated by ACTH, and inhibited by epinephrine.

Epinephrine and norepinephrine are inactivated by metabolizing them to inactive products using two enzymes, **COMT·** and **MAO**. COMT (catechol-O-methyltransferase) in liver and kidney methylates the catecholamines. MAO (monoamine oxidase, monamine oxidase) has a broad distribution. The enzyme, whose function is oxidative deamination, is found on the outsides of mitochondria and in catecholamine-secreting nerve endings. VMA (vanilmandelic acid) is the common urine product and small amounts of catecholamines are conjugated to form glucuronides and sulfates.

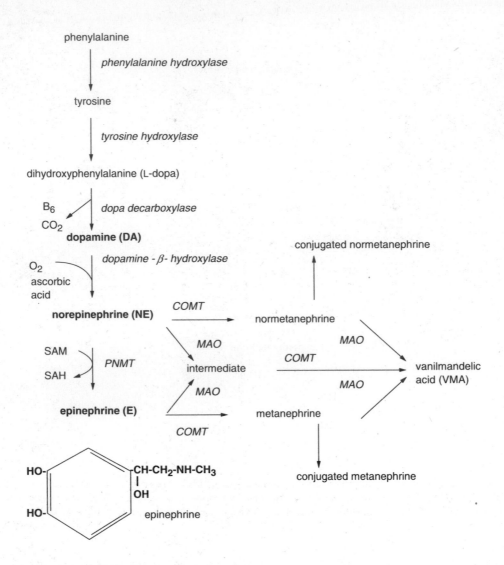

Figure 16.3 The figure shows the pathway for catecholamine synthesis from amino acids, metabolism by enzymes, and the structure of epinephrine. Names of catecholamines are boldface, names and abbreviations of enzymes are italicized. MAO = monoamine oxidase; COMT = catechol-O-methyltransferase; SAM = S-adenosylmethionine, a methyl donor; SAH = S-adenosylhomocysteine; PNMT = phenylethanolamine-N-methyltransferase.

Catecholamines conjugated as glucuronides and sulfates have also been obtained from adrenal glands perfused *in vitro*, and it seems that the CAs may therefore be produced for reasons other than elimination. CAs are produced, for example, by the adrenals of eels. All of black bear catecholamines are conjugated in plasma which also argues for an active role for these metabolites. Epple and colleagues speculate about the possible functions of conjugated catecholamines as hormones, cardiovasular and blood pressure regulators, and transport forms.[4]

Table 16.1 Plasma Catecholamines in People

	Norepinephrine pg/ml	Epinephrine pg/ml
HEALTHY		
basal	150–400	25–100
ambulatory	200–808	30–100
exercise	800–4000	100–1000
symptomatic hypoglycemia	200–1000	1000–5000
PATIENTS		
hypertension	200–500	20–100
surgery	500–2000	100–500
myocardial infarction	1000–2000	800–5000

Notice how "stress" is associated with increases in norepinephrine and epinephrine.   Data are from Goldfien, A. Adrenal Medulla. In Greenspan, F.S., editor. Basic and Clinical Endocrinology, Third Edition. Norwalk, CT: Appleton & Lange; 1991; p. 394.

AMOUNTS OF CATECHOLAMINES

The ratios of epinephrine and norepinephrine that are synthesized vary with species and age. In man, urine production of epinephrine is 10–70 µg/24 hours, and norepinephrine production is 0–20 µg/24 hours. Circulating catecholamines are 0.2 ± 0.08 µg/liter and NE 0.05 ± 0.03 µg/liter. The adrenal medulla has 0.22–0.84 mg/g epinephrine and 0.04–0.16 mg/g norepinephrine.[5] Catecholamines have a 3–4 minute half-life in blood where they may be free, conjugated, or bound to blood protein. Most epinephrine circulates bound to serum albumin (Table 16.1). Catecholamines, like other hormones, exhibit daily cycles (Figure 16.4).[6] Norepinephrine levels were greater (28% day, 75% night) in older men who had less stage 4 and REM sleep and more wakefulness at night. The aging effect on sleep might be associated with increased sympathetic nervous system activity.[7]

The comparative endocrinology of the catecholamines has been studied. An interesting observation is that the cardiovascular system of humans is more sensitive to epinephrine that the cardiovascular systems of common laboratory animals.[8]

The ratio of epinephrine to norepinephrine (E/NE) varies among species. Humans have E/NE ratios of ten to one. Cats have equal amounts of epinephrine and norepinephrine. Whales have 90–100% norepinephrine and it also predominates in birds. Most mammals are like humans with 10–30% of catecholamine as norepinephrine.

The E/NE ratio also changes with age. There is no epinephrine early in human development. By about one year of age, however, there are equal amounts of NE and E and the E/NE ratio increases thereafter.

SECRETION AND CELLULAR ORIGIN

Chromogranins are proteins that associate with norepinephrine and epinephrine in the granulated vesicles.[9] ATP is also bound up to the hormones. Chromogranin A is the most common chromogranin, but neuropeptide Y is also found in some noradrenergic neurons, and chromogranins are widely distributed in endocrine tissue.[10] Active transport keeps the catecholamines in the granulated vesicles. Reserpine inhibits the transport. The granulated vesicles release their contents

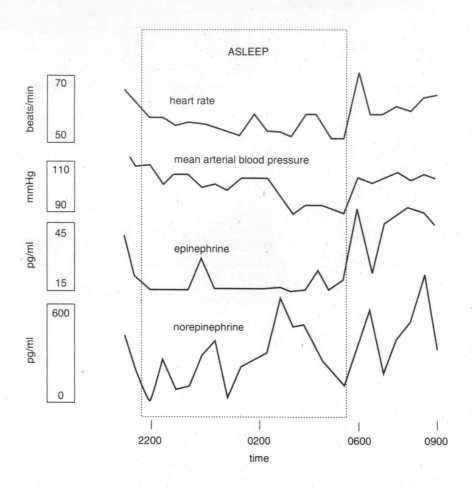

Figure 16.4 The graphs show the night changes of plasma catecholamines, heart rate, and blood pressure. The blood pressure correlated positively with plasma epinephrine (r = 0.54; p<0.01). The data are for one human subject sampled every two hours from 2100 (9 p.m.) to 0900 (9 a.m.). The subject was an older, hypertensive male. After Stern, N.; Beahm, E.; Sowers, J.; McGinty, D.; Eggena, P.; Littner, M.; Nyby, M.; Catania, R. The effect of age on circadian rhythm of blood pressure, catecholamines, plasma renin activity, prolactin, and corticosteroids in essential hypertension. In Weber, M.A.; Drayer, J.I.M., editors. Ambulatory Blood Pressure Monitoring. Darmstadt: Steinkopff; 1984; p. 157–162.

(catecholamines, chromogranins, ATP, and dopamine ß-hydroxylase) during secretion. Nerve cells that release norepinephrine as a neurotransmitter at their terminals also are able to recycle norepinephrine with an active reuptake mechanism.

Some cells in the brain and autonomic ganglia end catecholamine biosynthesis with dopamine which they then release to function as a neurotransmitter. There is a reuptake mechanism

for dopamine. Dopamine is metabolized by COMT and MAO and conjugated in a manner that parallels that for norepinephrine and epinephrine.

REGULATION OF ADRENAL MEDULLA

The adrenal medulla has been viewed as a modified sympathetic ganglion. The chromaffin

Table 16.2 Effects of Epinephrine Versus Norepinephrine

	Epinephrine	Norepinephrine
heart rate	increase	decrease
cardiac output	increase	variable
total peripheral resistance	decrease	increase
blood pressure	rise	greater rise
skin blood vessels	constriction	constriction
respiration	stimulation	stimulation
muscle blood vessels	dilation	constriction
bronchus	dilation	less dilation
eosinophil count	increase	no effect
metabolism	increase	slight increase
kidney	vasoconstriction	vasoconstriction
behavior	passive, tense	aggressive

Revised, with permission.   Bell, G.H.; Davidson, J.N.; Emslie-Smith, D. Textbook of Physiology, Eighth Edition. Churchill Livingston: Edinburgh; 1972; p. 868.

cells are considered to be modified postganglionic cells of the sympathetic nervous system.

The adrenal medulla is regulated by nerves. The chromaffin cells are innervated by nerve cells (preganglionic sympathetic neurons) whose cell bodies are located in the thoracic region of the spinal cord gray matter. The axons of these neurons pass though the vertebral ganglion and the celiac ganglion and synapse with chromaffin cells in the adrenal medulla. The nerve travelled by the axons to the adrenal is called the "splanchnic nerve."

The preganglionic nerve cells release acetylcholine (ACH, Ach, ACh) at their terminals in the adrenal medulla. Acetylcholine causes calcium to enter the chromaffin cells. The granule membranes fuse with the cell membrane and the contents of the granules are extruded into the capillaries (exocytosis).

Catecholamine secretion from the chromaffin cells is provoked when sympathetic nerves fire in response to an emergency. The norepinephrine and epinephrine are not always secreted in the same ratio. Certain stimuli (hemorrhage) preferentially increase the norepinephrine; other stimuli (hypoxia) increase the epinephrine.[11] Thus, there is selective secretion in the ratio of norepinephrine to epinephrine.

The accumulation of rough endoplasmic reticulum in the adrenal medulla cells of rats is reduced by pinealectomy. Kachi and coworkers speculate that the pineal hormone(s) cause an increase in RER aggregation which results in decreased catecholamine secretion.[12]

CARDIOVASCULAR FUNCTION OF EPINEPHRINE AND NOREPINEPHRINE

The most well known function of norepinephrine and epinephrine are their functions in the cardiovascular system, the heart and blood vessels (Table 16.2). In this system, epinephrine and norepinephrine may have similar effects, opposing effects, or only one may be effective.

Epinephrine stimulates the heart rate. The effects are direct because they can be obtained with hearts *in vitro*. Both contraction rate and force are stimulated. The catecholamines also increase myocardial excitability and can induce cardiac arrhythmias. Pulse rate is decreased by norepinephrine.

But the effects on the cardiovascular system are not limited to the heart. The blood vessels are also affected. The catecholamines control blood flow through individual organs. Norepinephrine is

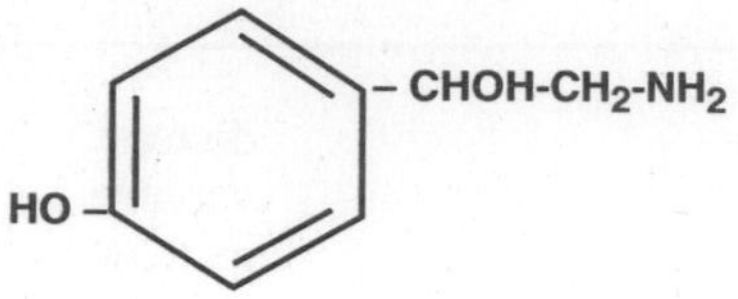

phenylephrine,
alpha agonist

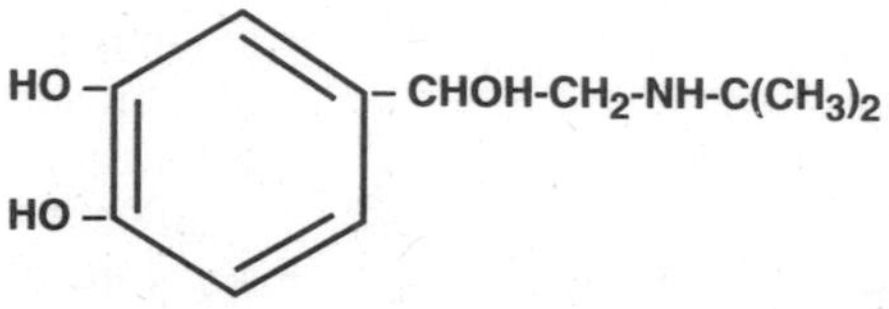

isoproterenol,
beta agonist

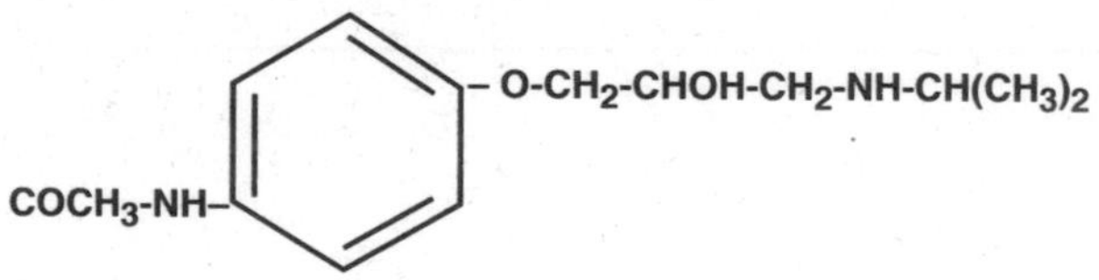

practolol,
beta antagonist

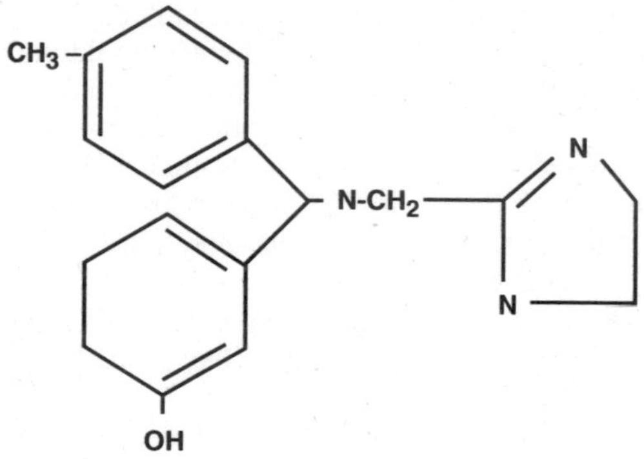

phentolamine,
alpha antagonist

Figure 16.5 The structures of catecholamine agonists and antagonists are shown.

a vasoconstrictor in most organs. Epinephrine, on the other hand, is a vasodilator for the liver and skeletal muscle; its vasodilating properties overshadow its vasoconstricting properties on other organs. Hypertension is a symptom of tumors of the adrenal medulla which usually secrete norepinephrine.

OTHER FUNCTIONS OF EPINEPHRINE AND NOREPINEPHRINE

The nervous system is a target of catecholamines.

Behavioral effects have been attributed to

Table 16.3 Catecholamine Receptors

Receptor name	Relative potencies	Mechanism of action
α_1	NE > E > ISO	calcium $^{2+}$, increase
α_2	NE > E > ISO	adenyl cyclase decrease
β_1	ISO > E = NE	adenyl cyclase increase
β_2	ISO > E > NE	adenyl cyclase increase
D_1	DA > E = NE	adenyl cyclase increase via G_s
D_2	DA > E = NE	adenyl cyclase decrease via G_i

For the most part, the receptor types are distinguished by the relative potencies of the catecholamines and catecholamine mimetics. The receptors are also distinguished by blocking agents. NE = norepinephrine, E = epinephrine, ISO = isoproterenol, DA = dopamine.

the catecholamines.[13] Both epinephrine and norepinephrine may increase alertness. Epinephrine may produce anxiety, restlessness, fatigue, and fear and passive tense behavior. Norepinephrine may be more associated with aggressive and hostile reactions. Some investigators consider the behavioral effects to be pharmacological.

The respiratory rate is increased by catecholamines. Again, epinephrine has twenty times the potency of norepinephrine. Epinephrine dilates the pupils of the eyes; it is fifteen times as strong as norepinephrine for the pupillary response.

Norepinephrine and epinephrine increase metabolic rate (calorigenic effect). The effects on metabolic rate require the thyroid (increases in beta receptors) and the adrenal cortex, but not the liver.

Thyroid hormone increases sensitivity to epinephrine in hyperthyroid individuals, whereas hypothyroid conditions decrease sensitivity to epinephrine. Thyroxine, a thyroid hormone, decreases the activity of MAO.

Epinephrine increases blood sugar (norepinephrine has one fourth the potency). It causes glycogenolysis (glycogen breakdown) in liver and muscle via a cAMP mechanism similar to that for glucagon. Epinephrine and norepinephrine are also lipolytic.

Plasma potassium first rises because K^+ is released from the liver, then falls because skeletal muscle takes up the K^+, after epinephrine or norepinephrine are injected.

Usually, catecholamines cause melanosome aggregation in the melanophores in the skins of lower vertebrates. The phenomenon has been called "excitement pallor." However, excitement darkening can also occur. Moreover, complex patterns of both lightening and darkening in different parts of the skin can result from catecholamines *in vivo*. An hypothesis of varying ratios of receptors on different melanophores has been used to explain the differing and dramatic effects of adrenal hormones on pigmentation.

Epinephrine and norepinephrine inhibit the intestines and uterine contractions (epinephrine is 100 times as potent as norepinephrine).

ALPHA AND BETA RECEPTORS

Sir Henry Dale's concept of adrenergic receptor sites on target tissues has been important to understanding the functions of catecholamines. Characterization of receptors is on the basis of pharmacological responses of target tissues. The relative potency of agonists (molecules that act like the hormone) can be measured. The receptors can also be distinguished by target cell responses to

Table 16.4 Catecholamine Alpha and Beta Effects

Alpha	Beta
arterioles vasoconstriction	adipose tissue lipolysis increase
cyclic AMP production decreased	arterioles vasodilation
cyclic GMP production increased	bone marrow erythropoiesis
insulin secretion decrease	cardiac (heart) muscle contraction
intestinal smooth muscle contraction	cyclic AMP production decreased
intestinal sphincters contraction	eye ciliary muscle contraction for near vision
liver glycogenolysis	heart A-V nodes conduction velocity increase
male sex organ ejaculation	heart S-A node rate increase
MSH secretion decrease	heart ventricles conduction velocity increase
pancreas acini decreased secretion	heart ventricles contractility increase
parathormone secretion decrease	hepatocyte glycogenolysis increase
radial muscle iris contraction (mydriasis)	insulin secretion increase
renin secretion decrease	intestinal motility and tone decrease
salivary gland potassium increase	lung bronchial muscle relaxation
salivary gland thick viscous secretion	MSH secretion increase
salivary gland water increase	parathormone secretion increase
skin pilomotor muscle contraction	pineal gland melatonin synthesis and secretion
skin sweat glands slight, localized secretion	renin secretion increase
spleen smooth muscle capsule contraction	salivary gland amylase secretion increase
stomach sphincters contraction	skeletal muscle glycogenolysis increase
systemic veins vasoconstriction	spleen smooth muscle capsule relaxation
ureter motility and tone increase	stomach gastrin secretion increase
urinary bladder smooth muscle contraction	stomach motility and tone decrease
urinary bladder trigone and sphincter contraction	systemic veins vasodilation
uterine smooth muscle contraction	urinary bladder detrusor relaxation
vascular smooth muscle contraction	urinary bladder smooth muscle relaxation
	uterine smooth muscle relaxation
	vascular smooth muscle relaxation

Ganong, W. Review of Medical Physiology, Fourteenth Edition. Norwalk, CT: Appleton & Lange; 1989.
Hadley, M. Endocrinology, Second Edition. Englewood Cliffs, NJ: Prentice-Hall; 1988.

antagonists (molecules that oppose the action of the hormone) or receptor blockers (Figure 16.5). Further, target tissues can be classified by their responses.

The receptors have been given letter names (Table 16.3). In the case of epinephrine and norepinephrine, the receptors were called alpha and beta receptors by Ahlquist. Subcategories of receptors are now indicated by numerical subscripts. The way in which the receptors respond to antagonists has revealed that a receptor-G protein interface may be the target for antagonists.[14]

Alpha receptors have the relative potency E > NE > PE > ISO. Isoproterenol (ISO, Isuprel), phenylephrine (PE, Neo-Synephrine), methoxamine, and clonidine are artificial agonists of catecholamines. Alpha responses are blocked by phenoxybenzamine (Dibenzyline), phentolamine, prazosin, yohimbine, and ergot alkaloids. Alpha receptors are found functioning in the iris, arterioles and veins (vasoconstriction), stomach, intestine, urinary bladder, ureter, uterus, skin, spleen capsule,

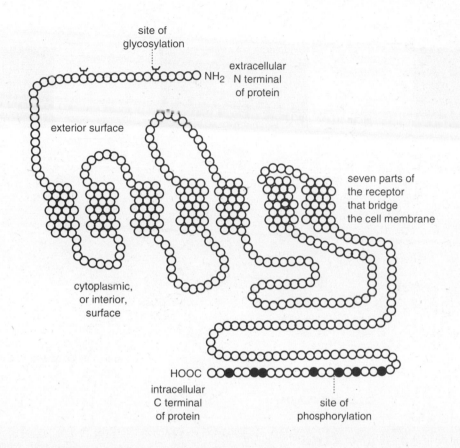

Figure 16.6 The diagram represents the structure of a beta-adrenergic receptor. Circles represent amino acid residues. The N-terminal, the C-terminal, and the seven membrane-spanning portions of the receptor have structures similar to rhodopsin. Modified, with permission. Benovic, J.L.; Mayor, F.; Somers, R.L.; Caron, M.G.; Lefkowitz, R.J. Light-dependent phosphorylation of rhodopsin by ß-adrenergic receptor kinase. Nature 321: 869–872; 1986; p. 871.

liver, pancreas, and salivary glands (Table 16.4). Alpha receptor stimulation decreases adenyl cyclase and Ca^{2+}.

Beta receptors have the relative potency ISO > E > NE > PE. Isoproterenol is the principal agonist. Beta blockers include propranolol, pronethalol, practolol, butoxamine, salbutamol, prenalterol, and atenolol. Beta receptors function to regulate smooth muscle, ciliary muscle, heart, arterioles and veins (vasodilation), lungs, stomach, intestine, urinary bladder, uterus, spleen capsule,

liver, pancreas, salivary glands, fat, and juxtaglomerular cells. Beta receptor stimulation increases adenyl cyclase. Most of the beta effects are consequences of epinephrine, except for the case of rat pineal melatonin synthesis which is increased more by NE.

Receptors for other molecules are similarly classified by their pharmacology. For example, acetylcholine's receptors are called muscarinic (respond to muscarine agonist) and nicotinic (respond to nicotine agonist). The acetylcholine ef-

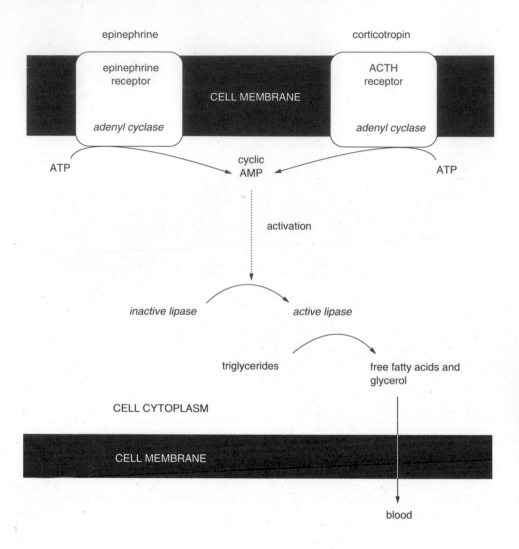

Figure 16.7 The mechanism of action for epinephrine (E) and ACTH on fat cells (adipocytes) via a hormone sensitive enzyme (lipase) is illustrated. In the cell membranes, receptors and transduction mechanisms differ for epinephrine (no calcium requirement) and ACTH (calcium required), but the receptors share a common adenyl cyclase. The mechanism of action for epinephrine's effects on glucose resembles the mechanism for glucagon.

fects on the adrenal chromaffin cells are via nicotinic receptors.

    Scientists visualize the alpha and beta receptors as residents of cell membranes of target tissue cells. The structure of the beta receptor has been proposed (Figure 16.6).

MECHANISM OF ACTION OF EPINEPHRINE

    Epinephrine stimulates glucose release from liver cells by a mechanism similar to that of glucagon. The epinephrine acts as the "first mes-

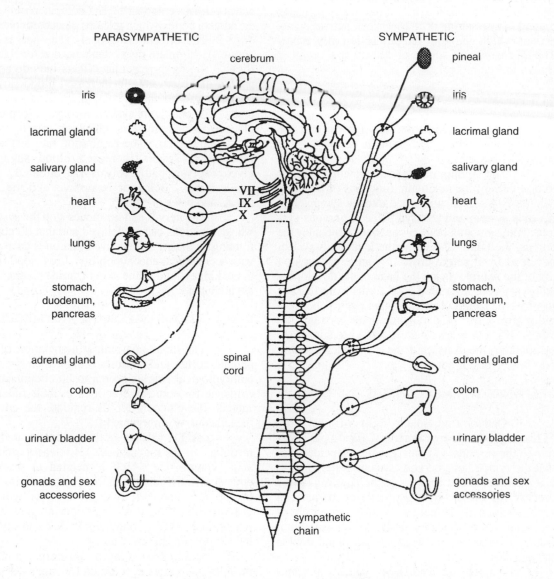

Figure 16.8 The diagram represents the autonomic nervous system which consists of the parasympathetic nervous system (left) and the sympathetic nervous system (right). The participants are the brain (cerebrum, midbrain, hindbrain), cranial nerves, ganglia (circles), sympathetic chains of ganglia (one chain is shown), the spinal cord (upper segments 1–12 thoracic spinal; middle segments 1–5 lumbar, and lower segments 1–5 sacral), and cells within some of the organs (e.g., adrenal medulla). Redrawn, with permission. Turner, C.; Bagnara, J. Endocrinology, Sixth Edition. Philadelphia, PA: W. B. Saunders; 1976; p. 316.

senger" and interacts with a receptor on the cell membrane, causing an increase in adenyl cyclase activity. The adenyl cyclase increases the synthesis of cyclic AMP which plays the part of the second messenger. The cyclic AMP allosterically activates protein kinase setting off a cascade of activation reactions which end with the production of glucose. The mechanism of action of epinephrine on fat is shown in Figure 16.7.

AUTONOMIC NERVOUS SYSTEM

The autonomic nervous system and the adrenal gland participate together in the response to stressful situations.

The autonomic nervous system functions to take care of the automatic functions of the body (Figure 16.8). It is subdivided into the sympathetic nervous system and parasympathetic nervous system. The sympathetic nervous system includes the adrenal medulla. The sympathetic nervous system develops from neural crest. Neural crest runs on top of the neural tube on the back of the developing embryo where the spinal cord forms from it. The top 15% of neural crest cells give rise to cholinergic neurons of the parasympathetic system, the middle 40–50% of neural crest cells yield adrenergic sympathetic neurons, and the remainder develop into both types of neurons.

RESPONSE TO EMERGENCIES

Cannon suggested a "fight or flight" array of responses involving the adrenal gland's participation in the responses to emergencies. His idea was that the sympathetic nervous system, responding to emergencies, elicits changes in the physiology that prepare the organism to do battle or to flee. In such a situation, it makes sense to suppose that reproductive and digestive functions can wait, but it is useful to increase the heart rate and blood flow to the muscles.

Events perceived physiologically as emergencies are emotional stress, cold, heat, burns, pH changes (acidosis, alkalosis), exercise, asphyxia and anoxia, hypotension, and hypoglycemia. Experimentally, stress responses can be induced by simple techniques such as exposing cats to barking dogs. Humans may exhibit the emergency responses in examinations and under stressful working conditions.

When an emergency occurs, the hypothalamic and amygdaloid regions of the brain are activated (by rage or fear). The brain regions stimulate the sympathetic nervous system which releases norepinephrine and epinephrine, the adrenal medulla which releases epinephrine and norepinephrine, and the adrenal cortex which releases glucocorticoids.

The effects are global. The nerves and hormones stimulate the systems needed for fight or flight. The cardiovascular effects include acceleration of heart rate and increased blood flow to coronary arteries and skeletal muscle and liver and brain. The endocrine system secretes epinephrine, glucocorticoids, insulin, glucagon, renin, melatonin, and ACTH. The respiration rate increases. Metabolism favors increased blood sugar so glycogenolysis and lipolysis are initiated. The pupils dilate. Behavior is anxious and the skin sweats and pales in color.

The nerves and hormones stop the systems whose functions can be delayed and that do not aid fighting or fleeing. Digestive function is decreased with decreased stomach mobility. Less blood flows to the kidneys and to the skin. Uterine contractions are inhibited.

INTERACTIONS OF CORTEX AND MEDULLA

The close anatomical association of the adrenal cortex and medulla despite their separate embryological origins seems to be circumstantial evidence for some interactions in their function. Indeed, the glucocorticoids regulate the adrenal medulla during embryonic life.

ACTH affects both the cortex and the medulla. In the medulla ACTH releases ascorbic acid (vitamin C) which is needed to preserve epinephrine and norepinephrine by preventing oxidation. It is also used by dopamine beta hydroxylase in biosynthesis of epinephrine and norepinephrine. ACTH stimulates PNMT activity and induces tyrosine hydroxylase.

Hormones of both the cortex and the medulla share roles in common functions—activity of the brain, glucose synthesis and mobilization, lipolysis, and responses to injury.

PINEAL MODEL FOR BETA RECEPTION

The pineal gland, especially the rat pineal gland, has served as a model for studying catecholamine function, particularly the actions of beta receptors and the cAMP mechanism of action of

Table 16.5 Catecholamine Receptor Agonists and Antagonists

Receptor	Agonists	Antagonists or blockers
beta receptor	isoproterenol (Isuprel®)	propranolol (Inderal®) atenolol (Tenormin®) butoxamine
alpha receptor	methoxamine (Vasoxyl®) phenylephrine (Neo-Synephrine®) clonidine (Catapres®)	phenoxybenzamine (Dibenzyline®) phentolamine (Regitine®) prazosin (Minipress®) yohimbine (Actibine®, Aphrodyne®, Yocon®, Yohimex®)

The table lists the generic name and some commercial name (in parentheses) of some of the alpha and beta receptor agonists and blockers. Beta receptors are found in most tissues—heart myocardium, blood vessels, kidney, gut, pancreas, liver, fat, bronchioles, and uterus. Alpha receptors are found in blood vessels, gut, pancreas, liver, skin, and uterus. Where both alpha and beta receptors are found in a tissue, they usually mediate opposing effects; however, alpha and beta receptors in liver both increase lipolysis.

norepinephrine.[15] The activity of the enzyme, N-acetyltransferase, can be stimulated in rat pineal glands with norepinephrine *in vitro* or with isoproterenol injections *in vivo*. In about four hours after beginning experimental treatment, rat pineal N-acetyltransferase activity rises from near zero activity to over 4 nmol/pineal/hr *in vitro* and over 30 nmol/pineal/hr *in vivo*.

The 30-fold stimulation can be increased to 100-fold by doing the experiment with rats whose pineal glands have been denervated by surgical ablation of the superior cervical ganglia. The increase is called "supersensitivity" or "superinduction" or "denervation hypersensitivity."[16] In contrast, if the pineal glands are repeatedly stimulated (e.g. by repeated isoproterenol injections *in vitro*), the glands become unresponsive. The terms "subsensitivity" or "exhaustion" have been used to denote this phenomenon. One possible cause of super- and subsensitivity responses is a change in the number or responsivity of the beta receptors.

Biochemicals, or drugs, can be tested by adding them to the culture media of rat pineal glands or by injecting them into rats. The compounds that stimulate pineal N-acetyltransferase activity similar to norepinephrine are classified as mimetics; the compounds that block the N-acetyltransferase stimulation are classified as antagonists. In a similar manner, lists of agonists and antagonists can be developed for any receptor system and have been constructed for catecholamine alpha and beta receptors (Tables 16.5, 16.6).

MEDICAL ASPECTS OF CATECHOLAMINES

Hyperfunction of the adrenal medulla, usually of chromaffin cell tumor origin, is called **pheochromocytoma**. Individuals with pheochromocytoma may produce 500 times normal epinephrine in the plasma. Symptoms include hypertension, raised metabolic rate, weight loss, psychosis, tremulousness, headache, nausea, epigastric pain, cutaneous flushing, visual disturbances, apprehension (sense of impending doom), increased respiratory rate, and lipemia. Eighty per cent of pheochromocytomas are adrenal, but 20% of them are found in other tissues that develop from neural crest. The disorder responds to treatments with surgery and alpha- and beta-adrenoceptor antagonists. Some of the symptoms can be caused by surgery.

Isoproterenol (along with epinephrine or atropine) is used clinically to increase heart rate

Table 16.6 Receptor Definition by Responses to Agonists and Antagonists

Receptor	Agonist	Antagonist	Agonist effect on adenyl cyclase activity
alpha$_1$	epinephrine slightly >norepinephrine >>isoproterenol	prazosin >phentolamine >yohimbine	none
alpha$_2$	epinephrine slightly >norepinephrine >>isoproterenol	phentolamine slightly >yohimbine >>prazosin	decrease
beta$_1$	isoproterenol >epinephrine =norepinephrine	metoprolol >butoxamine	increase
beta$_2$	isoproterenol >epinephrine >norepinephrine	butoximine >metoprolol	increase

Receptors in target cells are defined by their pharmacology. They are distinguished from one another by the differences of the relative potencies of their agonists and antagonists. In each cell, the chemicals are arranged in descending order of potency with the most potent agonist or antagonist at the top; the symbol > means greater than. Modified, with permission. Goldfien, A. The Adrenal Medulla. In Greenspan, F.; Forsham, P. Basic and Clinical Endocrinology, Second Edition. Los Altos, CA: Lange Medical Publications; 1986; p. 333.

(e.g., by infusing 4 micrograms/l). Beta adrenergic blockers, such as propranolol, are also used in cardiac care where they can help to control arrythmias.[17]

Monoamine oxidase metabolizes catecholamines and also can act on other substrates (serotonin, phenylethanylamine, dopamine, and tyramine). Monoamine oxidase inhibitors (MAOIs)—iproniazid, clorgyline, deprenyl, pargyline, phenelzine, isocarboxazid, tranylcypromine—have been used to treat mood disorders, depression, phobias, ulcers, sleep disorders, pain syndromes, attention, and obsessive-compulsive disorders.

REFERENCES

1. Deftos, L.J. Chromogranin A: Its role in endocrine function and as an endocrine and neuroendocrine tumor marker. Endocrine Reviews 12: 181; 1991.

2. Weiler, R.; Lassmann, H.; Fischer, P.; Jdllinger, K.; Winkler, H. FEBS 263: 337–339; 1990,

3. Epple, A.; Navarro, I.; Horak, P.; Spector, S. Endogenous morphine and codeine: Release by the chromaffin cells of the eel. Life Sciences 52: 117–121; 1993.

4. Epple, A.; Porta, S.; Nibbio, B.; Leitner, G. Release of conjugated catecholamines by the adrenal medulla equivalent of the American Eel, *Anguilla rostrata*. General and Comparative Endocrinology 90: (in press); 1993.

5. Williams, R. Textbook of Endocrinology. Philadelphia, PA: W. B. Saunders; 1987.

6. Brickman, A.S.; Stern, N.; Sowers, J.R. Circadian variations of catecholamines and blood pressure in patients with pseudohypoparathyroidism and hypertension. Chronobiologia 17: 37–44; 1990.

7. Prinz, P.N.; Halter, J.; Benedetti, C.; Raskind, M. Circadian variation of plasma catecholamines in young and old men: Relation to rapid eye movement and slow wave sleep. Journal of Clinical Endocrinology and Metabolism 49: 300–304; 1979.

8. Epple, A. Adrenomedullary catecholamines. The Endocrinology of Growth, Development, and Metabolism in Vertebrates. New York: Academic Press, Inc.; 1993; p. 327–343.

9. Weiler, R.; Meyerson, G.; Fischer-Colbrie, R.; Laslop, A.; Pahlman, S.; Floor, E.; Winkler, H. Divergent changes of chromogranin A/secretogranin II levels in differentiating human neuroblastoma cells. FEBS 265: 27–29; 1990.

10. Weiler, R.; Marksteiner, J.; Bellmann, R.; Wohlfarter, T.; Schober, M.; Fischer-Colbrie, R.; Sperk, G.; Winkler, H. Chromogranins in rat brain: Characterization, topographical distribution and regulation of synthesis. Brain Research 532: 87–94; 1990.

11. Martin, C. Endocrine Physiology. New York: Oxford University Press; 1985; p.277.

12. Kachi, T.; Takahashi, G.; Banerji, T.K.; Quay, W.B. Rough endoplasmic reticulum in the adrenaline and noradrenaline cells of the adrenal medulla: Effects of intracranial surgery and pinealectomy. Journal of Pineal Research 12: 89–95; 1992.

13. Ganong, W. Review of Medical Physiology, Fourteenth Edition. Norwalk, CT: Appleton & Lange; 1989; p. 164, 304

14. Luttrell, L.M.; Ostrowski, J.; Cotecchia, S.; Kendall, H.; Lefkowitz, R.J. Antagonism of catecholamine receptor signaling by expression of cytoplasmic domains of the receptors. Science 259: 1453–1457; 1993.

15. Binkley, S. The Pineal: Endocrine and Nonendocrine Function. Englewood Cliffs, NJ: Prentice-Hall; 1988; pp. 91–94.

16. Deguchi, T. Circadian rhythm of serotonin N-acetyltransferase activity in organ culture of chicken pineal gland. Science 203: 1245–1247; 1978.

17. Berkow, R. (ed) The Merck Manual, Fifteenth Edition. Rahway, NJ: Merck Sharp & Dohme;1987; pages 510–511.

CHAPTER 17

Pituitary Gonadotropins, Testicular Androgens

The masculinizing hormones are the androgenic steroids that are synthesized by the testes and other steroid secreting tissues. Testosterone is the principal androgen synthesized in testicular Leydig cells that functions in male reproduction. Regulation of androgens is by gonadotropins which are glycoprotein hormones from the pituitary gland. Reproduction has seasonal breeding cycles in many species, which are frequently governed using responses to photoperiod.

MALE REPRODUCTION

Peptide hormones from the hypothalamus, glycoprotein gonadotropin hormones from the anterior pituitary gland, and steroidal androgens from the gonads all are involved in the control of reproduction in males. The peptide hormones of the hypothalamus and the general steroidal natures of the androgens have been covered in previous chapters. The gonadotropins and the specific functions of the androgens in reproduction function are the subject of this chapter. The male gonad is called the testis and it has the dual function of producing hormones (endocrine function) and gametes (exocrine function).

Seasonal changes in hormone secretion are associated with many of the endocrine glands, but the seasonal changes have been particularly well studied in connection with male reproduction because of their well-defined breeding cycles which are amenable to experimentation. For example, the weight of the testis of the house sparrow increases 24-fold when the birds enter their breeding seasons. Changes in testicular anatomy and hormones follow the seasonal pattern of the testicular weight. Changes in testicular size are visible to the naked eye. Changes in gonad size are less apparent in those species, such as humans, that breed the whole year round.

GONADOTROPINS AND RELATED MOLECULES

The functional definition of "gonadotropin" is gonad-stimulating hormone. Broadly used, this definition includes glycoprotein hormones and prolactin (PRL) which has 198 amino acids and three disulfide bonds and is structurally similar to growth hormone. Prolactin has many functions in the reproduction of both sexes. However, most endocrinologists reserve the use of the word gonadotropin for a group of structurally related glycoproteins which include luteinizing hormone (LH), follicle-stimulating hormone (FSH), human chorionic gonadotropin (HCG), pregnant mare's serum (PMS), and human menopausal gonadotropin (HMG). Thyroid-stimulating hormone (TSH) is structurally related to the gonadotropins. In addition to around 204–211 amino acids reported for human TSH, FSH, and LH,[1] the family of glycoproteins contains carbohydrates: mannose, galactose, N-acetylgalactos-amine, N-acetylglycosamine, N-acetyl neuraminic acid, fucose, and sialic acid. The carbohydrates in the glycoprotein hormones may have the effect of lengthening their half-lives or may be involved in their recognition by target receptors.

The glycoproteins are composed of alpha (similar in FSH, LH, TSH) and active beta subunits (Figure 17.1). The subunit amino acid differences are responsible for immunological and biological specificity. During synthesis, it is believed that the subunit peptides are synthesized separately by transcription from two separate mRNAs. The peptides are joined together before addition of the carbohydrate groups. The addition of the carbohydrate moieties may utilize glycosyltransferase enzymes in the Golgi apparatus. The separate subunits (small amounts) and the completed hormones are secreted. Variation in the exact details of structure (molecular weight, number of amino acids, composition of carbohydrate moieties) varies with the scientific reference and species. For example, sheep and cows and humans have 70% homology in the alpha subunits.

REGULATION OF GONADOTROPINS

The secretion of the gonadotropins of the anterior pituitary gland is inhibited or stimulated by hypophysial neurohormones (Table 17.1). Anterior pituitary cells that make gonadotropins are targets of the releasing hormones. LRH (luteinizing hormone-releasing hormone = GnRH = gonadotropin-releasing hormone) releases LH from the anterior pituitary gland. A pulsatile pattern of LRH secretion is a requirement for stimulation of gonadotropin secretion because continuous application of LRH results in "desensitization" of the gonadotrops and gonadal suppression.[2] The LRH receptors are glycoproteins containing sialic acid residues.[3] Receptor synthesis, up-regulation prevention by inhibin, and a requirement for calcium oscillations have been studied.[4,5,6,7]

A mechanism of action for LRH stimulation of LH was proposed by Naor: (i) LRH binding to receptors on pituitary gonadotrops, (ii) stimulation of rapid phosphodiesteric hydrolysis of phosphoinositides, (iii) activation of PLC by GTP-binding protein, (iv) reduction of binding affinity of LRH to its receptor by activated G_p-GTP, (v) formation IP_3 which enhances calcium ion release from intracellular pools, and (vi) a 100 second burst

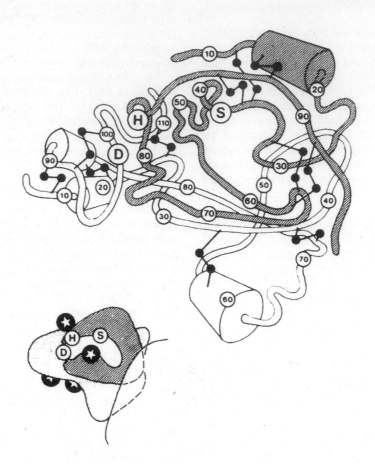

Figure 17.1 The diagram shows the proposed tertiary structure for human chorionic gonadotropin (HCG) upper right, and a space-filling model of a glycoprotein hormone at the receptor in the lower left. In HCG, the alpha subunit is hatched. The beta subunit is drawn underneath and has three helices. The letters (H, D, S) are putative active site residues (ser at 38, his at 83, asp at 99) and the stars designate glycosylated asparagine residues. Reproduced, with permission. Willey, K.P.; Leidenberger, F. Functionally distinct agonist and receptor-binding regions in human chorionic gonadotropin. Development of a tertiary structure model. J. Biol. Chem. 264: 19716; 1989.

of LH release by transient calcium rise.[8] Three calcium-binding proteins (calmodulin, CaM) have been identified for the gonadotrop: calcineurin, caldesmon, and spectrin.[9]

LH, FSH, TSH, HCG, PMS, HMG

     Luteinizing hormone (LH = ICSH = interstitial cell-stimulating hormone = lutropin) has two polypeptide subunits and MW28,000–30,000.

The alpha subunit of LH has 96 amino acids; the beta-three subunit has 120 amino acids. The hormone has disulfide bonds. 15.5% of the hormone molecule is carbohydrate. The half-life of LH is 30–60 minutes. LH functions as a gonadotropin in males and females (Table 17.2). LH is synthesized in the gonadotrops of the anterior pituitary gland.[10]

     Follicle-stimulating hormone (FSH = follitropin) has two polypeptide subunits (alpha and beta-two) and disulfide bonds and

Table 17.1 Release Hormones Change Pituitary Hormones

Releasing hormone	Group, age, pituitary hormone(s) measured	Response (mIU/ml)
	MEN, AGE RANGE	
LRH	18–40, ΔLH, ΔFSH	32, 3
LRH	>65, ΔLH, ΔFSH	23, 3
LRH	40–79, ΔTSH	>2
LRH	20–39, ΔPRL	15–40
LRH	40–59, ΔPRL	10–50
LRH	60–79, ΔPRL	5–90
	WOMEN, AGE OR MENSTRUAL PHASE	
LRH	follicular phase, ΔLH, ΔFSH	17, 3
LRH	LH peak, ΔLH at LH peak, ΔFSH	162, 8
LRH	luteal phase, ΔLH, ΔFSH	49, 3
TSH	<40, ΔTSH	>6
TSH	20–39, ΔPRL	30–120
TSH	40–59, ΔPRL	20–120
TSH	60–79, ΔPRL	10–100

The responses are given as changes (Δ). Modified, with permission. Findling, J.; Tyrrell, B. Anterior pituitary and somatomedins, I. Anterior pituitary. In Greenspan, F., editor. Basic and Clinical Endocrinology, Third Edition. Los Altos, CA: Lange Medical Publications; 1986; p. 92, 95.

MW30,000–34,000. The alpha subunit has 92 amino acid residues and the beta subunit has 118 amino acid residues. Sixteen percent of the molecule is carbohydrate and the half-life is 170 minutes. FSH is a gonadotropin in males and females. FSH is synthesized in the anterior pituitary gonadotrops.

Thyrotropin (thyroid-stimulating hormone, TSH) has two polypeptide subunits and MW28,000. It is synthesized by pituitary thyrotrops.[11] The alpha subunit has 89 amino acids and the beta-one subunit has 112 amino acids.[12] Sixteen percent of the molecule is carbohydrate. The half-life of TSH is 30–60 minutes. TSH function is to stimulate production of hormones by the thyroid thyrotrops. TSH is synthesized in the anterior pituitary gland. Concentrations of TSH in blood are 1–10 μU/ml. The thyroid gland has functions in female reproduction. The function of TSH is control of the thyroid gland.

Chorionic gonadotropin (CG, H C G = hCG = human chorionic gonadotropin) has two subunits. The alpha subunit (MW18,000) has five amino acids that differ from the alpha subunits of LH, FSH, and TSH. The beta subunit has MW28,000. HCG has activity similar to LH (luteotropic, luteinizing). HCG is synthesized by an embryonic layer, the syncytiotrophoblast, and is considered to be a placental hormone, a hormone of the chorionic villi. It can be detected in blood as early as 6 days after conception and in urine as early as 14 days after conception and is the basis of most pregnancy tests. Peak levels are 100,000 rat units. Urine from pregnant women is a source of clinically usable HCG. HCG is also found in males in pathological conditions where the HCG is

Table 17.2 Normal Values for Human Male Reproductive Hormones

Hormone	Amount per milliliter of blood
testosterone	3–10 ng
free testosterone	50–200 pg
dihydrotestosterone	0.6–3.0 ng
androstenedione	0.5–2.0 ng
estradiol	5–50 pg
estrone	30–170 pg
follicle-stimulating hormone	2–15 mIU
luteinizing hormone	2–15 mIU
prolactin	4–18 ng

Compiled from data in Braunstein, G. The testes. In Greenspan, F.; Forsham, P., editors. Basic and Clinical Endocrinology. Los Altos, CA: Lange Medical Publications; 1986; and Berkow, W. The Merck Manual, Rahway, NJ: Merck Sharp & Dohme Research Laboratories; 1987.

secreted by gastrointestinal and other tumors. A test of testicular endocrine function involves an injection of chorionic gonadotropin. If the testis is functioning, the CG binds to LH receptors on the Leydig cells and doubles androgenic steroid production. In males, CG causes differentiation of Leydig cells and it both induces and maintains testicular androgens. It causes the release of spermatozoa in amphibians which has been used as a biological pregnancy test.

Pregnant mare's serum (PMS) contains a hormone (MW23,000) that is found early in pregnancy but not during days 40–120 of pregnancy. Its site of synthesis is the uterine endometrial cups. But, unlike HCG, it is not excreted in urine. It has activity that is like follicle-stimulating hormone. PMS has provided a rich source of a hormone that has a long half-life so that it was used experimentally like FSH.

Human menopausal gonadotropin (HMG, hMG, menotropins) is in the urine of postmenopausal women and has MW31,000. It has FSH-like and LH-like activities and may be an altered mixture of pituitary gonadotropins.

Chorionic gonadotropin and menotropin can be used clinically to induce spermatogenesis and ovulation.

GONADOTROPIN MECHANISMS OF ACTION

The gonadotropins act upon the endocrine cells of the testis. In the testis, there are LH receptors that are induced by LH itself. Receptor induction is mediated by prolactin. The LH-receptor complex is internalized resulting in down regulation and probably is necessary in permitting the Leydig cells to recover their response to LH. FSH receptors have been localized to the Sertoli cells. The endocrine cells of the testes produce second messengers in response to stimulation by gonadotropins. "Multiple signaling pathways" have been proposed for the actions of single hormones (LRH, $PGF_{2\alpha}$, LH).[13] The FSH receptors in the testicular Sertoli cells are associated with a guanine nucleotide regulatory protein (G_s) which binds with GTP and activates adenyl cyclase. In the Leydig cells, LH increases phospholipase activity, increases cyclic AMP, mobilizes calcium ions, and

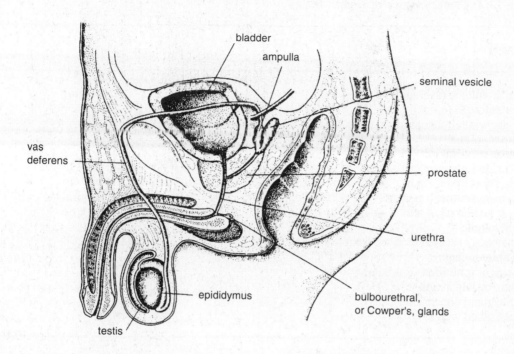

Figure 17.2 The diagram illustrates the anatomy of the human male reproductive system (primary organs and secondary accessory glands). Modified, with permission. Austin, C.R. Fertilization. In Austin, C.R.; Short, R.V., editors. Reproduction in Mammals, Book I: Germ Cells and Fertilization. New York: Cambridge University Press; 1972; p. 110.

increases testosterone production. Testicular endocrine cells also respond to other substances: adenosine, vasoactive intestinal peptide, GRF, LRH.

TESTICULAR ANATOMY

The testis (plural, testes) or testicle (adjective, testicular) is the male gonad. The testes of some mammals are located in a pouch called the **scrotum** (Figure 17.2, Table 17.3). It may surprise the reader to learn that birds, and some mammals (whales, armadillos, seals, rhinoceros), lack a scrotum. In the species that lack a scrotum, the testes can be found in the abdomen. In some species of mammals that do have a scrotum (e.g., laboratory rats), the testes can readily be pushed into the abdomen (Figure 17.3).

The purpose of housing the testes in a scrotum may be to provide a cooler **temperature** environment for the testes. When testes that normally reside in a scrotum are experimentally held in the abdomen of animals, or when the testes are bound closely to the body by clothing, degeneration of the seminiferous tubules occurs and sterility ensues. Insulated athletic supporters and hot baths (43–45C) have reduced sperm counts in humans. Human testes are normally a degree or two cooler (35°C) than internal body temperature (36.3–37.1°C in the morning). These observations about testicular temperature have lead endocrinologists to the idea that the testes cannot tolerate high body temperature. However, testicular cooling does not seem to be a requirement for species that possess intra-abdominal testes. The possibility that there is a natural functional significance to testicular mobility with concomitant changes in testicular temperature prompts the author to speculate that

Table 17.3 Characteristics of Human Males

Parameter	Value
testicular volume (average)	18.6 ± SD 4.8 ml
testicular length (range)	3.6–5.5 cm
testicular width (range)	2.1–3.2 cm
testicular volume	20–25 cubic cm
testicular temperature	35°C
time for spermatogenesis	74 days
blood testosterone, 8 a.m.	6.84 ± 2.11 ng/ml
blood testosterone, 8 p.m.	2.66 ± 0.52 ng/ml
blood testosterone, 4 a.m.	9.28 ± 1.17 ng/ml
semen volume	1–5 ml
spermatozoa in semen required for fertility	>20,000,000/ml
vas deferens length	35–50 cm
diameter of seminiferous tubules	165 μm
seminal vesicle length	10–20 cm
prostate gland dimensions	2x3x4 cm
prostate gland weight	20 g

Blood testosterone = mean plus or minus SEM. Braunstein, G. The testes. In Greenspan, F.; Forsham, P., editors. Basic and Clinical Endocrinology. Los Altos, CA: Lange Medical Publications; 1986; pp. 351–384. Barberia, J.M.; Giner, J.; Cortes-Gallegos, V. Diurnal variations of plasma testosterone in men. Steroids 22: 615–626; 1973; and Berkow, W. The Merck Manual, Rahway, NJ: Merck Sharp & Dohme Research Laboratories; 1987.

seasonal testicular mobility might contribute to seasonal cycles in testicular function.

The testis serves two functions—it produces sperm and it synthesizes hormones. This dual function is reflected in testicular histology (Figures 17.4). Spermatozoa are produced within seminiferous tubules by the germinal epithelium. The Sertoli cells provide structural support for the developing germinal cells. The endocrine cells of the testis that produce testosterone are the Leydig cells.[14]

SPERMATOGENESIS

Sperm production, spermatogenesis, is a maturation process taking 74 days in humans. Development of sperm occurs in the germinal epithelium. Spermatogonia near the basal lamina of the seminiferous tubules mature into primary spermatocytes. The primary spermatocytes divide to produce secondary spermatocytes and then spermatids which mature into spermatozoa (sperms, Figure 17.5). The sperm are freed into the lumen of the seminiferous tubule. During cell division and maturation, the complement of chromosomes is reduced to half (sperms have the haploid number 23 in humans). A spermatogonium can produce 512 spermatids.[15] The anatomy of spermatozoa varies among species (Figure 17.6). The cells—spermatogonia to spermatids—make up a germinal epithelium. In the testis, the germinal epithelium is organized into tubes, the **seminiferous tubules**, which are divided by fibrous septa into 250 pyramidal lobules of coiled seminiferous tubules.

ENDOCRINE TESTIS

The **Leydig** cells (interstitial cells of Leydig) are the steroidogenic endocrine cells of the

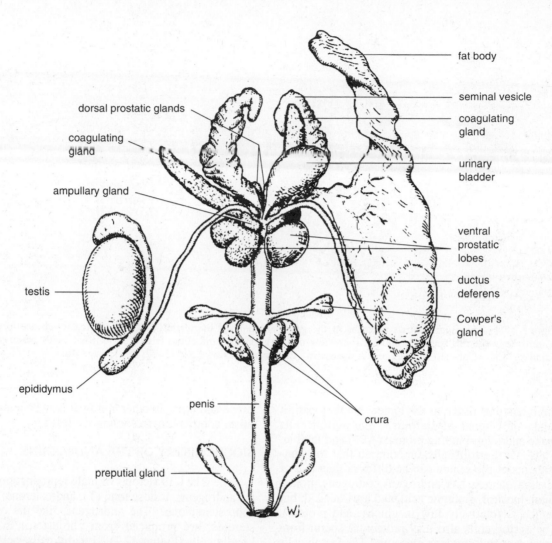

Figure 17.3 The diagram illustrates the anatomy of the rat male reproductive system (primary organs and secondary accessory glands). The fat body is not shown on the left side. On the left side, the coagulating gland is shown dissected free of the seminal vesicle. During a dissection or surgery, the rat's testes can easily be pushed back and forth through the inguinal canal between the abdomen and scrotum. Modified, with permission. Turner, C.; Bagnara, J. Endocrinology, Sixth Edition. Philadelphia, PA: W. B. Saunders; 1976; p. 422.

testis. The cells originate from mesenchyme (mesoderm) and synthesize steroids such as testosterone and estrogen. In seasonal breeders, there is a seasonal crop of Leydig cells. The Leydig cells are found outside and among the seminiferous tubules along with the blood vessels, lymphatic vessels, fibroblasts, and nerves.

The **Sertoli cells** of the seminiferous tubule also have endocrine function. In the germinal epithelium, the glycogen-rich Sertoli cells stretch from the basal lamina to the lumen and they are virtually folded around the maturing cells that become sperm. Damaged germ cells are consumed by the Sertoli cells (phagocytosis). The Sertoli cells maintain a blood-testicular barrier. They prevent large molecules (proteins) from passing from

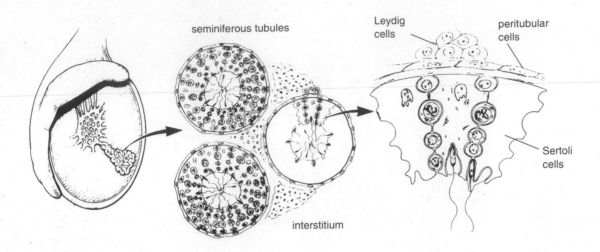

Figure 17.4 The figure shows sketches of the gross anatomy of the testis (left), histological cross sections of seminiferous tubules (center), and a closer view of the germinal epithelium (right). Modified, with permission. Skinner, M.K. Cell-cell interactions in the testis. Endocrine Reviews 12: 45–77; 1991; page 46.

the interstitial tissue to the lumen, but they permit ready movement of steroids. The Sertoli cells make androgen-binding protein (ABP) and inhibin. Thus, the Sertoli cells function so that the constituents of the semen can be different than that of plasma (semen has androgens, estrogens, potassium, inositol, glutamic acid, and aspartic acid; but semen is relatively low in glucose and protein). The Sertoli cells also may protect the sperm from causing an autoimmune response. The Sertoli cells may be responsible for transport of fluid to the lumen.

A blood supply reaches the testis from branches of the internal spermatic arteries called the testicular arteries. The testis contains a complex network of capillaries. Then the blood gathers in the pampiniform plexus, an anastomotic network of veins. Finally, the blood exits via the internal right spermatic vein which drains to the vena cava and the left spermatic vein which drains to the renal vein. The blood runs in parallel, but opposite, directions in the spermatic arteries and in the close-by pampiniform plexus of spermatic veins. Such an arrangement is called a "countercurrent" mechanism and may permit countercurrent exchange of testos-

terone and heat. In other words, it may be a mechanism contributing to cooling the testis.

BIOCHEMISTRY OF THE ANDROGENS

The C19 steroids of male reproduction are the androgens: testosterone (T), androsterone, and androstenedione. The androgens, like the other steroids, are produced from cholesterol in the Leydig cells (Figure 17.7). Leydig cells lack the 21-hydroxylase and 11-hydroxylase found in adrenal cortex, so the cells don't make mineralocorticoids and glucocorticoids. The cells have 17-α-hydroxylase which tracks pregnenolone to the pathway for the production of androgens. The Leydig cells can make progesterone because they have 3BDI, and a less important pathway for testosterone production is via this route. The adrenal cortex of both sexes can also make androgens.

LH stimulates production of androgens by increasing the conversion of cholesteryl esters to cholesterol. The mechanism of LH action uses cyclic AMP and activation of a protein kinase. Testosterone is the principal androgen. Plasma testosterone in normal men is about 0.5 μg/100 ml

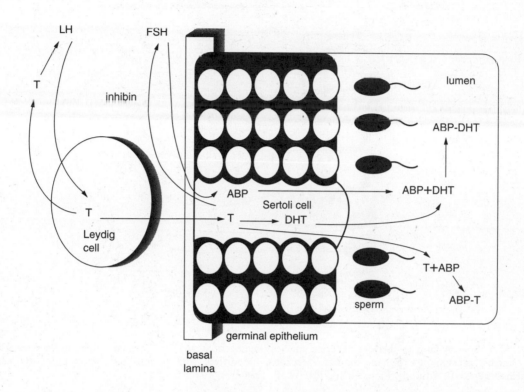

Figure 17.5 The diagram illustrates a Leydig cell and the germinal epithelium of a seminiferous tubule. Hormones of the male reproductive feedback system—testosterone (T), luteinizing hormone (LH), follicle-stimulating hormone (FSH), inhibin—regulate the Leydig and Sertoli cells. Sertoli cells produce androgen-binding protein (ABP) which they secrete into the seminiferous tubule lumen where it forms complexes with dihydrotestosterone (DHT) or testosterone. Spermatogenesis begins with spermatogonia by the basal lamina, continues in the germinal epithelium, and ends with the spermatids by the lumen into which the completed sperm are shed.

(3–12 ng/ml) and 95% of it comes from the testes; in normal women plasma testosterone comes from the ovaries and adrenals and is 0.2–0.7 ng/ml.[16]

  Androgen is transported in blood with the aid of binding globulins. Scientists variously suggest that 40–85% of testosterone travels bound to TeBG (**testosterone estradiol-binding globulin** = SHBG = sex hormone-binding globulin = GBG = gonadal steroid-binding globulin) whose precursor structure is known.[17] Albumin carries

testosterone (40%) as do other proteins (17%).

  An interesting aspect of androgenic function is that testosterone (T) is converted by its target tissues to a more active steroid, **dihydrotestosterone (DHT)**. The target tissues (embryonic genital tubercle, prostate, seminal vesicles, penis, skin, pituitary gland, liver, parts of hypothalamus) possess an enzyme, 5-α-reductase, that catalyzes the peripheral activation. In a target cell, testosterone is first converted to DHT. DHT binds

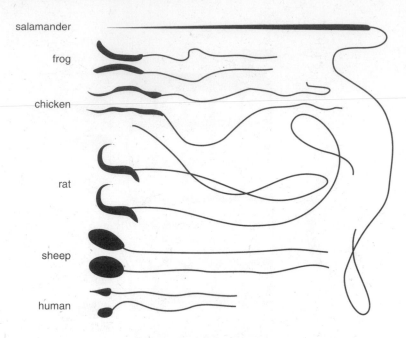

salamander

frog

chicken

rat

sheep

human

Figure 17.6 Sperms are sketched for different species (one spermatozoa for the salamander; two for each of the other species, presumably showing natural variation). Modified, with permission. Turner, C.; Bagnara, J. Endocrinology, Sixth Edition. Philadelphia, PA: W. B. Saunders; 1976; p. 437.

to a cytoplasmic receptor protein. The DHT receptor complex translocates to the nucleus where it changes its characteristics (transformation) and binds with nuclear chromatin. New mRNA synthesis directs new protein synthesis.

Males produce some **estrogens** in the testis and the adrenal gland. Plasma estrogen in males is one tenth of that in women on day of ovulation. The male adult secretes 0.05 mg/day[18] (13.9–31.2 nmol/day) and has circulating estradiol of 2 ng/dl or 5–50 pg/ml.[19] The lower normal levels in women are 6 ng/dl for early follicular phase of the menstrual cycle. Worry has been expressed that there has been an increase in male reproductive tract disorders in recent decades, and it has been suggested that this might be due to increased exposure to estrogen, especially in utero, because of changes in women's diets, oral contraceptive use, orally active anabolic estrogens in livestock feed, increased use of plants high in estrogen (soya), and environmental chemicals with estrogenic action.[20]

Androgen conjugates (e.g., glucuronides and sulfates) are formed from androgens in liver, and, possibly, in skin.[21] The main excretory products of testosterone are the **17-ketosteroids** (androsterone, epiandrosterone, etiocholanolone) formed by the liver and excreted in the urine. Two thirds of the 17-ketosteroids come from testicular androgen and some have biological activity (<20% of testosterone). Some testosterone is converted to estrogen in adrenal cortex, Leydig cells, and Sertoli cells.

TESTES, PENIS, AND SCROTUM

The testis is a target of testosterone. Testosterone acts on the seminiferous tubules. There it forms DHT which combines with androgen-binding protein (ABP) secreted by the Sertoli

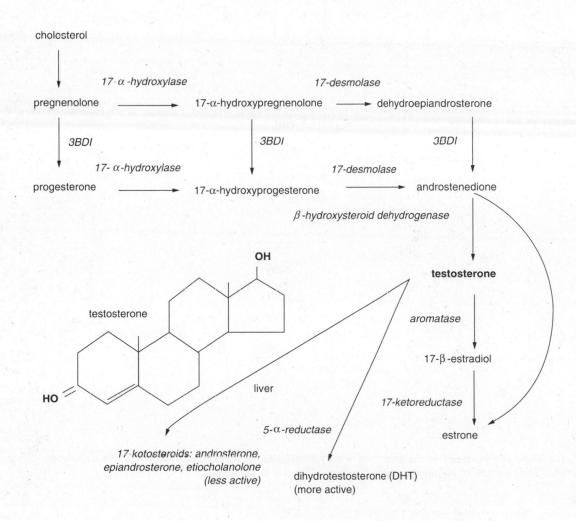

Figure 17.7 The biochemical pathway illustrates synthesis and metabolism of the androgens and the structure of testosterone. LH stimulates the conversion of cholesterol to pregnenolone. Testosterone is formed in the testis. Enzyme names are italicized. The liver produces 17-ketosteroids; some testosterone targets convert it to more potent dihydrotestosterone; the testis and other sites aromatize it to produce estrogen.

cells into the lumens of the seminiferous tubules. ABP is not the intracellular androgenic receptor. Instead, it may function to provide androgen in the seminal fluid. One possible role for luminal androgen is a function in the development of sperm or their maintenance or further maturation in semen. Androgen is required for spermatogenesis. It is also logical that semen could provide a route to androgenic targets giving them a high concentration of androgen while sparing the many structures the blood serves from effects of excess androgen.

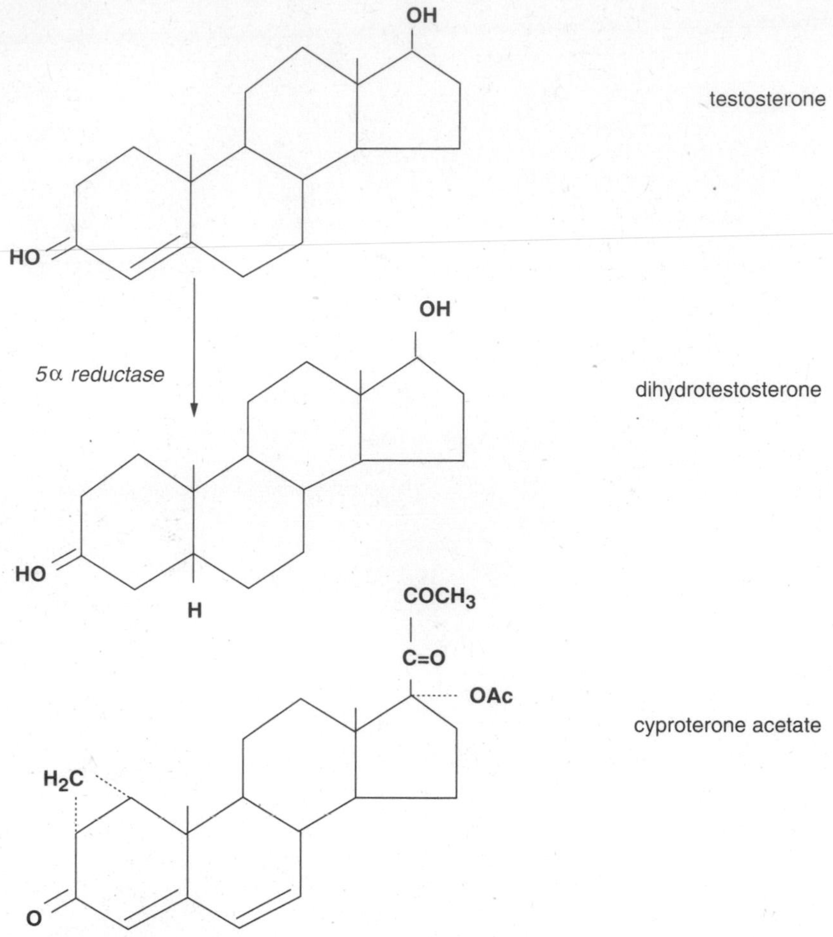

OH

testosterone

HO

5α reductase

OH

dihydrotestosterone

HO

H

COCH₃

C=O

OAc

cyproterone acetate

H₂C

O

Figure 17.8 The synthesis of the more active dihydrotestosterone (DHT) from the less active testosterone (T) is shown. The structure of an antiandrogen, cyproterone acetate is illustrated.

Androgens enlarge the penis and scrotum at the time of puberty. Testosterone causes the male accessory glands (prostate, seminal vesicles, bulbourethral glands) to function and produce seminal fluid. During puberty the growth of the scrotum, epididymus, vas deferens, seminal vesicles, prostate, and penis is dependent upon androgen.

ACCESSORY GLANDS

The **male accessory glands and organs** are the epididymus, vas deferens, the seminal vesicles, bulbourethral (Cowper's) gland, the prostate, and the ejaculatory duct. These structures are specialized for sperm storage and transport. The epididymus is a 20-foot long tube compressed into a mass that stores sperm. The vas deferens is a tube with muscles that help to move sperm. The seminal vesicles and prostate glands secrete the "vehicle" to carry the sperm.

Sperm from the seminiferous tubules enter the rete testis (plural, retia) which is a network of anastamosing ducts. From the rete testis, the sperm enter to the epididymus. The **epididymus** is a single duct into which the sperm are transported by the action of cilia, fluid pressure, and efferent ductule contraction. It takes the sperm 12 days to wend through the epididymus during which time they develop the capacity for fertiliza-

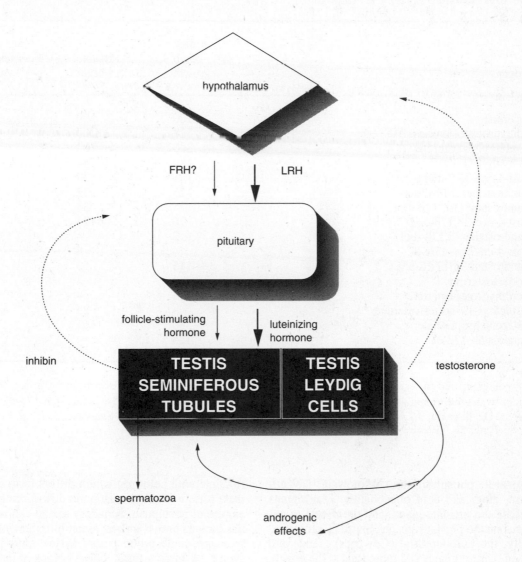

Figure 17.9 The diagram illustrates feedback regulation in the male reproductive system.

tion. The epididymus serves as a sperm storage site. When the sperm leave the epididymus, they traverse the vas deferens. Both vas deferens are severed during vasectomy. The tubes move sperm by peristalsis.

   Seminal vesicles produce 60% of the seminal fluid. They secrete the fluid into the ejaculatory duct and contribute fructose, phosphorylcholine, ergothioneine, ascorbic acid, flavins, and

prostaglandins. The prostaglandins were named because they were found in semen and thought to come from the prostate gland, but instead, the seminal vesicles are the major source. Androgens stimulate seminal vesicle secretion. Next in the journey of the sperms are the ejaculatory ducts which terminate in the prostatic urethra.

   The **prostate gland** secretes more fluid (20%) as well as spermine, citric acid,

Table 17.4 Relative Potency of Androgens

Androgen	Chick comb growth	Prostate weight	Seminal vesicle weight
testosterone	100	100	100
5-α-dihydrotestosterone (DHT)	228	268	158
17-α-methyltestosterone	300	103	100
17-α-methyl-5α-DHT	480	254	78
androst-4-ene-3,17-dione	121	39	17
5-α-androstane-3, 17-dione	115	33	13
5-α-androstane-3α, 17ß-diol	75	34	24
androst-4-ene-3ß,17ß-diol	76	124	133
5-α-androstane-3ß,17ß-diol	2	–	10
androst-4-en-3-on-17α-ol	–	8	2
5-α-androstan-3α-ol-17-one	115	53	8
19-nortestosterone	86	–	10
19-nordihydrotestosterone	118	–	–
17-α-methyl-19-nortestosterone	–	25	25
testosterone proprionate	380	161	146
5-α-androstan-17ß-ol	128	–	–

Potency is compared to testosterone whose value is arbitrarily set equal to 100. Tests on rats are by injection; inunction was used to apply the test substance in the comb test on chicks. DHT = 5-α-androstan-17ß-ol-3-one. Turner, C.D.; Bagnara, J.T. Endocrinology, Sixth Edition. Philadelphia, PA: W. B. Saunders; 1976; p. 413; and Liao, S.; Fang, S. Vitamins and Hormones 27: 17; 1969.

cholesterol, phospholipids, fibrinolysin, fibrinogenase, zinc, and acid phosphatase. Androgens stimulate the prostate gland, and the effects of androgens on the prostate are augmented by prolactin. Finally, the bulbourethral (Cowper's) glands and urethral (Littre) glands add more fluid to the semen. Androgens stimulate the bulbourethral glands.

SECONDARY SEXUAL CHARACTERISTICS

The male secondary sexual characteristics include those features that are associated with maleness, or virility. They vary depending on the species. Human secondary sex characteristics include larynx morphology, hair (axillary, chest, anal, pubic hair), body conformation (e.g., enlarged shoulder muscles), thickened skin sebaceous gland activity, and sex drive (sexual activity, libido). The male escutcheon is the male pattern of pubic hair (triangle with point up) which differs from the female pattern (triangle with point down). Some examples of nonhuman secondary sexual characteristics include horns, antlers, avian bill pigmentation, plumage, male brood patch, syrinx morphology (voice of birds), turtle claws, black thumbs of frogs, swordfish fins, and breeding behavior.

TARGETS OF THE ANDROGENS

As mentioned, males have "secondary sex characteristics" which depend on androgens, but which do not participate in actual semen production and transport. The virilizing effects of androgens appear at the time of puberty.

The **skeletal muscle growth** is stimulated by androgens. This function of androgens accounts for the more muscular bodies of males.

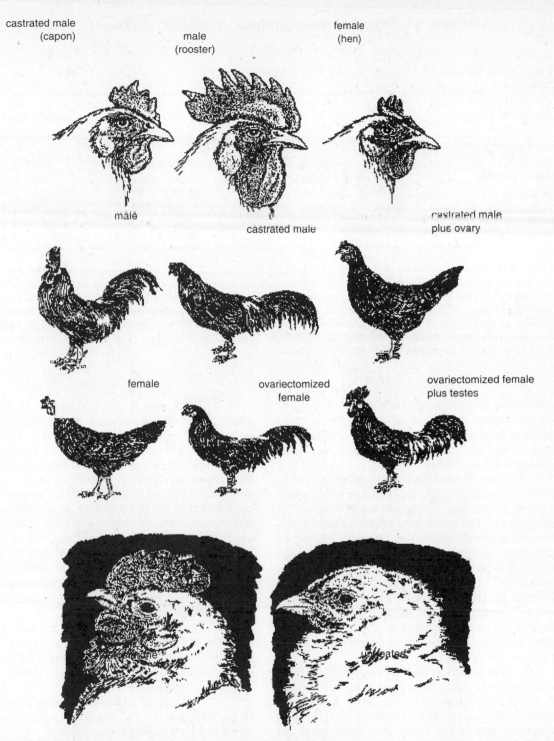

Figure 17.10 Reproductive hormones affect the appearance of fowl. The top row shows the heads of White Leghorn adult birds. Modified, with permission. Turner, C.D.; Bagnara, J. Endocrinology, Sixth Edition. Philadelphia, PA: W. B. Saunders; 1976; p. 423. The middle two rows show normal birds on the left, castrated birds in the center, and birds with gonads transplanted from the opposite gender on the right. Modified, with permission. Welty, J.C. The Life of Birds, Third Edition. Philadelphia: Saunders College Publishing; 1982; pp. 167–168. In summary, the presence of male characteristics such as enlarged combs, correlated positively with the presence of the testes or the administration of testosterone.

Table 17.5 Castration, Vasectomy, and Testosterone Therapy

Treatment group	Testes	Prostate	Seminal vesicles
intact	3010 ± 130	512 ± 85	841 ± 80
sham controls	3110 ± 98	457 ± 57	695 ± 63
castrated	–	202 ± 51	311 ± 52
vasectomized	2354 ± 207	362 ± 70	909 ± 116
castrated, testosterone	–	462 ± 79	1020 ± 167

The data in the table are weights in milligrams (± SEM) for organs of male albino laboratory rats. The data were collected one week after the operations were performed in the experimental groups. Sham controls had the entire castration operation except for the actual removal of the testes. Castration significantly reduced prostate and seminal vesicle size. The prostate and seminal vesicles of vasectomized rats were not significantly different from normal. Testosterone propionate, dissolved in oil vehicle (0.5 mg/day), was injected into a group of castrated rats; the replacement therapy maintained the prostate and seminal vesicle sizes. The endocrine experiment was done by a class of the author's endocrinology students.

Androgens also produce a pubertal "growth spurt" by stimulating the growth of the epiphyseal cartilaginous plates of the **bones**.[22] By affecting the muscles and bones, the androgens cause male body conformation to emerge. The skeletal muscles lack 5-α reductase, so the effects of testosterone must be direct. Paradoxically, the androgens also stop growth by causing the epiphyses to fuse in the long bones. The word "**anabolism**" is used to describe the growth-promoting effects of androgens and other compounds, so that is the reason for the term "anabolic steroids" (growth-promoting steroids). The androgens increase the synthesis and decrease the breakdown of protein.

Androgens stimulate growth of the **larynx**. The consequence of this stimulation is deepening of the voice. In birds there is a similar effect on the syrinx.

The skin is an androgen target. Male body **hair patterns** differ from the patterns of females in the pubic region, under the arms, on the face (beard and mustache), on the chest, on the abdomen, and on the back. Androgens stimulate the production of the male hair pattern and also stimulate the sebaceous glands of skin. Paradoxically, androgens also initiate baldness (alopecia). However, for androgen-induced baldness to occur, the individual must have inherited a genetic predisposition.

The **brain** is also a target of the androgens. While endocrinologists tend to waltz carefully around this subject, they variously attribute aspects of aggression and libido to androgens. Endocrinologists are more comfortable discussing the behavioral effects of androgens in nonhuman animals. For example, among "aggressive" behaviors they list perch calling, male dominance, and dominant mating behavior in birds. Castration usually eliminates the "aggressive" animal behaviors. Areas of the nervous system of some species have been identified as possible sites of androgen action, for example, the preoptic-anterior hypothalamus (AHPOA) of dove brains which regulates breeding behaviors.

The **kidney** is a target of the androgens. Mouse males have kidneys with different ultrastructure (different mitochondria and lysosomes in proximal tubules) and enzyme activities (lysosomal hydroxylases, cytochrome C oxidase).

Androgens stimulate **erythropoiesis**. In the bone marrow, red blood cell progenitors respond to 5-ß androgens and progestins.

In animals, observable changes in appearance related to the integument (skin) are a consequence of androgens. Skin coloration in fish and birds changes during the breeding season and the pigment changes usually involve changes in hormones. The nuptial pad formation in male am-

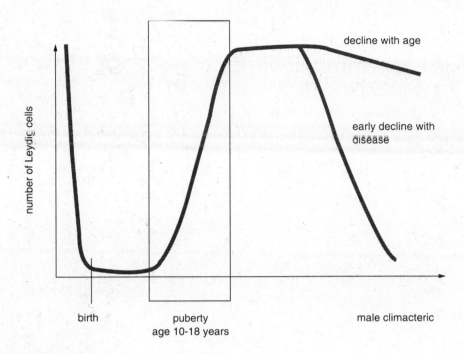

Figure 17.11 The graph illustrates the variation in Leydig cell populations over the course of the male human life.

phibians aids them in grasping the female during the mating act (amplexus). The bills of male house sparrows blacken with melanin during the breeding season. Antlers are another feature that exhibits a seasonal rhythm. Each year, testosterone stimulates loss of antler velvet, rutting odor, and growth of the neck mane in deer. The testosterone is controlled by day length (photoperiod). Birds also form brood patches. Feathers are lost from the abdomen and the skin changes to facilitate the transfer of heat from parents to incubating eggs. Several hormones participate in brood patch formation including estrogens, androgens, and prolactin.

Erection and ejaculation are viewed as events controlled by the brain. Erection is achieved by dilating the penis arterioles while compressing the veins so that the penis fills with blood. Erotic stimuli perceived by the brain are integrated in the spinal cord to cause efferent parasympathetic fibers of the pelvic splanchnic nerves to release transmitters (ACH, VIP) causing vasodilation. Ejaculation

involves several spinal reflexes. Afferent impulses from touch receptors in the glans penis are conveyed to the spinal cord by the internal pudendal nerves. The upper lumbar spinal cord integrates the signals and causes the hypogastric nerves to contract the smooth muscles of the vasa deferentia and seminal vesicles which moves the semen into the urethra. A second spinal reflex involving the upper sacral and lower lumbar spinal cord causes repeated 0.8-second contractions of the skeletal bulbocavernosus muscle to move the semen through the urethra. Sympathetic vasoconstriction terminates erection. Androgens are not viewed as playing a role in these events as they occur, but the androgens may function in the development of the spinal nervous apparatus for controlling penile reflexes.

RECEPTORS AND ANTIANDROGENS

Androgen receptors have been studied (e.g., in the intact human lymph node carcinoma of

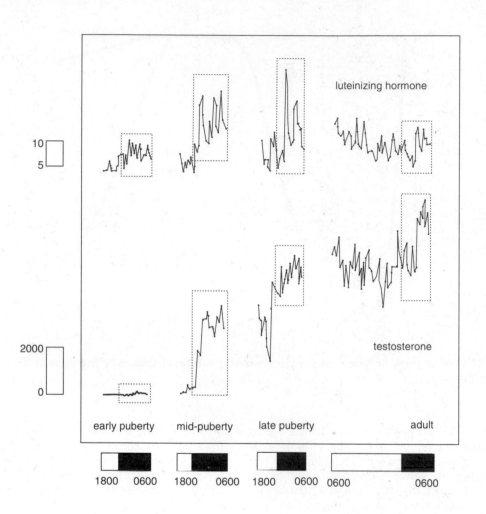

Figure 17.12 The graphs show the rhythms in LH and testosterone during puberty and in adult human males. The vertical bars on the left indicated 2000 pg/ml testosterone and 5 mIU/ml of luteinizing hormone (LH). The horizontal bars below the record are 12-hours long for the stages of puberty and 24-hours long for adults. The black bars and broken line boxes enclose the night time. Modified, with permission. Judd, H.L. Biorhythms of gonadotropins and testicular hormone secretion. In Krieger, D.T., editor. Endocrine Rhythms. New York: Raven Press; 1979; p. 305.

the prostate).[23] Synthetic compounds (cyproterone, cyproterone acetate = CTA) have been used to produce "chemical castration" (Figure 17.8). These compounds act on targets and prevent androgen from expressing its activity. The probable mechanism for the antiandrogens is competition with testosterone for receptor sites. In the prostate, CTA antagonizes formation of DHT-

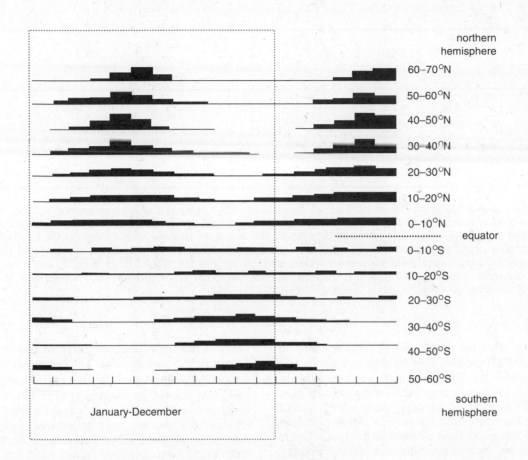

Figure 17.13 The graph shows the timing of breeding seasons of birds relative to north and south latitude. The lines represent different latitudes. The heights of the bars are proportional to the number of species that produce eggs during the month of the year at that latitude. The horizontal axis is time in months with 18 months shown beginning in January on the left and ending in June on the right. Note how the breeding season is reversed in northern versus southern temperate latitudes. The breeding season is spread throughout the year in latitudes near the equator. Modified, with permission. Baker, J.R. The relation between latitude and breeding season in birds. Proc. of the Zoological Society of London, Series A 108: 557–582; 1938.

receptor proteins. The compounds have been controversial for their use in treating sexual deviates among the prison and priestly populations.[24]

REGULATION OF THE TESTIS

Models for the regulation of the testis include feedback inhibition (Figure 17.9). The models usually include two feedback loops which may function separately.

In the model for regulation of testosterone, the hypothalamus secretes **LRH**. Luteinizing hormone, **LH**, was named for its function in the female, but it has another name, which was given for its function in males—interstitial cell-stimulating hormone. LRH causes the anterior pituitary gland to secrete LH. The LH causes the Leydig cells to produce testosterone. Testosterone acts on targets and feeds back negatively on the hypothalamus.

Table 17.6 Photoperiod Modifies Testis Size in Sparrows

Treatment	DD constant dark	LD6:18 short days	LD16:8 long days
blind	17 ± 20	15 ± 12	404 ± 106
unoperated		10 ± 4	426
initial control		7 ± 4	

Sparrows (house sparrows, *Passer domesticus*) were treated with surgery and with environmental lighting. DD = constant dark; LD6:18 is a short photoperiod with six hours of light per day; LD16:8 is a long photoperiod with 16 hours of light per day. Except for initial controls, the data were obtained after 61 days in the lighting regimens. The experiment shows that the sparrows were able to respond to lengthening photoperiod and that the sparrows have extraretinal light perception. Values are mean weights for pairs of testes in milligrams ± one standard deviation. Menaker, M.; Keatts, H. Extraretinal light perception in the sparrow, II. Photoperiodic stimulation of testicular growth. Proc. Nat. Acad. Sci. 60: 146–151; 1968.

A more controversial feedback loop involves **FSH** produced by the pituitary gland. FSH stimulates the Sertoli cells to produce **inhibin**. Inhibin feeds back negatively on the pituitary gland to inhibit FSH production. Molecular structures have been proposed for several inhibins obtained from the antral fluid of ovarian follicles. The inhibins are various combinations of three polypeptide subunits, two of which are similar to transforming growth factor-ß (TGFß). The subunits alone stimulate FSH secretion. Some models incorporate a hypothetical FSH-RH, but it has not been found and LRH causes the pituitary to secrete both FSH and LH.

LRH is intriguing because it has been proposed as a "natural aphrodisiac."

BIOASSAYS FOR ANDROGENS

Bioassays of androgens can be used to illustrate the relative potency of various natural and synthetic androgens (Table 17.4)

Comb's of domestic fowl are used to bioassay testosterone. Testosterone (or unknown) is dissolved in oil and either injected into the birds or rubbed directly on the combs (inunction). The area of the comb size or comb weight can be used as a measure of amount of hormone.

The importance of barnyard fowl to endocrinology should not be underestimated. According to Hadley,[25] the first endocrinological study was done by Berthold in 1849.[26] The experiment involved ablation which caused a deficit and replacement therapy which restored function. Berthold observed that removing both testes (castration) from cockerels (young male fowl) resulted in their failure to develop the comb and wattles characteristic of roosters (Figure 17.10). Moreover, the castrated males lacked interest in hens, had weak crows, fought listlessly compared to normal roosters, and generally did not behave as males. Transplanting testes (of the same or different bird) into the abdomen of castrated animals restored normal male behavior and normal combs and wattles. This meant that the testes did not require anatomical connections (i.e. nerves) to produce their masculinzing effects. Hadley summarizes: "Berthold concluded that the testes secreted something that conditioned the blood, and he speculated that the blood then acted on the body of the cockerel to cause the development of male characteristics."[27]

Bioassays involving rodent reproductive systems involve measuring the effects of androgens on ventral prostate or seminal vesicle weight (Table 17.5). Androgen causes increases in prostate and

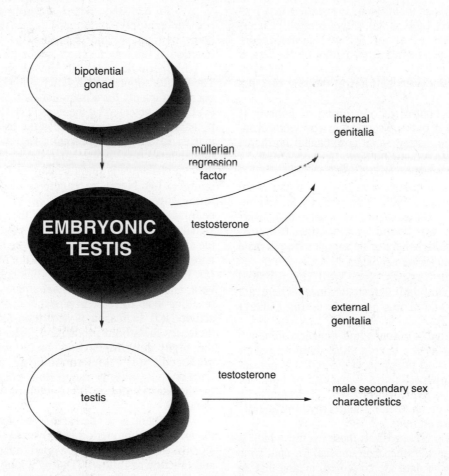

Figure 17.14 The diagram illustrates the hormonal control of the development of the anatomy of the male reproductive system. Müllerian regression factor prevents the formation of female internal genitalia by causing the müllerian ducts to regress.

seminal vesicle weights. Castration by surgical removal of both testes results in reduced prostate and seminal vesicle weights.

LIFE CYCLE, SIX-WEEK CYCLE, DAILY RHYTHM, AND EPISODIC RELEASE

The reproductive system is an endocrine system where cyclic changes are particularly noticeable. Cyclic changes in endocrine reproductive function attracted endocrinologists to seek and find cyclic changes in other endocrine systems.

Testicular function has a **life cycle.** Testicular function changes with age in both non-human animals and man. Testicular function can be measured by the number of Leydig cells (Figure 17.11) which is high in developing embryos but drops by the time of birth to low levels. The onset of reproductive maturation is called "puberty." Puberty occurs in all male animals. In humans it happens between ages 10 and 15 years of age.[28] During puberty, the number of Leydig cells increases for about four years. From that time, the Leydig cell numbers plateau or slowly decline with age. Cessation, or decline in, male reproductive function has been called the male climacteric. Testosterone exhibits great variability in human males over the course of their lives.

LRH, as mentioned, is secreted in a pulsatile pattern. LRH is naturally secreted in intermittent pulses of about 1 per 3 hours before puberty and the rate increases to about 1 per hour at the time of puberty. Puberty can be induced in monkeys with pulses of LRH at the rate of 1 per hour.[29]

The control of the timing of puberty is not established, but as discussed in a previous chapter, melatonin, acting as an antigonadal hormone, may function to prevent puberty from occurring.

The question has been asked as to whether human males have any cycles that are similar to the monthly menstrual cycles possessed by female human beings. The evidence is scanty, but a **six-week cycle** was found in the urine 17-ketosteroids in a study where urine samples from a male were collected for sixteen years.[30]

Daily cycles are well established rhythms in circulating testosterone. There are rhythms in luteinizing hormone during puberty (Figure 17.12).

Steroid hormones and gonadotropins are also noteworthy for having short duration peaks. When these short peaks occur, secretion is considered to be "**pulsatile**," as if packets of hormone were being periodically released. If the pulsatile peaks are rhythmic, then ultradian rhythms (shorter than a day) are present.

The presence of all these cycles, which is becoming typical rather than unusual for endocrine system as more data are collected, means that an endocrine parameter, such as the amount of testosterone, is not held constant, and that a single measurement is insufficient for an understanding of the function.

SEASONAL CYCLES

In humans and some other animals, breeding is continuous, a year round event. But in many species, the testis is an organ with a marked annual cycle, or seasonal cycles, in many species of animals (**seasonal breeders**). In many species, for example in hamsters, seasonal rhythm of reproductive function is controlled by the length of light in the day. Functions that are subject to control by daylength (or nightlength) are **photoperiodic**. William Rowan concluded, based on pioneering experiments with testis size of juncoes, that "daily increases of illumination are conducive to developmental changes in the sexual organs."[31]

In hamsters, which are **long day breeders** for example, photoperiods greater than 12 hours of light per day stimulate the growth and function of the testes. The neuroendocrine control of photoperiodic reproduction has been studied. The results support the following hypothetical sequence of events for a mammal such as a hamster: (1) Light is detected by the eyes. (2) The retinohypothalamic nerve tract conveys the lighting information to the suprachiasmatic region of the hypothalamus. (3) A circadian biological clock in the hypothalamus is stimulated by dark or inhibited by light. (4) Nerve tracts convey the information to the superior cervical ganglia. (5) Adrenergic neurons whose cell bodies are in the ganglia send signals via the nervii conarii to the pineal gland. If the signal is "dark," then the nerve endings release norepinephrine from terminals in the pineal gland. (6) Pinealocytes respond to norepinephrine with a beta adrenergic cAMP mechanism of action, resulting in an increase in pineal N-acetyltranferase activity. (7) Increasing N-acetyltransferase activity increases melatonin production. The duration of the night determines how much melatonin is produced. (8) Melatonin is an antigonadal hormone, it inhibits the testes, possibly via a mechanism involving the regulation of pituitary prolactin.

There is a "**duration hypothesis**" for the way that photoperiod is converted to endocrine signals. Photoperiod is converted to testicular size and function as follows: During a long night (e.g., 16 hours of dark, LD8:16), lengthy melatonin production inhibits the testes. During a short night (e.g., 8 hours of dark, LD16:8), less melatonin is produced and the testes grow and function. As the seasons of the year progress, the hamsters develop large active testes (testicular recrudescence) in the spring and their testes become small and quiescent in the fall. The cycle repeats year after year. It is a natural, reversible method of seasonal birth control used by seasonal breeders.

In the fall, the gonads regress in response to long nights. However, if long nights are maintained, **spontaneous recrudescence** occurs. In other words, the animals become insensitive to light. There is a "**refractory period**" which must pass before the system again becomes sensitive to the inhibitory effect of long nights.

The description is for long day breeders. Long day, or spring breeders, include most animals: birds, horses, donkeys, ferrets, cats, raccoons. But there are also fall, or short day, breeding animals: sheep, goats, badgers, grey seals, and deer. In equatorial zones, some species breed all year round (Figure 17.13). Nonetheless, even in the Galapagos, where photoperiod varies annually by only 18 minutes, some animals are seasonal breeders such as the sea lions.

Seasonal reproductive cycles, like many other annual rhythms, have been shown to depend upon an inherent annual clock.[32] The clock for **circannual rhythms** can be influenced by environmental factors; possibly it can be entrained by annual photoperiodic changes. Social isolation reduces the period length of the testicular size cycle in starlings. Moreover, subjecting organisms to unusual light-dark regimens whose period length is not 24 hours can alter the length of their rhythms. For example, the starling testicular cycle can be shortened to as little as 2.4 months.

In animals that possess **extraretinal light perception**, such as birds, photoperiod can exert its effects in the absence of the eyes (Table 17.6). Pineal photoreceptors may participate in the nonretinal light detection, but experiments have indicated that there are yet other unidentified extraretinal light receptors (ERRs) localized in the head region.[33]

The question arises as to whether there are seasonal cycles in the reproductive function of human males. In this regard, it has been pointed out that there are seasonal cycles of conception and birth. Anecdotes about early Eskimos living in arctic photoperiodic extremes tell of a phenomenon, "furor sexualis," that recurred with the lengthening days of springtime.

Not all of the issues in seasonal breeders are resolved by the melatonin hypothesis. There may be pineal antigonadal hormones other than melatonin. Temperature may contribute to the detection of changes in season in lizards. The location of the extraretinal receptor is not established. The eyes make melatonin which may contribute to the control of seasonal breeding.

MÜLLERIAN-INHIBITING SUBSTANCE

In both genders, the primitive gonad develops from the genital ridge (Figure 17.14). The cortical region of the gonad becomes a testis during weeks seven and eight of gestation. TDF (testis-determining factor) from a gene on the short arm of the Y chromosome is necessary for the development of the testis from the bipotential gonad. When the testis develops, the Leydig cells appear. The Leydig cells produce testosterone and the Sertoli cells produce müllerian regression factor (MRF, MIS = müllerian-inhibiting substance). The factor is a protein related to inhibin that has 535 amino acids.

MRF causes the müllerian ducts to regress on the side it is secreted. Testosterone causes development of the male genitalia. In some species, the brain is a target of androgens. In rats, for example, the presence of androgens during the first few days after birth results in (1) the development of the male behavioral sex pattern and (2) the male pattern of hypothalamic gonadotropin secretion after puberty.

SPERM TRANSPORT, CAPACITATION, AND COPULATORY PLUGS

Several hormones increase the motility of the female reproductive tract (e.g., oxytocin and nonapeptides, prostaglandins, catecholamines). It is possible that contractions produce rapid transport of sperm in the female system in this manner. However, the contractions are expulsive rather than propulsive so that this possibility, however intriguing, may not work. Also arguing against a role for oxytocin is the fact that hypophysectomy does not affect the pregnancy rate of rodents.

Sperm gain their ability to be mobile as they pass through the epididymus and the female reproductive tract. The improvements of sperm performance in the female reproductive tract appear to be due to substances in the fluids in the female reproductive tract which improve the attraction of sperm and ova. The change in the sperm resulting from their sojourn in the female reproductive tract is called "sperm capacitation."

Following mating, rodent semen coagulates forming a copulatory plug in the vagina of the female. The copulatory plug remains for a day or so. Females can be visually examined for the presence of the copulatory plugs as evidence that copulation has taken place.

MALE CONTRACEPTION

Condoms provide a barrier method of contraception that can be used by males. Condoms work by simply preventing sperm from entering the female reproductive tract. There are also biological methods of male birth control.

The only biological method of male contraception in wide use is sterilization by vasectomy. Vasectomy is a surgical procedure in which the two vasa deferentia are cut and/or ligated. Since vasectomy does not remove the testes, the testes are still able to function and produce male hormones. In some but not all cases the operation is reversible. Ganong gives a reversibility rate of 50% as measured by subsequent pregnancies.[34] About 50% of vasectomized men develop antibodies to their own spermatozoa which may be a factor in the reversibility of the operation. After the operation, sperms are still made for years, but they cannot get to the exterior so they degenerate and are resorbed. Variations in human libido have been reported after vasectomy, and increased libido and aggressiveness have been reported in vasectomized bulls.

Theoretically, chemical and endocrine methods of male contraception should be possible. Antiandrogens (e.g., cyproterone acetate) produce chemical castration by acting as androgenic receptor antagonists. An inhibitor of androgen-synthesizing enzymes could be used. Immunological castration could be achieved with antibodies to testosterone, gonadotropins, or LRH. LRH receptor antagonists or inhibin could be used. Gossypol, a phenolic chemical from the cotton plant, inhibits lactate dehydrogenase (LDH isozyme) of sperm cells. But none of these have so far produced a widely usable male contraceptive method.

CLINICAL ASPECTS OF MALE ENDOCRINOLOGY

Malnutrition and **vitamin B deficiency** have similar effects in man and experimental animals—the male accessory organs involute (as they do after castration or hypophysectomy) which is attributed to hypofunction of the Leydig cells.[35]

The consequences of deficiencies of Leydig cells is deficient androgenic production (hypogonadism). When castration or Leydig cell deficiency (due to deficiencies of LRH, LH, or FSH) starts in childhood, **eunuchoidism** occurs. Typically, eunuchs are tall because androgen is needed to close the epiphyses of the bones. They have narrow shoulders, small muscles, feminized body configuration, small genitalia, underdeveloped prostate glands, anosmia, high-pitched voices, nonpigmented scrotum without rugal folds, sparse axillary hair, and female pubic hair distribution (triangle with the base up).

The consequences of Leydig cell deficiency are less drastic if the hypogonadism occurs after puberty. Castrated men experience loss of libido, hot flashes, irritability, passivity, and depression. But the voice remains low and the secondary sex characteristics regress only slowly.

Hormone replacement therapies involving LRH, LH, FSH, and androgens are used to treat deficiencies in male reproductive function. HCG (3000 to 4000 I.U. injected intramuscularly three times a week for three months) has been used to stimulate puberty onset in cases of delayed puberty. If spermatogenesis is a goal of the treatment, then HCG or LH are not sufficient, but instead FSH (or menotropins which contain high levels of LH and FSH) are required.

Hypergonadism can result from androgen-secreting tumors. Precocious pseudopuberty is one consequence. However, Leydig cell tumors are rare. Apparently, excess testosterone is not viewed as a medical problem (!). Ganong says about male hypergonadism: "Hyperfunction of the testes in the absence of tumor formation is not a recognized entity. Androgen-secreting testicular tumors are rare and cause detectable endocrine symptoms only in prepuberal boys, who develop precocious pseudopuberty."[36]

Males can suffer from anomalies of the sex chromosomes. A **chromosome anomaly** (XXY, XXXY, XXYY, XXXXY) that is a common cause of male hypogonadism is **Klinefelter's syndrome**, in which the individual has an extra X chromosome (0.2% of male live births). The defect shows up during puberty where the testes do not develop seminiferous tubules and the Leydig cells are abnormal. Symptoms may include gynecomastia (breast development), low testosterone, elevated FSH and LH, azoospermia, delayed puberty, diminished hair growth, eunuchoid personality characteristics, abnormal growth of lower extremities, lack of ambition, difficulty in maintaining permanent employment, rambling conversations, and mental retardation. Treatments include androgen therapy and mastectomy (for gynecomastia).

Investigators have suggested that there are more **XYY** individuals (4 times the normal population in prison populations and 20 times normal in combined penal-mental institutions) associated sometimes with symptoms of taller than normal

Table 17.7 Symptoms of Prostate Enlargement or Anabolic Steroids

Benign prostate hypertrophy	Excess synthetic steroids
bladder outlet obstruction	prostate hypertrophy
progressive urinary frequency	cholesterstatic jaundice
urination urgency	hepatoma (liver tumor)
nocturia (frequent night urination)	premature epiphyseal fusion
decreased size and force of urine stream	water retention
sensations of incomplete emptying	hypertension
terminal dribbling	erythrocytocis
almost continuous overflow	inhibition of spermatogenesis
incontinence	gynecomastia (breast enlargement)
complete urinary retention	acne
enlarged prostate (rectal examination)	aggressive behavior
renal failure	changes in thyroid function
urinary tract infections (burning urination, chills, fever)	changes in adrenal function
azotemia (excess blood nitrogen, uremia; retention of excretory products in blood due to failure to excrete them)	priapism (persistent penile erection usually without desire)

Prostate hypertrophy is found by age 50 in half of human males and by age 80 in 100% of human males.

height, aggressive behavior, mental retardation, and/or bad acne; however, these results are controversial. XYY occurs in 1/1000 male live births.

During development, the testes normally descend from abdominal position to scrotal position. When the testes do not descend, the term used is **cryptorchidism**. In 1/20,000 males there are no testes (bilateral anorchia). About 3% of full-term males have cryptorchidism at birth, but the testes descend spontaneously during the first year so that the incidence of cryptorchidism is 0.2–0.8% by age one year. The condition is treated with surgery and hormone therapy (HCG).

Endocrinologists have sought endocrine causes for human sexual preferences (e.g., **homosexuality**) and human sexual behavior. Fetal androgens may play a role in preparing the brain for later sexual activity. The Merck Manual states: "Some support for this hypothesis is to be found in the higher-than-expected prevalence of homosexual fantasies and behavior in men and women whose mothers received diethylstilbestrol (DES) during pregnancy."[37] According to the same source, homosexuality occurs in about 5% of the male population. Scott F. Gilbert discusses the development of sexual behaviors:

> When newborn male rats are castrated [they] display female sexual behaviors such as lordosis when they mature. Conversely, when newborn female rats are given a single dose of testosterone during the neonatal period, they develop masculine endocrine and sexual behaviors. . . . . [M]asculine behavior patterns could be permanently induced with a single dose of the female sex hormone estradiol [giving rise to] the conversion hypothesis [where estrogen, which can be derived from testosterone in males, is responsible for defeminization]. Neonatal estradiol appears to be responsible for 'defeminizing' the brain, whereas the actual masculinization of behavior is probably due to testosterone or dihydrotestosterone [so that] the development of the male nervous system involves both defeminizing and masculinizing steps...Extrapola-

ting from rats to humans is a risky business, as no stereotypic sex-specific human behavior has yet been identified. What is 'masculine' behavior in one society may be 'feminine' behavior in another (much to the embarrassment of naive travelers). Although the popular press publicizes research that finds biologically determined differences in skills or behaviors between the sexes, these papers have been widely criticized. Moreover, the overlap in behaviors precludes these from being considered sex-specific.[38]

Less well known deleterious effects on male reproductive endocrinology may be associated with drug and substance abuse. Athletes, especially weight lifters, have taken to using **anabolic steroids** to increase weight and muscle gain. However, androgen therapy can have adverse effects (Table 17.7). Lowered testosterone and gynecomastia have been reported as side effects of long term use of **marihuana** (cannabis). **Alcoholism** is listed among the causes of male impotence.[39] Other causes of impotence that may have endocrine components are low testosterone and drugs that may affect hormones (hypertensives, sedatives, tranquilizers, amphetamines). The common view expressed in the *Merck Manual* that male impotence is "almost always due to intrapsychic factors" has not spurred research on the effects of alcohol on the reproductive system.

A usual concomitant of aging in male humans is the enlargement of the prostate gland. Bladder outlet obstruction symptoms derive from such **benign prostate hypertrophy** (BPH). BPH is common in men and is found in about 20% of men >60 years old in an unreferred medical clinic; the incidence in patients visiting a urologist is higher yet, >50%.[40] The etiology of BPH is unknown, but it is possible that the endocrine changes in association with aging are involved.[41] About 122,000 cases of prostate adenocarcinoma were estimated for the USA in 1991 with a history of increases in each decade. Here again, the etiology is not known but is suspected to be hormone related.[42]

Puberty can occur too early or too late. Children with precocious puberty have been treated successfully with a long-acting analogue of LRH (once daily, subcutaneous injections, 4 µg/kg of body weight). LRH analogue treatment reverses premature sexual development, slows rapid growth, and delays skeletal maturation. By preventing early epiphyseal closure, the treated children are expected to attain normal adult heights. The treatment is believed to work because the LRH is not pulsatile and the gonadotropin release is inhibited.[43]

REFERENCES

1. Norman, A.; Litwack, G. Hormones. Orlando, FL: Academic Press; 1987; pp. 184–185.

2. Conn, P.M.; Crowley, W.F. Gonadotropin-releasing hormone and its analogues. The New England Journal of Medicine 324: 93–103; 1991.

3. Hazum, E.; Conn, P.M. Molecular mechanism of gonadotropin releasing hormone (GnRH) action: I. The GnRH receptor. Endocrine Reviews 9: 379–386; 1988.

4. Braden, T.D.; Conn, M.P. Altered rate of synthesis of gonadotropin-releasing hormone receptors: Effects of homologous hormone appear independent of extracellular calcium. Endocrinology 126: 2577–2582; 1990.

5. Braden, T.D.; Farnworth, P.G.; Burger, H.G.; Conn, P.M. Regulation of the synthetic rate of gonadotropin-releasing hormone receptors in rat pituitary cell cultures by inhibin. Endocrinology 127: 2387–2392; 1990.

6. Huckle, W.R., Conn, P.M. Molecular mechanism of gonadotropin releasing hormone action. II. The effector system. Endocrine Reviews 9: 387–395; 1988.

7. Stojilkovic, S.S.; Catt, K.J. Calcium oscillations in anterior pituitary cells. Endocrine Reviews 13: 256–289; 1992.

8. Naor, Z. Signal transduction mechanisms of Ca2+ mobilizing hormones: The case of gonadotropin-releasing hormone. Endocrine Reviews 11: 326–353; 1990.

9. Janovick, J.A.; Natarajan, K.; Longo, F.; Conn, P.M. Caldesmon: A bifunctional (calmodulin and actin) binding protein which regulates stimulated gonadotropin release. Endocrinology 129: 68–74; 1991.

10. Gharib, S.D.; Wierman, M.E.; Shupnik, M.A.; Chin, W.W. Molecular biology of the pituitary gonadotropins. Endocrine Reviews 11: 177; 1990.

11. Magner, J.A. Thyroid-stimulating hormone: Biosynthesis, cell biology, and bioactivity. Endocrine Reviews 11: 354–385; 1990.

12. Hadley, M. Endocrinology, Second Edition. Englewood Cliffs, NJ: Prentice-Hall; 1988; pp. 100–101.

13. Leung, P.C.K.; Steele, G.L. Intracellular signalling in the gonads. Endocrine Reviews 13: 476–498; 1992.

14. Skinner, M.K. Cell-cell interactions in the testis. Endocrine Reviews 12: 45–77; 1991.

15. Ganong, W. Medical Review of Physiology, Fourteenth Edition. Norwalk, CT: Appleton & Lange; 1989; p. 363.

16. Goldfien, A.; Monroe, S.E. Ovaries. In Greenspan, F.; Forsham, P., editors. Basic and Clinical Endocrinology. Los Altos, CA: Lange Medical Publications; 1986; p. 471.

17. Hammond, G.L. Molecular properties of corticosteroid binding globulin and the sex-steroid binding proteins. Endocrine Reviews 11: 65; 1990.

18. Ganong, W.; Op. cit.; p. 368.

19. Braunstein, G.D. The testes. In Greenspan, F.; Forsham, P., editors. Basic and Clinical Endocrinology. Los Altos, CA: Lange Medical Publications; 1986; p. 360.

20. Sharpe, R.; Skakkebaek, N.E. Are oestrogens involved in falling sperm counts and disorders of the male reproductive tract? The Lancet 341; 1392–1395; 1993.

21. Rittmaster, R.S. Androgen conjugates: Physiology and clinical significance. Endocrine Reviews 14: 121–132; 1993.

22. Bourguignon, J. Linear growth as a function of age at onset of puberty and sex steroid dosage: Therapeutic implications. Endocrine Reviews 9: 467–488; 1988.

23. Ort, E.; Bodwell, J.; Munck, A. Phosphorylation of steroid hormone receptors. Endocrine Reviews 13: 105–129; 1992.

24. Toufexis, A. What to do when priests stray. Time; September 24; 1990; p. 79.

25. Hadley, M. Endocrinology, Second Edition. Englewood Cliffs, NJ: Prentice-Hall; 1988; p. 100–101.

26. Berthold, A. A. Transplantation der Hoden. Arch. Anat. Physiol. Wiss. Med. 16: 42–46; 1965.

27. Hadley, M.; Op. cit.; p. 2.

28. Berkow, R., editor. Merck Manual, Fifteenth Edition. Rahway, NJ: Merck Sharp & Dohme Research Laboratories; 1987; p.1283

29. Bourguigon, J. Time-related neuroendocrine manifestations of puberty: A combined clinical and experimental approach extracted from the 4th Belgian Endocrine Society Lecture. Horm. Res. 30: 224–234; 1988.

30. Luce, G.G. Biological Rhythms in Psychiatry and Medicine. Washington, D.C.: US Government Printing Office; 1970.

31. Rowan, W. Relation of light to bird migration and developmental changes. Nature 115: 494–495; 1925.

32. Gwinner, E. Circannual Rhythms: Endogenous Clocks in the Organization of Seasonal Processes. New York: Springer-Verlag; 1986

33. Underwood, H.; Groos, G. Vertebrate circadian rhythms: Retinal and extraretinal photoreception. Experientia 38: 1013–1021; 1982.

34. Ganong, W.; Op. cit.; p. 366.

35. Turner, C.; Bagnara, J. Endocrinology, Sixth Edition. Philadelphia, PA: W. B. Saunders; 1975, p. 436.

36. Ganong, W.; Op. cit.; p. 370.

37. Berkow, R., editor. Merck Manual, Fifteenth Edition. Rahway, NJ: Merck Sharp & Dohme Research Laboratories; 1987; p. 1501.

38. Gilbert, S.F. Developmental Biology, Second Edition. Sunderland, MA: Sinauer Associates, Inc. Pub.; 1988; p. 759.

39. Berkow, R., editor.; Op. cit.; p. 1655.

40. Wasson, J.H.; Bruskewitz, R.C. Disorders of the lower genitourinary tract: Bladder, prostate, and testicles. In Berkow, R., editor. Merck Manual, Fifteenth Edition. Rahway, NJ: Merck Sharp & Dohme Research Laboratories; 1987; p. 611.

41. Berkow, R. The Merck Manual, Sixteen Edition. Rahway, NJ: Merck & Co.; 1992; p. 1736.

42. Berkow, R.; Ibid.; p. 1750.

43. Gonzalez, E.R. For puberty that comes too soon, new treatment is highly effective. JAMA 248: 1149–1158; 1982.

CHAPTER 18

Estrogens and Progesterone and the Ovary

The female gonads, the ovaies, produce feminizing steroid hormones (estrogens and progestins) and eggs (ova). Female reproduction is characterized by estrous, menstrual, and seasonal cycles. The ovary is regulated by feedback loops involving the pituitary gonadotropins. In addition to its function in female reproductive cycles, the ovary has endocrine functions in pregnancy and lactation.

ENDOCRINOLOGY OF FEMALE REPRODUCTION

The endocrinology of female reproduction is a subject that includes the anatomy of the gonads and associated organs, hormones of the ovary, and the gonadotropins that control them.

The subject of female reproduction is noteworthy for the same multiplicity of cycles—life cycle from menarche to menopause, seasonal cycles, daily cycles, and episodic release—that cause fluctuations in the hormones and the physiological events that they control in males. In addition, in female mammals, there are menstrual or estrous cycles. In this chapter topics are first introduced and then their cyclic nature is revisited in more detail. The chapter ends with a number of topics relating to human female reproduction (libido, menstrual irregularities, oral contraceptives, menopause, abortion, artificial control of ovulation) that involve hormones.

ANATOMY OF FEMALE REPRODUCTIVE SYSTEMS

The human female reproductive system consists of internal and external organs. The human female gonad is the **ovary**. The ovary has two functions: the ovary produces eggs (ova) and the ovary synthesizes hormones. Eggs travel from the ovary through the **oviducts** (Fallopian tubes, uterine tubes) where they are fertilized. When fertilized eggs reach the **uterus** (womb), they implant and development begins. Entrance of sperm and delivery of the offspring from the uterus occurs through the **cervix**. The cervix is at the juncture of the uterus and the **vagina**. All of these organs are internal (Figure 18.1). The vagina ends at the exterior structures (**major labia, minor labia, hymen, clitoris**). The external structures are portrayed in Figure 18.2.

Ovaries are paired in most species, but, in birds, the right ovary and oviduct do not persist into adult life; adult birds have only the left ovary and left oviduct. Reproductive systems of other species have some differences from that in the human. For example, the rat uterus has two uterine horns (Figure 18.3). The internal reproductive systems of female birds, reptiles, amphibians, and fish end externally in the **cloaca**. The cloaca of birds, for example, is a receptacle for the feces from the intestines, a depository for the excretions of the

kidneys through the ureters, and has the genital organs. The dorsal wall of the cloaca contains the bursa of Fabricus which is involved in antibody responses.

ANATOMY OF THE OVARY

The ovarian tissue is made up of the follicles and the stroma. The outer ovarian zone is a cortex containing the follicles and stroma; the remaining ovary is an inner medulla. The histology of the ovary shows the events in the production of ova (Figure 18.4). The outer margin of the mammalian ovary is an ovarian capsule. Immature ova are present in the ovary at birth in individual **primordial follicles**.

The rest of this discussion of the ovarian anatomy applies to adults with time spans referring to women. The ovary goes through changes that have been called the ovarian cycle. The cycle is also discussed later in this chapter in the sections on cyclicity in female reproduction.

During a follicular phase that lasts about two weeks, follicles begin to mature. The **antrum** (a cavity or lumen) forms in the follicle and fills with fluid. A mature follicle is called a **graafian follicle**. The cells that form the walls of the graafian follicle are called the **theca interna**. Follicle enlargement is followed by **ovulation**, the release of the ovum. Ovulation is accomplished by rupturing the follicle. However, ovulation is not supposed to involve the violent burst of the follicle. Instead, an area of the wall of the graafian follicle and overlying ovarian cortex becomes thin by shedding or phagocytosis of cells and loss of capillary blood supply. The resulting thin translucent spot, the stigma, first becomes raised, then tears (possibly with the aid of proteolytic enzymes), and finally releases fluid containing the egg from the follicle. **Atretic follicles** (degenerating follicles) are those that develop but do not ovulate.

Following ovulation, the follicle enters a **luteal phase** that lasts another two weeks. After ovulation, blood fills the follicle and it is called a **corpus hemorrhagicum**. Lower abdominal pain that accompanies ovulation (mittelschmerz, German for middle pain) may be due to minor bleeding from the follicle into the abdomen. The cells that form the follicle (granulosa cells, theca cells) proliferate to fill the follicle with **luteal cells**. The luteal cells are yellow in color and rich

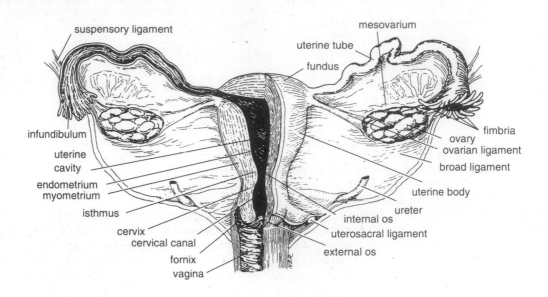

Figure 18.1 Internal anatomy of the reproductive organs of the human female is shown in frontal view. The left side of the diagram has been cut away to show the lumens of the uterine tube (oviduct), uterus (uterine cavity, internal os, cervical canal, external os), and vagina. The organs are suspended by ligaments—the mesovarium ligament attaches the ovary to the broad ligament. The fundus, endometrium, and myometrium are parts of the uterus. Redrawn, with permission. Tortora, G.J.; Anagnostakos; N.P. Principles of Anatomy and Physiology, Sixth Edition; New York: Harper & Row; 1990; p. 894.

in lipids. The corpus luteum persists throughout pregnancy, or, if no pregnancy occurs, the corpus luteum degenerates about ten days after ovulation. Scar tissue replaces the follicle resulting in a white body called the **corpus albicans**.

The newly ovulated ovum rides ciliary currents to enter the oviduct through the fimbria (finger-like projections at the opening to the oviducts which massage the ovary). Cilia in the upper oviduct and muscular peristalsis of the oviduct move the ovum through the oviduct. Fertilization takes place in the oviduct. The embryo is thought to require a sojourn in the oviduct for viability, possibly while the uterus is prepared. In humans, the ovum enters the uterus in 3 days; but in other species, from 2–8 days elapse before the embryo enters the uterus. Implantation, the attachment of the human embryo to the maternal organs in a fixed place, occurs 8–13 days after fertil-

ization. Here again, the time of implantation varies from 4–35 days in different species of animals.

The ovary consists of follicles in which the eggs develop and **stroma**, the interstitial (interfollicular) cells outside the follicles. Preovulatory events and atresia are accompanied by infiltration of the stroma by white blood cells (mast cells). Later in the ovarian cycle, eosinophils and T lymphocytes migrate into the corpus luteum, possibly attracted by a prostaglandin. Noncycling macrophages are a major component of the stroma and are present near the perifollicular capillaries. Adashi has proposed that macrophages communicate with ovarian cells in paracrine "encounters of the third kind" where the macrophages secrete cytokines (IL-1 and TNFa) that act on the ovarian cells as in situ modulators of

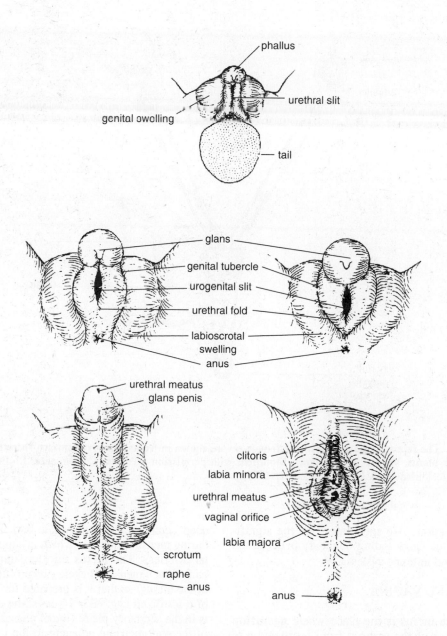

Figure 18.2 The development of human external genitalia is drawn. The diagrams show the "indifferent" (upper), seven-eight–week (middle), and twelve-week (lower) stages. The embryo is initially "bipotential" because it has the possibility of developing into either a male or a female. Redrawn, with permission. Ganong, W. Medical Review of Physiology, Fourteenth Edition. Norwalk: CT: Appleton & Lange; 1989; p. 356.

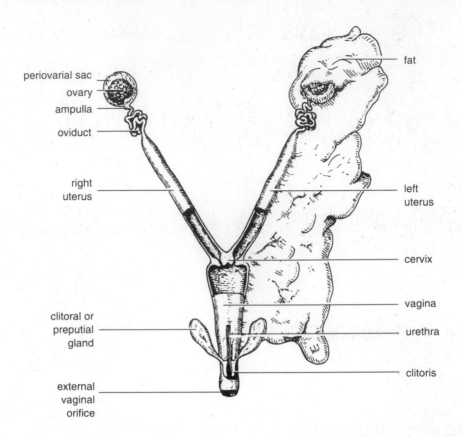

Figure 18.3 The reproductive organs of the female rat are shown in frontal view. Cutaways show the cavities in the bicornate uterus, vagina, and urethra. Modified, with permission. Turner, C.; Bagnara, J. Endocrinology, Sixth Edition. Philadelphia: W. B. Saunders; 1976; p. 471.

ovarian function. He speculates that the significance is in the "now fading boundary between the endocrine and immune systems."[1]

UTERUS AND VAGINA

The uterus is the place where **gestation** (development of the embryo from fertilization to birth) takes place. The anatomical structure of the uterus is not fixed, but varies as its function changes during reproductive cycles and pregnancy in the human (Figure 18.5). The layers that make up the uterine walls, the endometrium, consist of **uterine glands** and **arteries**. The uterus has a deep layer, the stratum basale which is not shed during menstruation and which is supplied by basilar arteries. The uterus thickens during the first half of each menstrual cycle (the proliferative phase of the uterus) so that it is prepared for implantation of a fertilized egg. For 14 days, the endometrium is in the secretory phase (luteal phase). Two thirds of the endometrium adjacent to the uterine lumen are shed during menstruation including the secretory stratum functionale which is supplied by the spiral arteries.

The vaginal histology also varies with the normal changes in reproductive function. Different cells are present and shed in the vagina during dif-

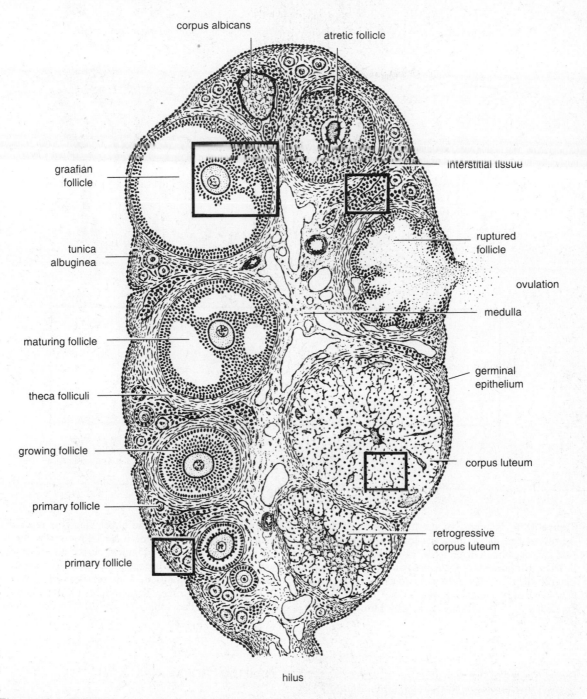

Figure 18.4 The anatomy of the mammalian ovary is shown in an idealized drawing. The follicles are shown in various stages of development with events of the ovarian cycle shown in clockwise sequence beginning lower left near the hilus. Boxes enclose (clockwise from lower left) a primary follicle, the ovum in a graffian follicle, a region of stroma, and luteal cells. Modified, with permission. Turner, C.; Bagnara, J. Endocrinology, Sixth Edition. Philadelphia: W. B. Saunders; 1976; p. 371.

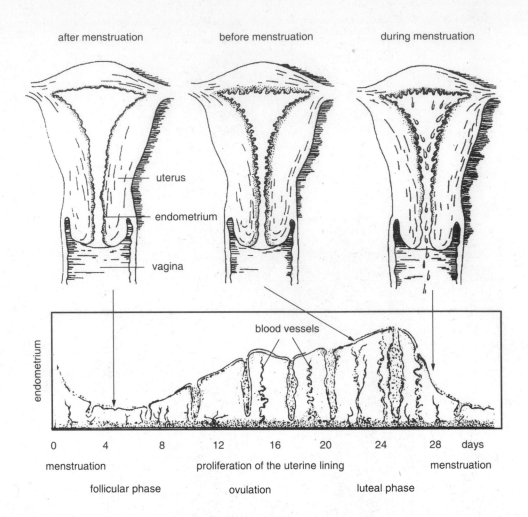

Figure 18.5 Anatomy of the uterus changes during the human menstrual cycle. The upper diagrams represent the uterus and its cavities; the lower diagram represents the endometrium which is the inner lining of the uterus. The endometrium changes (thickness, histology) during the menstrual cycle and is sloughed during menstruation. If fertilization occurs, then menstruation does not follow, and the endometrium becomes secretory (not shown). In this diagram, day zero coincides with the first day of menstruation. Modified, with permission. (Upper) Kogan, B.A. Health: Man in a Changing Environment. Harcourt, Brace, Jovanovich; 1970. (Lower) Postlethwait, S.N. Human Sexuality Minicourse Development Project. Philadelphia, PA: W.B. Saunders; 1976; p. 7.

ferent phases of the reproductive cycle; they can be easily seen in smears of the vaginal lining and fluid as in rodents (Figure 18.6). At times the vagina is thin with a cornified epithelium and at other times the epithelium proliferates and has leucocytes.

OVARIAN HORMONES

The ovary is the source of steroid hormones (estrogens, progestens, androgens) and peptide hormones (relaxin).

Estrogens are synthesized in the ovary

proestrus   estrus

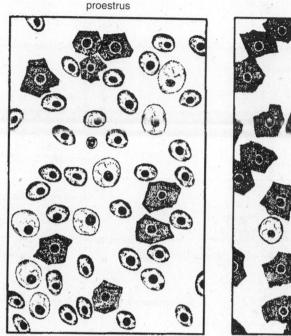
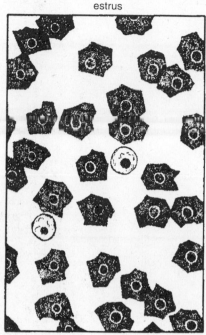

Figure 18.6 Sketches of cells obtained in smears obtained by scraping rodent vaginas (e.g., rats, mice, or hamsters) with a toothpick. The smears representing proestrus and estrus are distinctive and can be easily used to follow rodent female reproductive cycles. (Left) During proestrus, "fried egg" shaped nucleate epithelial cells, which are oval cells with prominent nuclei, are obtained in abundance. The cells stain readily with methylene blue and can be inspected, while still wet, with light microscopy. (Right) During estrus, cornified cells (squames, squamous cells), which may lack nuclei, are observable in the same way. During other phases of the cycle, metestrus and diestrus, fewer cells may be obtained; the cells that are obtained are predominantly leucocytes. Cornified cells also appear in human vaginal smears. The diagrams are reproduced from Sadleir, R.M.F.S. Cycles and seasons. In Austin, C.R.; Short, R.V., editors. Reproduction in Mammals, Book 1: Germ Cells and Fertilization. New York: Cambridge University Press; 1972; page 89.

from cholesterol and cholesteryl esters (Figure 18.7, Table 18.1). The theca interna cells of the follicles, the granulosa cells of the follicles, the corpus luteum, and the placenta secrete estrogens. Estradiol (ß-estradiol, E_2) is the major and most potent estrogen produced. A group of enzymes that makes estrone from androstenedione, and estrogen from testosterone, is called the aromatase system in the microsomal fraction of the cells. The aromatase system catalyzes three steps: (1) hydroxylation of the C19 methyl group, (2) oxidation of the C19 hydroxyl group, and (3) hydroxylation at the 3-α position. In the blood, 17-ß-estradiol and estrone are in equilibrium. Sex hormone-binding globulin carries 37% of circulating estradiol, 60% rides on serum albumen, and 3% circulates free.

LH stimulates theca interna cell enzymes that synthesize androstenedione from cholesterol. The LH effect is via LH receptors on the theca interna cells and a cyclic AMP mechanism. The theca cells secrete circulating estradiol. The androgens from the theca cells enter the granulosa cells; the granulosa cells then make estradiol from the androgens and secrete the estradiol into the follicular fluid. So the antral fluid estrogens come from granulosa cells, whereas blood estrogens come from

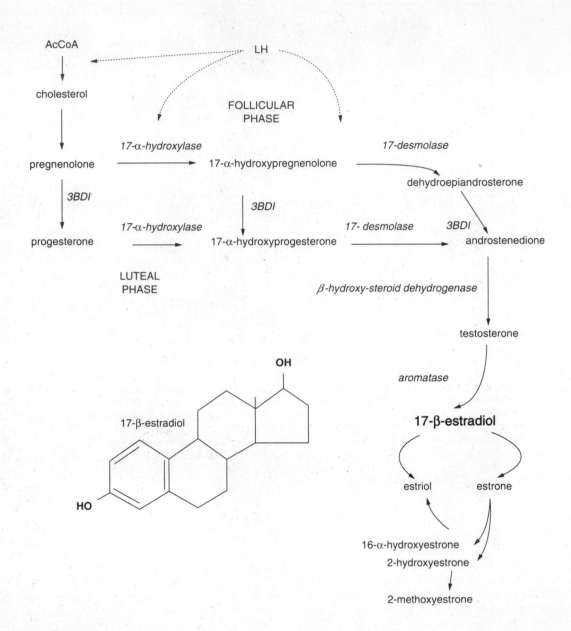

Figure 18.7 Synthesis of estrogens from cholesterol is illustrated. Enzyme names are italicized. LH stimulates conversion of cholesterol to androgen. The upper pathway is used in the follicular phase of the menstrual cycle; the lower pathway is used in the luteal phase of the menstrual cycle.

Table 18.1 Estradiol in Women Peaks in the Late Follicular Menstrual Cycle Phase.

Estradiol	Early follicular phase	Late follicular phase	Midluteal phase
plasma concentration µg/dl	0.006	0.033–0.07	0.02
production rate µg/day	81	445–945	270
secretion rate µg/day	70	400–800	250

Ovulation occurs at the end of the follicular phase of the menstrual cycle. Lipsett, M.B. Steroid hormones. In Yen, S.S.C.; Jaffe, R. B., editors. Reproductive Endocrinology. Philadelphia, PA: W. B. Saunders; 1978; p. 84.

the theca interna.

The role for FSH is an action on granulosa cells. The FSH may induce and activate aromatase activity which may covert androgen (made in the thecal cells) to estrogens. The action is mediated by cyclic AMP. Thus there is a two-cell hypothesis: thecal cells ⇒ androgen ⇒ granulosa cells ⇒ estrogen.

Other estrogens are also produced. Liver uses 17-ß-hydroxysteroid dehydrogenase to convert estradiol to estrone. Metabolites of estrone and estradiol include 16-α-hydroxyestrone, 2-hydroxyestrone, estrone sulfate, estriol, and estriol 3-sulfate-16-glucuronide. Estrogen metabolites (glucuronide and sulfate conjugates) are excreted into the bile (from which they can be reabsorbed and recycled) and urine.

Progesterone is synthesized from cholesterol in the corpus luteum during the menstrual cycle and the placenta during pregnancy (Figure 18.8). The hormones that prolong gestation are grouped and variously called progestens, progestins, progestagens, progestogens, or gestagens. Progestin and Progestone are brand names for progesterone. Amounts of progesterone correlate with menstrual phase (Table 18.2). Plasma progesterone concentration, progesterone production rate, and progesterone secretion rate are all highest during the luteal phase of the menstrual cycle. In the blood, CBG (transcortin) transports 18% of progesterone, but serum albumin carries 80%.

Progesterone has a short half-life of 5 minutes. In the category "gestagens," Borth includes hormones (progesterone and pregnanediol), a drug (medroxyprogesterone), and a metabolite (6-α-methyl-17-α-acetoxy-6-ß,21-dihydroxy-4-pregnene-3-20-estagen).[2]

The ovary, in order to make estrogens, must first produce **androgens** which, from the viewpoint of female reproduction, act as precursors for estrogen. So females have androgen secretion that is ovarian in origin (Table 18.3). Androgens in women also come from the adrenal cortex. Androgens are high in atretic follicles.

Synthetic estrogens and progestens have been widely investigated and used for contraception. The problem encountered in attempts to use natural steroids for contraceptives was that they were not orally potent. So the chemical achievement was to produce orally potent synthetic steroids with various steroidal effects. Ethinyl estrogen has oral potency. Norethindrone, an ethinyl derivative of estrogen, is a synthetic progestational agent (Figure 18.9). Ethinyl estrogen and norethindrone have sometimes combined in contraceptive pills. Progestin implants, inserted under the skin, have been used to prevent pregnancy for long periods of time (up to 5 years).

Relaxin is a hormone of the ovary that is not a steroid. Relaxin is a polypeptide with amino acid similarities to human insulin and to IGF-I and IGF-II (insulin-like growth factors).

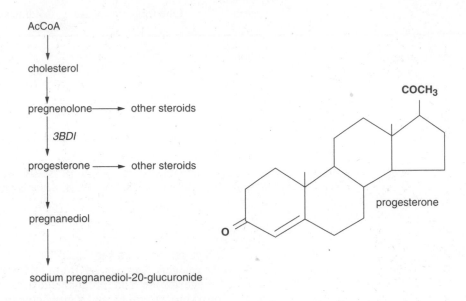

Figure 18.8 Synthesis of progesterone from cholesterol and metabolism is shown in the pathway chart.

GONADOTROPINS

As they do in males, the gonadotropins play important roles in controlling reproduction in females. The structures of LH and FSH in the female are the same as the structures of LH and FSH in the male. Without the pituitary, ovaries, like testes, atrophy.

There appears to be only one releasing factor, **LRH** (GnRH, LH-FSH-RH), from the hypothalamus that is capable of releasing both FSH and LH from the pituitary. A separate FSH-RH has been hypothesized but remains the subject of controversy.

FSH is responsible for the maturation of follicles in the ovaries. FSH is inhibited by estrogen and inhibin. Antral fluid from the follicles inhibits FSH production. The follicular fluid contains polypeptide subunits with molecular weights of 18,000 and 14,000. Depending how the subunits are combined and linked by disulfide bonds,

they can form **inhibin** A, inhibin B, two activins, or TGFß (transforming growth factor). The inhibins inhibit FSH production; the activins and TGFß stimulate FSH secretion. FSH receptors are found on the granulosa cells; FSH causes the granulosa cells to produce estradiol from androgens.

LH secretion precedes ovulation and completes maturation of ovarian follicles. Prolactin, on the other hand, inhibits ovulation. As mentioned, LH also stimulates production of androgens by the theca interna cells. LH is usually inhibited by estrogen, except just before ovulation when high estrogen levels appear to have a positive feedback effect resulting in episodic LRH (GnRH) secretion and the LH surge. Progesterone feedback may block the secretion of LH by decreasing the rate of LH pulses. LH receptors appear in the granulosa cells as a consequence of FSH and estrogen, but LH receptors are also in theca cells, interstitial cells, and luteal cells.

Table 18.2 Progesterone in Women Is Highest During the Luteal Phase of the Menstrual Cycle

Progesterone	Follicular phase	Luteal phase
plasma concentration (μg/dl)	0.095	1.113
production rate (μg/day)	2.1	25
secretion rate (μg/day)	1.5	24

Lipsett, M.B. Steroid hormones. In Yen, S.S.C.; Jaffe, R. B., editors. Reproductive Endocrinology. Philadelphia, PA: W. B. Saunders; 1978; p. 84.

PUBERTY

As in males, the reproductive hormones of females exhibit a time course of changes over a lifetime (Figures 18.10, 18.11). Tanner[3] described and classified the various stages of the human female reproductive life based on externally visible characteristics—breast development (thelarche), appearance of pubic hair (pubarche), and maturation of the external genitalia. During the **prepubertal** stage (Tanner Stage I) the breasts are undeveloped and pubic hair is absent. Episodic gonadotropins, steroid hormones, and pituitary sensitivity to LRH rise to peaks several months after birth up to age two. From age 2 years old to 9–10 years old, the gonadotropins, steroid hormones, and sensitivity to LH decrease to low levels (e.g., FSII and LH <1 ng/ml; 17-ß-estradiol < 7 pg/ml in girls).

With the approach of **puberty** (the point of development when reproduction is first possible), there are endocrine changes that precede the onset of sexual development. The early endocrine events include decrease in sensitivity to negative feedback, initiation of episodic gonadotropin secretion in sleep, concomitant increases in plasma reproductive steroids, and increased pituitary sensitivity to LRH (Table 18.4). In girls the sequence of appearance of signs of approaching puberty is (i) breast development, (ii) appearance of pubic hair, and (iii) onset of menstruation (**menarche**). Puberty before age 8 (girls) or age 9 (boys) is considered precocious; puberty after age 13 (girls) or age 14 (boys) is considered to be delayed. Several factors contribute normal variation to the age of

puberty in women: individual variation, geographical region, and, maybe, variation with decade in which the puberty occurs.

First, there is **individual** variation. A classification scheme used to quantitatively assess the individual variation in puberty was established by Tanner. Puberty in female women is divided into three Tanner stages (II, III, IV); prepuberty childhood is Tanner stage I; and adults provide a fifth stage (V). In 1969, the breast stage II occurred at 12.15 years of age while breast stage V occurred at 15.33 years of age. The onset of menarche was given as 12.8 ± SD 1.2 years which was closely correlated to skeletal age 13 years.[4] Onset of reproductive development occurs between ages 8–13 years in 98.8% of American girls (9–14 years of age for boys).[5]

Second, Tanner proposed that there has been variation with **decade** over the past 175 years. The age of onset of puberty has been declining in the United States and other countries at the rate of 1–3 months per decade (Figure 18.12). Speculations as to the cause of the decline include better diet or a stimulatory effect of increased lighting due to the development and augmented use of bright artificial light sources.[6] The ideas have been challenged by Bullough.[7]

Third, there is **geographical variation** in the onset of puberty (Table 18.5). British girls develop 6 months later (menarche 10–16.6) than American girls.

Fourth, there is **racial variation** in the onset of puberty in girls; black girls develop earlier than other racial groups. The geographical and ra-

Table 18.3 Androgens in Women

Androgen	Plasma concentration μg/dl	Production rate mg/day	Secretion rate μg/day
testosterone	0.038	0.26	—
dihydrotestosterone	0.020	0.05	0.01–0.02
dehydroepiandrosterone	0.490	8.00	0.3–3
androstenedione	0.159	3.20	0.8–1.6

Lipsett, M.B. Steroid hormones. In Yen, S.S.C.; Jaffe, R. B., editors. Reproductive Endocrinology. Philadelphia, PA: W. B. Saunders; 1978; p. 84.

cial variations are not apparent in boys.

Fifth, the onset of menarche in girls has been associated with body weight and exercise. Mishell summarized the findings:

> The mean time of onset of menarche was previously thought to occur when a critical body weight of about 48 kg or 106 lb was reached. However, it is now believed that the body composition is more important than total body weight in determining the time of onset of puberty and menstruation. Thus the ratio of fat to both total body weight and lean body weight is probably the determining factor in the time of onset of puberty and menstruation. Individuals who are moderately obese, between 20% and 30% above the ideal body weight, will have an early onset of menarche. Malnutrition is known to delay the onset of puberty, and well-nourished individuals with prepubertal strenuous exercise programs resulting in less total body fat have also been shown to have a delayed onset of puberty...[B]allet dancers, swimmers, and runners had menarche delayed to about age 15 if they began exercising strenuously before menarche ...[S]tress is not the cause of the delayed menarche in these exercising girls, as girls of the same age with stressful musical careers did not have a delayed onset of menarche...[F]or girls engaged in premenarcheal athletic training, menarche was delayed 0.4 years for each year of athletic training.[8]

DAILY CYCLES

In the night-active (nocturnal) rats, events in the estrous cycle have daily timing so that, on the night of estrus, mating behavior begins before midnight and ovulation occurs after midnight. Hamsters began estrus at 5 hours after noon in LD16:8.   The rhythm persisted with a period longer than 24 hours when the hamsters were placed in constant light.[9]   In pubertal girls, estradiol peaks around 1–3 o'clock in the afternoon, and the LH surge occurs twelve hours later at 1–4 o'clock in the morning (Figure 18.13).

EPISODIC RELEASE

There are "pulsatile" or "episodic" patterns of hormone release in the circulating gonadotropins which are especially apparent during the ascending limb of the midcycle surge (Figure 18.14). The importance of pulsatile LRH has been related to re-

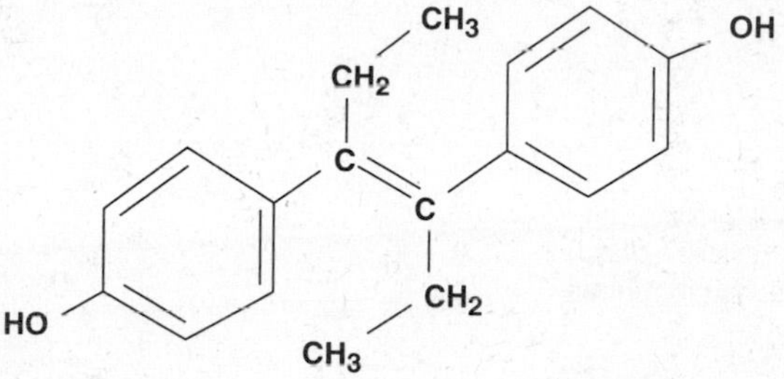

diethylstilbestrol,
synthetic estrogen

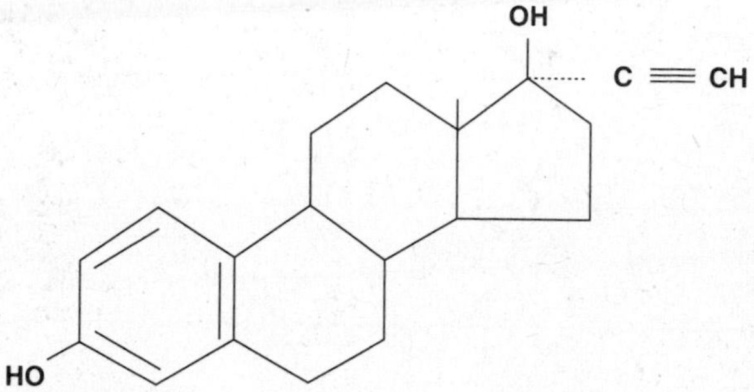

ethinyl estradiol,
synthetic estrogen

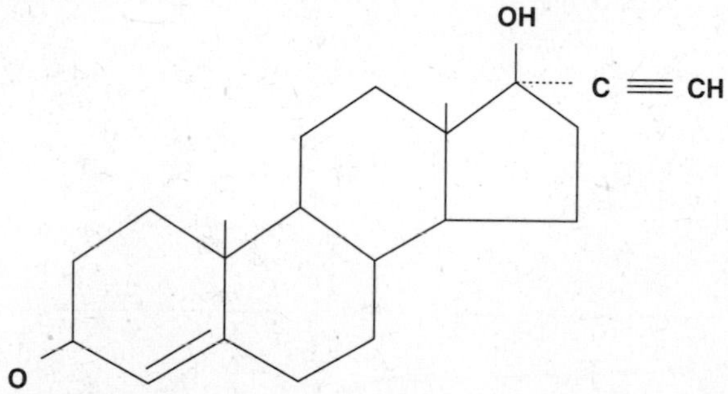

norethindrone,
synthetic progestin

Figure 18.9 Examples of synthetic reproductive steroids are shown.

ceptors. If LRH is infused constantly, there is down regulation in pituitary LRH receptors and LH declines. However, if LRH is applied in pulses (e.g., one per hour), LH secretion is stimulated. Frequency of pulses is increased by estrogen and catecholamines; but pulse frequency is decreased by progesterone, testosterone, enkephalins, and ß-endorphin. Therefore, pulse frequencies are high late in the follicular phase just before ovulation and probably contribute to the stimulation of ovulation.

MENSTRUAL CYCLE

The human female reproductive cycle has a length of about a month, and so it was named the menstrual cycle. The menstrual cycle is conspicuously marked by periodic bleeding from the vagina in primates (menses, menstruation, or menstrual period). However, there are also remarkable but less visible menstrual cycle changes in hormones (gonadotropins, estrogen, progesterone), in anatomy (ovary, uterus, vagina), and in body temperature. In the menstrual cycle, the reproductive organs prepare for fertilization (follicular phase), re-

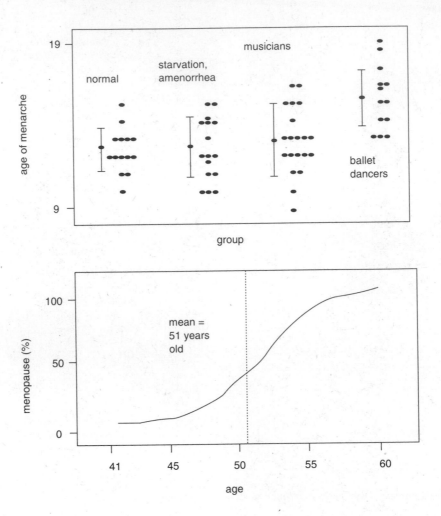

Figure 18.10 The graphs show (upper) ages at menarche and (lower) ages at the time of menopause for women. In the upper graph, individual data points are shown, and the vertical lines show means and standard deviations for each group. In the lower graph, the frequency distribution of the time of the age of menopause is shown. Redrawn, with permission. (Upper) Warren, M.P. The effects of exercise on pubertal progression and reproductive function in girls. J. Clin. Endocrinol. Metabol. 51; 1150; 1980. (Lower) Jaszmann, L.J.B. Epidemiology of the climacteric syndrome. In Campbell, S., editor. Management of the Menopause and Post-menopausal Years. Lancaster, England: MTP Press Ltd.; 1976; p. 12.

lease the egg (ovulation), and prepare for pregnancy (luteal phase).

    The mode (most common) length of the menstrual cycle is 28 days, but there are several numbering systems. Usually, day one is assigned to be equivalent to the first day of menstruation. For a 28-day cycle, the use of equating day one to

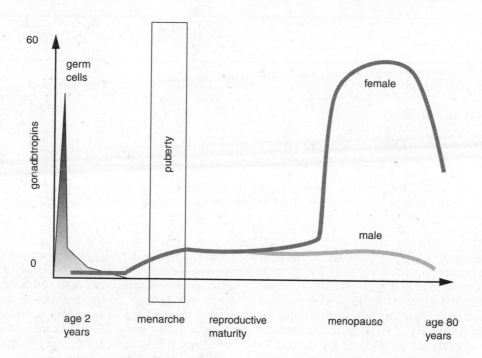

Figure 18.11 The graphs represent the variation in total urinary gonadotropins (rat units/24 hours) over the course of the human female lifetime. Male levels are shown for the later years for comparison. The number of germ cells in the human ovaries peaks before birth, then drops to less than 3 million at birth, and declines slowly to less than one million by the reproductive years. The age of onset of menstruation (menarche) is 12.8 years (ages 8-13) in the United States; the age of onset of menopause is 42–60 years. Data reported for the ages of menarche and menopause vary among sources. Menarche has been occurring earlier and menopause has been occurring later in recent times so that the length of the female reproductive life has increased.

the first day of menses normally estimates ovulation for the fourteenth day of the cycle. A disadvantage of this numbering system comes from the fact that the luteal phase is a relatively constant (14 ± 2 days). Thus, when there is variation in the menstrual cycle length, the variation is mostly in the follicular phase. So counting out 14 days from the first day of menses can be a poor way of estimating the day of ovulation. There is an alternative numbering system. Some scientists number the days starting with day zero as the LH peak which coincides with the day of ovulation. When that is done, menstruation occurs on the fifteenth day.

The length of the menstrual cycle is variable. The mode length of the menstrual cycle is 28 days, but cycle lengths vary dramatically both within an individual woman and between women (Figure 18.15). The average length of the human menstrual cycle is 33 ± 0.6 days. The temporal pattern of the menstrual cycle of an individual can be visualized by plotting the cycle using the raster graphing method (Figure 18.16). The menstrual cycle length of an individual varies with age (Figure 18.17). Irregular cycles produce long period lengths just after menarche and as menopause approaches. For most of a woman's reproductive life, however, the length of her menstrual cycle gradually shortens.

The body temperature of women has a cycle that corresponds to the menstrual cycle (Figure 18.18). Body temperature rises from less than 97.9°F to more than 98.3°F (about 0.6°F) just after ovulation. The body temperature cycle has

Table 18.4 Hormone Increase at the Time of Puberty in Women

	Prepubertal	Puberty
plasma LH, FSH (ng/ml)	0.5–0.7	2–3
plasma 17-ß-estradiol (pg/ml)	<7	60
LH (ng/ml) response to LRH	1–2	4–5

Grumbach, M.M. Onset of puberty. In Berenger, S.R., editor. Puberty. H.E. Stenfert Kroese, Martinus Nijhoff; 1975; Grumbach M.M. et al. Control of the Onset of Puberty. In Grumbach, M.M.; Grave, G.D.; Mayer, F.E., editors; Wiley: New York; 1974.

been used as an indicator of ovulation. It has been used in attempts to predict fertility in order to achieve conception or to improve the ability of the "rhythm" method to reduce fertility. Ganong suggests that the temperature increase is due to the increase in progesterone: "Progesterone is thermogenic and is probably responsible for the rise in basal body temperature at the time of ovulation."[10]

Scientists and nonscientists have wondered whether there is any importance to the correlation between the length of the menstrual cycle and the 29.5-day lunar month. It is logical to consider the possibility that our foremothers' reproductive cycles might have been synchronized by the light of the full moon alternating with the dark of the new moon. As evidence for the idea, Dewan claimed that a night of light on days 14–17 of the menstrual cycle regularized the irregular menstrual cycles of women toward a 29.5-day average.[11] Other primates provide some evidence against the lunar idea since chimpanzee menstrual cycles are 35 days long and gorillas have 39-day menstrual cycles.

Consider the hormone changes that occur during the menstrual cycle in humans (Figure 18.19). First, during the follicular phase, estradiol levels increase in response to stimulation of the cells of the developing follicle of the ovary by the gonadotropins. Estrogen secretion climbs to a peak that precedes ovulation. Second, an enormous spike of LH, the **LH surge**, preceeds ovulation. Ovulation separates the follicular and luteal phases. Third, once ovulation has taken place, the follicle becomes a corpus luteum producing **proges-terone**. Similar sequences of hormone changes occur in the estrus cycles of rats (Figure 18.20) and other species. A great many correlations have made the menstrual cycle an important consideration in clinical applications. For example, breast cancer excision during the follicular phase resulted in a recurrence risk of 43%, recurrence risk for surgery later in the cycle was only 29%.[12]

ANATOMICAL CHANGES IN THE MENSTRUAL CYCLE

In humans, an **ovarian cycle** of anatomy correlates with the changes in hormones during the menstrual cycle (Figure 18.21). The ovarian changes were also mentioned in the discussion of the anatomy of the ovary earlier in this chapter. In the follicular phase, there are dramatic follicle size changes that correlate with estrogen production. The primordial follicle is small; the egg, or oocyte, is <25 μm in diameter and enlarges before ovulation to 80–100 μm. But the graafian follicle reaches a diameter of 2–2.5 cm just before ovulation. Estradiol causes proliferation of granulosa cells in small follicles. Steroid hormones are secreted into the follicular fluid and the levels of androgens and estradiol in follicular fluid can be up to 40,000 times blood concentrations (e.g., estradiol 1500 ng/ml in follicular fluid). After ovulation, the follicle becomes a corpus luteum in the luteal phase.

Moreover, in humans and mammals, a **uterine cycle** also occurs (Figure 18.22). At the end of menstruation the uterus is at a starting point

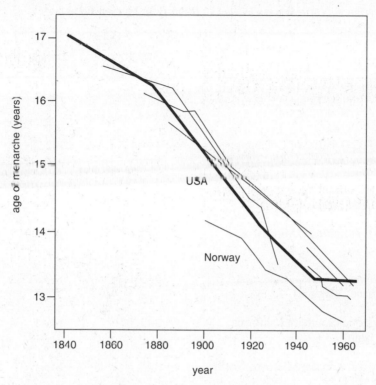

Figure 18.12 The graphs show a remarkable decline in the age of menarche in eight countries in the temperate northern hemisphere: USA, Denmark, Germany, Sweden, United Kingdom, Finland, Holland, and Norway. Redrawn, with permission. The age of menarche was reduced by about four years. Tanner, J.M. Growing up. Scientific American; September; 1973; p. 22.

with only a thin basal endometrial layer. The uterine changes are divided into two parts: (i) the **proliferative phase**, where the uterus grows during the follicular phase, and (ii) the **secretory phase** which is coincident with the luteal phase. Noyes, Hertig, and Rock[13] further classified the changes in the endometrium: (i) Gland mitoses (the growth phase lasts from days 4–14 after the first day of menstruation). (ii) Pseudostratification of nuclei. (iii) Basal vacuolation (after ovulation; the phase lasts five days; subnuclear glycogen-rich vacuoles appear and these vacuoles herd the epithelial cell nuclei into the center of their cells). (iv) Secretion (visible secretion of acidophilic intraluminal glandular material occurs days 3–11 after ovulation; secretion peaks day 21 after the last day of menstruation). (v) Stromal edema. (vi) Pseudodecidual reaction. (vii) Stromal mitoses (many mitoses during proliferation, decline in numbers of mitoses after ovulation, reappearance of mitoses during predecidual formation). (viii) Leukcocytic infiltration (lymphocyte infiltration begins about 2 days before menstrual-flow onset and peaks on the day of menstrual-flow onset). During the menstrual phase, the entire functional layer of the endometrium sloughs off.

The cervix is located where the vagina meets the uterus and it exhibits a **cervical cycle**. The cervix secretes cervical mucus (98% water, 1% inorganic salts; sodium chloride, simple sugars, polysaccharaide, proteins, glycoproteins, alkaline pH. The mucus changes throughout the menstrual cycle, and, because the changes result from changes in estrogen and progesterone, the cervical mucus is an indicator of hormone status (Figure 18.23). In the follicular phase, estrogen stimulates production of clear watery mucus, up to 700 mg/day. The patterns of dried cervical mucus are fern-like

Table 18.5 Geographical Variation in the Age of Puberty in Human Females

Region	Breast	Hair	Menarche
EAST CENTRAL (Illinois, Kentucky, Ohio, West Virginia)	141.0	141.7	149.1
MIDDLE ATLANTIC (District of Columbia, Maryland, New Jersey, New York, Pennsylvania)	141.4	142.2	151.0
NEW ENGLAND (Connecticut, Massachusetts, New Hampshire, Rhode Island, Vermont)	142.1	143.1	151.5
NORTH CENTRAL (Michigan, Minnesota, Wisconsin)	142.1	143.6	152.1
SOUTHEAST (Alabama, Florida, Louisiana, Mississippi, Tennessee, Virginia)	143.4	143.4	152.3
SOUTHWEST (Arizona, Southern California, Oklahoma, Texas, Utah)	142.3	143.1	152.5
MIDCENTRAL (Iowa, Kansas, Missouri, North Dakota)	143.7	143.4	152.9
NORTHWEST (Northern California, Montana, Oregon, Washington)	143.9	143.7	153.0
AVERAGE	142.5	143.0	151.8

Ages for breast budding, pubic hair appearance, and menarche are in months. Zacharias, L., Wurtman, R.J.; Schatzoff, M. Sexual maturation in contemporary American girls. Amer J. Obstet. Gynecol. 108: 833; 1970.

("ferning") when estradiol is high. Progesterone reduces mucus secretion (to 20–60 mg/day) during the luteal phase and pregnancy, making the mucus scanty, thick, and cellular. The nature of the mucus may affect the performance of spermatozoa.

The **vaginal cells** also vary with the changes in reproductive steroid hormones. The vagina, like the uterus, is a target of estrogen. In the vagina during the follicular phase (i) estrogen stimulates the proliferation and maturation of epithelial cells, (ii) thickens the vaginal mucosa, (iii) increases glycogen in epithelial cells, and (iv) increases exfoliated superficial cells. The exfoliated cells are the ones that can be examined in vaginal smears. Estrogen causes the sloughed cells to have the following characteristics: mature, flat, polygonal, squamous, pyknotic nuclei, hyperchromatic nuclei. In the luteal phase, when progesterone levels are high, the exfoliated cells are intermediate cells distinguished by possession of a nonpyknotic nucleus.

In estrogen deficiency (prepubertal and postmenopausal) in human females, the exfoliated cells are basal-parabasal cells that have the following characteristics: small, oval or round, immature, large vesicular nuclei, cyanophilic cytoplasm. A "maturation index" based on the ratios of these cells in vaginal smears can be used clinically as a

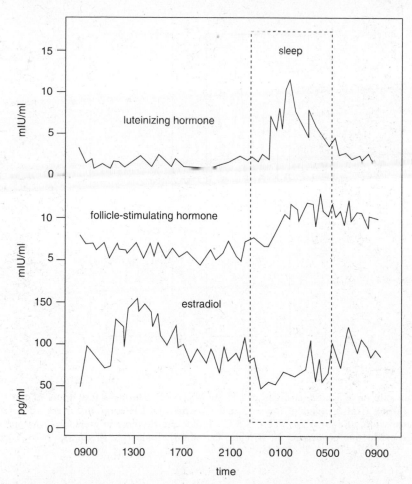

Figure 18.13 Daily cycles occur in human female hormones. Redrawn, with permission. Rebar, R.W.; Yen, S.S.C. Endocrine rhythms in gonadotropins and ovarian steroids with reference to reproductive processes. In Krieger, D., editor. Endocrine Rhythms. New York: Raven Press; 1979; p. 264.

qualitative indicator of the presence or absence of estrogen.

In rodents, it is useful and easy to diagnose stage of reproductive cycle from the cells in vaginal smears. Removing the ovaries reduces the incidence of estrus; estrogen injections increase the incidence of estrus in ovariectomized rats (Table 18.6).

ESTROUS CYCLES

Only primates have menstrual cycles. Other female mammals have estrous cycles (estrous or estrual, adjective; estrus or oestrus, noun). There is no menstruation in estrous cycles. Estrous cycles are named for a period of **heat**, or sexual receptivity ("mad desire"[14]). According to Sadlier:

> The word 'oestrus' derives from the Greek *oistros*, a gadfly, and was used to describe the erratic and nervy behavior of a cow when being attacked by such flies. A similarly nervous and touchy disposition characterizes many females when in heat, so that oestrus now refers to this stage of the reproductive cycle.[15]

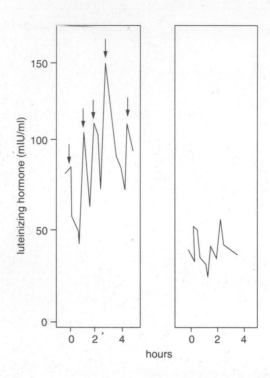

Figure 18.14 Pulsatile, or episodic, changes in LH are observed. During a few hours of the rising (left) there are 5 pulses and falling (right) nights of days 13 and 14 when the LH surge occurred. 0 hours = sleep onset. Redrawn, with permission. Rebar, R.W.; Yen, S.S.C. Endocrine rhythms in gonadotropins and ovarian steroids with reference to reproductive processes. In Krieger, D., editor. Endocrine Rhythms. New York: Raven Press; 1979; p. 271.

The cycles are easily studied in laboratory rodents (rats, mice, hamsters) because estrus coincides with the appearance of cornified cells in vaginal smears, ovulation occurs during estrus, and the cycles are only four or five days long. The cycles have been divided into stages—diestrus, proestrus, estrus, and metestrus—which can be determined from vaginal smears. Day one of an estrous cycle is arbitrarily set at the first day of heat. The lengths of estrous cycles vary among species (Table 18.7). The laboratory rat has hormone cycles that are similar to those in humans—peaks in LH and estradiol precede ovulation during proestrus, and progesterone rises after ovulation during diestrus. The external genitalia of some animals exhibit visible changes during estrus.

Dogs have two or more cycles per year in which bleeding occurs. But the bleeding is not true menstruation. It is called diapedesis bleeding and involves the passage of red blood cells through vessel walls into the tissues, rather than sloughing of the uterine lining which characterizes menstruation.

SEASONAL CYCLES

Female animals have seasonal breeding patterns that match the seasonal breeding patterns of their male counterparts. So the female hamster has changes in the function of its ovaries, just as does the male hamster in the function of its testes. Reproductively active females exhibit their estrous cycles, reproductively quiescent females do not exhibit estrus. Animals that have only one estrous cycle per year (foxes, bears, cows, sheep, pigs) are monestrus. Seasonally breeding grey squirrels have two breeding and birth seasons per year; they are

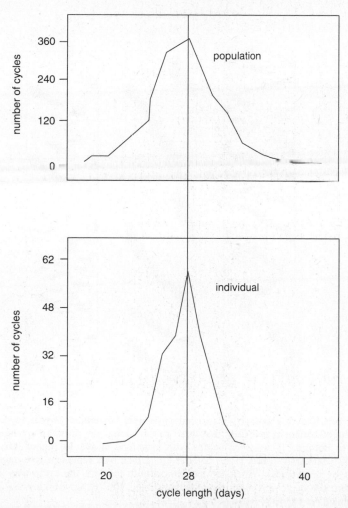

Figure 18.15 The graphs illustrate variation in menstrual cycle lengths in women. (Upper) The frequency distribution for menstrual cycle length for a population of women is graphed. The data are from 2460 cycles. 77% of the cycles fall between 25 and 31 days in length. Redrawn, with permission. Haman, J.O. The length of the menstrual cycle. A study of 150 normal women. Am. J. Obstet. Gynecol. 43: 870–843; 1942. (Lower) The frequency distribution for the menstrual cycle length in the least variable woman in a study of 592 women. 61 of the woman's 225 cycles (27.1%) were 28 days long. Redrawn. Hartman, C.G. The irregularity of the menstrual cycle. In Hartman, C.G., editor. Science and the Safe Period. Huntington, NY: Robert E. Krieger, Pub. Co.; 1972; p. 128. Data are from Vollman's most regular subject. Vollman, R.F. Degree of variability of the length of the menstrual cycle in correlation with age of woman. Gynaecologia 142: 310–314; 1956.

diestrous. Dogs also come into heat twice a year but they lack breeding seasons (possibly because of their exposure to artificial lighting which prevents them from experiencing short days in their association with humans). Other animals that have two or more cycles per year are seasonal polyestrus species (goats, ewes, mares). Some organisms breed all year round (humans, gorillas, chimpanzees,, laboratory rats and mice and hamsters, captive monkeys, captive lemurs). Bright constant light (LL) causes some rodents to go into constant estrus. Yet other animals (camels, rabbits) have continuous estrus

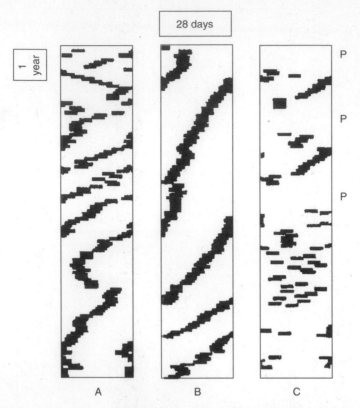

Figure 18.16 A raster plot shows a woman's menstrual cycle over her entire 32-year reproductive life. In a column, the data were arranged on horizontal lines that were 28 days long; the lines are arranged vertically in chronological order from top to bottom. The record begins with menarche at age 14 (upper left, column A), continues (column B), and ends 32 years later (lower right, column C). Black bars represent five days of menses; P = interruption of menstruation by pregnancy. When the pattern drifts to the left, the cycle was less than 28 days long; when it drifts to the right, the cycle was more than 28 days long. Reilly, K.; Binkley, S. The menstrual rhythm. Psychoneuroendocrinology 6: 181–184; 1981.

interrupted by pregnancy or pseudopregnancy.

The same route and sequence for control of seasonal breeding by photoperiod and the pineal gland that has been hypothesized for males is hypothesized for females (long dark ⇒ eyes ⇒ retinohypothalamic tract ⇒ suprachiasmatic nuclei ⇒ superior cervical ganglia ⇒ nervii conari ⇒ norepinephrine ⇒ cAMP ⇒ N-acetyltransferase ⇒ melatonin ⇒ prolactin inhibition ⇒ suppressed ovaries).

Is there **seasonal breeding** in human women? There is anecdotal evidence that humans may have the capacity for seasonal breeding cycles. Before exposure to modern civilization and lighting, Eskimo women were reported to cease men-

strual cycles during the winter. There are seasonal cycles in conceptions, testosterone, and menstrual cycle length. In Finland, where daylength varies greatly with changes in season because of the high latitude, summer (June to September) had the highest rates of conception and the conception rate dropped in winter (November to February).[16]

TARGETS OF ESTROGENS AND PROGESTERONE

The first function of the ovary is to produce eggs. But the second function of the ovary is to produce hormones.

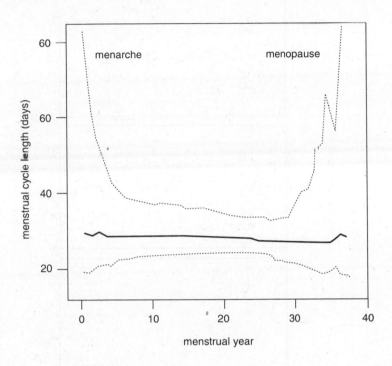

Figure 18.17 The graph shows the variation in menstrual cycle length that occurs over the lifespan of women. The center line shows the median menstrual cycle lengths from menarche (left, menstrual year 0) to menopause (right). The upper and lower broken lines bracket 90% of all cycles. Redrawn, with permission. Treolar, A.E.; Boynton, R.; Behn, B.; Brown, B. Variation of the human menstrual cycle through reproductive life. Int. J. Fert. 12: 77–176; 1967.

Targets of estrogen include the gonads (ovarian follicles) and the accessory organs: vagina, uterus, oviducts. Yet other targets are in the skin (mammary glands, axillary and pubic hair growth, sebaceous gland secretion). There are targets in the brain (libido, sexual receptivity, mating behavior) and on the hypothalamus (feedback on LRH secretion), and in the pituitary gland (feedback on LH secretion). Estrogen causes the liver to produce angiotensinogen and thyroid-binding globulin, decreases plasma cholesterol production, deposits minerals in bone, causes water and sodium retention, produces anabolic weight gain, and determines the female pattern of fat distribution.

Targets of progesterone also include the oviducts, uterus, cervix, vagina, mammary glands, brain, and hypothalamus. Progesterone also raises basal metabolic rate. Estrogen is accorded a major role in promotion of cell proliferation, while progesterone is concerned with preparation of the uterus for ovum implantation and causes the glandular components of the mammary gland to differentiate.[17]

REGULATION OF THE OVARY

Regulation of the ovary involves classical negative feedback loops (Figure 18.24). In the model shown, two negative feedback loops are envisioned, one for estrogen during the follicular phase and another for progesterone during the luteal phase. In this model, the woman must oscillate between the two loops at ovulation and menstruation. But women are spontaneous periodic ovulators. That is, they apparently ovulate without any stimulatory external signal. Spontaneous

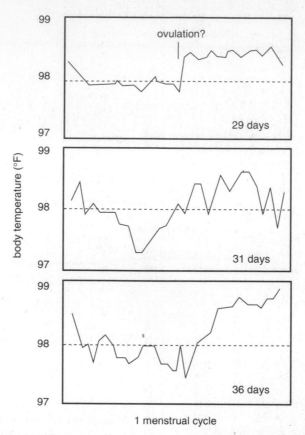

Figure 18.18 The graphs show body temperature changes during the human menstrual cycle. The data, measured by taking the body temperature once a day, have been replotted and normalized to the same horizontal axis (representing one cycle beginning with the first day of menstruation at the left). A decrease in body temperature has been used by women to guess the date of ovulation; ovulation usually occurs two weeks before the menses. (Top) Burt, J.B.; Brower, L.A. Education for Sexuality. Philadelphia, PA: W. B. Saunders; 1970. (Middle and bottom). Hartman, C.G., editor. Mechanisms Concerned with Conception. London: Pergamon; 1963; p. 267.

ovulators also include cows, goats, sheep, pigs, horses, dogs, foxes, hamsters, mice, rats, and rhesus monkeys.

The key event upon which scientists have focussed is the induction of ovulation. Hadley[18] describes a **"prostaglandin model"** for ovulation in which an influx of calcium ions causes production of prostaglandin $PGF_{2\alpha}$. A consequence of the prostaglandin change in the local environment is the contraction of the smooth muscle cells in the theca interna. Contractions of the theca interna smooth muscle cells squeeze the follicle contents. The apical layers of follicle cells respond to the pressure first by thinning and finally by rupturing.

Alternatively, Ganong[19] discusses an **"estrogen positive feedback model"** for ovulation in which high concentrations of estrogen produced in the follicular phase have a positive feedback effect stimulating LH secretion leading to the LH surge. Exogenous estrogens given at high levels to monkeys for 36 hours produce an LH surge. Throughout the rest of the cycle, estrogen and progesterone have negative feedback effects on gonadotropins.

However, not all animals are spontaneous ovulators. Some animals are **reflex ovulators** (induced ovulators). For the reflex ovulators, the sequence of events is clearcut. In the reflex ovulators, the act of copulation (mating, coitus) provides stimuli for ovulation. The stimuli are perceived by the genitals, eyes, ears, and nose. The perceptions are collected in the brain and signal the ventral hypothalamus to secrete LRH causing the pituitary to secrete LH which in turn causes the ovary to ovulate. The reflex ovulation system is especially efficient because it insures that the sperm are there waiting to fertilize the egg. Ovulation in reflex ovulators occurs 8–50 hours after mating, depending on the species. The reflex ovulators include animals notorious for their fertility: domestic cats, ferrets, mink, ground squirrels, and rabbits.

The sequence of events in a reflex ovulator, such as the rabbit, is as follows: Light information is perceived by the eyes. ⇒ Light information is transmitted to the pituitary via the hypothalamic hormones. ⇒ The pituitary secretes FSH. ⇒ The FSH causes growth of ovarian follicles. ⇒ The ovary secretes estrogen. ⇒ Estrogen produces estrous characteristics in the uterus, vagina, and brain. ⇒ Sexual receptivity and mating behavior culminates in copulation. ⇒ Copulation stimulates the cervix. ⇒ Sensory signals from the cervix are carried by the spinal cord to the brain where they stimulate the hypothalamic release of LRH. ⇒ LRH causes the pituitary to secrete LH. ⇒ LH causes the ovary to ovulate. ⇒ The ovarian follicle luteinizes. ⇒ The corpus luteum secretes progesterone. ⇒ Progesterone produces a progestational uterus. ⇒ Progesterone maintains gestation for fertilized embryos. ⇒ Lactogenic hormones (e.g., prolactin) are secreted. ⇒ Lactogenic hormones, estrogen, and progesterone cause the the mammary glands to grow and function. In reflex ovulators, then, copulation provides a signal for ovulation and initiates the sequence.

Women are not generally believed to be reflex ovulators. But the "fertile" period of women should be viewed as being quite broad. Ganong describes it:

> The ovum lives for approximately 72 hours after it is extruded from the follicle, but it is probably fertilizable for less than half this time. Sperms apparently survive in the female genital tract for no more than 48 hours. Consequently the 'fertile period' during a 28-day cycle is no longer than 120 hours, and it is probably much shorter. Unfortunately for those interested in the 'rhythm method' of contraception, the time of ovulation

is rather variable even from one menstrual cycle to another in the same woman. Before the ninth and after the twentieth day, there is little chance of conception; but there are documented cases of pregnancy resulting from isolated coitus on every day of the cycle.[20]

Motile sperm have been seen up to a week after intercourse although they are believed capable of fertilization for a shorter period of time. The rhythm method of fertility reduction has a 10–25% failure rate.

BIOASSAYS OF ESTROGEN, FSH, AND LH

Vaginal cornification, easily observed with a light microscope in vaginal smears, can be used to bioassay estrogens. Using ovariectomized rats, estrogen can be injected or introduced into the vagina with subsequent appearance of cornified cells in vaginal smears as a positive sign of estrogen. Estrogen also increases weight of ovariectomized animals; the uterus increases its weight in 6–8 hours by taking up water and in 21–30 hours by hypertrophy and hyperplasia (growth by increasing the cells). FSH increases ovarian weight of hypophysectomized rats. LH depletes ascorbic acid from the luteinized rat ovary and so ovarian ascorbic acid depletion can be used as a measure of LH.

FEMALE LIBIDO

As noted above, in animals there are variations in sexual behavior that correlate with the reproductive cycles. The role of hormones in human female libido was discussed by Ganong:

> In adult women, ovariectomy does not necessarily reduce libido (defined in this context as sexual interest and drive) or sexual ability. Postmenopausal women continue to have sexual relations, often without much change in frequency from their premenopausal pattern. This persistence is probably due to secretion of steroids from the adrenal cortex that are converted to circulating estrogens but may also be due to the greater degree of encephalization of sexual function in humans and their relative emancipation from instinctual and

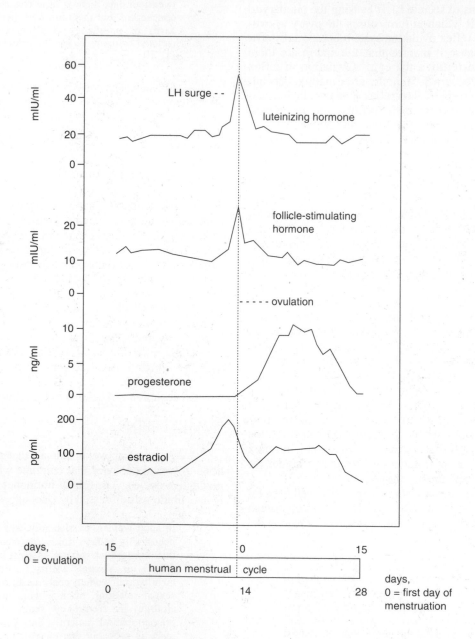

Figure 18.19 The graphs show the changes in some gonadotropins (LH and FSH) and steroids (progesterone, estradiol) during the human menstrual cycle. Redrawn, with permission. Thorneycroft, I.H. et. al. Am. J. Obstet. Gynecol. 111: 947; 1971.

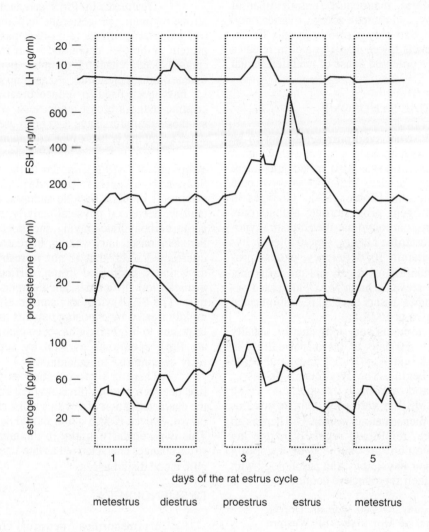

days of the rat estrus cycle

metestrus   diestrus   proestrus   estrus   metestrus

Figure 18.20 Gonadotropins and steroids change during the rat estrous cycle and are dependent upon time of day. Rectangles enclose daily 14-hour light phases (0500–1900) of the light-dark cycle, LD14:10, in which the rats were kept. Redrawn, with permission. Schwarz, N.B. The role of FSH and LH and their antibodies on follicle growth and ovulation. *Biology of reproduction* 10: 236–272; 1974.

hormonal control. Treatment with sex hormones increases sexual interest and drive in humans.[21]

In human females, libido is increased by exogenous estrogen. During the menstrual cycle, most reports are that there is more spontaneous female-initiated sexual activity at about the time of ovulation when estrogen would be high and, in other species, would cause heat. There arc a number of conditions in which female hormones are known to be altered in which there are changes in libido as symptoms—oral contraceptives, menopause, postmenopausal estrogen therapy, cyproterone acetate, ovariectomy. Androgen may also play a role in female libido. Testosterone levels lower than 10 ng/dl in females are considered a potential cause of inhibited sexual desire.[22]

PREMENSTRUAL SYNDROME

Premenstrual syndrome (PMS, not to be confused with pregnant mare's serum with which it shares an abbreviation) is also called late luteal phase dysphoric disorder. Premenstrual syndrome has many symptoms (Table 18.8). Changes in hormones (estrogen, progesterone, aldosterone, ADH, prolactin), carbohydrate metabolism, hypoglycemia, progesterone allergy, steroid allergy, hypoglycemia, vitamin B_6 deficiency, excess prolactin, fluid retention, estrogen and progesterone, prostaglandins, elevated brain MAO, increased endorphins, and other factors have all been implicated as possible causes of PMS.

The symptoms vary individually, usually occur the last 7–10 days of the menstrual cycle, may last a few hours to 10–12 days, and cease when menses begin. The syndrome worsens as women age and approach menopause. The incidence of PMS has variously been reported as 5% to 95% of menstruating women.[23] There is an entrenched idea, reinforced regularly in the lay press, that women are subject to crippling variations in their physiology and psychology with the changes of their reproductive hormones.

In a study of 200 women, Doreen Kimura, a University of Western Ontario psychology professor, found that when the levels of estrogen were high, the women showed greater verbal fluency and used their hands more skillfully than when levels were low. In one test of verbal dexterity, the women were asked to say 'A box of mixed biscuits in a biscuit mixer' as fast as possible five times. Their average time was 14 sec. on high-estrogen days, vs 17 sec. when hormone levels were low. On the other hand, the women's spatial abilities—picking a shape out of a complex pattern, for example—were stronger on low-estrogen days.[24]

Treatments for PMS have included progesterone regimens, progesterone implants, birth control pills, tranquilizers (e.g., diazepam), increased protein in the diet, decreased sugar in the diet, increased dietary vitamin B complex (pyridoxine), and magnesium supplements. Potassium-saving diuretics have been used to reduce bloating. Bromocriptine reduces breast tenderness. Prostaglandin synthesis inhibitors have also been used, especially when cramping is part of the complaint.

Sack and coworkers[25] pointed out that the symptoms of PMS are similar to the symptoms of **Seasonal Affective Disorder** (SAD). The symptoms of SAD include sadness, anxiety, irritability, decreased physical activity, increased appetite, carbohydrate craving, increased weight, earlier sleep onset, later waking, increased sleep time, interrupted sleep that is not refreshing, daytime drowsiness, decreased libido, difficulties around menses, work difficulties, and interpersonal difficulties. The SAD symptoms can be effectively and rapidly treated by exposing patients to bright light. Exposure to bright light has been claimed to alleviate PMS symptoms as well by suppressing an early evening rise in melatonin.[26]

There is some question as to where the line between normal physiological variations and the characterization of PMS as a disorder should be drawn, or even if such a line should be drawn at all. This is particularly murky in the area of premenstrual changes characterized as late-luteal phase-specific mood disturbances.[27]

DYSMENORRHEA

Dysmenorrhea (menstrual cramps) is due to uterine contractions caused by prostaglandin released when the endometrium breaks down. The symptoms can be severe and include pain radiating to the back and thighs, diarrhea, and vomiting. Other symptoms (sweating, tachycardia, headaches, nausea, diarrhea, tremulousness) may accompany the abdominal cramps that occur just before and during menstruation. The incidence of dysmenorrhea has variously been reported as 3% to 90%.[28] Once the relationship with prostaglandins was discovered, nonsteroidal anti-inflammatory compounds such as aspirin and other NSAIDS (naproxen,

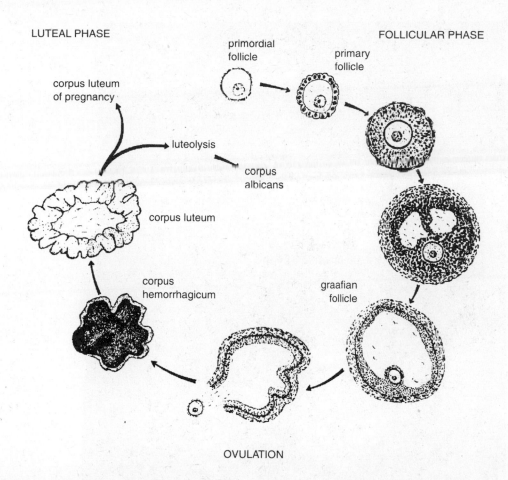

LUTEAL PHASE

FOLLICULAR PHASE

primordial follicle

primary follicle

corpus luteum of pregnancy

luteolysis

corpus albicans

corpus luteum

graafian follicle

corpus hemorrhagicum

OVULATION

Figure 18.21 Changes are visible in a follicle of the ovary with the progression of the menstrual cycle. The ovarian cycle proceeds through the follicular phase which ends with ovulation. The luteal phase follows ovulation. If pregnancy occurs, the corpus luteum persists through gestation. If pregnancy does not happen, the corpus luteum undergoes luteolysis leaving a corpus albicans in the ovary. Modified, with permission. Hadley, M. Endocrinology, Second Edition. Englewood Cliffs, NJ: Prentice-Hall; 1988; p. 430.

ibuprofen, and indomethacin, mefenamic acid) that inhibit prostaglandin synthesis, provided effective treatment when used before the pain begins. Dysmenorrhea was reduced (from 38% to 21% in one study) by oral contraceptive use.

AMENORRHEA

Amenorrhea (amenorrhoea) is the absence of menstruation. There are numerous types of amenorrhea. Lack of menarche, primary amenorrhea, can be due to numerous causes (Turner's syn-

drome, hypogonadism, thyroid insufficiency, adrenal insufficiency, testicular feminization, absent or abnormal female reproductive organs, failure to develop the olfactory lobe, deficiency of LRH, etc.). In women in whom menarche has occurred, secondary amenorrhea can also be due to a variety of causes.

The first kind of amenorrhea is the normal amenorrhea of **pregnancy**. Amenorrhea of pregnancy is due to the progestational action of progesterone.

A second kind of amenorrhea is

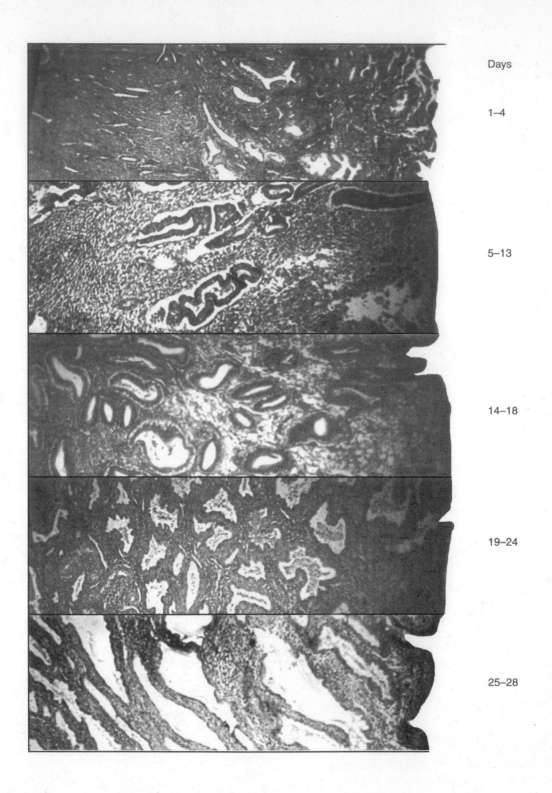

Days

1–4

5–13

14–18

19–24

25–28

Figure 18.22 (Facing page) A composite of five sections of uterus show anatomical changes during the menstrual cycle. From top to bottom, the sections are from days 1–4, 5–13, 14–18, 19–24, and 25–28. The lumen of the uterus is on the right. The figure was made by photographing portions of transparencies. Eichler, V.B. Histology of the Endocrine System; Slide Set #617; Educational Images, Ltd.; Lyons Falls, NY.

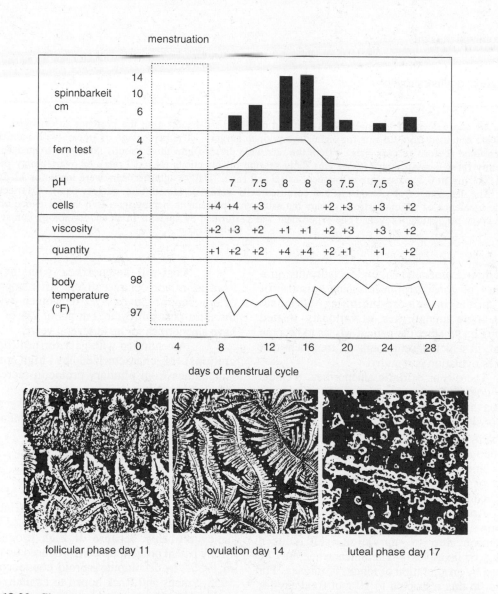

follicular phase day 11   ovulation day 14   luteal phase day 17

Figure 18.23 Changes occur in cervical mucus as the menstrual cycle proceeds. (Upper) Modified, with permission. Modhissi, K. Composition and function of cervical secretion, Chapter 31. In, Greep, R.O., editor. Handbook of Physiology, Section 7: Endocrinology, Volume Two. American Physiological Society; 1973. (Lower) The three pictures show smears of cervical mucus. Reprinted, with permission. Ingelman-Sundberg, A.; Wirsen, C. A Child is Born. New York: Delacorts Press; 1965.

Table 18.6 Dependence of Estrus on the Ovaries of Rats

	Before surgery	After surgery
sham	34%	20%
ovariectomized plus oil	28%	6%
ovariectomized plus estrogen	32%	62%

The data are the percent of vaginal smears that had cornified cells indicating the presence of estrogen. Vaginal smears were obtained from 26 rats for eight days prior to surgery. The percentage of smears with cornified cells was determined (before surgery data). Then the rats were divided into three groups that were treated with sham ovariectomy (N = 7 rats), ovariectomy plus daily sesame oil injections (N = 10 rats), or ovariectomy plus daily estradiol (0.1 mg in 0.2 ml sesame oil) injections (N = 9 rats). Daily vaginal smears were made for 12 days after surgery. The percentages of smears that had cornified cells were determined (after surgery data). Ovariectomy reduced the incidence of vaginal estrous smears but estrogen replacement therapy increased the incidence of vaginal estrus to twice pretreatment levels. The experiment was performed by students in an endocrinology course.

hypothalamic amenorrhea, undoubtedly due to a deficiency of gonadotropin-releasing hormone or excess prolactin release-inhibiting hormone. Hypothalamic amenorrhea is variously treated depending on whether the patient wishes to become pregnant, in which case a course of treatment that stimulates ovulation is required.

There is an **athletic** amenorrhea. Female athletes commonly develop amenorrhea (it occurs in about a third of long-distance runners) which correlates positively with weight loss and negatively with the percentage of body weight that is fat. Spontaneous LH pulse frequencies decrease.[29] Athletic amenorrhea is usually reversible with a reduction of physical activity, increase in body weight, and increase in body fat.

Another cause of amenorrhea is **anorexia nervosa** (an eating disorder of malnutrition due to starvation, self-induced vomiting, or laxatives). The amenorrhea may be explained by an alteration of female hormones. For example, in rats restricted to 10 g of food/day for 60 days, there is a decrease in pituitary gonadotropins and estradiol. The hormones can be increased with LRH.[30] The positive role of fat in female fertility is believed due to the high solubility of estrogen in fat.

Post-pill amenorrhea sometimes follows use of oral contraceptives. After stopping use of oral contraceptives, 97% of women ovulate by the third post-pill cycle, but about 2% of women have amenorrhea for up to several years.

Amenorrhea with galactorrhea (breast secretions) is characterized by high prolactin (sometimes from pituitary prolactin secreting tumors).

Amenorrhea with androgen excess has a variety of causes (ovarian, adrenal, menopause, etc.).

ORAL CONTRACEPTIVES

The antiovulatory properties of progesterone were recognized many years ago (Haberlandt, 1929). After all, ovulation is suppressed in pregnancy probably because of high progesterone. Orally potent progestens were produced by Djerassy in 1956. In developing steroid contraceptives in 1958, Pincus and Rock hoped to capitalize on the antiovulatory properties of progesterone. A variety of oral contraceptives (birth control pills) have since been developed which consist of synthetic estrogen and progesten (given daily for three weeks on, one week off) or progesten only (given daily).

Table 18.7 Estrous Cycle Lengths

Common name of animal	Species	Days
cow	*Bos taurus*	20–21
goat	*Capra hircus*	20–21
elephant	*Elephas maximus*	21
sheep	*Ovis aries*	14–20
pig	*Sus scrofa*	21
horse	*Equus caballus*	19–23
camel	*Camelus bactrianus*	10–20
dog	*Canis familiaris*	60
mink	*Mustela vison*	8–9
fox	*Vulpes vulpes*	90
ground squirrel	*Citellus tridecemlineatus*	16
guinea pig	*Cavia porcellus*	16–17
golden hamster	*Mesocricetus auratus*	4
mouse	*Mus musculus*	4–5
rat	*Rattus norvegicus*	4–5
shrew	*Sorex araneus*	13–19
platypus	*Ornithorhynchus anatinus*	60
opossum	*Didelphis marsupialis*	28
mouse lemur	*Microcebus murinus*	45–55

Van Tienhoven, A. Reproductive Physiology. Philadelphia, PA: W. B. Saunders; 1968; Sadleir, R. Cycles and seasons. In Austin, C.; Short, R., editors. Reproduction in Mammals Book 1: Germ Cells and Fertilization. Cambridge University Press; 1972; p. 90; Gorbman, A.; Dickhoff, W.; Vigna, S.; Clark, N.; Ralph, C. Comparative Endocrinology. New York: John Wiley and Sons; 1983; p. 502.

The pills are effective and reduce pregnancy to <0.2% by the end of the first year. Pregnancy rates for most of the oral contraceptives are only 0.1 to 1.0 per 100 woman years of use.[31]

The pills inhibit ovulation but also have other effects on the female reproductive system which may contribute to the prevention of pregnancy. The pills can alter oviduct contractions, cause endometrial atrophy, alter cervical mucus so that it may become impermeable to sperm (cervical hostility), block sperm capacitation, produce semiatrophic vaginal smears, and depress hormones (estrogen, pregnanediol, LH surge).

Because the pills are used by large numbers of women, there have been serious concerns about side effects of the oral contraceptives. Mild side effects (breakthrough bleeding, nausea, mastalgia, excessive withdrawal bleeding, transient psychologic changes, irritability, depression, fatigue) usually do not prevent women from using birth control pills. However the contraceptives may be discontinued for moderately severe side effects (headaches, worsened migraine, weight gain, increased skin pigmentation, acne, hirsutism, vaginal infections, etc.). Severe side effects include vascular disorders (venous thromboemboli disease, myocardial infarction, cerebrovascular disease), gastrointestinal disorders (cholestatic jaundice, symptomatic gallbladder disease), and depression (enough to cause 5% of patients to stop taking some types of pills).

In women on birth control pills, the menstrual body temperature cycle is lost. For contraception, progesten implants inserted under the skin prevent pregnancy for up to five years; they also can produce amenorrhea. Some synthetic pro-

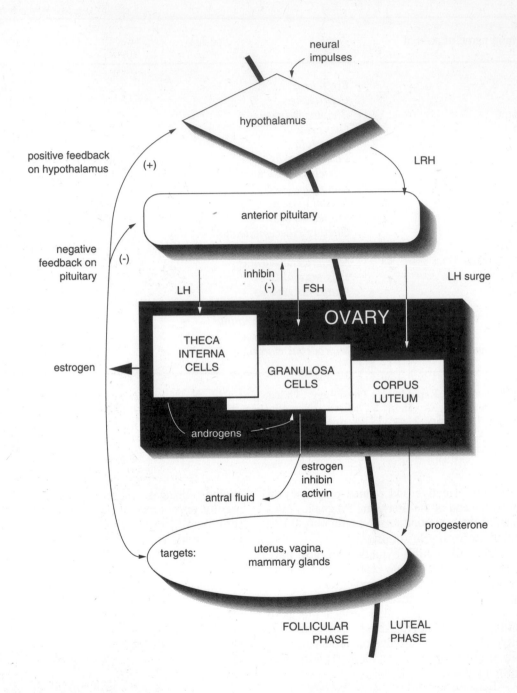

Figure 18.24 The diagram shows the regulation of female reproductive cycles. Negative feedback of estrogen and inhibin regulates pituitary secretion of LH and FSH; positive feedback of estrogen on the hypothalamus leads to the LH surge shifting the ovary from the follicular phase (left) to the luteal phase (right).

Table 18.8 Premenstrual Syndrome (PMS) Symptoms

MOOD ALTERATION, PSYCHOLOGICAL COMPLAINTS irritability nervousness lack of control agitation anger, aggression insomnia difficulty concentrating lethargy, severe fatigue depression tension	CARDIOVASCULAR easy bruising cardiac palpitation (fast beating heart) GASTROINTESTINAL SYMPTOMS bloating constipation nausea vomiting changes in appetite
SYMPTOMS RELATED TO FLUID RETENTION edema (swelling), bloated feeling transient weight gain oliguria (decrease in amount of urine) breast fullness, pain, tenderness thirst	SKIN PROBLEMS acne neurodermatitis (localized scratch dermatitis) aggravation of other skin disorders MISCELLANEOUS aggravation of epilepsy pelvic heaviness, pressure, pain backache worsening of respiratory allergies
NEUROLOGICAL SYMPTOMS headache vertigo syncope (fainting) paresthesias (sensations of tingling, crawling, or burning of skin) of the extremities hot flushes	worsening of respiratory infections visual disturbance conjunctivitis crying changes in libido poor coordination, clumsiness, accidents

O'Brien, K. PMS: The premenstrual syndrome: A review of the present status of therapy. Drugs 24: 140; 1982; and Berkow, R., editor. The Merck Manual, Fifteenth Edition. Rahway, NJ: Merck Sharp & Dohme Research Laboratories, Inc.; 1987; p. 1711.

gestens even inhibit sperm production in male animals.

MENOPAUSE

Menopause (climacteric) is the cessation of menstrual cycles. It begins gradually with shortened follicular phase, then the cycles become irregular, and finally, ovulation stops. The timing of the onset of menopause has been attributed to ovarian depletion of eggs and to alterations in LRH patterns.[32]

The endocrinological events surrounding menopause have been studied. In the ovary, the follicles are depleted and there is degeneration of the theca and granulosa cells. The cells stop responding to gonadotropins and produce less estrogen. The reduction in estrogen, due to the decrease in negative feedback, causes an increase in gonadotropins. This process precedes menopause by about five years. FSH levels increase and prolactin levels decrease in the premenopausal years. At menopause, LH levels increase causing the ovaries and adrenal glands to produce androgens. Postmenopausal women produce large amounts of androstenedione of which 95% comes from the

Table 18.9 Menopause Symptoms

REPRODUCTIVE SYSTEM cessation of menstruation cessation of ovulation reduction in ova number in ovary dyspareunia (painful intercourse) vaginitis vaginal atrophy (thinning of epithelium) vulvar skin thinning decrease in size of labia minora, clitoris, uterus, and ovaries	**CARDIOVASCULAR SYMPTOMS** cardiac palpitations tachycardia (rapid heart rate) **URINARY SYMPTOMS** increased pelvic relaxation urinary incontinence cystitis (bladder inflammation)
MOOD ALTERATION, PSYCHOLOGICAL COMPLAINTS fatigue irritability insomnia nervousness lack of sleep intermittent dizziness depression forgetfulness inability to concentrate paresthesias (sensations of tingling, crawling, or burning of skin)	**GASTROINTESTINAL SYMPTOMS** nausea flatulence constipation or diarrhoea weight gain **SKIN PROBLEMS** thinning skin hair loss **MISCELLANEOUS** hot flushes osteoporosis arthralgia (joint pain) myalgia (muscle pain) cold hands and feet
HORMONES high FSH and LH low estrogen, slightly reduced androgen	

Berkow, R., editor. The Merck Manual, Fifteenth Edition. Rahway, NJ: Merck Sharp & Dohme Research Laboratories, Inc.; 1987; p. 1687.

adrenal glands. Peripheral body fat converts the androstenedione to estrone. The estrone production depends on the weight of the woman—lean women may convert 1.5% of the androgen to 40 mg estrone/day while obese women convert 7% of the androgen to produce 200 mg of estrone/day.[33]

Menopause has variable symptoms which are also symptoms of ovariectomy (Table 18.9). Hot flushes (menopausal flushes, hot flashes) and sweating occur in 75% of women during menopause, usually for less than one year. The hot flushes are correlated with LH pulses, but occur in hypophysectomized women, so the flushes probably involve an LRH mechanism. Hot flushes were vividly described by Goldfien and Monroe:

> The hot flush often starts with a sensation of pressure in the head, followed by a feeling of warmth in the head and neck and upper thorax. It may be associated with palpitations and gradually spreading waves of heat over the entire body. The feeling of warmth and flushing is quickly followed by sweating. The sweating and vasodilatation lead to heat loss and a decrease in core temperature of approximately 0.2°C. These episodes last 10–20 minutes.[34]

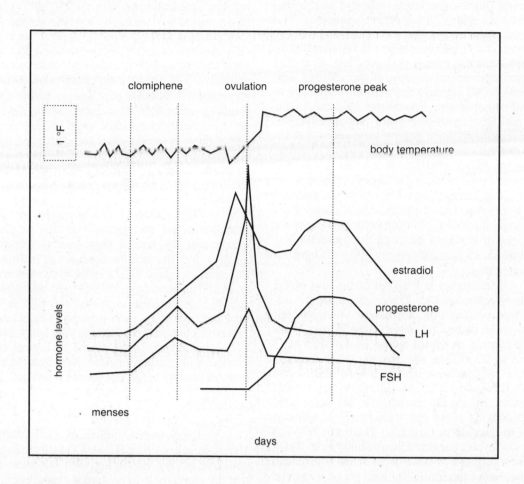

Figure 18.25 Treatment with the fertility drug clomiphene causes a sequence of female hormone changes (here shown for 32 days). The clomiphene treatment begins the fifth day after the onset of spontaneous menstruation or five days after the onset of withdrawal bleeding induced with progesterone. An LH surge and ovulation ensues 5–9 days after the last clomiphene tablet. Modified, with permission. Mishell, D.R.; Davajan, V. Infertility, Contraception, and Reproductive Endocrinology, Second Edition. Oradell, NJ: Medical Economic Books; 1986.

Serious problems are increases in heart disease and osteoporosis (enlargement of bone marrow at expense of solid bone parts making the bones more fragile). **Osteoporosis** in post-menopausal women can mean a loss of 0.75–2.5% bone mass per year. The consequence of the bone loss is an increase in fractures of the vertebrae (resulting in stooping posture and backache), hip fractures, and wrist fractures with little or no trauma. For example, a ten-fold increase in fractures of the carpal end of the radius occurs in 35–55 year old women; the increase is not seen in men. Factors that increase the risk of osteoporosis are white or Oriental race, slenderness, early menopause, family history of osteoporosis, diet (low calcium, low vitamin D, high caffeine, high alcohol, high protein), smoking, and sedentary life-style.

Estrogen replacement therapy relieves hot flushes, restores a feeling of well being, and relieves many of the other symptoms. The estrogen replacement also prevents skin thinning and dermal collagen loss that follow menopause, and, consequently, retards skin wrinkling. Extended estrogen replacement therapy, dietary calcium supplements (1000 mg/day) and vitamin D are used to combat osteoporosis. Treatments for osteoporosis with estrogen replacement are proved effective. Other treatments have been disappointing but include oral calcium supplements, estrogens, fluoride, androgens (men), sunlight (to increase vitamin D formation in the skin), back supports, physical exercise, phosphate supplements, calcitonin, parathyroid hormone, and diphosphonate compounds (etidronate disodium). No compelling evidence for an effect of estrogen on cognitive function was found in 65–95 year old women given estrogen replacement therapy.[35]

Menopause is a signal of the end of the female reproductive life. The cessation of menstruation is associated with, and believed by many scientists to be caused by, the **decline in ova** in the female ovaries. A pair of human fetal ovaries has 7 million to 20 million oocytes, but this number is reduced to 2 million by the time of birth, and further reduced to 200,000–400,000 by the time of menarche. During the reproductive life, some 8000 of the oocytes begin development (3–30 follicles begin to develop per cycle). There are 300-400 ovulatory cycles per reproductive lifespan in which one (or more rarely two) ova are actually ovulated. The number of primordial follicles per ovary can be 100,000 in a ten-year-old female but drops to 10–1000 in women nearing menopause who have had irregular cycles for a year. Less than one primordial follicle is found in postmenopausal women who have had no menses (menstrual periods) for one year.[36]

At the same time, the ovaries stop secreting 17-ß-estradiol and progesterone so that the target organs (uterus, vagina) atrophy. The reduction in negative feedback by the reproductive steroids causes large increases in gonadotropins, FSH, and LH. Animals don't have menopause, but old female mice and rats have sustained diestrus and high gonadotropins that resemble the human female climacteric.

The **age of menopause** in women is reported as 51 years, but menopause may begin as early as age 40.[37] The age span for spontaneous menopause is 42–60 years.[38] Variation in age of menopause, like the age of menarche, differs in different countries.[39] A factor in predicting the age of menopause is the age of menopause of the individual's mother, and this observation has led to the view that the age of menopause is determined genetically. The age at which menopause occurs is increasing.[40] Smokers may have an earlier spontaneous menopause.[41] Menopause before the age of 40 is medically considered to be premature. The age of onset is *not* believed to be affected by oral contraceptive use, age of menarche, pregnancies, lactation, failure to ovulate spontaneously, race, socioeconomic conditions, education, height, or weight.

The effect of the increase in age of menopause and the decrease in age of puberty means that the female reproductive lifespan is lengthening. Further, the median age of first marriage has increased dramatically in the last century (it is still increasing; between 1980 and 1988 the age of first marriage increased from 25 to 26 in men and from 22 to 24 in women). Social changes in reproductive patterns (teenage pregnancy, premarital sexual activity) may be the biological consequence of increasing the time span from the earlier onset of puberty to the later age of marriage.

ABORTION

Drugs used to induce abortion outside the United States, such as **RU-486** (Mefipristone) and epostane, act by interfering with progesterone so that the uterus fails to prepare for pregnancy. The drugs, which are sometimes combined with a prostaglandin, are effective 95% of the time during the first five weeks of pregnancy.[42] Other postcoital contraceptives ("morning-after pills") include conjugated estrogens, ethinyl estradiol, and DES. Intrauterine exposure to **DES** (diethylstilbestrol), which was formerly used to prevent miscarriages, has been linked to an increased incidence in vaginal cancer.

INHIBITION AND STIMULATION OF OVULATION

Various drugs affect female reproduction. Ovulation can be prevented in rats with pentobarbital administered 12 hours before the expected time of ovulation. Prevention of ovulation by pentobarbital is called **barbiturate blockade**.

Problems of infertility that are due to failure to ovulate in women with otherwise functional reproductive organs can be treated with **clomiphene citrate** (Clomid®). The drug is a weak estrogenic compound which stimulates ovulation in 80% of treated women by causing secretion of gonadotropins (Figure 18.25). A typical treatment is 50 mg/day for five days beginning 5 days after the onset of menses or withdrawal bleeding (induced with progesterone or oral progestin).[43] Side effects are those of menopause (hot flushes). Another "side effect" is a 5% increase in multiple gestations, usually twins. To achieve its effects in stimulating fertility, clomiphene citrate competes for estrogen-binding sites in the hypothalamus, blocks the negative feedback of endogenous estrogen, LRH is released, FSH and LH are released, the oocyte matures, estradiol levels increase exponentially, and finally there are LH and FSH surges resulting in ovulation and luteinization.

Other treatments induce fertility. **Menotropins** (Pergonal®, human menopausal gonadotropins) and HCG also stimulate ovulation. The treatment is more expensive than Clomid® and has a high probability of producing multiple births (25–40% of treated women become pregnant, 10–20% have twins, 5–10% have triplets). **LRH** also has potential for induction of ovulation. Pulsatile administration of 1–10 mg every 60–120 minutes causes ovulation. **Bromocriptine** mesylate, (Parlodel®, an ergot alkaloid) binds to dopamine receptors in the pituitary gland and thereby inhibits prolactin secretion. Bromocriptine treatment of amenorrhea with galactorrhea causes menses in 3–5 weeks and can be used to improve fertility.

REFERENCES

1. Adashi, E.Y. The potential relevance of cytokines to ovarian physiology: The emerging role of resident ovarian cells of the white blood cell series. Endocrine Reviews 11: 456; 1990.
2. Borth, R. Generic names for steroid hormones and related substances. Contraception 12: 373; 1975.
3. Tanner, J. M. Growth and endocrinology of the adolescent. In Gardner, L.I., editor. Endocrine and Genetic Diseases of Childhood, Philadelphia, PA: W.B. Saunders, Philadelphia; 1969; pp. 19–69.

4. Styne, D. Puberty. In Greenspan, F.; Forsham, P., editors. Basic and Clinical Endocrinology, Second Edition. Norwalk, CT: Appleton & Lange;1987; p. 462.
5. Styne, D.; Ibid.; p. 456.
6. Tanner, J.M. Growing up. Scientific American, September; 1973; p. 22.
7. Bullough, V.L. Age at menarche: A misunderstanding. Science 213: 365–366; 1981.
8. Droegemueller, W.; Herbst, M.D.; Mishell, D.R.; Stenchever, M.A. Comprehensive Gynecology. St. Louis, MO: C.V. Mosby; 1987; pp. 967–968.
9. Alleva, J.; Waleski, M.; Alleva, F. A biological clock controlling the estrous cycle of the hamster. Endocrinology 88: 1368–1379; 1971.
10. Ganong, W. Review of Medical Physiology, Fourteenth Edition. Appleton & Lange, Norwalk, CT; 1989; p. 380.
11. Dewan, E. On the possibility of a perfect rhythm method of birth control by periodic light stimulation. Am. J. Obstet. Gyn. 99: 1016–1019; 1967.
12. Senie, R.T., et al. Timing of breast cancer excision during the menstrual cycle influences duration of disease-free survival. JAMA 266: 3276; 1991.
13. Noyes, Hertig, and Rock. In Benson, R. editor. Current Obstetric and Gynecologic Diagnosis and Treatment, Fifth Edition. Lange; 1984.
14. Hadley, M. Endocrinology, Second Edition, Prentice-Hall, Englewood Cliffs, NJ; 1988; p. 443.
15. Sadlier, R. Cycles and seasons. In Austin, C.; Short, R., editors. Reproduction in Mammals Book 1: Germ Cells and Fertilization. Cambridge University Press; 1972; p. 87.
16. Reiter, R. Chronobiologia 1: 365–396; 1974.
17. Clarke, C.L.; Sutherland, R.L. Progestin regulation of cellular proliferation. Endocrine Reviews 11: 266–302; 1990.
18. Hadley, M. Endocrinology, Second Edition, Englewood Cliffs, NJ: Prentice-Hall: 1988; p. 431.
19. Ganong, W.; Op. cit.; p. 380.
20. Ganong, W. Review of Medical Physiology, Volume Fourteen. Appleton & Lange, Norwalk, CT; 1989; p. 374.
21. Ganong, W.; Op. cit.; p. 214.
22. Berkow, R., editor. The Merck Manual, Fifteenth Edition. Rahway, NJ: Merck Sharp &

Dohme Research Laboratories of Merck & Co., Inc.; 1987; p. 1655.

23. Droegemueller, W.; Herbst, M.D.; Mishell, D.R.; Stenchever, M.A. Comprehensive Gynecology. St. Louis: C.V. Mosby; 1987; p. 945.

24. Are your hormones up? Time. November 28; 1988.

25. Sack, D.; Rosenthal, N.; Parry, B.; Wehr, T. Biological rhythms in psychiatry. In Meltzer, H., editor. Psychopharmacology. New York: Raven Press, New York; 1987; p. 669–85.

26. Parry, B.L.; Berga, S.L.; Kripke, D.F.; Gillin, J.C. Melatonin and phototherapy in premenstrual depression. In Chronobiology: Its Role in Clinical Medicine, General Biology, and Agriculture, Part B, Wiley-Liss; 1990; pp. 35–43.

27. Rubinow, D.R. The premenstrual syndrome. Journal of the American Medical Association 268: 1908–1912; 1992.

28. Droegemueller, W.; Herbst, M.D.; Mishell, D.R.; Stenchever, M.A.; Op. cit.; p. 942.

29. Cumming, D.; Vickovic, M.; Wall, S; Fluker, M. Defects in pulsatile LH release in normally menstruating runners. J. Clin. Endocrinol. Metab. 60: 810–812; 1985.

30. Kotsuji, F.; Hosokawa, K.; Topinaga, T. Effects of the daily administration of gonadotropin-releasing hormone on the anterior pituitary gland of rats with restricted feeding. Journal of Endocrinology 134: 177–182; 1992.

31. Baird, D. T.; Glasier, A.F. Hormonal contraception. New England Journal of Medicine 328: 1543–1549; 1993.

32. Marx, J. Sexual responses are—almost—all in the brain. Science 241: 903-904; 1988.

33. Droegemueller, W.; Herbst, M.D.; Mishell, D.R.; Stenchever, M.A.; Op. cit.; p. 1085.

34. Goldfien, A.; Monroe, S. The ovaries. In Greenspan, F.; Forsham, P.; editors. Basic and Clinical Endocrinology, Third Edition. Norwalk, CT: Appleton & Lange; 1992; p. 479.

35. Connor, E. B.; Silverstein, D.K. Estrogen replacement therapy and cognitive function in older women. Journal of the American Medical Association 269: 2637–2641; 1993.

36. Richardson, S.; Senikas, V.; Nelson, J. Follicular depletion during the menopausal transition: Evidence for accelerated loss and ultimate exhaustion. J. Clin. Endocrinol. Metab. 65: 1231; 1987.

37. Berkow, R.; Op. cit.; p. 1687.

38. Goldfien, A.; Monroe, S., The ovaries. In Greenspan, F.; Forsham, P. Basic and Clinical Endocrinology, Second Edition. Norwalk,CT: Appleton & Lange; 1987; p. 419.

39. Gray, R. The menopause—epidemiological and demographic considerations. In Beard, R., editor. The Menopause. Lancaster, England: MTP Press Ltd; p. 25–40.

40. Flint, M. Is there a secular trend in age of menopause? Maturitas 1: 133–139; 1978.

41. Droegemueller, W.; Herbst, M.D.; Mishell, D.R.; Stenchever, M.A.; Op. cit.; p. 1082.

42. Regelson, W.; Loris, R., Kalimi, M. Beyond abortion: RU-486 and the needs of the crisis constituency. Journal of the American Medical Association 264: 1026–1027; 1990.

43. Droegemueller, W.; Herbst, M.D.; Mishell, D.R.; Stenchever, M.A.; Op. cit.; p. 1048.

CHAPTER 19

Pregnancy Hormones, Oxytocin, and Prolactin

The hormones of pregnancy include estrogen, progesterone, prolactin, oxytocin, human chorionic gonadotropin, somatomammotropin, prostaglandins, and relaxin. The pituitary, ovaries, and placenta secrete the hormones of pregnancy. Oxytocin from the hypothalamus functions in parturition and in milk ejection by a positive feedback system involving responses to sensory stimuli. Prolactin from the anterior pituitary gland has far-ranging effects on the reproductive organs, lactation, parental behavior, skin, osmoregulation, growth, and metabolism. During pregnancy in mammals, estrous and menstrual cycles cease, ovulation stops, and the uterus specializes to support the pregnancy.

HORMONES AND REPRODUCTION

Hormones are key players in all aspects of reproduction—in the production of the gametes (ova and sperm) by the gonads, in fertilization, in early development, in parturition, and in care of the young. During pregnancy in mammals, a placenta forms. The placenta must be viewed, along with the gonads, as an endocrine gland. It produces more than 30 hormones—protein hormones, glycoprotein hormones, cytokines, and growth factors.[1] The main steroid hormones secreted by the placenta are progesterone and the estrogens.[2]

Some of the cast of characters (the ovaries, hypothalamus, and pituitary and their hormones) may be the same as already discussed, but, during pregnancy, their concentrations and secretory patterns change dramatically in ways that transform the entire female reproductive system—estrous and menstrual cyclic hormone releases stop, ovulation ceases, and the uterus specializes to support the pregnancy.

FERTILIZATION

In mammals, the act of **coitus** (mating) consists of the male inserting his penis into the female where he ejaculates semen containing sperm into the upper vagina near the cervix. The **sperm** migrate through the cervix and uterus and into the oviducts, a process that takes 4–5 hours. Fertilization of the ovum by a spermatozoan takes place in the oviduct. Martin and Hoffman describe the time course of fertilization in humans:

> Following intercourse, sperm that are to survive penetrate the cervical mucus within minutes and can remain viable there until the mucus character changes [to be copious, nonviscous, and slightly alkaline], approximately 24 hours following ovulation. Sperm begin appearing in the outer third of the uterine tube (the ampulla) 5–10 minutes after coitus and continue to migrate to this location from the cervix for about 24–48 hours. Fertilization normally occurs in the ampulla.[3]

A membranous structure, the zona pellucida, encloses the ovum. Many sperms bind to the zona using a reaction between zona sperm receptors and an egg-binding protein on the sperm plasma membrane. The successful binding of a sperm causes the sperm receptor to trigger the acrosomal reaction. In the **acrosomal reaction**, the acrosome, which is an organelle on the sperm's head likened to a lysosome, disintegrates releasing enzymes (e.g., acrosin, a protease). Using the acrosin, the sperm is able to penetrate the zona. The sperm also interacts with the ovum membrane. The sperm fuses with the ovum membrane. The union of the sperm and membrane results in reduced ovum membrane potential, and then the zona pellucida changes structure. Once these events take place, the ovum is protected against fertilization by a second sperm. The fusion of the membranes of ovum and sperm causes the beginning of the sequence of embryonic development.

CONTRACEPTION

Contraception is used to prevent fertilization for the purpose of family planning (Table 19.1). Methods such as the diaphragm and the condom depend on a physical barrier between sperm and uterus. Others, such as spermicides, depend upon killing the spermatozoa. **Oral contraceptives** are based on antiovulatory properties of progesterone. The phrase "the pill" has come to refer to oral contraceptive pills. Contraceptive pills may have effects on the female reproductive organs that hinder the process of fertilization of the ovum or implantation of the fertilized egg (e.g., altered rate of travel of the ovum through the fallopian tubes, endometrial atrophy in the uterus, thickening of cervical mucus to produce cervical impermeability or "hostility" to sperm). However, the actions of oral contraceptives are summarized:

> The action of [oral contraceptives] results from a negative feedback on the hypothalamus, inhibiting gonadotropin-releasing hormone; therefore, the pituitary does not secrete gonadotropins at midcycle to stimulate ovulation. The endometrium of the uterus becomes thin, and the cervical mucus becomes thick and impervious to sperm.[4]

Morning-after pills are designed to block implantation, or in the case of Mifepristone and epostane, cause the uterine lining to slough. The idea of postcoital remedies is not new.

Table 19.1 Contraceptive Hormones, Physical Barriers, and Surgeries

Contraceptive	Failure rate	Possible side effects
oral contraceptives (female)	2–8% progestogen alone <0.2% combinations	depression, migraine headache, oligomenorrhea, undiagnosed amenorrhea, heavy cigarette smoking, temporary inhibition of ovulation, hemorrhagic stroke, thrombotic stroke, nausea, vomiting, fainting, sleep disturbances, hypertension
levonorgestrel in polysiloxone capsule subdermal implants	<1%	irregular uterine bleeding, amenorrhea
diaphragm, cervical cap with contraceptive cream or jelly (female)	3%, properly used 15% overall	
periodic abstinence (couple)	10%	
condom (male)	3–4%	
intrauterine devices (female)	<2%	bleeding, pain, expulsion, uterine perforation, bacterial contamination of endometrial cavity, spontaneous abortion
vasectomy (male)	0% once sperm-free ejaculates have been produced	up to 5% complications including hematoma, inflammatory responses to sperm leakage, spontaneous reanastomosis
tubal ligation (female) by laparoscopic fulguration	1 per 1000 procedures, some ectopic	0.6–6% complications including hemorrhage or bowel injury
elective vaginal hysterectomy (female)	0%	100% permanent sterility

Use of oral contraceptives is contraindicated by pregnancy, active liver disease, hyperlipidemia, uncontrolled hypertension, diabetes mellitus with vascular change, thrombophlebitis, thromboembolic history, coronary artery disease, stroke, sickle cell disease, estrogen dependent cancer, liver adenoma, cholestatic jaundice of pregnancy, prolonged immobilization of lower extremity. Failure rate is pregnancy rates per year of use, except tubal ligations. Berkow, R., editor. The Merck Manual, Sixteenth Edition. Rahway, NJ: Merck Sharp & Dohme Research Laboratories of Merck & Co., Inc.; 1992; pp. 1773–1780.

For generations, pregnant women have dosed themselves with unpalatable, hazardous potions in desperate, largely unsuccessful efforts to rid their bodies of unwanted fetuses. Among the dubious household remedies: swallowing narcotics made from hempseed, douching with the caustic

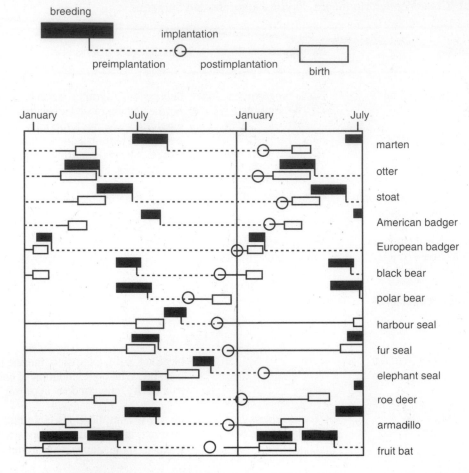

Figure 19.1 The figure illustrates times of breeding, birth, and implantation versus month of the year. A generalized example of the means of representation used is shown at the top: breeding (black bar), preimplantation (dashed line), implantation (circle), postimplantation (solid line), and birth (white bar). Modified, with permission. Sadleir, R. Cycles and Seasons. In Austin, C.; Short, R., editors. Reproduction in Mammals, I. Germ Cells and Fertilization. Cambridge University Press; 1972; p. 100.

disinfectant potassium permanganate, and even quaffing gin laced with iron filings.[5]

Intrauterine devices (IUDs) are inserted into the uterus for contraceptive purposes. The devices are usually plastic and/or copper, and they may act in a number of ways. IUDs may cause a sterile tissue reaction in the endometrial cavity yielding neutrophil breakdown in the uterus which produces products that are toxic to the sperm. Or IUDs may disturb the normal uterine

sequence of events so that the conditions for implantation are not appropriate when the blastocyst arrives for implantation.

Another alternative for family planning, especially when families are completed, is sterilization. Surgical sterilization of males for family planning is by **vasectomy** which involves cutting and tying the vas deferens. Female sterilization for family planning is by **tubal ligation**. In the female sterilization, the oviducts can be disrupted by fulguration (destruction of tissue by means of electric sparks), or by blocking the tubes with

Table 19.2 Durations of Pregnancies

Organism	Species scientific name	Gestation (days)
Indian elephant	*Elephas maximum*	623
black rhinoceros	*Diceros bicornis*	540
camel	*Camelus dromedarius*	390
blue whale	*Sibbaldus musculus*	365
southern fin whale	*Balaenoptera physalus*	365
Pacific grey whale	*Eschrichtius glaucus*	365
horse	*Equus cabullus*	336
cow	*Bos taurus*	280
human	*Homo sapiens*	280
chimpanzee	*Pan satyrus*	227
caribou	*Rangifer tarandus*	230
white-tailed deer	*Odocoileus virginianus*	204
baboon	*Papio conatus*	187
rhesus monkey	*Macaca mulata*	163
goat	*Capra hircus*	151
sheep	*Ovis aries*	150
pig	*Sus scrofa*	114
chinchilla	*Chinchilla laniger*	111
tiger	*Panthera tigris*	105
guinea pig	*Cavia porcellus*	63–70
cat	*Felis cattus*	63
dog	*Canis domesticus*	63
ferret	*Mustela furo*	41–43
wallaby	*Protemnodon bicolor*	35
red kangaroo	*Megaleia rufa*	33
rabbit	*Oryctolagus cuniculus*	31
dormouse	*Muscardinus avellanarius*	23
rat	*Rattus norvegicus*	21–23
mouse	*Mus musculus*	19–23
hamster	*Mesocricetus auratus*	14–18
opossum	*Didelphis virginianus*	13

Sadleir, R.M.F.S. Cycles and Season. In Austin, C.; Short, R., editors. Reproduction in Mammals Book 1: Germ Cells and Fertilization, Cambridge University Press; 1972; p. 96; and Martin, C. Endocrine Physiology. New York: Oxford University Press; 1985; p. 708.

bands or clips, or by ligation and partial excision.

Choice of the method to be used for contraception is not just a relatively simple matter of which contraceptive has the least side effects or which contraceptive has the lowest failure rate. For example, the condom has no side effects for a woman, and a higher failure rate, but it affords some protection against sexually transmitted diseases. Vasectomy has no side effects for a woman and it is totally effective, but it provides no protection against sexually transmitted diseases.

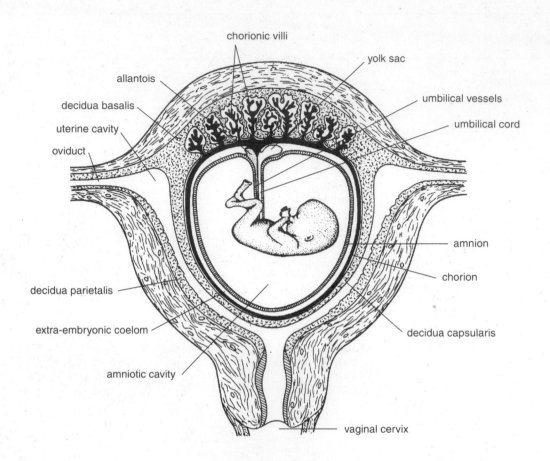

Figure 19.2 The simplified diagram shows the fetal membranes, fetus, and uterus. Modified, with permission. Huettner, A. F. *Comparative Embryology of the Vertebrates.* New York: MacMillan; 1949.

IMPLANTATION, DELAYED IMPLANTATION, AND DURATION OF GESTATION

Implantation is the event in which the embryo and uterus attach to each other. The fertilized egg, or conceptus, divides during the four to six days it spends in the oviduct and uterus before implantation. Thus, the developing embryo is at the blastocyst stage when it implants in the uterus. In the process of implantation, the layers surrounding the embryo (the syncytiotrophoblast and cytotrophoblast, cells from the embryo) interact with the endometrium so that the endometrium is invaded by the blastocyst which embeds itself in the endometrium. In humans, implantation starts days 5–8 after fertilization and is completed by day 9 or 10.[6] The blastocyst has 1000 to 10,000 cells at the time of implantation. The absence of the immunological rejection reaction is important for the process of implantation to take place. The immunological relationship of the fetus to the mother is that of a transplant or parasite, because the mother and fetus are genetically distinct:

> Like a successful parasite, the fetal-placental unit manipulates the maternal 'host' for its own gain but normally avoids imposing excessive

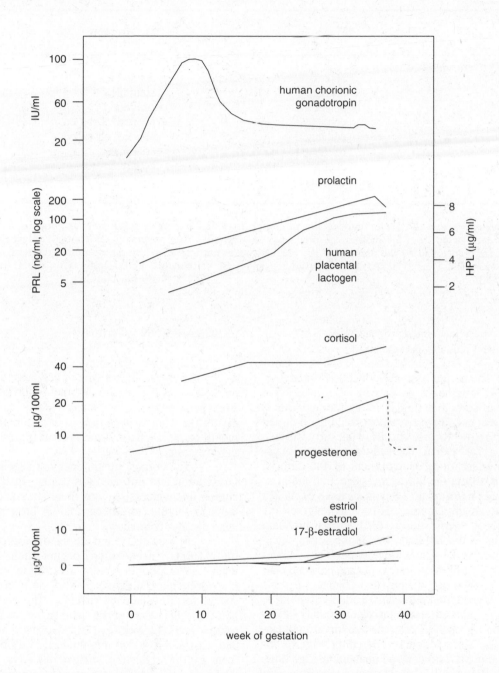

Figure 19.3 Some hormone changes during pregnancy are shown. Progesterone decreases precipitously at the time of parturition. Replotted form data published in Aragona, C.; Friesen, H.G. Lactation and galactorrhea. In DeGroot, L.J.; Cahill, G.F.; Martin, L.; Nelson, D.H.; Odell, W.D.; Potts, J.T.; Steinberger, E.; Windgrad, A. I., editors. Endocrinology, Volume 3. New York: Grune & Stratton; 1979; pp. 1614–1617.

Table 19.3 Pregnancy Maintenance

Organism	Hypophysectomy	Ovariectomy
rabbit	aborted	aborted
dog	aborted	continued
guinea pig	continued	continued
mouse	continued	aborted, absorbed
rat	continued	aborted, absorbed
sheep	continued	continued
rhesus monkey	continued	continued
woman	continued	continued

The table shows the effect of removing the pituitary gland or the ovaries from pregnant organisms. If the embryos are ejected from the mother, the pregnancy is "aborted." The pregnancy is "aborted, absorbed" if the embryos are reabsorbed by the mother. If the pregnancy was not terminated by the operation, the designation is "continued." Van Tienhoven, A. Reproductive Physiology of Vertebrates. Philadelphia, PA: W. B. Saunders; 1968; p. 336.

stress that would jeopardize the 'host' and thus the 'parasite' itself.[7]

The period of time from conception to parturition is lengthened as part of the reproductive strategy of some mammals. In one strategy that is usually associated with seasonal breeding, **delayed implantation** occurs. In the wild, only the tree mouse has "aseasonal" delayed implantation. In delayed implantation, development of the embryo stops, usually at the blastocyst stage, and the blastocyst does not implant. Scientists have explained that delayed implantation is used to lengthen the period from fertilization to birth so that breeding can occur in the fall and birth in the spring when conditions for the young are optimal. Other strategies for adjusting the duration of time between mating and birthing are delayed fertilization (in some bats), delayed development (extended gestation, in some bats), and embryonic diapause (delay of implantation by suckling in some marsupials and lactating laboratory rodents). Breeding patterns for some mammals with delayed implantation are illustrated in Figure 19.1. **Gestation durations** vary in mammals from as little as 14 days in the hamster to almost two years in the elephant (Table 19.2).

PREGNANCY IN WOMEN

Pregnancy duration in women is estimated as 266 days from the the date of conception or 280 days (40 weeks) from the first day of the last menstrual period (assumes a 28–day cycle).[8] Clinicians divide the human gestation period into three 3-month parts: first trimester, second trimester, and third trimester.

The corpus luteum does not degenerate if fertilization and implantation occur. Instead, the corpus luteum persists into pregnancy and functions to secrete hormones, mainly progesterone, that influence pregnancy.

In humans, in the uterus, the formation of the placenta (placentation) occurs about day 10 when the trophoblast cells invade the maternal blood vessels. Blood seeps into the intercellular spaces forming lacunae (lakes). The embryo is nourished by blood in the lacunae. First the placenta is around the embryo and exchanges nutrients and wastes across cell membranes. Villi begin to form in the chorionic surface on days 11–12. About day 19, the placenta develops its own blood vessels and establishes the "villar pattern of transfer from maternal blood to fetal blood."[9] During week 12, the placenta becomes discoid and by weeks 18–20 has reached its final form, though it continues

Table 19.4 Pregnancy Tests

Test	Sensitivity for HCG (mIU/ml)
Gravindex®	3500
Prognosticon Dri-Dot®	1000–2000
e.p.t.®	1250
Pregnosticon®	700–750
RIAs, ß-HCG antibody tests	10–15

Gravindex® and Prognosticon Dri-Dot® detect pregnancy approximately two weeks after the first missed menses; RIA and ß-HCG antibody tests detect pregnancy as early as ten days after fertilization. The table was made from information in Berkow, R., editor. The Merck Manual, Fifteenth Edition. Rahway, NJ: Merck Sharp & Dohme Research Laboratories of Merck and Co., Inc.; 1987; p. 1745.

to grow for the rest of the nine months to a weight of one pound (about 500 grams). Some of the anatomical relationships between the fetus and the uterus are shown in Figure 19.2.

The vagina also changes during pregnancy. For example, in the rat, the surface cells become columnar and the middle cell layers become vacuolated and the epithelium secretes mucus (mucification reaction). The mucus-secreting vagina can be induced experimentally in rats by injecting progestens or androgens.[10]

CHORIONIC GONADOTROPIN

Hormones, from the pituitary and ovary and placenta, are important in the events and maintenance of pregnancy (Figure 19.3). But pregnancy maintenance does not require the presence of the ovaries and pituitary glands in all species. Experiments, removing the ovaries or the pituitary during pregnancy, have been done to determine whether the pituitary or the ovary is necessary for the persistence of a pregnancy. The results vary depending on the species—both glands may be necessary or neither gland may be required (Table 19.3).

Chorionic gonadotropin (CG, HCG = hCG = human chorionic gonadotropin) functions to maintain the corpus luteum. Chorionic gonadotropin is considered to be a hormone product of the placenta. The gonadotropin is a glycoprotein with 237 amino acids that is similar to the pituitary glycoproteins. It contains about 30% carbohydrate by weight and sialic acid contributes 10% of the weight of the molecule. It is believed that the sialic acid stabilizes the hormone against degradation. Because of its similarities to pituitary glycoproteins, HCG has LH and TSH activities.

During early pregnancy, the doubling rate for HCG concentration is every 1.7 to 2 days, so HCG provides an early indication of the occurrence of a pregnancy.

The hormone HCG is the basis for most urine and blood pregnancy tests. Peak maternal HCG (about 100,000 mIU/l) occurs during the tenth week of pregnancy. Thereafter the hormone concentration gradually declines to about 10,000 mIU/l in the third trimester.

The cells of the embryonic layers (cytotrophoblast) may make a releasing-factor (hCGnRH = human chorionic gonadotropin-releasing hormone) that is biologically and immunologically similar to LRH. In turn, the hCGnRH releases HCG from the syncytiotrophoblast.

Human chorionic gonadotropin is normally produced only in pregnant women, but HCG has other effects. Chorionic gonadotropin causes differentiation of Leydig cells and increases androgen production in males. The effect of HCG in males may be because of HCG's structural similarities to LH. Chorionic gonadotropin causes release of spermatozoa in lower vertebrates. Chorionic gonadotropin can be used in replacement therapy where it substitutes for FSH and LH.

Table 19.5 False Positives and False Negatives

Sample	Frog test pregnant	Frog test not pregnant	Agglutination pregnant	Agglutination not pregnant
pregnant	55%	45%	73%	27%
HCG	44%	56%	73%	27%
nonpregnant	7%	93%	24%	76%
male	18%	82%	23%	77%
Ringer's solution	11%	89%	20%	80%

The Galli-Mainini frog test (sperm in urine is positive) and a latex agglutination-inhibition test were performed by novices (endocrinology laboratory students) on samples of urine (from pregnant women, women who were not pregnant, or men) or were performed on standard solutions (HCG, 12.5 IU/ml in amphibian Ringer's solution and amphibian Ringer's solution). The samples were provided to the students as unknowns. The percentages are calculated from the reported results and the total number of tests done. In other words, when the students tested urine from pregnant women with the frog test, 55% of the students reported a correct positive (pregnant) result and 45% of the students reported a false negative result. Overall, the agglutination test produced fewer false negatives; the Galli-Mainini test produced fewer false positives. Data collected by students in the author's endocrinology class.

ESTROGEN AND PROGESTERONE

The placenta also produces large quantities of **estrogen**. Estrogen in human maternal urine rises to 20,000 mU/day in comparison to 300 mU/day for urine from nonpregnant women. Fetal and maternal steroid precursors (e.g., fetal DHEA sulfate from the fetal adrenal gland) are converted to androgens and aromatized in the placenta to make estrogens (estrone, estradiol, estriol, estetrol). Estradiol and estrone in pregnancy rise to 50 times their prepregnancy levels; estriol rises to 1000 times its prepregnancy level. Estriol provides an indicator of fetal function; a drop greater than 50% indicates fetal jeopardy.

The placenta begins producing **progesterone** from maternal cholesterol by the second month of human gestation. Before that, progesterone comes from the ovaries. Progesterone inhibits uterine contractions, prepares the uterus structurally for the embryo, prevents ovulations, and may prevent immunological rejection of the embryo. By the third trimester, amounts of progesterone are 250–350 mg/day.

SOMATOMAMMOTROPIN

The placenta makes somatomammotropin whose 191 amino acid structure is similar to human growth hormone. Other names for somatomammotropin include placental lactogen; hPL = HPL = human placental lactogen; chorionic growth hormone prolactin = CGP; and human chorionic somatomammotropin = HCS. Somatomammotropin has little effect on growth, but it is diabetogenic, it stimulates the pigeon crop sac growth, and it has some lactogenic activity. The amount of somatomammotropin circulating in maternal blood is proportional to the size of the placenta; low amounts are indicative of placental insufficiency. The function of somatomammotropin in pregnancy is debated, but has been summarized: "HCS has most of the actions of growth hormone and apparently functions as a 'maternal growth hormone of pregnancy' to bring about the nitrogen, potassium, and calcium retention and decreased glucose utilization seen in this state."[11]

Other hormones secreted by the placenta or

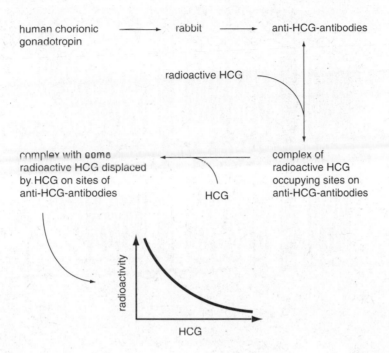

Figure 19.4 The principles of RIA (radioimmunoassay) for HCG (human chorionic gonadotropin) are presented diagrammatically. (i) A rabbit forms antibodies to injected HCG. (ii) The antibodies, harvested from the rabbit's blood, are mixed with radioactive HCG which occupies the binding sites for HCG on the antibodies. (iii) Then, the radioactive HCG-antibody complex is reacted separately with a series of unknown and standard samples containing HCG. For each sample, the resulting solution is centrifuged and the radioactivity of the pellet containing the antibody is counted. A standard curve is plotted for the standard samples. The more HCG in the standard, the greater the displacement of radioactive HCG from antibody sites, and the lower the radioactivity that is counted. The radioactivity of unknowns is determined by reading HCG corresponding to the radioactivity of the unknown from the standard curve.

isolated from the placenta include a TSH-like thyrotropic glycoprotein, an ACTH-like peptide, a lipotropin-like peptide, an endorphin-like peptide, and an FSH-like protein.[12] The placenta may also make relaxin and renin.

CORPUS LUTEUM OF PREGNANCY

During pregnancy, the corpus luteum of the ovary makes progestens (progesterone, 17-hydroxyprogesterone) and estradiol. In humans, the corpus luteum is required for early pregnancy until 42 days of gestation. Before that time, removal of the corpus luteum causes serum progesterone and estradiol to plummet, and the pregnancy is aborted.

Abortion after corpus luteum removal can be prevented by administration of progesterone. After 42 days of gestation, removing the corpus luteum does not result in abortion, presumably because by then the placenta is producing sufficient progesterone.

The ovary also produces **relaxin** during pregnancy. Relaxin (molecular weight 6000) is a polypeptide hormone whose structure has similarities to insulin. Relaxin is made by the corpus luteum. During pregnancy, it rises in maternal circulation to 1 ng/ml. Relaxin from the ovary is not essential for pregnancy maintenance. During pregnancy, relaxin functions to make mechanical alterations of the reproductive organs—cervical ripening, pubic symphysis softening, uterine con-

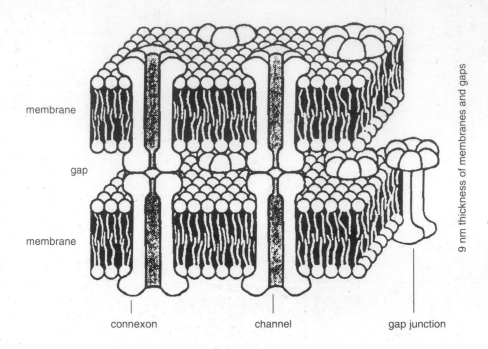

membrane

gap

membrane

9 nm thickness of membranes and gaps

connexon   channel   gap junction

8nm between gap channels

Figure 19.5 The diagram shows a hypothetical representation of gap junctions. The junctions bridge the 2-nm space, or gap, between two membranes (e.g., the presynaptic and postsynaptic membranes). Six subunits, connexons, in hexagonal arrays, surround a channel through which low molecular weight solutes (ions, amines, sugars) can pass without entering the extracellular fluid. Voltage and calcium and pH regulate the diameter of the channel. Redrawn, with permission. Kandel, E.R.; Schwartz, J.H., editors. Principles of Neural Science, Second Edition. New York: Elsevier; 1981; p.65.

traction inhibition, increased myometrial glycogen synthesis, increased myometrial water uptake, and mammotropism.

Hormones from the corpus luteum are responsible for the early symptoms of pregnancy: absence of menstruation, softening of the uterus, elevated basal body temperature, breast tenderness, fatigue, and so-called "morning sickness" (nausea).

OTHER ENDOCRINE FUNCTIONS DURING PREGNANCY

The **pituitary gland** gets about 33% larger during pregnancy because of lactotrop hyperplasia and concomitant increase in prolactin secretion. The pituitary becomes unresponsive to LRH so that LH and FSH levels fall; this goes together with the suppression of ovulation and the men-

strual or estrous cycles during gestation. Responses of GH to hypoglycemia and arginine infusion first increase, then decline during pregnancy.

The **thyroid gland** also enlarges in pregnancy and takes up and clears more iodine and makes more thyroxine. Hyperthyroidism is mimicked by pregnancy, and hypothyroidism during pregnancy is usually harmful to the fetus. In areas with endemic goiter, iodine supplements and thyroid hormone treatment of the mother may prevent cretinism.[13] Thyroid hormones are necessary for normal development in most species. Radioactive iodine administered to pregnant women can destroy the fetal thyroid.

The maternal **parathyroid gland** has to increase parathyroid hormone production to meet

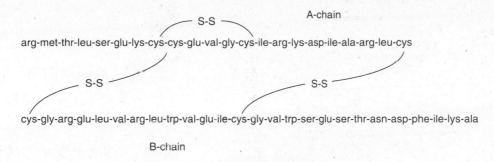

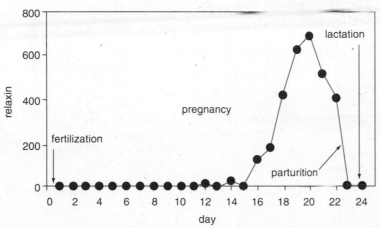

Figure 19.6 The structure of relaxin is shown at the top. Below the structure is a graph of relaxin immunoactivity levels (mg/g equivalent) in extracts of ovaries from pregnant and lactating rats. Sherwood, O.D.; Crnekovic, V.E.; Gordon, W.L.; Rutherford, J.E. Radioimmunoassay of relaxin throughout pregnancy and during parturition in the rat. Endocrinology 107: 691–698; 1980.

the fetal calcium requirement for development of its skeleton (about 30 grams of calcium).

The **pancreas** increases insulin secretion, and increased concentrations of insulin are found in blood. There are changes in metabolism in which the fetus is protected at the expense of the mother. Maternal glucose levels drop as fetal glucose needs are met. Maternal energy requirements are met by peripheral metabolism of fatty acids. Even moderate fasting can injure the fetus. Oral hypoglycemics taken by pregnant women can lower fetal blood glucose.

Increased estrogen doubles CBG (corticosteroid-binding globulin) and thereby raises circulating glucocorticoids three-fold by lengthening the half-life of plasma cortisol, even though **adrenal cortex** production of glucocorticoids drops 20%. The fetus also contributes glucocorticoids which cross the placenta. The appearance of

striae (so-called stretch marks) is attributed to the increase in adrenal hormones.

The zona glomerulosa produces 8–10 times as much **aldosterone**. Renin substrate, renin, renin activity, and **angiotensin** increase. But renin and aldosterone do not appear to be involved in late pregnancy edema or in pregnancy-induced hypertension.

Maternal-circulating **testosterone** rises into the male range in the first trimester; as for glucocorticoids, the rise appears to be related to the testosterone binding to a carrier globulin (SHBG, sex hormone-binding globulin).

PREGNANCY TESTS

The technology for pregnancy testing has a long tradition and has undergone an evolution from bioassay to techniques that depend on

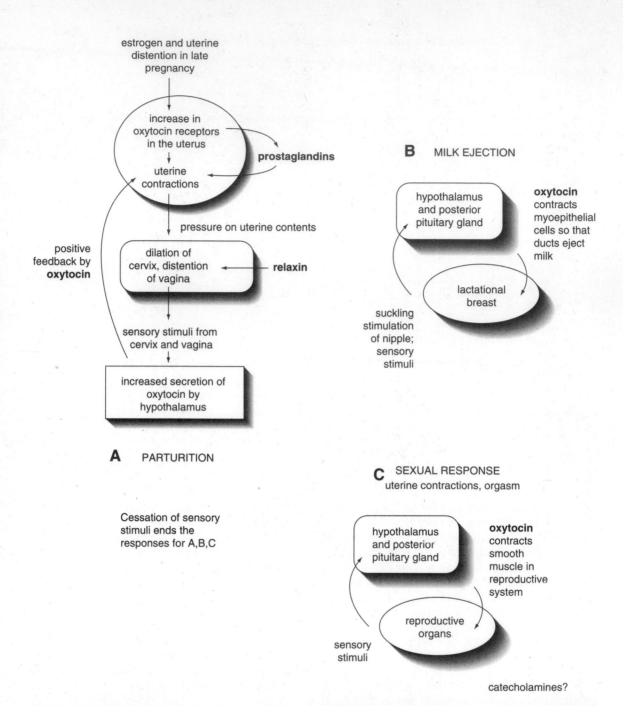

Figure 19.7 The diagrams represent the regulation of oxytocin in parturition (A) and suckling (B). In the model for parturition, the initiating event is the increase in oxytocin receptors in the myometrium and decidua (pregnancy endometrium). The process stops when the uterine contents are expelled, removing the sensory stimuli from the cervix and vagina. The model in the lower right illustrates the suckling reflex (milk-ejection reflex) that is initiated when the nipples and areolas are touched. Note the presence of positive feedback for regulation of oxytocin. There is also possible role for oxytocin in sexual responses (C).

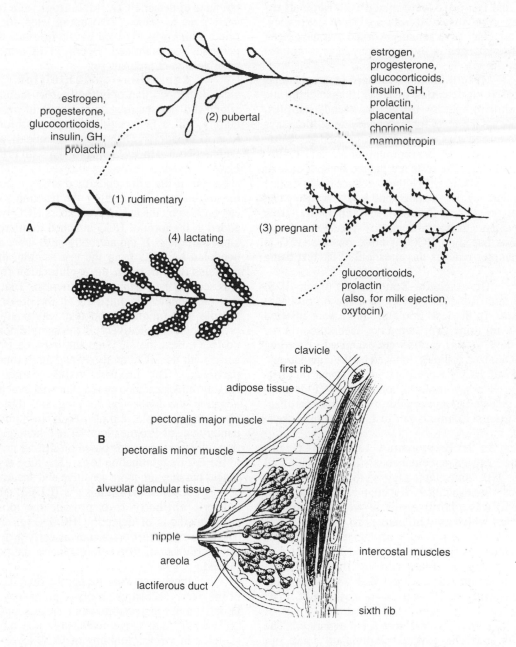

Figure 19.8 The diagrams represent (A) the sequence of development of the ducts of the mammary glands and (B) the anatomy of the human female breast. The events of development from the rudimentary childhood stage are under control of the hormones listed between them. Redrawn, with permission. Ganong, W. Review of Medical Physiology, Fourteenth Edition. Norwalk, CT: Appleton & Lange; 1989; p. 386; and Norman, A.W.; Litwack, G. Hormones. Orlando, FL: Academic Press; 1987; p. 570.

the use of antibodies.

Three to four thousand years ago, barley seed and test urine were mixed with earth. If the barley grew faster, it was a sign of pregnancy. This test may have actually worked to some extent, because estrogen in the urine may have stimulated barley growth.

Most of the more modern pregnancy tests are based on detection of HCG, human chorionic gonadotropins, in urine or blood samples. Originally the tests for pregnancy were bioassays that required rats, mice, frogs, or rabbits. More recently the tests are radioimmunological or immunological. The tests are judged on their ease of use, the degree to which they produce false positive and false negative results, and how early they can detect pregnancy (Tables 19.4 and 19.5). How early can pregnancy be detected? The answer to that for tests based on HCG, is how soon the HCG in the samples reaches the threshold of the test being used.

The **Ascheim-Zondek test** (circa 1928) used mice to detect HCG in urine of pregnant women. In the test, immature mice were injected with 2 ml urine over two days, then killed on the fifth day. Their ovaries were examined. Bleeding and luteinized follicles, induced by the gonadotropic action of HCG, were positive evidence of pregnancy. The test took 96 hours, was 98% dependable, detected pregnancy three weeks after fertilization, used six animals per test, and required fresh urine.

In the **Kupperman test** for HCG, immature rats were subcutaneously injected with 2 ml urine. Six hours later they were killed and their ovaries were examined. Hyperemia (increased blood content) was a positive sign of pregnancy. In another test which used immature rats, pregnancy was indicated by the presence of vaginal estrus 72–96 hours after test substance was introduced.

The **Friedman test** for HCG used rabbits. A rabbit was injected with 10–15 ml urine intravenously and killed 24–48 hours later. The rabbit's ovaries were examined for signs of ovulation as a positive test for pregnancy. The rabbits must be isolated individually and not stressed to avoid stimulating ovulation with signals other than test urine.

The **Hogben test** used female toads (South African clawed toads, *Xenopus laevis*) to detect HCG. The dorsal lymph sacs were injected with urine. Release of eggs, ovulation, 6–12 hours later was positive evidence of pregnancy.

The **Galli-Mainini test** also used amphibians to detect HCG. Male frogs were injected with 5 ml of urine. Two hours later, the frog's urine, which was excreted by the frog in a dry fingerbowl, was examined. Sperm in the urine was a positive sign of pregnancy.

Agglutination-inhibition tests were developed that only took a few minutes and which did not require maintenance of an animal colony. In a latex agglutination inhibition test (e.g., Gravindex®, Ortho Pharmaceutical), a liquid with antibodies to HCG was mixed with urine on a black microscope slide and allowed to react for 30 seconds. If the urine contained HCG, it bound to the antibodies. To visualize the reaction so that it can be seen by the naked eye, excess HCG was then added in the form of HCG attached to microscopic latex particles. If the antibody sites were already occupied by HCG from the test sample, then the particles did not react, no agglutination response was seen in the ensuing two minutes. That meant that the sample contained HCG, the donor of the sample was pregnant, the test was positive for pregnancy. Alternatively, if the sample contained no HCG, then the HCG on the latex particles reacted with the HCG antibody and agglutinated the particles. The mixture visibly turned more "grainy" in appearance on the slide and indicated the negative, the donor was not pregnant. Urine tube tests (for example, e.p.t.®, early in-home pregnancy test, or Pregnosticon®) use hemagglutination inhibition reactions based on similar principles to the latex agglutination tests. The tube tests take longer but they are more sensitive and accurate.

Radioimmunoassays (RIAs) and **beta subunit antibody tests** provide the most sensitive methods of detecting HCG (Figure 19.4). The tests can detect pregnancy as early as ten days after fertilization, even before a menstrual period is missed.

Pregnancy tests are not the final indicators of pregnancy. Positive proofs of pregnancy are fetal heart tones (detectable with a stethoscope at 18-20 weeks), fetal movements, presence of a fetal skeleton in x-rays, doubling of HCG levels, ultrasound detection of a fetus with cardiac motion and an intrauterine sac, and delivery of a fetus. Other signs of pregnancy are (i) missed menstruation for two weeks, (ii) changes in the appearance of the vagina and cervix (more bluish to purple), and (iii) softer cervix and uterus.

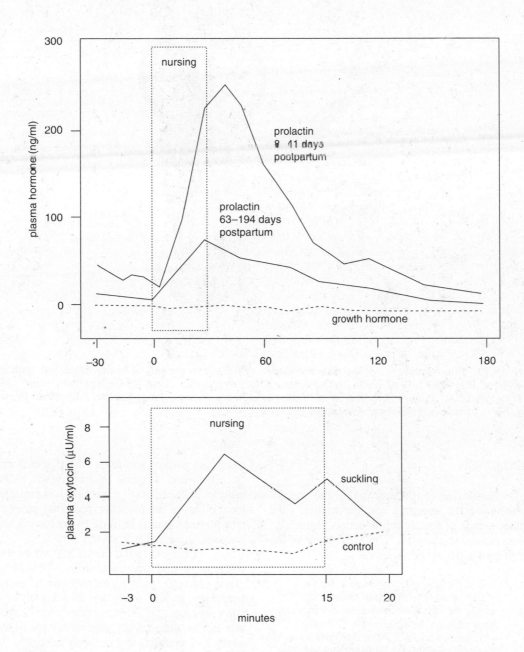

Figure 19.9 The figure shows the changes in hormones during episodes of nursing (suckling) in lactating women. The figures have been redrawn, with permission. Noel, G.L.; Suh, H.N.; Frantz, A.G. J. Clin. Endocrinol. Metab. 36: 1255; 1974; and Weitzman, R.E.; Leake, R.E.; Rubin, R.T.; Fisher, D.A. The effect of nursing on neurohypophyseal hormone and prolactin secretion in human subjects. J. Clin. Endocrinol. 51: 836–839; 1980.

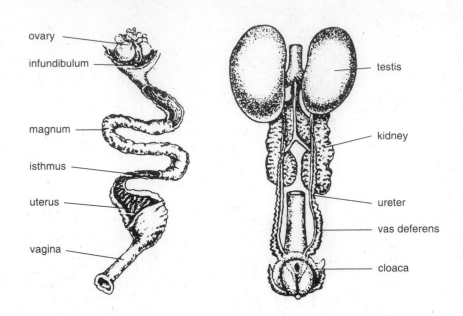

ovary

infundibulum

magnum

isthmus

uterus

vagina

testis

kidney

ureter

vas deferens

cloaca

Figure 19.10 The diagrams show the male and female reproductive systems of birds. Modified, with permission. Welty, J.C. The Life of Birds, Third Edition. Philadelphia, PA: Saunders College Publishing; 1982; pp. 160–163; Jull, M.A. Poultry Breeding. New York: John Wiley & Sons; 1952; Sturkie, P.D. Avian Physiology. Ithaca, NY: Comstock Publishing Associates; 1965.

PARTURITION

Parturition (birth, delivery) is the process by which the fetus separates from the mother. Like the other events of female reproduction, parturition involves hormone changes. The exact cause of the onset of parturition is not known:

> The difficulty in identifying a single initiating event in human labor may simply be that there is more than one. Approaching the matter in a different way, one could ask: What are the factors responsible for maintenance of pregnancy, and how can they fail?[14]

One reason that the initiating event has been difficult to pin down is that removing suspected signals has not blocked labor from occurring. Delivery occurs without increased maternal oxytocin, without the fetus (the placenta delivers on time), and without bearing down (voluntary muscle contractions). Onset of labor might be a local effect of the placenta (secreting progesterone into uterine tissues) because twins having separate placentas can have independent births.

Changes in the uterus happen as the final weeks of normal pregnancy arrive. The changes include painless uterine contractions of increasing frequency, and softening and thinning of the cervix and lower uterus effacement (ripening). Labor usually has an abrupt onset, uterine contractions recur every 2–5 minutes, and delivery normally follows within a day.

One idea about the initiation of labor involves progesterone, the **progesterone block** hypothesis. Progesterone maintains pregnancy and if progesterone is not present, the pregnancy is terminated. Progesterone also declines precipi-

```
NH2-
leu-pro-ile-cys-pro-gly-gly-ala-ala-arg-      (10)
cys-gln-val-thr-leu-arg-asp-leu-phe-asp-      (20)
arg-ala-val-val-leu-ser-his-tyr-ile-his-      (30)
asn-leu-ser-ser-glu-met-phe-ser-glu-phe-      (40)
asp-lys-arg-tyr-thr-his-gly-arg-gly-phe-      (50)
ile-thr-lys-ala-ile-asn-ser-cys-his-thr-      (60)
ser-ser-leu-ala-thr-pro-glu-asp-lys-glu-      (70)
gln-ala-gln-gln-met-asn-gln-lys-asp-phe-      (80)
leu-ser-leu-ile-val-ser-ile-leu-arg-ser-      (90)
trp-asn-glu-pro-leu-tyr-his-leu-val-thr-      (100)
glu-val-arg-gly-met-gln-glu-ala-pro-glu-      (110)
ala-ile-leu-ser-lys-ala-val-glu-ile-glu-      (120)
glu-gln-thr-lys-arg-keu-leu-glu-gly-met-      (130)
glu-leu-ile-val-ser-gln-val-his-pro-glu-      (140)
thr-lys-glu-asn-glu-ile-tyr-pro-val-trp-      (150)
ser-gly-leu-pro-ser-leu-gln-met-ala-asp-      (160)
glu-glu-ser-arg-leu-ser-ala-tyr-tyr-asn-      (170)
leu-leu-his-cys-leu-arg-arg-asp-ser-his-      (180)
lys-ile-asp-asn-tyr-leu-lys-leu-leu-lys-      (190)
cys-arg-ile-ile-his-asn-asn-asn-cys-        (199)
-COOH
```

Figure 19.11 The structure of prolactin is shown. It has three disulfide bonds. Modified, with permission. Li, C. H. Chemistry of ovine prolactin. In Greep, R.O. Section 7: Endocrinology, IV. The Pituitary Gland and Its Neuroendocrine Control, Part 2; Washington, D.C.: American Physiological Society; 1974; p. 106.

tously at the time of parturition. So one idea is that a decline in progesterone is the initiating event. However, even if this is true, we then face the question, "What causes the decline in progesterone?"

Catecholamines affect uterine contractions. The uterine contracting effect involves α_2 receptors; labor inhibition, or uterine relaxation, involves β_2 receptors. The action of progesterone may involve uterine catecholamine receptors. The ratio of beta to alpha receptors is increased by progesterone. Another idea is that stretch-induced hypertrophy of the uterus may lead to degeneration of the nerves removing a beta "neural inhibitor influence" of catecholamine neurotransmitters.

Another idea is based on an **increase in myometrial gap junctions**. Gap junctions (nexuses, low resistance electrical pathways) form between cells that make up tissues such as the myometrium of the uterus (Figure 19.5). Intercellular spaces are narrowed from 25 nm to 3 nm at the location of a gap junction. In addition, there is a characteristic hexagonal array of protein units called connexons which surround a 2-nm channel. Channels of adjacent cells are aligned. Dissolved substances smaller than MW1000 (sugars, ions, amino acids) can cross rapidly through the channel from one cell to the next without going through the intracellular fluid. Channel diameter is subject to regulation by calcium, pH, and voltage. The gap junctions allow exchange of chemical messages and aid propagation of electrical activity. The

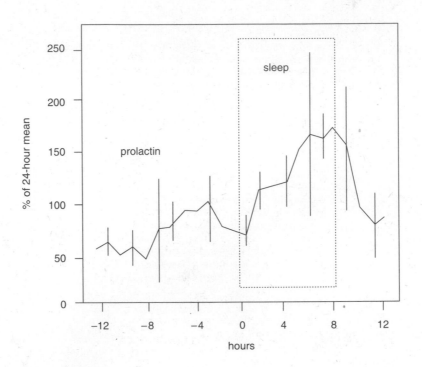

Figure 19.12 The figure illustrates the average daily cycle in prolactin in six male and female human subjects. The data are plotted with time 0 = the beginning of the sleep time. Standard deviations are represented by vertical lines for some, but not all, of the points to give an indication of variability. Redrawn, with permission. Frantz, A.G. Rhythms in prolactin secretion. In Krieger, D.K., editor. Endocrine Rhythms. New York: Raven Press; 1979; p. 177.

numbers of gap junctions present between uterine muscle cells increases just before, during, and after delivery, and the junctions are otherwise absent in pregnant or nonpregnant animals. In the gap junction model for parturition initiation, an increase in the estrogen to progesterone ratio occurs preceding birth. The change in the estrogen to progesterone ratio, or the increase in progesterone, increases the number of gap junctions in the myometrium of the uterus. The gap junction increase is supposed responsible for the contractions of true labor.

Prostaglandins may play a role in par-

turition. Arachidonic acid, a precursor of prostaglandins, is found in high concentration in chorion and amnion. Prostaglandin synthetase is active in decidua. Prostaglandins were identified for their ability to cause uterine contractions. Exogenous prostaglandins can induce labor or produce abortions; prostaglandin synthetase inhibitors block premature labor and prolong labor; and oxytocin increases prostaglandin formation in the decidua.

Somatomammotropin, or placental prolactin, is another hormone that increases in the fetus and amniotic fluid in late gestation. It is possible that this hormone also plays a role in parturition.

ACTH or glucocorticoids induce delivery. Thus, the onset of parturition initiated by the fetal pituitary-adrenal axis is a possibility. The placenta makes placental progestogens, progesterone, and pregnenolone; the fetus uses placental progestens to synthesize the androgens DHEA and 16-hydroxy-DHEA; the placenta forms estradiol and estriol from the fetal androgens. The ACTH could change the estrogen to progesterone ratio by inducing 17,20-desmolase and 17-α-hydroxylase in the placenta.

Increased levels of **relaxin** are found in some animals at the time of parturition (Figure 19.6). Relaxin promotes uterine contractility, so that relaxin could have a role in the initiation of the birth process in some species. Relaxin, synergistic with estrogen, lengthens the inter pubis symphysis. Relaxin is made by the corpus luteum of the ovaries, by the placenta, and by the uterus.

Oxytocin (Pitocin™) induces labor. Some models for an oxytocin role in labor initiation have been suggested. Both fetal and maternal oxytocin increase during labor. Oxytocin effects may involve increased uterine sensitivity to oxytocin rather than increases in circulating levels (about 25 pg/ml before labor) because there is a greater than 100-fold increase in oxytocin receptors, possibly in response to estrogen and uterine distention, during pregnancy. The number of oxytocin receptors peaks during early labor. Inhibition of oxytocin secretion prolongs labor. Evidence for the role of oxytocin would be inability to deliver in women with diabetes insipidus, but some have normal deliveries prompting proponents of oxytocin models for the initiation of birth to suppose that the disease resulted in defective vasopressin secretion but spared oxytocin-secreting neurons.

Once labor has been initiated, a **positive feedback loop** involving oxytocin takes place (Figure 19.7). Uterine contractions dilate the cervix (by increasing pressure on the cervix?) which causes the cervix to signal the brain via afferent nerves. The brain in turn increases oxytocin secretion. Oxytocin increases uterine contractions by contracting smooth muscle in the uterus and by stimulating prostaglandin formation (prostaglandins cause uterine contractions). Increased uterine contractions and bearing down further stimulate the cervix.

The positive feedback model for oxytocin initiation of uterine contractions has similarities to the coital induction of ovulation model for induced ovulators. There are seasonal, estrous, and daily cycles in oxytocin. Oxytocin's seasonal changes were observed in the female goat stimulated by vaginal distention; oxytocin was high (about 160 mU/ml plasma) in February–April and low (<20 mU/ml plasma) from March–November.[15] As evidence of estrous cycling, neurophysin doubled from 4 ng/ml to 8 ng/ml in monkeys just after ovulation.[16] Oxytocin has a circadian rhythm which increases during the day (to about 20 µU/ml) and declines during the night (to about 5 µU/ml) in the cerebrospinal fluid of monkeys.[17]

LACTATION

The process of lactation (the formation or secretion of milk) requires mammary glands. The possession of mammary glands is the attribute for which mammals are named. Mammary glands are one of the characteristics that distinguish mammals from other vertebrates (birds, reptiles, amphibians, and fish) that do not possess mammary glands. Lactation can be divided into four stages: mammogenesis, lactogenesis, galactopoiesis, and milk ejection. Each of these stages has its own array of endocrine changes. In childhood the mammary glands are rudimentary. Mammogenesis produces adult mammary glands during puberty. During pregnancy the mammary glands become lactational (lactogenesis). After birth, with suckling stimuli, the mammary glands continue to be lactational (galactopoiesis and milk ejection).

Mammogenesis is the development of the mammary glands. The hormones involved in mammogenesis are estrogen, progesterone, prolactin, GH, and glucocorticoids. Estrogen promotes growth of the duct system at the time of puberty. Progesterone is necessary for full development of the mammary glands. Other hormones that have some effect on mammogenesis include gonadotropins, somatotropin, corticotropin, thyrotropin, insulin, and human placental lactogen.

Lactogenesis is the name given to milk secretion during pregnancy (as early as month five) and lactation by the mammary glands. The principal hormones required for lactogenesis are prolactin and hormones of the adrenal cortex. Lactogenesis

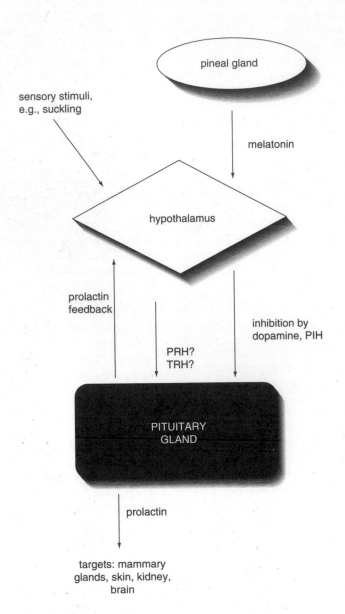

Figure 19.13 The figure illustrates the regulation of prolactin.

is inhibited by estrogen and progesterone in late pregnancy but facilitated by somatotropin and thyrotropin. After delivery, increased prolactin and declining progesterone and estrogen stimulate copious milk secretion.

Galactopoiesis is the maintenance of lactation. It requires a suckling stimulus. The main hormone involved is prolactin, but there are also effects of corticotropin, somatotropin, thyrotropin, and oxytocin.

Milk ejection is the process of milk removal from the mammary glands. Milk ejection involves a suckling reflex (touch stimulating of nipples and areolas) and the hormone oxytocin (Figure 19.8). Oxytocin causes the myoepithelial cells lining the duck walls of the mammary glands to contract which results in milk being ejected through the nipple (Figure 19.9). Other hormones contribute to milk ejection, including vasopressin, histamine, acetylcholine, pilocarpine, serotonin. Stress blocks milk ejection and epinephrine can block it via vasoconstriction. In the absence of suckling, the breasts become engorged with milk. Animals are able to secrete milk a few hours after delivery. Humans secrete colostrum just after parturition and milk secretion follows in 1–3 days. Milk secretion is associated with the postpartum decline in estrogen. Estrogen administration stops lactation.

Without nursing, menstrual cycles resume so that the first menstruation occurs about six weeks after parturition. In women who nurse, prolactin is stimulated by suckling and prolactin inhibits LRH secretion and thereby inhibits ovulation. About 50% of women who nurse do not ovulate spontaneously. Ovulation and menstrual cycling resume at weaning when nursing is ceased. Despite this, breast-feeding should not be taken as a method of birth control.

BIRDS

Reproduction in birds does not involve a pregnancy. Instead, the eggs are laid by the female, incubated by their parents, and hatched by the developing chicks.

Male and female reproductive tracts in birds differ from those in mammals (Figure 19.10). In birds, there is no scrotum; the testes are in the abdomen. Welty attempts to explain the temperature problem using observations of Riley and Wolfson:

> In many birds whose body temperature are too high for the production of spermatozoa by day, the nocturnal drop in body temperature makes sperm production possible at night [and] the caudal storage region of the vas deferens in some species swells into a cloacal protuberance whose temperature... may be 4°C cooler.[18]

The reproductive and excretory organs empty into the cloaca. The female has only the left ovary in most birds (raptors have a pair). The single ovary may be an adaptation to reduce weight for flight, or, to keep two mature eggs from cracking each other during hard landings. Photoperiod usually controls the ovarian and testis cycles with long days increasing gonadotropin release. Photoperiod effects on the testes are dramatic so that the testes in breeding condition are sometimes 200–300 times as large as in the nonbreeding condition. Male reproductive function in birds can be impressive. Duck testes in breeding season can be a tenth of the body weight; the male chicken can ejaculate 8 billion sperm; a sperm can travel the length of a hen's oviduct in 26 minutes.[19]

Chickens have cycles of egg laying. They lay eggs in a sequence called a **clutch**. The chicken lays one egg every 26 hours for 3–5 days, then does not lay eggs for 40–48 hours. Various stimuli (light, food, temperature) influence clutch timing. Egg production is also an impressive phenomenon for the large amount of growth that is achieved in a short time. For example, a rook follicle matures from 3.5 mm in diameter to 14.6 mm in diameter in four days.[20] Posterior pituitary injections stimulate a hen to lay an egg in 3–4 minutes.[21]

Estrogen causes chicken livers to form calcium-binding phospholipoprotein for egg formation, and estrogen stimulates oviduct growth and differentiation. During the breeding season, the avian oviduct is 10–50 times as heavy as when the birds are sexually inactive or ovariectomized. Progesterone causes the chick oviduct to secrete avidin and ovalbumen. The chick oviduct has provided a model for investigating the mechanism of action of steroids in general and progesterone in particular.[22] Most of the time that an egg is in the oviduct (18–20 hours in the hen), it is in the uterus or shell gland where its watery albumen, limy shell, and eggshell pigments are added. Laying hens have physiological changes that adapt them for egg production. They must do this because, in the domestic hen for example, 250 eggs can be laid per year. Blood sugar and calcium provide examples of physiological adaptations for egg laying. Blood sugar concentration in laying birds is twice that in males or nonlaying females. Blood calcium rises (i.e., from 10 mg/100 cc to 19 mg/100 cc) in the ovulating pigeon.

To improve the contact between the bird's blood stream and the shell of the egg during incubation, **brood patches** (incubation patches) form. Brood patches are defeathered areas on the bird's abdomen. When the brood patch forms, the bird loses down and the skin vascularization increases so that the skin appears to be inflamed. A bird can increase its ability to apply warmth to eggs by almost 6°C. Estrogen, androgen, prolactin, and progesterone variously induce one to three brood patches depending on the species.

Birds do not have mammary glands and must fetch food for their young. In some birds, a part of the digestive system is the crop. The crop stores food for a day or more until there is space in the stomach. Pigeons have a crop that is a large double sac. The pigeon crop can store food, and it can also secrete a "**crop milk**" or "pigeon milk" for feeding the young. Formation of crop milk is controlled by the hormone prolactin. The milk is produced in both sexes by desquamation of the inner cell layers of the paired crop sacs. The cells are regurgitated to feed the young. The effect of prolactin to increase the weight of the crop sacs of pigeons was the basis for the bioassay of prolactin. Another bioassay is to measure the increase in height of the crop sac epithelium in the white squab pigeon.

Secondary sex characteristics of birds are dependent upon hormones. Plumage, color, combs, wattles, spurs, size, song (crowing), and reproductive behavior constitute the secondary sex characteristics. Some male characteristics depend on testosterone and intact testes (combs, wattles, plumage, song, sex instincts); some male characteristics are inhibited by estrogens (spur, penis, maletype syrinx). Castrated roosters (capons) lose male characteristics and can be feminized with ovarian transplants or restored to masculinity with testis transplants. Castrated hens (poulards) can be masculinized by implanting testes.

PROLACTIN

Prolactin is also called "galactin," "mammotropin," "luteotrophic hormone (LTH)," "lactogenic hormone," and "pituitary lactogen." The molecule is a protein with three disulfide bonds and prolactin's molecular weight is 23,000 (Figure 19.11). Prolactin's 199 amino acids bear similarities to growth hormone. Sixteen percent of amino acids differ between prolactin and growth hormone; 13% of amino acids are different between prolactin and human chorionic somatotropin. Animal prolactins are not active in humans despite the similarity of 141 of the 199 amino acids. Prolactin is synthesized from preprolactin (MW 40,000-50,000) which is also secreted and which accounts for 8–20% of plasma immunoreactivity.

In human plasma, prolactin is 5 ng/ml in men and 8-9 ng/ml in nonpregnant women. The upper normal range is 15–30 ng/ml. About 400 mg/day are secreted. Prolactin has a daily cycle with its peak at the end of the night (4 a.m. to 7 a.m.) and its nadir in the morning (Figure 19.12). However, the prolactin secretion is tied to sleep per se, whenever sleep occurs. Prolactin is produced episodically by the anterior pituitary gland lactotrops which are acidophils.

The number of lactotrops increases to 50% of the acidophils during pregnancy and lactation. Prolactin is also secreted by choriondecidual tissue (placental prolactin). Prolactin does not follow a reproducible pattern of changes during the menstrual cycle but averages higher in the preovulatory and luteal phases. During pregnancy prolactin rises steadily. Kidney and liver remove prolactin from the circulation. The half-life of prolactin is about 15–50 minutes.

Prolactin secretion is inhibited by PIH (prolactin-inhibiting hormone) which appears to be dopamine (from tuberoinfundibular dopaminergic neurons secreted into the hypophysial portal veins). The cell bodies of the neurons are in the arcuate nuclei and the terminals of the neurons are mostly in the external layer of the median eminence in the same area as LRH endings. Feedback, stimulation of dopamine secretion by prolactin, in the median eminence is a probable means of prolactin regulation (Figure 19.13). Hypothalamic extracts, however, also have prolactin-releasing factors. Potential prolactin-releasing factors include TRH, VIP (vasoactive intestinal peptide), and serotoninergic pathways. Prolactin can be depleted experimentally from the anterior pituitary gland by cysteamine.[23] Bird prolactin may be regulated by a stimulatory mechanism.

There are many stimuli that increase prolactin, including L-dopa, melatonin, exercise, sexual intercourse (women), surgical stress, psychological stress, hypoglycemia, acute myocardial infarction, sleep, pregnancy (peaks at parturition), drugs that block dopamine receptors (chlorpromazine, phenothiazines, haloperidol, metoclopramide, reserpine, methyldopa, amoxapine, or opiates), TRH, putative PRH, estrogens, oral contraceptives, VIP (from the hypothalamus), opioids, MAO inhibitors, cimetidine, verapamil, intraventricular histamine or melatonin, and licorice. But the most potent stimulation is that of the nipple (suckling, nursing). Prolactin secretion is inhibited by dopamine agonists (bromocriptine, levodopa, apomorphine, pergolide, or ergot alkaloids), GABA, and cholinergic pathways.

Prolactin has been called the "hormone of maternity."[24] Prolactin acts on the breast to cause milk secretion. Prolactin finds receptors on the plasmalemma of mammary gland alveolar secretory cells. The numbers of receptors are increased by prolactin and estradiol, but decreased by progesterone. In the mechanism of action, prolactin stimulates phospholipase A2 activity. The consequence of the phospholipase activity increase is production of arachidonic acid from phosphatidylcholine. Prostaglandins that stimulate mRNA transcription are produced from the arachidonic acid. The further action on mammary glands involves mRNA, increasing casein and lactalbumin, and microtubules. Prolactin inhibits ovulation in lactating women. One idea is that the ovary is believed to be the target of this effect and prolactin may inhibit the actions of gonadotropins at the ovary. Another idea is that PRL surges act on the hypothalamus to inhibit LRH. In some organisms (rodents), prolactin maintains the corpus luteum.

Prolactin may function in males to control the testis. Prolactin appears to be necessary for maintaining testicular LH receptors on Leydig cells. Hypophysectomy results in a loss of the receptors; prolactin treatment augments the receptor numbers. Inhibition of prolactin secretion (ergot alkaloids) decreases testicular LH receptors. Prolactin stimulates growth of the prostate gland of the castrated rat when it is also given testosterone.

Sites of prolactin action in the brain include neurons in the dorsomedial nuclei, ventromedial nuclei, tuberoinfundibular dopaminergic neurons, and ependyma of the choroid plexus. Moreover, prolactin may act on the liver to stimulate **synlactin** production. Synlactin is a somatomedin-like factor that synergizes the action of prolactin.[25]

Prolactin is noteworthy for its bewildering array of functions in a variety of species. Bern and Nicoll classified these functions into actions related to reproduction, integument and derivatives, osmoregulation, growth, and metabolism (Table 19.6). One of the most interesting aspects of prolactin function has to do with its regulation of fat. Prolactin is responsible for the premigratory fattening that occurs in migrating species of birds. According to Cincotta, Schiller, and Meier, prolactin plays a central role in the regulation of lipogenesis and body fat stores in species representing all the vertebrate classes. Timed prolactin injections can increase (or decrease) body fat stores in two weeks, and a prolactin inhibitor, bromocriptine, can reduce body fat in nonhuman animal subjects.[26,27] Morning bromocriptine administration reduced body fat stores more 12% in obese human subjects and reduced weight 2.5% in the obese subjects.[28]

MISCARRIAGES

Spontaneous abortions, or miscarriages, are usually due to abnormality of the fetus, absence of the fetus, or a damaged placenta. Spontaneous abortion is viewed clinically as a natural mechanism for rejecting an abnormal fetus or terminating an abnormal pregnancy. In the second trimester, miscarriages may have more contribution from maternal factors—a problem with the cervix, disorders of the uterus, endocrine disorders (hypothyroidism, diabetes mellitus), viruses, and even emotional shock. The events leading to the abortion usually include a drop in progesterone. High LH secretion may be a predictor of miscarriage in some women:

> Of the 147 women with LH concentrations of less than 10 IU/l (normal LH group) 130 (88%) conceived, whereas only 31 (67%) of the 46 women with LH values of 10 IU/l or more (high LH group) did so. . . . These data indicate an important role for hypersecretion

Table 19.6 The Many Functions of Prolactin

PROLACTIN ACTIONS RELATED TO REPRODUCTION AND PARENTAL CARE

1. Nest building and fin-fanning in teleost fish
2. Skin mucus secretion and discus milk secretion in teleost fish
3. Reduction of toxic effects of estrogen in fish
4. Growth and secretion of seminal vesicles in teleost fish
5. Preparation for prespawning migration in teleost fish
6. Stimulation of eft water drive and skin changes in amphibians
7. Secretion of oviducal jelly in amphibians
8. Spermatogenic and antispermatogenic activities in amphibians
9. Termination of cyclic male sexual activity in amphibians
10. Secretion of crop milk in pigeons
11. Formation of brood patches in birds
12. Lipogenesis and deposition of premigratory fat in birds
13. Antigonadal activity in birds
14. Premigratory restlessness (Zugunruhe) in birds
15. Feeding of young birds
16. Setting on eggs in domestic fowl
17. Synergism with steroids on female reproductive tract in birds
18. Stimulation of mammary gland development and lactation in mammals
19. Synergism with androgen in male sexual accessory growth in mammals
29. Maintenance and secretion of corpus luteum in mouse, rat, ferret, possible synergism in other species of mammals
21. Increased fertility of dwarf mice
22. Retrieval of young by laboratory rats
23. Decrease in copulatory activity in male rabbits

PROLACTIN ACTIONS ON INTEGUMENT AND DERIVATIVES

1. Maintenance of hypophysectomized euryhaline teleost fish in fresh water
2. Skin mucus secretion and secretion of discus milk in teleost fish
3. Melanogenesis and proliferation of melanocytes (synergist with MSH) in teleost fish
4. Stimulation of eft water-drive including skin changes in amphibians
5. Proliferation of amphibian melanophores
6. Regulation of reptile skin molting
7. Shedding of crop sac epithelium in secretion of crop milk
8. Brood patch formation in birds
9. Stimulation of feather growth in birds
10. Stimulation of mammary gland development and lactation in mammals
11. Sebaceous gland size and activity in mammals
12. Rat preputial gland size and activity
13. Mammalian hair maturation

Table 19.6 The Many Functions of Prolactin (cont.)

PROLACTIN ACTIONS RELATED TO OSMOREGULATION
1. Maintenance of hypophysectomized euryhaline teleost fish in fresh water
2. Skin mucus secretion in teleost fish
3. Gill mucus-cell physiology in teleost fish
4. Renal excretion in teleost fish
5. Preparation of prespawning migration in teleost fish including preadaptation to fresh water
6. Stimulation of eft water drive and skin changes in amphibians
7. Renotropic in mammals

PROLACTIN ACTIONS RELATED TO GROWTH
1. Thyrotropin stimulation in teleost fish
2. Stimulation of eft water-drive during the second metamorphosis in amphibians
3. Stimulation of larval growth and possible peripheral thyroxine antagonism in amphibians
4. Stimulation of somatic growth in reptiles
5. Stimulation of caudal regeneration in reptiles
6. Hyperphagia in reptiles
7. Stimulation of growth in birds
8. Stimulation of growth in mammals

PROLACTIN ACTIONS RELATED TO METABOLISM
1. Thyrotropin stimulation in teleost fish
2. Lipid deposition in teleost fish
3. Resistance to high temperature stress in teleost fish
4. Hyperglycemic-diabetogenic in amphibians
5. Goitrogenic in amphibians
6. Reduction in lipid deposition in reptiles
7. Hyperphagia in reptiles
8. Lipogenesis and deposition of premigratory fat in birds
9. Stimulation of growth in birds
10. Hyperglycemic-diabetogenic in birds
11. Hyperglycemic-diabetogenic in mammals
12. Lipid deposition in mammals
13. Stimulation of growth in mammals
14. Erythropoietic in mammals

After Turner, C.P.; Bagnara, J.T. Endocrinology, Sixth Edition. Philadelphia, PA: Saunders; 1976; p. 106–107; compilation based on Bern, H.A.; Nicoll, C.S. The taxonomic specificity of prolactins. In Fontaine, M., editor. La specificite zoologique des hormones hypophysaires et de leurs activites. Paris: Centre Naional de la Recherche Scientifique; 1969; p. 193.

of LH before conception in miscarriage. This finding offers the possibility of a simple predictive test for women before pregnancy.[29]

GYNECOMASTIA

Gynecomastia is breast development in the male and is seen commonly in neonatal males and in about 70% of males during puberty. In adult males, the occurrence is about 1% (visible) with up to 40% upon histological examination. Gynecomastia is induced by drugs (amphetamines, anrogens, CG, cimetidine, digitalis, estrogens, hydoxyzine, isoniazid, marijuana, meprobamate, methadone, methyldopa, phenothiazines, reserpine, spironolactone).[30] Gynecomastia is a symptom of endocrine disorders (hypogonadism, hyperprolactinemia, hyperthyroidism, hypothyroidism). The causes of gynecomastia involve reduced testosterone, estrogen effects on the breast, or prolactin effects on the breast. In the case of marijuana, gynecomastia results from interaction with breast estrogen receptors.

HYPERPROLACTINEMIA

Hyperprolactinemia, increased prolactin levels, may be a symptom of chromophobe adenoma. Other symptoms associated with hyperprolactinemia may include galactorrhea (excessive flow of milk) and amenorrhea (failure to menstruate) in women. Prolactin excess causes testosterone reduction, decreased spermatogenesis, impotency, infertility, and decreased libido in men. Other consequences of hyperprolactinemia include glucose intolerance, hyperinsulinemia, anxiety, and depression. In animals, secretion of prolactin can be prolonged by coitus, cervical stimulation, or foster litter suckling; the condition is called pseudopregnancy. Women who imagine themselves pregnant when they are not (pseudocyesis, false pregnancy) can have symptoms of pregnancy such as morning sickness, abdominal enlargement, and changes in the breast.

MATERNAL-FETAL HORMONE EXCHANGES

The subject of the exchange of hormones between the mother and the fetus can be conveniently considered from two perspectives: (1) hormones from the fetus that influence the mother, (2) hormones of the mother that influence the fetus.

During pregnancy, the placenta functions as an endocrine gland producing more than 30 hormones (Figure 19.14). Some of the hormones are steroidal hormones.[31] The placenta carries on the reactions from cholesterol to pregnenolone; and the placenta converts two fetal steroid products to estradiol and estriol. For the steroids then, the mother provides cholesterol to the placenta, the fetus returns estrogens to the mother. The placenta becomes a source of progesterone by weeks 6–8 of human pregnancy. By the third trimester, women produce 210 mg/day of progesterone which is ten times the amount of the luteal phase of the menstrual cycle. Circulating levels of progesterone are 150–175 ng/ml at term. The placenta also produces protein hormones, glycoprotein hormones, cytokines, and growth factors. The placenta is a target possessing receptors for a variety of hormones including thyronines, steroids, protein hormones, etc. Placentas have served as a natural source for isolation of hormones and receptors. Placental function has been studied using perfusion, organ culture, explant culture, and dispersed placental cells in culture.[32]

The fetal adrenal glands also produce steroids. The fetus produces androgen precursors DHEAS (dehydroepiandrosterone sulfate) and 16-OH-DHEAS, which are necessary for the placenta to produce estrogen. In the early fetus, when there is an intermediate lobe, MSH and CLIP-like peptides dominate the fetus during gestation. There is a switchover to ACTH production just before parturition.[33] Urinary estriol is not usually great in women, but urinary estriol is the principal estrogen formed by the fetus. Therefore, maternal estriol is indicative of fetal status. The fetus also makes glucocorticoids and they may play a role in initiating parturition in some species. The physiological significance of the fetal adrenal has been summarized by Pepe and Albrecht:

> Products of the fetal adrenal gland appear to play an important role in regulating maturation of various organ systems in the fetus, providing the fetus homeostatic mechanisms to respond to stress, and initiating and/or participating in the cascade of events culminating in the birth of a newborn....[C]ortisol, presumably of fetal adrenal origin, is one of the

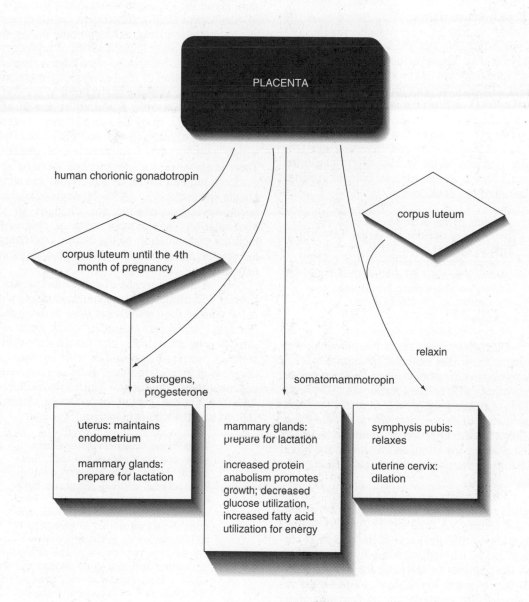

Figure 19.14 The figure illustrates the endocrinology of pregnancy. Redrawn, with permission. Tortora, G.J.; Anagnostakos, N.P. Principles of Anatomy and Physiology, Sixth Edition. New York: Harper & Row; 1990; p. 940.

chemical messengers involved in the stimuli to lung maturation, deposition of glycogen in the liver, and induction of several enzymes in the fetal brain, retina, pancreas, and gastrointestinal tract.[34]

It is possible that the fetal endocrine system plays a role in parturition. Fetal oxytocin rises before an increase can be measured in maternal oxytocin. Thus, it is possible that very early in labor, the fetus secretes a hormone, oxytocin, which, if it reached the decidua (the portion of the endometrium of the uterus that is cast off in parturition and menstruation) and myometrium (the muscular portions of the uterus) might cause the uterus to contract. A role for fetal cortisol in parturition has also been considered:

> Ablation of the fetal adrenal in sheep prevents parturition, whereas infusion of cortisol or ACTH to the fetus induces premature delivery [but the] evidence that the fetal adrenal of the human or nonprimate participates in the initiation of labor is less convincing.[35]

Other hormones cross the placenta For example, to show that maternal melatonin reaches the embryos, investigators injected pregnant female baboons or rats with tritiated melatonin (3H-acetyl-melatonin). Subsequently they were able to show the appearance of the radioactivity in the plasma at 3 minutes after the injection, in amniotic fluid 3–8 minutes after the injection, and finally in the blood (12–21-fold increase) and cerebrospinal fluid of the fetuses.[36,37]

Teratogens are agents that produce abnormalities in anatomy, even "monsters," in embryos and fetuses. A fetus can be harmed directly by diffusion of the agent across the placental barrier, or it can be harmed indirectly by an agent's effect on the placenta or uterus or the maternal-placental physiological interactions. Teratogens include some drugs: methotrexate, 6-mercaptopurine, cyclophosphamide, chlorambucil, busulfan, colchicine, vinblastine, vincristine, actinomycin D, thalidomide. Hormones can also be teratogenic in animals and humans though only in pharmacologically high concentration. Whether or not an agent has a harmful effect depends upon dose and stage of pregnancy. Teratogenic hormones include corti-

sone, sex hormones including contraceptive pills, androgenic hormones, and synthetic progestins.

Agents given to mothers can also act as carcinogens for the fetus. When pregnant women were given the synthetic nonsteroidal estrogen diethylstilbestrol (DES), subsequent female offspring had an increase in vaginal carcinoma during their teen years and other abnormalities of reproductive function. Male offspring were also vulnerable, having constriction of urethra opening or abnormal locations for the opening of the urethra.

Hormones are produced by the placenta that appear in the maternal blood stream. These include HCG (with its LH-like and FSH-like effects) which contributes to suppression of ovulation. There is also a thyroid-stimulating hormone and a corticotropin that stimulate the thyroid and adrenal glands, respectively. A melanocyte-stimulating hormone is responsible for changes in skin pigmentation. **Melasma**, "mask of pregnancy," includes pigmentation of the head. Darkening of the areolae and a dark line down the midabdomen may occur.

A final sequence of endocrine changes ensues as the mother and neonates interact, which culminates in the events associated with **weaning**. For example, in rats and mice which wean about three weeks after birth, the intestines exhibit a series of morphological and enzyme changes (e.g., decrease in lactase, maltase, alkaline phosphatase, and peptidase activities). The changes correlate with the natural period of weaning; Henning, Ballard, and Kretchmer comment:

> There is now considerable evidence to show that the changes are under hormonal rather than dietary control. The adrenal cortical hormones have been strongly implicated since adrenalectomy interferes with the normal pattern of development, and administration of glucocorticoids during the first two weeks of life causes precocious appearance of sucrase and alkaline phosphatase as well as rapid disappearance of lactase and the capacity for pinocytosis.[38]

The mother and the fetus are genetically distinct. Because of this, there is potential for rejection because of immune responses. Changes in cell-mediated immune responses have been observed during pregnancy. Progesterone reduces the *in vitro* responses of maternal lymphocytes and is a candidate for mediating the immunosuppression of pregnancy preventing fetal rejection.[39]

CHROMOSOME ANOMALIES

The primary determining factor for gender is the complement of sex chromosomes—normally XX in the human female and XY in the human male. There are anomalies of the sex chromosomes that occur: **Turner's syndrome** or ovarian agenesis (XO), **Klinefelter's syndrome** or seminiferous tubule dysgenesis (XXY), superfemale (XXX), and XYY. Reproductive abnormalities accompany some of these conditions including failure of puberty in Turner's syndrome and abnormal seminiferous tubules in Klinefelter's syndrome. There are also other problems such as increased occurrence of mental retardation or acne. Development of a testis requires a Y chromosome which carries a testis-determining factor (TDF). It has been suggested that bearing an extra Y chromosome has further implications:

> The XYY pattern has...been observed in males who tend to be tall and have severe acne. This karyotype has attracted considerable attention because its incidence was initially reported to be high in prison populations. However, it is also relatively common in the general population, and there is little solid evidence that individuals with the XYY pattern are predisposed to aggressive behavior.[40]

HERMAPHRODITES

The word "hermaphrodite" is used to denote a bisexual being in which the characteristics of both sexes are combined. The word derives from a Greek legend where Hermes and Aphrodite became united in a single body while they were bathing.

Some individuals have an XX/XY mosaic pattern and, in this condition, it is possible for the individual to develop both ovaries and testes so that the individual is a **true hermaphrodite**. But, not all disorders of the reproductive system are subsequent to genetic abnormalities. Some of the disorders are hormonal disorders that have their origins in development.

Normal development of the male reproductive system requires that the bipotential gonad be-come an embryonic testis due to the Y chromosome testis-determining factor. The embryonic testis then secretes MRF (müllerian regression factor) and testosterone which cause the male internal and external genitals to form from bipotential primordia; further development of the testes at puberty result in testosterone secretion which provokes the male secondary sex characteristics. On the other hand, in the female, the bipotential gonad develops into an embryonic ovary, the bipotential primordia develop into female internal and external genitalia, and at puberty the ovarian hormones stimulate female secondary sex characteristics. Abnormal development due to hormones usually has to do with deficiency or excess androgens.

Pseudohermaphrodites have reproductive organs that do not match their sex chromosomes. In some disorders, a hormonal dysfunction is responsible for aberrant development of the reproductive system.

Female pseudohermaphroditism is the condition where male genitals develop in XX females. This can happen because of exposure of female fetuses to exogenous androgens while the reproductive organs are forming from weeks 8–13 of gestation. Still later, after the organs are formed, androgen can cause clitoral hypertrophy. The excess androgen can come from the fetal adrenal gland or maternal androgen excess.

Male pseudohermaphroditism is the condition where female genitalia and female internal genitals develop in XY males. The cause may be failure of the embryonic testes to secrete müllerian regression factor.

FEMINIZING TESTIS

Feminizing testis can be due to $5-\alpha$-reductase deficiency where testosterone fails to be converted to its more active form by target organs. Feminization in males can also be due to deficiency of androgen receptors in the target organs or in the receptor-binding ability. The disorders, collectively called androgen resistance, where female characteristics occur in the presence of testosterone, are accompanied by failure to menstruate because the uterus and ovaries are absent.

AMBIGUOUS GENDER

In cases of ambiguous gender, a gender assignment is made. In so-called "sex change operations" the individual is treated with appropriate plastic surgery and hormone therapy to make the physical characteristics match the individual's gender preference. In making gender assignments, which is done when children are born with ambiguous sex organs, Conte and Grumbach make the curious suggestion: "In recommending male sex assignment, the adequacy of the size of the phallus should be the most important consideration."[41] Estrogen and progesterone are administered cyclically in individuals reared as females; testosterone is used to virilize assigned males.

REFERENCES

1. Ringler, G.E.; Strauss, J.F. In vitro systems for the study of human placental endocrine function. Endocrine Reviews 11: 105–123; 1990.

2. Albrecht, E.D.; Pepe, G.J. Placental steroid hormone biosynthesis in primate pregnancy. Endocrine Reviews 11: 124–150; 1990.

3. Martin, M.C.; Hoffman, P. The endocrinology of pregnancy. In Greenspan, F.; Forsham, P., editors. Basic and Clinical Endocrinology, Second Edition; Norwalk, CT: Appleton and Lange; 1987, p. 476.

4. Berkow, R., editor. The Merck Manual, Fifteenth Edition. Rahway, NJ: Merck Sharp & Dohme Research Laboratories of Merck & Co., Inc.; 1987; pp. 1734–1735.

5. Langone, J. After-the-fact birth control. Time; October 10, 1988; p. 103.

6. Berkow, R., editor; Op. cit.; p 1743.

7. Martin, M.C.; Hoffman, P.; Op. cit.; pp. 481–482.

8. Berkow, R., editor; Op. cit.; p. 1746.

9. Berkow, R., editor; Op. cit.; pp. 1743–1744.

10. Gorbman, A.; Dickhoff, W.; Vigna, S.; Ralph, C. Comparative Endocrinology. New York: John Wiley and Sons; 1983; p. 495.

11. Ganong, W. Review of Medical Physiology, Fourteenth Edition. Norwalk, CT: Appleton and Lange; 1989; p. 383.

12. Martin, M.C.; Hoffman, P.; Op. cit.; p. 480.

13. Martin, M.C.; Hoffman, P.; Op. cit.; p. 561.

14. Martin, M.C.; Hoffman, P.; Op. cit.; p. 486.

15. Seif, S.M.; Robinson, A.G. Rhythms of the posterior pituitary. In Krieger, D.T. Endocrine Rhythms. New York: Raven Press; 1979; pp. 187–201.

16. Seif, S.M.; Robinson, A.G.; Ibid.; pp. 187–201.

17. Reppert, S. M.; Perlow, M. J.; Artman, H. G.; Ungerleider, L., G.; Fisher, D. A.; Klein, D. The circadian rhythm of oxytocin in primate cerebrospinal fluid: Effects of destruction of the SCN. Brain Research 307: 384–387; 1984.

18. Welty, J.C. The Life of Birds. Philadelphia, PA: Saunders College Publishing; 1982; p. 160.

19. Welty, J.C.; Ibid.; p. 159.

20. Benoit, J. Organes uro-genitaux; reproduction-characteres sexuels et hormones determinisme du cycle sexuel seasonier. In Grasse, P., editor. Traite de Zoologie. Tome XV, Oiseaux. Paris: Masson et Cie; 1950.

21. Welty, J.C.; Op. cit.; p. 163.

22. O'Malley, B.; Buller, R. Mechanisms of steroid hormone action. The Journal of Investigative Dermatology 68: 1-4; 1977.

23. Weinstein, L.A.; Landis, D.M.D.; Sagar, S.M.; Millard, W.J.; Martin, J.B. Cysteamine depletes prolactin (PRL) but does not alter the structure of PRL-containing granules in the anterior pituitary. Endocrinology 115: 1543–1550; 1984.

24. Hadley, M. Endocrinology, Second Edition. Englewood Cliffs, NJ: Prentice-Hall; 1988; p. 95.

25. Mick, C.; Nicoll, C. Prolactin directly stimulates the liver in vivo to secrete a factor (Synlactin) which acts synergistically with the hormone. Endocrinology 116: 2049–2053; 1985.

26. Cincotta, A.H.; Schiller, B.C.; Meier, A. Bromocriptine inhibits the seasonally occurring obesity, hyperinsulinemia, insulin resistance, and impaired glucose tolerance in the Syrian hamster, Mesocricetus auratus. Metabolism 40: 639–644; 1991.

27. Cincotta, A.H.; Meier, A. Reductions of body fat stores and total plasma cholesterol and triglyceride concentrations in several species by bromocriptine treatment. Life Sciences 45: 2247–2254; 1989.

28. Meier, A.; Cincotta, A.H.; Lovell, W.C. Timed bromocriptine administration reduces body fat stores in obese subjects and hyperglycemia in type II diabetics. Experientia 48: 248–253; 1992.

29. Regan, L.; Owen, E.J.; Jacobs, H.S. Hypersecretion of luteinising hormone, infertility, and miscarriage. The Lancet 336: 1141–1144; 1990.

30. Braunstein, G. D. Testes. In Greenspan, F.S. Basic and Clinical Endocrinology, Third Edition.

Norwalk, CT: Appleton & Lange; 1991; p. 435.

31. Albrecht, E.D.; Pepe, G. J. Placental steroid hormone biosynthesis in primate pregnancy. Endocrine Reviews 11: 124–150; 1990.

32. Ringler, G.E.; Strauss, F.; Op cit.; pp. 105–123.

33. Pepe, G.J.; Albrecht, E.D. Regulation of the primate fetal adrenal cortex. Endocrine Reviews 11; 151–176; 1990.

34. Pepe, G. J.; Albrecht, E.D.; Ibid.; 1990.

35. Pepe, G. J.; Albrecht, E.D.; Ibid.; 1990.

36. Klein, D. Evidence for the placental transfer of 3H-acetyl-melatonin. Nature (New Biol.) 237: 117; 1972.

37. Reppert, S. A source of melatonin for the immature animal. In Klein, D., editor. Melatonin Rhythm Generating System. Basel, Switzerland: Karger; 1981; pp. 182–192.

38. Henning, S.J.; Ballard, P.L.; Kretchmer, N. A study of the cytoplasmic receptors for glucocorticoids in intestine of pre- and postweanling rats. The Journal of Biological Chemistry 250: 2073–2079; 1975.

39. Szekeres-Bartho, J. Endocrine regulation of the immune system during pregnancy. Archivum Immunologiae et Therapiae Experimentalis 38: 125–140; 1990.

40. Ganong, W.; Op. cit.; p. 357.

41. Conte, F.A.; Grumbach, M.M. Abnormalities of sexual differentiation. In Greenspan, F.; Forsham, P., editors. Basic and Clinical Endocrinology, Second Edition. Norwalk, CT: Appleton and Lange; 1987; p. 455.

SECTION V

OTHER ENDOCRINE TOPICS

The section covers some endocrine topics that do not fit neatly into the previous coverage of the hormones and the classical endocrine glands. This section provides a broader perspective of chemical messenger function in integrating the physiological events within an organism and between organisms.

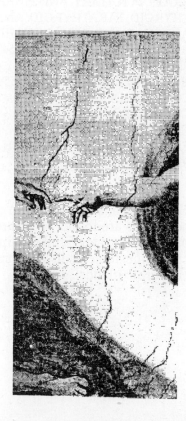

CHAPTER 20

Aging, Hibernation, Sleep, Cytokines, Chalones, Erythropoietin

Hibernation, sleep, and aging are physiological events in which noteworthy changes in hormones are found. The three events are also intriguing for the potential that hormones offer for their artificial manipulation. Cytokines, chalones, and erythropoietin are endocrine subjects in vertebrates that don't fit easily into discussion of the classical endocrine glands.

AGING

Arking defines aging as "those series of cumulative, universal, progressive, intrinsic, and deleterious functional and structural changes that usually begin to manifest themselves at reproductive maturity and eventually culminate in death" for which there is a mnemonic (CUPID).[1] The correlation (r values) of some physiological variables with chronological age was measured (here arranged in order of declining correlation with increased age): accommodation of the eye 0.88, vital capacity -0.77, forced expiratory volume -0.70, systolic blood pressure 0.69, height -0.68, hearing loss 0.66, creatinine clearance -0.60, visual acuity -0.57, weight 0.56, reaction time 0.52, grip strength -0.52, diastolic blood pressure 0.51, and tapping -0.44; serum albumin -0.36; basal metabolic rate -0.34; plasma glucose 0.30; serum globulin 0.09.[2] Men actually lose about five centimeters of height and five kilograms of weight between the ages of 30 and 80.[3] Age at natural menopause is inversely associated with longevity.[4] It is immediately apparent that some of these physiological variables that change with age have endocrine components in their regulation.

Many aspects of physiology have been considered for their possible roles in the aging process,[5] for example, enzyme inducibility,[6,7] cell capacity to survive,[8] change from cycling to non-cycling cells,[9] cell division rates (Table 20.1),[10] free radical accumulation, collagen fiber cross-linking, autoimmunity, immune function decline,[11] diet, accumulation of DNA copying errors, etc. Robert Arking arrayed the various theories of the causation of aging and assessed their current status: DNA damage and DNA repair (proved), error catastrophe (disproved), dysdifferentiation (possible), free radical (probable), waste accumulation (possible), cross-linkage (proved), wear and tear (incorporated into other theories), metabolic theories (disproved), genetic theories (probable), selective death (probable), neuroendocrine (proved for female reproductive aging and other specialized cases), immunological (probable).[12]

HORMONE DECLINE IN AGING

Not unexpectedly, changes in almost all aspects of the endocrine system are characteristic of aging.[13]

The daily cycles of the hormones probably change because the circadian activity rhythms alter with aging. Aging reduces amplitude and changes in period length of circadian rhythms.[14] For example, the circadian rhythms of mice freerun (persist in constant conditions) with shorter period lengths as the mice progress from puberty to old age.[15]

Humans decrease their sleep durations from 12 hours at 1 year of age to less than 8 hours over 30 years of age.[16]

Even more intriguing, given the observed endocrine changes, is the possibility of thwarting aging by preventing or reversing endocrine changes. Hormones as droplets sprayed from the fountain of youth are not a remote fantasy; estrogen replacement therapy in women after menopause is a current reality. Gregerman and Bierman, however, throw a "wet blanket" on the idea that aging is due to endocrine failure:

> ...aging was thought by some scientists to be the direct result of deficiency states resulting from age-related failure of the endocrine glands to secrete their hormones. Such thinking now seems naive as the complexities of the processes of aging have become more apparent....Nonetheless, although mastery of the organs of internal secretion can no longer be viewed as the key to longevity, normal aging does produce a variety of effects on hormone production, secretion, and action.[17]

During aging, serum concentrations of many hormones decrease and histological changes are observed in endocrine glands. For example, there is a drop in the percentage of anterior pituitary chromophobes from 40% in the young to 25% in adulthood and a <20% decrease in pituitary weight.[18] The hormone and histological changes led investigators to view aging, for the most part, as a damping of endocrine function. Although reports disagree, producing some discrepancies, the majority of hormones decline in amount with old age (Tables 20.2 and 20.3). In the aged, not only do levels of hormone production change, but there are also changes in sensitivity of target organs to the hormones, the response time, and the receptor

Table 20.1 Lifespan Correlation with the Lifetime of Cultured Fibroblasts

Subject	Mean maximum lifespan (years)	Fibroblast doublings
human, young donors	rapid aging	2–10
mouse, embryos	3.5	14–28
mink, embryos	10	30–34
chicken, embryos	30?	12–35
human, embryos	110	40–60
Galapagos tortoise, young donors	175	90–125

The table shows doubling rates (finite number of population doublings before death) for cultured normal fibroblasts. Accelerated aging is characteristic of Werner's syndrome and progeria. Hayflick, L. Cell biology of aging. Bioscience 25: 629-637; 1975; p. 631.

mechanisms. If we can't explain the "why" of aging, at least we can describe "how" endocrinology changes on a hormone-by-hormone basis.

HYPOTHALAMUS, PITUITARY, AND AGING

Antidiuretic hormone (ADH) and, possibly, atrial natriuretic factor (ANF) production increases with aging. The plasma ADH level is larger in 54–92-year-old persons in comparison to 21–29-year-old persons given the same osmotic stimulus. At the same time, with aging, the kidney's ability to conserve sodium and to concentrate urine is impaired and the elderly have a reduced subjective awareness of thirst. There are disorders associated with the changes in the ability to regulate salt and water balance (syndrome of inappropriate ADH secretion or SIADH, dehydration, serum sodium <136 mEq/l or hyponatremia, and serum sodium >146 mEq/l or hypernatremia).

Growth hormone and growth hormone responses to challenges are variously claimed as unchanged or reduced in aging men. It has been noted that growing juveniles have more peaks of GH during the day and during the last two thirds of a night of sleep. GH has recently been the subject for popular press articles on aging. *Longevity* and *Time* magazines have brought Daniel Rudman's provocative studies (in which older men given human growth hormone reduced body fat by 14.4%, increased muscle mass 8.8%, and increased skin thickness 7.1%) to the attention of the general public.[19,20]

THYROID AND AGING

There is an age-related decline of the basal metabolic rate from 0.24 l/min (oxygen consumption) in 20-year-old men to 0.18 l/min in 90-year-old men. The decreased BMR is attributed to the age-related decrease of muscle mass.[21] Thus, a decline in thyroid hormones is not blamed for the effect on metabolic rate. However, thyroxine production drops 50% from young adults to advanced old age, and serum T_3 decreases in humans.[22] Paradoxically, serum TSH rises. Hypothyroidism and nodule formation increase with aging, but hyperthyroidism incidence remains constant.

PARATHORMONE, CALCITONIN, AND AGING

The disorders of mineral metabolism also increase in frequency in the aged. Disorders involv-

Table 20.2 Aging Changes Hormones in Humans

Hormone	Blood concentration	Response to a challenge	Disposal by metabolism	Target sensitivity
ADH	o	+		
gonadotropins	+	-		
TSH	+	-	o	o
GH	o	-		
thyroxine	o	o	-	
triiodothyronine	o			
PTH	-			
cortisol	o	o	-	
adrenal androgens	-	-		
aldosterone	-	-	-	
insulin	-	-	-	-/o
glucagon	o	o		
testosterone	-/o	-	-	-
estrogen, women	-			-
estrogen, men	-/o			

The table shows changes that occur in hormones with aging. Plus (+) means increased in the aged, minus (-) means decreased in the elderly, and open symbol (o) means no change with aging. Except for ADH, gonadotropins, and TSH, all the values are no change or negative. After Table 29-3 in Gregerman, R.I.; Bierman, E.L. Chapter 29: Aging and hormones. In Williams, R.D., editor. Textbook of Endocrinology, Sixth Edition. Philadelphia, PA: W. B. Saunders; 1981; p. 1208.

ing calcium include osteoporosis, osteomalacia, Paget's disease, hypercalcemia, and hypocalcemia. Low phosphate and magnesium are common in the elderly.

Parathormone levels may increase slightly with age. Calcitonin drops during the third decade of life, but calcitonin has not been proven to be linked with the aging increase in osteoporosis.[23] Following ovariectomy or menopause, women lose bone mass. The bone loss is due to reduced levels of circulating estrogen. Fatter women, whose adipose tissue converts steroids to estrogen, have some protection against the osteoporosis and tendency to fracture that is observed more in slender women. Estrogen replacement therapy slows the bone losses. In older women, there is also an increase in osteocalcin (bone Gla protein, BGP) which inhibits calcification.[24]

PANCREAS AND AGING

In response to a meal or ingested glucose, blood glucose increases 20–50 mg/dl. Aging increases the meal response by about 5 mg/dl cach decade. Fasting blood glucose increases only 1–2 mg/dl each decade. The decline in glucose tolerance with age has been explained several ways—there is a 16% increase in the proportion of the body mass that is fat by age 70; the insulin produced in older subjects contains a higher proportion of less potent proinsulin; etc. Moreover, glucose induction of hepatic glucokinase via insulin is slower in the aged.[25] The disorders of carbohydrate metabolism in the elderly include, of course, diabetes mellitus. Accelerated aging is described for diabetics.

Not all hormones decrease with aging. Pancreatic polypeptide (PP) in 30-year-old-humans

Table 20.3 Aging, Hormones, and Rhythms

Aging change	Hormones
reduced amplitude or amount in older people	growth hormone, thyrotropin, epinephrine, norepinephrine, testosterone, estradiol, 17-hydroxy-progesterone, dehydroepiandrosterone sulfate, renin, aldosterone, cortisol, ß-endorphin, somatostatin, ACTH, melatonin, prolactin, LH, potent insulin, calcitonin, T_3, T_4
increased amplitude or amount in older people	norepinephrine, aldosterone, pancreatic polypeptide, ADH, ANF, PTH, female gonadotropins
phase shifted in older people	corticosterone, cortisol, testosterone, aldosterone, melatonin
unchanged in older people	ß-endorphin, GH, epinephrine, aldosterone

Data from Brock, M.A. Chronobiology and aging. Journal of the American Geriatric Society 39: 74–91; 1991 and from other sources. Note that there are conflicting reports about the effects of age on some hormones.

is about 54 pg/ml. The values of pancreatic polypeptide increase to 297 pg/ml in 70-year-olds.[26]

ADRENAL FUNCTION AND AGING

The adrenal cortex exhibits histological changes (e.g., fragmentation of mitochondria) despite minimal declines in ACTH with aging. Plasma cortisol is maintained despite a 30% decline in secretion rate. As for the thyroid hormones, the idea is that levels are maintained by a decline in catabolism. Cortisol, cortisol metabolites, dehydroepiandrosterone, DHA, and hepatic glucocorticoid receptors decline (numbers or affinity?) with age.[27] Urinary 17-ketosteroids drop to about half the levels of young individuals. Induction of enzymes (e.g., tyrosine aminotransferase) by glucocorticoids stimulated by ACTH may take longer in the elderly.[28]

Aldosterone concentrations are variously reported to either not change much with aging or to decline 30–50%; plasma renin declines 30–50% with aging. The aged are thus more susceptible to factors that alter renin (upright posture, salt restriction, diuretics). They have increased risks of hyperkalemia (too much potassium).

Epinephrine levels are supposedly maintained in the elderly. Plasma norepinephrine increases. Animal and human studies support the hypothesis of diminished sensitivity to the catecholamines for stimuli such as blood vessel contractility, lipolysis, and liver gluconeogenesis. Meites comments on the role of hypothalamic catecholamines in aging in rats:

The decline in hypothalamic catecholamine (CA) activity with age in rats leads to a reduction in hormone secretion by the neuroendocrine system, and results in decreased reproductive function, a reduction in protein synthesis, development of numerous mammary and pituitary tumors, and probably contributes to the decline in immune function. Some of these same effects can be produced in young rats by administration of drugs that lower hypothalamic CA activity. Administration of drugs to old rats that elevate hypothalamic CA activ-

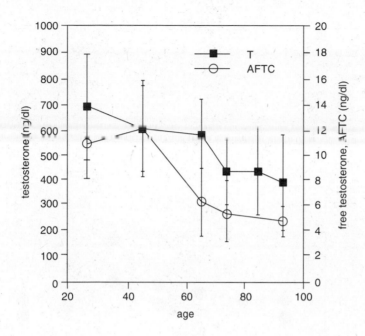

Figure 20.1 The graph shows the effect of age on testosterone in men. T = testosterone; AFTC = free testosterone; points represent means; and vertical lines represent standard errors of the mean. Data are from a table in Abrams, W.B.; Berkow, M.D., editors. The Merck Manual of Geriatrics. Rahway, NJ: Merck & Co.: 1990; p. 1187.

ity can inhibit or reverse the reproductive decline, increase protein synthesis, induce regression of mammary and pituitary tumors, decrease disease incidence, probably elevate immune function, and significantly extend the life span.[29]

GONADS AND AGING

As stated by S. G. Korenman, "spermatogenesis is remarkably sustained despite advanced age in the presence of adequate testicular androgen synthesis."[30] Elderly men suffer from hypo-gonadism (decreased testicular androgen production, Figure 20.1) which is characterized by blunting the 6–8 a.m. peak of testosterone. A rise in LH accompanies the reduced testosterone. As mentioned, prostate hypertrophy is characteristic of aging in humans, dogs, and lions.[31]

The cessation of menses, which occurs in all elderly women, has been discussed in the chapter including estrogens and progestogen and menopause. With aging in women, estrogen declines, estrogen production stops at menopause. Low estrogen means that the negative feedback on the hypothalamus is reduced, and the consequence is that gonadotropin concentrations soar. Martin comments on the control of female aging:

The normal decline in reproductive functions [in rats] has been linked with changes in the arcuate nuclei and the associated ability to release sufficient quantities of LRH....estrogens play a role in hypothalamic aging, since females gonadectomized soon after achieving reproductive competence can support the functions of ovaries implanted at a later time,

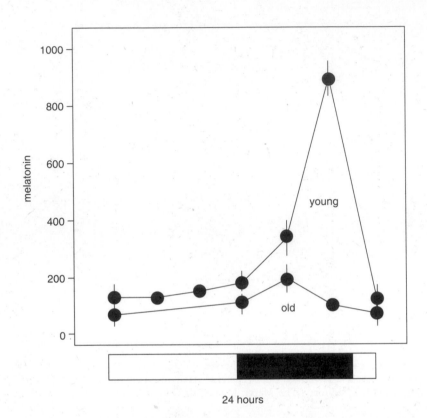

Figure 20.2 Aging reduced the dark-time melatonin (pg/gland) peak in two-month-old and eighteen-month-old hamsters. The upper (young) graph is for the melatonin [pg/gland] in two-month-old hamsters. The vertical bars indicate standard errors where they exceeded the size of the plotted symbols. The horizontal bar indicates the light-dark cycle in which the hamsters were housed. After data in Reiter, R.; Richardson, B.; Johnson, L.; Ferguson, B.; Dinh, D. Pineal melatonin rhythm: Reduction in aging Syrian hamsters. Science 210: 1372–1374; 1980.

whereas those permitted to retain their own gonads into "middle age" cannot do this.[32]

Estrogen therapy is a treatment for elderly women to combat the symptoms of menopause. Usually nonsynthetic estrogen (e.g., CEE or conjugated equine estrogen) is administered orally to achieve a level of 30–40 pg/ml of serum estradiol which is comparable to the premenopausal early follicular phase. However, estrogen is also effec-

tive when it is administered vaginally, implanted in subdermal pellets, applied in skin patches, or when it is injected subcutaneously. Progestin is also commonly administered as part of the hormone replacement regimen.

CAUSES OF AGING

Causes of aging are still a matter of speculation. Some ideas that have been offered to explain aging are (i) random DNA mutations in so

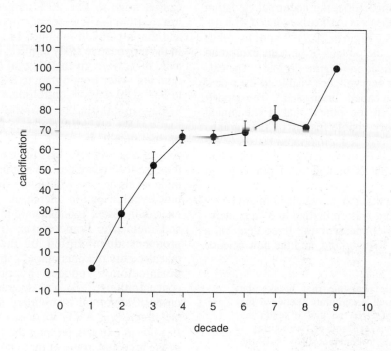

Figure 20.3 Pineal calcification increases as humans age. The percentage of individuals with pineal calcium deposits is shown for ages ten years (decade one) to 90 years (decade nine). Data are from Table 53 in Kitay, J.; Altschule, M. The Pineal Gland. Cambridge, MA: Harvard University Press; 1954.

matic cells which causes an accumulation of abnormalities, (ii) nonenzymatic combination of glucose with amino groups which results in detrimental cross linkages between collagen, proteins, and DNA, (iii) that there is a cumulative formation of tissue damaging free radicals, or (iv) that aging is preprogrammed by a biological aging clock.[33] There is considerable evidence for the clock idea; after all, each species possesses a characteristic average lifespan. But the hypothesis that there is an aging clock does not explain how aging is accomplished.

Reduction in the efficacy of the endocrine system may contribute to aging. Endocrine decrements with aging include decreased hormone production, increased time lag for enzyme induction, and decreased target sensitivity. As regards the targets, there is evidence that there are decreases in hormone-sensitive adenyl cyclase with age. Such a decline would provide a global mechanism for re-

duction of the effectiveness of many hormones. As noted by Gergerman and Bierman:

These reports....clearly indicate that endocrine related membrane function, i.e. the AC [adenyl cyclase] system, is involved in the aging process, and they provide an important clue to the explanation of age-related alterations of hormone sensitivity.[34]

IMMORTALITY

Notwithstanding our uncertainties as to the cause(s) of aging, hormones offer hope for improving the quality of life of the elderly as promoted in the popular press and as stated by David H. Solomon: "The endocrine and metabolic control systems of the body offer many of the greatest opportunities for preventing the disabilities associated with aging."[35]

Pineal function exhibits several interesting changes with aging. First, the nocturnal elevation of melatonin synthesis is markedly reduced with aging in hamsters (Figure 20.2)[36] and in other species. Second, the pineals of humans exhibit an increase in calcification (Figure 20.3).[37] The calcium deposits, or acervuli, are visible to the naked eye and have been called "brain sand." The deposition of calcium in the pineal makes the pineal gland a remarkably visible feature of radiographs and CAT (computer-aided tomography) scans of the head. Calcification of the pineal gland is not a sign of degeneration but is indicative of pineal gland activity.

The idea that the pineal gland might be responsible for aging was embodied in a "a contemporary work of fiction involving three couples, a chateau-clinic in Switzerland, and the new science of rejuvenation":

> ...the chief enzyme that breaks the links which accumulate [between the helices of DNA so that it sends the wrong message and causes aging] -- what one might fancifully call the Methuselah Enzyme, because it really determines longevity -- begins to disappear from the body...It's at this point that true aging begins. And as time goes on, it slowly accelerates until, as we all know, the body is completely metamorphosed into the state we call senility, at which point death occurs. But if the Methuselah Enzyme could be isolated, if it could be synthesized in the laboratory, if it could be reintroduced into the body by shots, then there is no reason why the cross-links could not continue to be destroyed, the cell maturation stopped, and the disease of aging prevented or cured. In short, there's no reason why man could not stay young forever....Now we know the pineal secretes a hormone called melatonin, as well as the enzyme hydroxyindole-O-methyltransferase, which regulates the synthesis of melatonin....After four years of work, I finally isolated an enzyme secreted by the pineal, which I named Mentase.[38]

The concept that melatonin might fight aging was reiterated in a popular magazine article[39] which cited the studies showing that melatonin caused mice to live 20% longer, that melatonin lowered human low-density lipoprotein 15–30%, and that melatonin inhibited breast cancer in rats. In the provocative study of mice, when 575-day-old male mice were given 10 µg/ml melatonin in their drinking water from 6 p.m. to 8:30 a.m., they lived to 931 ± 80 days. Control mice only lived 755 ± 81 days ($p < 0.01$).[40]

So, scientific evidence for a possible role of the pineal in aging has followed fictional conjectures. Sandyk lists the evidence supporting the case for melatonin: (i) nocturnal plasma melatonin levels decline with aging; (ii) the incidence of pineal calcification increases with aging; (iii) melatonin resets hypothalamic-mediated hormonal and metabolic homeostasis; (iv) pinealectomy produces disinhibition of the HPA-axis; (v) pinealectomy disrupts opioid peptide rhythms; (vi) pinealectomy reduces hypothalamic opioid concentrations; (vii) pinealectomy facilitates the onset of abnormal involuntary movements; (viii) melatonin (via AVT) increases slow-wave sleep; (ix) pineal extracts prolong the lifespan of rats.[41] While arguable, some of these points do establish a model for consideration of hormone function in the regulation of aging.[42]

One theory of the way melatonin retards aging is that it acts as an antistress agent via the brain opioid system.[43] A second suggestion is that melatonin enhances immune responses.[44] A third mechanism for melatonin delaying aging might be that a well defined melatonin rhythm prevents detrimental internal temporal disorder.[45]

The pineal gland is not the only gland singled out by fiction authors to play a role in the aging process. The thymus gland is prominent early in development but later on it is reduced. The writer, John Saul, made use of this endocrine fact in his book *Darkness*. He writes:

> "They're doing something," Barbara said. "They're doing something with our children, and its keeping them young. They're taking something from them, Craig. I don't understand it, and I can't prove it, but I know it's true. They stole our daughters, Craig."[46]

However appealing, it seems too much to hope for one hormone to be the solution to

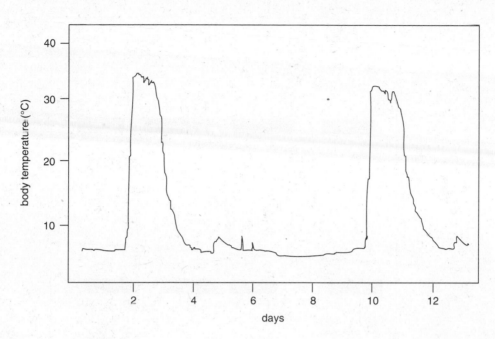

Figure 20.4 Body-temperature record of a hibernating marmot. The air temperature was 5°C. Courtesy, Dr. Gregory Florant.

extending the quality and duration of life. In general, most hormone levels decline with aging. So it seems obvious that an array of hormone replacements might fend off the infirmities of old age. Estrogen has already been used extensively to ameliorate the consequences of menopuase in women. Now, the use of hormones to abrogate the effects of aging are being explored—e.g., estrogen, DHEA, testosterone, RU-486, melatonin, and GH.

Death and aging are being challenged with new optimism, especially for improved quality of life in the later years.[47] Immortality is still only a dream, but it seems that we may be on a threshold for increasing useful lifespan with a combination of hormone treatments, dietary restrictions, and genetic approaches.[48]

HIBERNATION

Hibernation is the physiological process in which some mammals adapt to winter cold extremes by lowering their body temperatures. Some animals that hibernate are woodchucks, marmots, hedgehogs, bats, dormice, hamsters, and ground squirrels. Myrsovsky described some of the facts about hibernators: (i) hibernators are not thermally passive; (ii) they have a highly developed mechanism for heat production; (iii) hibernation can occur in a warm, lighted room; (iv) hibernators consume enormous amounts of food in fall but are only weakly motivated to obtain food; (v) during hibernation water is conserved.[49] Hibernation can be subdivided into preparation, entry, maintenance, and arousal phases.

The preparation period prior to hibernation is characterized by fattening, gonad regression, and reduced activity of most endocrine glands. Hibernation may occur in a den, the hibernaculum, in some species. During hibernation the animal curls in a characteristic pose. In entering the state of hibernation, the animal's body temperature may drop to only a few degrees above freezing (Figure 20.4).

As an animal enters into and remains in deep hibernation, the physiological processes of hibernating animals all slow down—the heart rate drops, the respiratory rate decreases, and the deep body temperature (T_b) remains a few degrees above

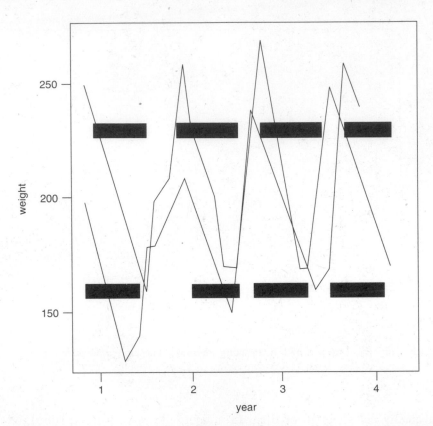

Figure 20.5 The figure illustrates the circannual cycles of body weight (lines, in grams) and hibernation (bars) that freerun in two golden mantled ground squirrels (*Citellus lateralis*) over a period of more than three years. After Pengelley, E.; Asmundson, S. Free-running periods of endogenous circannian rhythms in the golden-mantled ground squirrel *Citellus lateralis*. Comp. Biochem. Physiol. 30: 177-183; 1969.

the ambient temperature (T_a). The animal does not remain in the state of hibernation through the entire winter season, but instead arouses periodically. During the arousals, when the body temperature is high, the animal may urinate, defecate, eat, fix the nest, and sleep. After an **arousal**, the animal then returns to the hibernating state. The episodes of hibernation—entry into hibernation to arousal from hibernation—are called **bouts**. Hibernation is characterized by repeated entries and arousals. Early investigators used a simple technique to detect hibernation—they sprinkled sawdust on a hibernator. The next time the animal was examined, the sawdust was gone if it had aroused. Implanted transmitters can be used to record body temperature continuously.

Hibernation ends for the winter season

with the final arousal or emergence from hibernation in spring. One of the great remaining mysteries of physiology is how hibernation is controlled.

In the laboratory, hibernation can be initiated with cold temperatures and removal of the food supply. Early arousals can be stimulated by handling or warming the hibernating animal. One of the most dramatic events for a physiologist to watch is arousal of an animal from hibernation. Some years ago, Dr. Bruce Goldman of the University of Connecticut demonstrated the arousal of a Siberian hamster (*Phodopus sungorus*) to the author in the laboratory. The hibernating hamster was curled, stiff, and cold to the touch. Its tiny nose and the digits of its forepaws were pale and bluish. Its eyes were tightly closed. The hibernating hamster could easily have been mistaken for dead. When the hamster was warmed by handling, its paws began to tremble and gradually, over a period of an hour, its nose and paws became pink as it emerged from the hibernating state. It was as if a dead animal was restored, reluctantly, to life.

CIRCANNUAL RHYTHMS AND CUES FOR HIBERNATION

In the laboratory, hibernation recurs on a near annual basis (e.g., with a period of 298–314 days in ground squirrels kept at 3°C) so that it is considered that hibernators have innate "circannual" rhythms (Figure 20.5).[50] A rhythm meets criteria for being "circannual" if it persists for two or more years when the subjects are exposed to unchanged lighting and temperature conditions.

We know there are some external cues for synchronizing circannual rhythms because woodchucks transferred from Pennsylvania to Australia reverse their annual body weight cycles. The obvious potential cues for synchronization of annual cycling are ambient temperature and light, but the issue of the method by which circannual rhythms are synchronized with the 365-day year is still unsettled. Colder temperatures lengthened the circannual periods of ground squirrels by two months and temperature can phase shift the circannual rhythm.

Preventing hibernation in ground squirrels with high temperature (30°C) treatments for six weeks in December and January advanced testicular recrudescence by 4–5 weeks but did not alter the timing of events the subsequent autumn.[51] But Gwinner considers there to be some evidence for temperature independence of circannual rhythms, and he considers the evidence for photoperiod changes as a synchronizing cue to be equivocal.[52]

Annual cycles involve physiological changes other than hibernation in mammals; annual cycles are also seen in feeding, molting, plasma androgens, reproductive condition, nest building, locomotor activity, antler replacement, milk production, and water consumption. But in nature, the annual cycles are not shorter than 365 days, instead they are synchronized with the 365-day year. The annual rhythms recur when light-dark cycles are held constant. For example, the molting rhythm persisted for ten years in chickadees and warblers kept in LD10:14.[53] In the chickadees and for other rhythms, the fact that they persist in the absence of obvious external time cues has been considered evidence that they are timed by innate, or endogenous, biological clocks.

ENDOCRINE GLANDS AND HIBERNATION

From the outset, physiologists have been interested in the roles of the endocrine glands during hibernation.[54,55] During hibernation, the endocrine glands become smaller, or "involute." The view that the endocrine glands ceased activity during hibernation, "polyglandular involution," has dominated perception of the endocrine role in hibernation. The endocrine system suppression is seen experimentally as smaller gland weights, histological changes, and reduced hormone production. The regression is most obvious in the glands controlled by the pituitary—the gonads, the thyroid, and the adrenal glands. Suppression of the endocrine glands is not constant throughout hibernation. Some time after the middle of the hibernation season most of the endocrine glands begin to resume their activities. Peak endocrine activities of most glands occur near the time of the spring emergence from hibernation.

The way hormones function qualifies them as prime candidates for the regulators of the process of hibernation, so the interest in the hormone changes in hibernation has been more than academic. Here, the endocrine changes in hibernation are presented in a gland-by-gland account beginning with the brain.

BRAIN, PITUITARY, AND PINEAL IN HIBERNATION

The brain exhibits endocrine-associated changes during hibernation. Neurosecretion is "slight" in summer. The amount of neurosecretory material increases in the hypothalamus and pituitary during January and February in ground squirrels as if neurosecretory material is being stored during hibernation. Lesions of the suprachiasmatic nuclei of the hypothalamus do not abolish the hibernation cycle, but they do shorten the circannual period length.[56]

Biogenic amines (serotonin, norepinephrine) in the brain have been suggested for roles in body temperature control in some species.[57] Entry into and continuation of hibernation may involve serotonin. Injection of serotonin decreases body temperature in ground squirrels. Hibernation can be prevented by disrupting serotonin synthesis (with parachlorophenylalanine, PCPA, or midbrain median raphe lesions).[58] Nor-epinephrine injected into brain ventricles increases body temperature and may be involved in arousal from hibernation. But the effects of biogenic amines are not always consistent when various species are considered which has prevented the formulation of a general hypothesis.

Antidiuretic hormone has been measured in the posterior pituitary through the hibernating season in the garden dormouse and was 1.4 I.U. in December (just before hibernation onset), 6.35 I.U. in January and February (mid-hibernation), 4.19 I.U. in April (just before arousal), and 2.10 I.U. in April (just after arousal). The data are consistent with the idea that ADH is released in conjunction with arousal.

Pituitary changes in weight and histology recur annually. In ground squirrels the pituitary weight decreases to a minimum in December–January (early hibernation), rapidly increase January–March (late hibernation), and peaks in April–May (after emergence from hibernation). Histologically, high activity of basophils, which are the source of gonadotropins and TSH, is associated with the spring.

Since the pineal appears to inhibit the go-nads by increasing melatonin production in re-sponse to long photoperiods, its role in hibernation has been investigated. First, there is evidence from several species that the pineal is involved in ther-moregulation. The pineal and the retina make me-latonin each night from its indole precursor, sero-tonin. Body temperature drops at night in day-ac-tive animals such as house sparrows, and the rhythm is abolished by pinealectomy. Injected me-latonin lowers body temperature in sparrows and some other species which is consistent with the hypothesis that night melatonin production lowers body temperature.[59] Second, there is evidence that the pineal and/or melatonin are involved in hiberna-tion. Melatonin injections increase the frequency and duration of hibernation in ground squirrels.[60] Increases in melatonin correlated with arousals irre-spective of time of day. Pinealectomy shortens the circannual period of ground squirrels.[61] During hibernation the daily cycle of plasma melatonin is abolished[62] and pinealocyte size is reduced. Full evaluation of the role of melatonin in hibernation is complicated by the fact that it is synthesized in both the pineal and the eyes; animals can hibernate

without their pineal glands.

THYROID, PARATHYROID, AND PANCREAS IN HIBERNATION

Because the thyroid hormones are associ-ated with control of body temperature and basal metabolic rate, the thyroid has been a focus of study for hibernation physiologists. Generally, thyroid activity is considered to be low prior to hibernation and during early hibernation, increasing in late hibernation, and finally resuming activity at the end of hibernation. Thyroid hormone levels de-crease as hibernators enter a bout of hibernation and increase during periodic arousals. Hyperthyroidism delays hibernation.

Hypercalcemia (blood, heart, skeletal mus-cle) is a characteristic of hibernation. Para-thormone, which increases blood calcium, increases during early hibernation and decreases during late hibernation. Parafollicular cells, which secrete calcitonin which lowers blood calcium, are more abundant in some hibernators. Some species have osteoporosis during hibernation which reverses upon arousal in association with a burst of parafol-licular cell activity. The roles of calcium in hiber-nation include not only the bones, but also the maintenance of membranes and energy metabolism.

Blood glucose decreases during hibernation in nonfeeding hibernators, is maintained in hiberna-tors that feed during periodical arousals, and rises to 350% of normal in hibernating bats. Circulating insulin, which lowers blood sugar, is lower in fall and winter but rises during arousals. Insulin in-creases in the pancreas during hibernation which may mean that it is stored. Glucagon secretion is probably lower during hibernation.

ADRENAL AND GONADS IN HIBERNATION

Adrenal weights and catecholamines are highest in the fall (October–November) and lowest in the spring (March–May). Adrenalectomy pre-vents hibernation in ground squirrels and some hamsters.[63]

There may be a role for adrenal glucocorti-coids in the control of hibernation. An adrenal cor-tex graft or injections of deoxycorticosterone re-stores the ability to hibernate. Histological varia-tion in adrenal cortex cells suggests that the cortex peak activity occurs after hibernation (May), drops

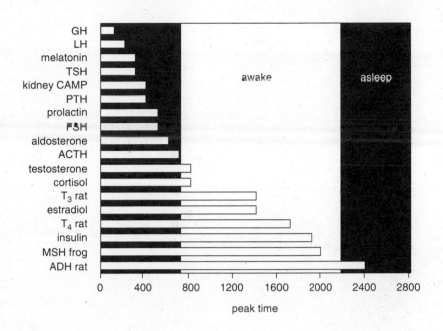

Figure 20.6 The figure shows the timed sequence of daily hormone rhythm peaks. The approximate times of hormone peaks (right ends of bars) have been plotted overlaying the sleep-wake cycle. The data are for humans except for T3, T4, and ADH, which are from rats, and the MSH data which are for amphibians. The graph was made from graphs of hormone rhythms in this book. The graph does not show the width of various peaks. The figure is intended to illustrate the concept that the hormones come into play in a temporal sequence. Note that for the humans, the hormones of the pineal and pituitary glands peak at night, whereas the hormones of the glands driven by the pituitary gland peak in the awake time.

in summer (July), and is lowest in hibernation (January). Plasma ACTH is low during hibernation. Increases in circulating glucocorticoids correlate with arousals.

Zona glomerulosa function during hibernation is characterized by increases in width, cell nuclei size, aldosterone concentration, and renal aldosterone secretion. Renin and angiotensin II levels are maintained or increased during hibernation. The physiological consequence is to conserve electrolytes during hibernation.

Catecholamines appear to play a major role. Ten hours prior to hibernation, catecholamine turnover stops.[64] There are lower norepinephrine turnover rates during hibernation. Norepinephrine secreted by the adrenal medulla and sympathetic nervous system increases more than 30-fold during arousal, and epinephrine increases more than 100-fold during arousal.[65] The norepinephrine stimulates thermogenesis (heat production) for arousals. Removing the adrenal medulla does not prevent entry into nor arousal from hibernation, but catecholamines are synthesized elsewhere than in the adrenal medulla.

Seasonal hibernators may also be seasonal breeders. In spring breeders, the gonads regress in the fall, and the gonads remain quiescent through the short days of autumn and early winter. Finally, as spring approaches, the gonads grow (spontaneous recrudescence). Then breeding takes place. In hibernators, the cycle parallels hibernation with growth of the gonads preceding the final

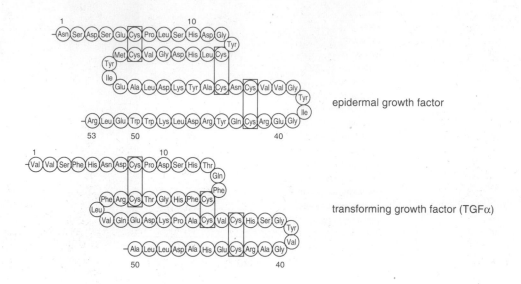

epidermal growth factor

transforming growth factor (TGFα)

Figure 20.7 Structures of two cytokines. Modified, with permission. Fisher, D.A.; Lakshmanan, J. Metabolism and effects of epidermal growth factor and related growth factors in mammals. Endocrine Reviews 11: 419; 1990.

arousal from hibernation. Fall breeders may have delayed fertilization or implantation to extend the time from the fall breeding to spring parturition. Castration facilitates entry into hibernation and increases hibernation bout durations. But cyclic hibernation occurs in castrated animals. Actively functioning gonads prevent hibernation. Stimulating the gonads (e.g., by injecting pituitary gonadotropins) causes arousal, and in the case of females, ovulation.

HIBERNATION TRIGGER

There are still some other hormones whose potential role deserves investigation. First, there are seasonal color changes in pelage (fur, feathers) that might make it worth investigating the role of the molecules derived from pro-opiomelanocortin. Second, preparation for hibernation involves both fattening and a decrease in food supply,

so prolactin and gastrointestinal hormones should play roles. Clearly, one way of organizing hibernation is by a sequence of endocrine events which act in concert to control seasonal breeding at the same time.

An exciting "endocrine" idea is that there is a "hibernating hormone" or "trigger" that is secreted into the blood. Investigators have obtained tantalizing evidence for such a trigger by inducing hibernation in a nonhibernating individual animal using the blood obtained from another individual animal while it was hibernating. Dawe and Spurrier describe their experiment:

> Natural mammalian hibernation was continuously maintained under laboratory conditions throughout spring and summer seasons in a colony of thirteen-lined ground squirrels by serial transfusional passage of blood from hibernating animals to active

animals. This procedure successfully produced hibernation in animals until late summer, at which time naturally occurring (spontaneous) hibernations occurred in the colony, thus terminating the experiment.[66]

Efforts to isolate and characterize a chemical hibernation "trigger" or hibernation hormone signal from blood of hibernating animals have so far not succeeded.

SLEEP CHARACTERISTICS

Sleep is another of the nagging remaining mysteries of physiology. Characteristics of sleep have been determined by studying sleeping subjects in laboratory settings. Onset of sleep is concomitant with a decrease in neck muscle tone which causes the head to drop. Locomotor movements are reduced during sleep. In most species, body temperature drops when the individuals are asleep. In humans, the nightly decrease in body temperature is less than 1°C, but in other species it can be much larger. For example, individual house sparrows displayed a 5°C night-time decrease in body temperature.

The description of sleep includes the interesting subdivision of sleep into two phases: **slow-wave sleep** (SWS) and paradoxical or rapid-eye-movement sleep (REM). REM sleep is called **"paradoxical" sleep** because some of its EEG (electroencephalogram) characteristics are more similar to the EEG of waking than to other states of sleep. Dreaming, rapid eye movements, penile erections, a drop of tonic chin muscle activity, depression of spinal reflexes, low amplitude EEG waves, blood pressure increases, and blood pressure variability are associated with the REM phase of sleep.[67] The SWS and REM phases of sleep alternate at about 90-minute intervals. Some investigators believe the 90-minute (ultradian) rhythm represents a basic rest activity cycle (BRAC) present throughout the day and night in humans.

Sleep disorders have received attention. In the laboratory, sleep researchers have investigated various aspects of sleep such as insomnia, snoring (sleep apnoea), narcolepsy (inappropriate sleeping), sleep deprivation, and napping. The investigators have identified disorders of sleep that contribute to fatigue.

HORMONES AND SLEEP

When it comes to endocrinology, the levels of most hormones have well-defined daily cycles (e.g., melatonin and growth hormone peak at night, testosterone peaks in the morning in human subjects). The hormone cycles have been illustrated in their associate chapters. Sleep, or a rest-activity cycle, correlates with daily cycles in hormone levels (Figure 20.6). The growth hormone rhythm was shown in a previous chapter. Growth hormone has low levels in the morning (<3 ng/ml) but spurts during naps, after meals, and to 40 ng/ml during the slow-wave sleep episodes. The relationship of hormones and sleep can be viewed as arraying the hormone changes in a temporal sequence. In other words, endocrine function is organized by time of day or night. An interesting pattern emerges on inspection of this distribution of peak times of day for various hormones: most pituitary and pineal rhythms peak at night when subjects are normally asleep and the hormones of the glands, driven by the pituitary hormones, peak in the day-time. And there seems to be an alternation of the times of steroid versus peptide and amine hormone production. More data may reveal a general time pattern of well ordered endocrine events.

The thyroid hormones seem to be an exception but for the thyroid, the data are from nocturnal rats. It should not be assumed that nocturnal and diurnal animals have the opposite timing of their daily hormone rhythms. For example, melatonin peaks at night in all species so far studied whether they are nocturnal or diurnal.

The discovery and elucidation of hormone rhythms has given new meaning to our understanding of endocrine regulation as suggested by Dr. Dorothy Krieger:

> The recognition and description of rhythmicity of hormonal secretion has led to important insights in clinical and experimental endocrinology and neuroendocrinology. The appreciation of such rhythmicity has had major applications to the delineation of "normal" values of hormonal concentrations (which in many instances are dependent not only on time of day but on frequency of sampling), to determination of treatment schedules,

Table 20.4 Cytokines

Group or factor	Members
interleukins	IL1-IL11
colony-stimulating factors	M-CSF, G-CSF, GM-CSF
tumor necrosis factors	TNFα, TNFß
interferons	IFNα, IFNß, IFNγ
transforming growth factors	TGFα, TGFß 1-5
activin	
inhibin	
chemotactic factors	
growth factors	epidermal growth factor
	fibroblast growth factor
	insulin-like growth factor
	nerve growth factor

Tabibzadeh, S. Human endometrium: An active site of cytokine production and action. Endocrine Reviews 12: 272–290; 1991.

and to understanding the pathophysiology of disease states characterized by altered rhythmicity. The increased knowledge of rhythmicity has led to altered concepts of the nature and scope of hormonal secretion, hormonal interrelationships, hierarchies of hormonal control, and neural regulation of hormonal function.[68]

CONTROL OF SLEEP

An interesting question is whether there is any role for chemical messengers in controlling the sleep-wake cycle. The pineal gland, hypothalamus, serotonin, muramyl peptides, cytokines, and sleep dialysates provide some clues.

Removing the pineal gland abolishes the circadian body temperature[69] and rest-activity rhythms in house sparrows.[70] The sparrows become active all the time; whether or not they exhibit sleep in this state, as measured by EEG, is not known. Melatonin is produced by the pineal and retina in the dark-time in various species whether or not they are nocturnal (night active), like rats and hamsters, or diurnal (day active) like humans and house sparrows. Therefore melatonin can not simply be the "sleep hormone" that causes

sleep in all vertebrate species. Injection of melatonin into sparrows, however, did cause the birds to assume their "roosting" posture characteristic of sleep and reduced the sparrows' body temperatures by amounts similar to the night-time body temperature decrease.[71] Sedation, reduced sleep onset latency, increased rapid-eye-movement sleep, and increased sleep have been reported in studies where melatonin was administered to humans.[72,73] On the other hand, melatonin is derived from serotonin, which has been implicated in sleep, and the dynamics of the serotonin-to-melatonin conversion that proceeds in the pineal and retina may play a role in the control of the sleep-wake rhythm. Moreover, melatonin is precisely regulated by light and dark. For example, when animals or humans are exposed to light which interrupts their normal dark-time, melatonin plummets to low levels.

Electrolytic lesions of the hypothalamic suprachiasmatic nuclei (SCN) abolish circadian rhythms in rats[74] and in many other species. In mammals, the signals that control the pineal gland originate in the SCN and are conveyed to the pineal via the sympathetic nervous system and its superior cervical ganglion (SCG). It is likely that the timing rhythm for the rest-activity cycle in humans also has its origins in the hypothalamus.

Just as with hibernation, serotonin is implicated in the onset of REM sleep. For example, parachlorophenylalanine (PCPA) inhibits the synthesis of serotonin and causes insomnia. Jouvet[75] has suggested that the "priming serotonergic mechanisms that are located in the caudal part of the raphe system act, probably, through deaminated metabolites on cholinergic mechanisms, which in turn...may trigger the final noradrenergic mechanism of REM sleep located in the nucleus locus ceruleus." The raphe system and nucleus locus coruleus are located in the brain.

A link between infectious diseases, muramyl peptides, cytokines, and sleep has been proposed by Toth and Krueger:

> There is a common observation that many people experience feelings of increased 'sleepiness' during infectious disease and . . . bed rest has been prescribed by physicians for centuries as an aid in recuperation . . . . sleep, like fever . . . is a cardinal sign of infectious disease, and . . . biological systems involved in the modulation of immune responsiveness, sleep, and body temperature are closely interrelated.[76]

Injections of some of the cytokines and muramyl peptides (microbial somnogens) and combinations of them induced sleep or increased the amount of time spent in SWS (slow-wave sleep).

There has also been the possibility of a "sleep hormone." Using the same strategy as was used with hibernators, injection of blood from sleeping animals (e.g., goats, rabbits) into waking ones (e.g., rats, rabbits) has induced sleep, supporting the idea that there is a blood-borne factor(s) that is responsible for sleep.[77] Attempts have been made to isolate the "sleep-inducing factor delta" by dialysis of cerebral venous blood obtained from rabbits during sleep.[78]

CYTOKINES

Cytokines are proteins that are involved in cell-to-cell communication (Figure 20.7). To the extent that they are soluble and can move through fluid, they qualify as chemical messengers even if they do not meet classical definitions of hormones (Table 20.4).

When there is an injury or an infection, leucocytes and other cells secrete proteins that act on other leucocytes. These proteins were called interleukins. There are now eight of them and they have been found to come from both immune and nonimmune cells that participate in the process of inflammation. The role of interleukin has been expanded. Interleukin-1 (IL-1), for example, is now responsible for parts of the fever syndrome, pituitary-adrenal activation, increased slow-wave sleep, and behavioral changes. Interleukin-1 is pyrogenic and anorexic. One idea about how interleukin works is that it acts on circumventricular organs of the brain where it causes production of prostaglandins. Rats injected intracerebroventricularly with IL-1ß were conditioned to develop a taste aversion for saccharin.[79] Biological therapy with IL-2 had antitumor effects in patients with renal cell cancer or metastatic melanoma.[80] This immunologic antitumor activity is achieved by stimulation of host immune reactions and therefore holds promise for treatments of other cancers.

Proinflammatory cytokines are involved in the endometrial reactions (proliferation, differentiation, menstrual shedding), stimulation of prostaglandins, and body temperature elevation.[81]

CHALONES

"Chalones" is the name given to a group of local hormones that inhibit the growth of epithelia.[82] The name "chalone" comes from the Greek word *chalan* meaning to slow down. Because they are believed to inhibit mitosis, they have been of particular interest in seeking clues to controlling cancers. Hadley wonders:

> Are some cancers, disease states characterized by uncontrolled mitotic activity, the result of a deficient chalone mechanism? Will injections of the tissue-specific chalone lead to restoration of cell division of the normal state?[83]

An example of one of the growth factors has been called **epidermal chalone**, or epithelial chalone, which has been found in extracts of epidermis. When the epidermis is wounded, the loss of inhibitory factors from the cells of the wound causes the adjacent cells to proliferate.[84] The extracted mitotic inhibitor lacks species specificity. Skin extracts inhibit human epidermoid tumor growth.[85]

There is another example in the testis. DHT forms a complex with a receptor. DHT or the complex stimulates cell proliferation and one idea is that it does so by removing a chalone.[86]

Chalones have also been proposed for control of cell division of granulocytes, fibroblasts, liver, and lymphocytes.

ERYTHROPOIETIN AND HIGH ALTITUDE

Erythropoiesis is the formation of erythrocytes (red blood cells, RBCs).[87] An individual weighing 70 kg has 2.3×10^{13} red blood cells. The rate of red blood cell synthesis is 2.3×10^6 per second. A factor that comes from the kidney (95%), but also a little from liver, and stimulates erythrocyte production was discovered in transfusion experiments. It is called erythropoietin (EP, Ep) or erythrocyte-stimulating factor (ESF). Erythropoietin is a sialo-protein (MW variously reported 39,000 to 46,000). Its half-life is five hours. In human plasma, erythropoietin levels range 4–26 mU/ml.

Erythropoietin comes from precursors, erythrogenin and globin. Erithrogenin is mainly produced in the kidney. Renal erythropoietic factor (REF), an enzyme released by kidney cells, may covert a plasma protein from the liver to erythropoietin.[88,89]

Renal tissue hypoxia is the signal for erythropoietin production. The kidney "renal oxygen sensor" detects the intrarenal tissue oxygen tension. Erythropoietin increases when the oxygen supply is low and decreases when the oxygen supply is high. Other things besides low oxygen that stimulate erythropoietin are increased metabolic rate, thyroid hormones, dinitrophenol, red blood cell destruction, somatotropin, and androgen. Erythropoietin is reduced by hypophysectomy. The kidney produces 95% of adult human erythropoietin but there are, in addition, extrarenal sources such as liver. Erythropoietin is also reduced when the kidneys are removed and restored with transplants.

Erythropoietin has three actions: (i) increases the number of erythrocytes, (ii) increases erythrocyte hemoglobin content, and (iii) early release of erythrocytes from marrow. Erythropoietin acts on red bone marrow cells to cause a two-to three-fold increase in proliferation of erythrocyte precursor cells in the bone marrow and stimulates the formation of erythroblasts. Erythropoietin has similar actions on fetal liver.

Erythropoietin deficiency is associated with anemia. Excess erythropoietin production is associated with erythrocyte proliferation (polycythemia). Erythropoietin is stimulated by conditions of low oxygen such as hemorrhage and anemia. An increase in red blood cells is a normal response made in the adjustment to high altitude.

REFERENCES

1. Arking, R. Biology of Aging. Englewood Cliffs, NJ: Prentice Hall; 1991; 420 pages.
2. Arking, R.; Ibid.; 69.
3. Arking, R.; Ibid.; p. 55.
4. Arking, R.; Ibid.; p. 75.
5. Arking, R.; Ibid.; p. 9.
6. Adelman, R.; Freeman, C.; Cohen, B. Enzyme adaptation as a biochemical probe of development and aging. Advances in Enzyme Regulations 10: 365–382; 1972.
7. Adelman, R.C.; Britton, G.W. The impaired capability for biochemical adaptation during aging. Bioscience 25: 639–643; 1975.
8. Hayflick, L. Human Cells and Aging. Scientific American 218; no. 3; 32–37; 1968.
9. Gelfant, S.; Graham Smith, J. Aging: Noncycling cells an explanation. Science 178: 357–368; 1972.
10. Hayflick, L. Cell biology of aging. Bioscience 25: 629–637; 1975.
11. Adler, W.H. Aging and immune function. Bioscience 25: 652–657; 1975.
12. Arking, R.; Ibid.; p. 285.
13. Abrams, W.B.; Berkow, M.D., editors. The Merck Manual of Geriatrics. Rahway, NJ: Merck & Co.; 1990; 1267 pages.
14. Brock, M.A. Chronobiology and Aging. Journal of the American Geriatrics Society 39: 74–91; 1991.
15. Pittendrigh, C.; Daan, S. Circadian oscillations in rodents: A systematic increase in their frequency with age. Science 186: 548–550; 1974.
16. Webb, W. Twenty-four hour sleep cycling. In Kales, A., editor. Philadelphia, PA: J. B. Lippincott; 1969; p. 53–65.
17. Gregerman, R.I.; Bierman, E.L. Chapter 29: Aging and hormones. In Williams, R.D., editor. Textbook of Endocrinology, Sixth Edition. Philadelphia, PA: W. B. Saunders; 1981; p. 1192.
18. Martin, C.R. Endocrine Physiology. New

York: Oxford University Press; 1985; p. 828.

19. Lawren, B. The hormone that makes your body 20 years younger. Longevity, New York: Longevity International, Ltd., October 1990; pp. 31–33.

20. Dorfman, A. Getting a shot of youth. Time Magazine, July 16, 1990; p. 53.

21. Tzankoff, S.P.; Norris, A.H. Effect of muscle mass decrease on age-related BMR changes. J. Appl. Physiol. 43: 1001; 1977.

22. Finch, C.E. Neuroendocrinology of aging. Bioscience 25: 645–650; 1975.

23. Martin, C.R. Endocrine Physiology. New York: Oxford University Press; 1985; p.481.

24. Martin, C.R.; Ibid.; 1985; p. 16.

25. Adelman, R.C. Loss of adaptive mechanisms during aging. Fed. Proc. 38: 1968; 1979.

26. Martin, C.R.; Op. cit.; p. 192.

27. Finch, C.E. Neuroendocrinology of aging: A view of an emerging area, Bioscience 25: 645–650; 1975.

28. Adelman, R.C. Loss of adaptive mechanisms during aging. Fed. Proc. 38: 1968; 1979.

29. Meites, J. Aging: Hypothalamic catecholamines, neuroendocrine-immune interactions, and dietary restriction, Proceedings of the Society for Experimental Biology and Medicine 195: 304-311; 1990.

30. Korenman, S.G. Male hypogonadism and impotency. In Abrams, W.B.; Berkow, M.D., editors. The Merck Manual of Geriatrics. Rahway, NJ: Merck & Co.; 1990; p. 841.

31. Martin, C.R. Endocrine Physiology. New York: Oxford University Press; 1985; p. 603.

32. Martin, C.R.; Op. cit.; p. 671.

33. Ganong, W. Review of Medical Physiology, Fourteenth Edition. Norwalk, CT: Appleton & Lange; 1989; p. 35.

34. Gergerman, R.I.; Bierman, E.L. Chapter 29: Aging and hormones. In Williams, R.D., editor. Textbook of Endocrinology, Sixth Edition. Philadelphia, PA: W. B. Saunders; 1981; p. 1207.

35. David H. Solomon, Section, 68, Introduction. In Abrams, W. B.; Berkow, M.D., editors. The Merck Manual of Geriatrics. Rahway, NJ: Merck & Co.; 1990; p. 774.

36. Reiter, R.; Richardson, B.; Johnson, L.; Ferguson, B.; Dinh, D. Pineal melatonin rhythm: Reduction in aging Syrian hamsters. Science 210: 1372–1374;1980.

37. Kitay, J.; Altschule, M. The Pineal Gland. Cambridge, MA: Harvard University Press; 1954.

38. Stewart, F.M. The Methuselah Enzyme. New York: Arbor House; 1970; pp. 29, 175.

39. Mcauliffe, K. Live 20 years longer, look 20 years younger. Longevity, Longevity International, Ltd., New York, October 1990; pp. 22–28.

40. Pierpaoli, W.; Maestroni, G.J.M. Melatonin: A principal neuroimmunoregulatory and anti-stress hormone: Its anti-aging effects. Immunology Letters 16: 355–362; 1987.

41. Sandyk, R. Possible role of pineal melatonin in the mechanisms of aging. Intern. J. Neuroscience 52: 85–92; 1990.

42. Kloeden, P.E.; Rossler, R.; Rossler, O.E. Does a centralized clock for aging exist? Gerontology 36: 314–322; 1990.

43. Maestroni, G.J.M.; Conti, A.; Pierpaoli, W. Melatonin antagonizes the immunosuppressive effect of acute stress via an opiatergic mechanism. Immunology 63: 465–469; 1988.

44. Pierpaoli, W.; Op. cit.

45. Armstrong, S.M.; Redman, J.M. Melatonin: A chronobiotic with anti-aging properties. Medical Hypotheses 34: 300–309; 1991.

46. Saul, J. Darkness. New York: Bantam Books; 1991; p. 329.

47. Darrach, B. The war on aging. Life 15 (October): 32–45; 1992.

48. Meites, J. Aging: Hypothalamic catecholamines, neuroendocrine-immune interactions, and dietary restriction. Proc. Soc. Exp. Bio. Med. 195: 304–311; 1990.

49. Myrsovsky, N. The adjustable brain of hibernators. Scientific American 218: 110–118; 1968.

50. Pengelley, E.T. Circannual Clocks: Annual Biological Rhythms. Academic Press: New York; 1974; 523 pages.

51. Barnes, B.M.; York, A.D. Effect of winter high temperatures on reproduction and circannual rhythms in hibernating ground squirrels. Journal of Biological Rhythms 5: 119–130; 1990.

52. Gwinner, E. Circannual Rhythms: Endogenous Annual Clocks in the Organization of Seasonal Processes. New York: Springer-Verlag; 1986; 154 pages.

53. Gwinner, E.; Ibid.

54. Hudson, J.W.; Wang, L.C.H.. Hibernation: endocrinologic aspects. Ann. Rev. Physiol. 41: 287–303; 1979.

55. Lyman, C.P.; Willis, J.; Malan, A.; Wang, L.

Chapter 12: Hibernation and endocrines. In Hibernation and Torpor in Mammals and Birds. San Diego: Academic Press; 1982; pp. 207–236.

56. Zucker, I.; Bosches, M.; Dark, J. Suprachiasmatic nuclei influence circannual and circadian rhythms of ground squirrels, Am. J. Physiol. 13: R472–R480; 1983.

57. Feldberg, W.; Myers, R.D. Effects on temperature of amines injection into the cerebral ventricles. A new concept of temperature regulation. J. Physiol. (London) 173: 225–326; 1964.

58. Spafford, D.C.; Pengelley, E.T. The influence of the neurohumor serotonin on hibernation in the golden-mantled ground squirrel, *Citellus lateralis*. Comp. Biochem. Physiol. 38(2A): 239–250; 1971.

59. Binkley, S. Pineal and melatonin: circadian rhythms and body temperature. In Scheving, L.; Halberg, F.; Pauly, J., editors. Chronobiology. Tokyo: Igaku Shoin; 1974; pp. 582–585.

60. Palmer, D. L.; Riedesel, M.L. Responses of whole-animal and isolated hearts of ground squirrels, *Citellus lateralis*, to melatonin. Comp. Biochem. Physiol. 53C: 69-72; 1976.

61. Zucker, I. Pineal gland influences period of circannual rhythms of ground squirrels. Am. J. Physiol. 249: 111–115; 1985.

62. Florant, G.; Rivera, M.; Lawrence, A.; Tamarkin, L. Plasma melatonin concentrations in hibernating marmots: Absence of a plasma melatonin rhythm. Amer. J. Physiol. 247: R1062–R1066; 1984.

63. Popovic, V. Endocrines in hibernation. Bull. Bus. Comp. Zool. 124: 104–130; 1960.

64. Draskoczy, P.; Lyman, C.P. Turnover of catecholamines in active and hibernating ground squirrels. J. Pharmacol. Exp. Ther. 155: 101–111; 1967.

65. Florant, G. L.; Weitzman, E. D. Diurnal and episodic pattern of plasma cortisol during fall and spring in young and old woodchucks (*Marmota monax*). Comp. Biochem. Physiol. A 66A: 575–581; 1981.

66. Dawe, A.; Spurrier, W. A. Hibernation induced in ground squirrels by blood transfusion. Science 163: 298–299; 1969.

67. Snyder, F.; Hobson, J.A.; Goldfrank, F. Blood pressure changes during human sleep. Science 142: 1313–1314; 1963.

68. Krieger, D.T., editor. Endocrine Rhythms. New York: Raven Press; 1979, 332 pages.

69. Binkley, S.; Kluth, E.; Menaker, M. Pineal and locomotor activity: Levels and arrhythmia in sparrows. J. Comp. Physiol. 77: 163–169; 1972.

70. Gaston, S.; Menaker, M. Pineal function: The biological clock in the sparrow? Science 160: 1125–1127; 1968.

71. Binkley, S. Op. cit.

72. Penny, R. Episodic secretion of melatonin in pre- and postpubertal girls and boys. J. Clin. Endocrinol. Metab. 60: 751–756; 1985.

73. Vaughan, G. Melatonin in humans. In Reiter, R., editor. Pineal Research Reviews II, New York: Alan R. Liss; 1984; pp. 141–201.

74. Stephan, F.; Zucker, I. Circadian rhythms in drinking behavior and locomotor activity of rats are eliminated by hypothalamic lesions. Proc. Nat. Acad. Sci. USA 69: 1583–1586; 1972.

75. Jouvet, M. Neurophysiological and biochemical mechanisms of sleep. In Kales, A., editor. Sleep. Philadelphia, PA: J. B. Lippincott; 1969; pp. 89–100.

76. Toth, L.A.; Krueger, J.M. Infectious disease, cytokines, and sleep. In Mancia, M., Marini, G., editors. The Diencephalon and Sleep. New York: Raven Press, Ltd.; 1990; pp. 331–341.

77. Pappenheimer, J.R.; Miller, T.B.; Goodrich, C.A. Sleep-promoting effects of cerebrospinal fluid from sleep deprived goats. Proc. Nat. Acad. Sci. (Wash.) 58: 513–517; 1967.

78. Monnier, M.; Hosli, L. Dialysis of sleep and waking factors in blood of the rabbit. Science 146: 796–798; 1964.

79. Tazi, A.; Crestani, F.; Dantzer, R. Aversive effects of centrally injected interleukin-I. Neuroscience Research Communications 7: 159–165; 1990.

80. Rosenberg, S.A.; Yang, J.C.; Topalian, S. L.; Schwartzentruber, D.J.; Weber, J.S.; Parkinson, D.R.; Seipp, C.A.; Einhorn J. H.; White, D.E. Treatment of 283 consecutive patients with metastatic melanoma or renal cell cancer using high-dose bolus interleukin 2. JAMA 271; 907-913; 1994.

81. Tabibzadeh, S. Human endometrium: An active site of cytokine production and action. Endocrine Reviews 12: 272–290; 1991.

82. Patt, L.M.; Houck, C. The incredible shrinking chalone. FEBS Lett. 120: 163–170; 1980.

83. Hadley, M.E. Endocrinology, Second Edition. Englewood Cliffs, NJ: Prentice Hall; 1988; p. 288.

84. Bullough, W.S. Mitotic control in adult mammalian tissues. Biol. Rev. 50: 99–127; 1975.

85. Finkler, N., Acker, P. Chalones: A mini-review. Mt. Sinai J. Med. 45: 258–64; 1978.

86. Martin, C.R. Endocrine Physiology. New York: Oxford University Press; 1985; p. 609.

87. Adamson, J.W.; Kaushansky, K.; Powell, J.S.; Segal, G.M. Hormones and blood production. In, DeGroot, L.J. Endocrinology, Volume 3. Philadelphia, PA: W. B. Saunders; 1989; pp. 2612–2631.

88. Telford, I.R.; Bridgman, C.F. Introduction to Functional Histology. New York: Harper & Row, Pubs.; 1990; p. 165.

89. Tortora, G.J.; Anagnostakos, N.P. Principles of Anatomy and Physiology. New York: Harper & Row, Pubs.; 1990; p. 551.

CHAPTER 21

Phytohormones, Invertebrate Hormones, and Pheromones

Plants use chemical messengers—phytohormones or plant hormones—such as auxins and gibberellins. Invertebrates also have chemical messengers (invertebrate hormones such as ecdysone) which move through their circulation regulating development. Chemical messengers between individuals of a species are the pheromones—used as sex attractants and alarm signals. These odd bedfellows are grouped in this chapter because, except for some of the pheromones, these subjects do not involve vertebrates.

PHYTOHORMONES

Since plants do not have blood, their chemical messengers cannot meet the classical definition of hormones. Nonetheless they do have chemical messengers which may move in the plant vasculature or from cell to cell.

"Phytohormone" (literally meaning "plant hormone") is the word that some plant physiologists use to refer to chemical messengers in plants. Plants make use of many chemical messengers in their physiology whether or not they qualify as hormones or even as phytohormones. A few of them—auxins, gibberellins, cytokinins, inhibitors, ethylene—will be discussed briefly here. Plants also produce substances that act on other species. For example, there is a volatile principle emanating from oak leaves that is necessary for the mating of polyphemus moths.[1]

Some endocrinologists bristle at the heresy of even including plants in an endocrinology textbook. Plants are included here to provide a broader perspective of chemical messengers, because some of them are chemically related to some mammalian hormones (e.g., auxin is an indole as is melatonin), and because they are involved in functions that are regulated by hormones in vertebrates (growth, reproduction).

AUXIN IN PLANTS

"Auxin" is the name given to a plant growth hormone, indoleacetic acid (IAA), isolated and identified in the 1930s. Synthetic auxins include phenylacetic acid and chlorinated IAAs. According to Bandurski and Nonhebel (Table 21.1), auxin is involved in "stimulation of cell division, stimulation of shoot growth, inhibition of root growth, control of vascular system differentiation, control of tissue culture differentiation, control of apical dominance, delay of senescence, promotion of flowering and fruit setting and ripening."[2] Auxin has a variety of actions (Table 21.1) and some effects of auxin are illustrated by auxin bioassays (Figure 21.1).

The *Avena* curvature test makes use of oat (*Avena*) sprouts (coleoptiles). The seedling is decapitated and the substance to be assayed is applied to the stump in an agar block. The agar block is placed on the stump asymmetrically for two hours. Auxin causes growth, so the seedling grows on the side near the block if auxin is present.

Curvature of the seedling is proportional to the amount of auxin in amounts up to five micromolar, so the amounts of auxin can be quantified. The *Avena* **straight growth assay** also uses oat coleoptiles. The sprouts are decapitated and incubated in a solution containing the compound to be assayed. Incubation lasts 12 hours. A few millimeters lengthening of the coleoptile is proportional to the log of IAA concentration. IAA can also be measured with 75 other bioassays, colorimetric assays, fluorometric assays, mass spectrometry, gas chromatography, an immobilized enzyme assay, and radioimmunoassays. The chemistry of IAA may vary depending on which part of the plant is examined. Synthesis of IAA involves tryptophan as a precursor (Figure 21.2); IAA is metabolized to other indole products by reactions including oxidation.

Even a human or animal endocrinologist has probably noticed the way that plants turn toward the sun for light. **Phototropism** provides another example of an auxin function. Dennison defines phototropism as "the developing curvature of a growing organ in response to some asymmetric external light source....the bending of the organ is oriented in relation to the direction of the illumination, usually approximately towards it or away from it."[3] Auxin is involved in phototropism since bending is accomplished by elongation of the cells on the side of the plant away from the light. Plant physiologists view the bending effect as due, not to destruction of auxin on the sunny side, but rather to "lateral auxin redistribution" in which the plants auxin moves to the shady side. Blooming sunflowers turn their heads throughout the day to follow the the sun as it arcs through the heavens; when they do this together in synchrony in a farmer's field, the effect is dramatic. But the effects may not be due to auxin since sunflower seedlings (*Helianthus*) appear to achieve phototropism with some other substance.

Plants lack blood but nevertheless transport chemicals through their vascular tissue, from cell to cell, and within the cell cytoplasm. For example, auxin is transported in the plant's vascular tissue (phloem) and in the cytoplasm. IAA concentrations in phloem sap are 4–13 ng/l. Transport velocities in phloem sap are 100–240 mm/hour. IAA transport is estimated in pea seedlings as 11 mm/hour. The system is described as "rapid and specific downward polar transport." Transport of

Table 21.1 Responses to Auxin in Plants

Physiological event	Effect of auxin
cell division	stimulation of cell division in cambial cells
cell elongation	stimulation of shoot growth; inhibition of root growth
cell differentiation	stimulation of differentiation of xylem and phloem; promotion of initiation of roots by cuttings, callus tissue morphogenesis regulation
seedling morphology	red-light inhibition of mesocotyl elongation reversed
geotropism	IAA transported to underside of shoot
phototropism	IAA transported to dark side of shoot
apical dominance	apical bud replacement
leaf senescence	delayed
leaf abscission	inhibits abscission when applied to leaves, but promotes abscission when applied near the abscission layer
flowering	may promote flowering
fruit setting	permits parthenocarpic fruit development
fruit ripening	ripening delayed

The global effects of exogenously applied auxin are shown. Modified, with permission. After Table 1.1 in Bandurski, R.S.; Nonhebel, H.M. Chapter 1: Auxins. In Wilkins, M.B. Advanced Plant Physiology. Marshfield, MA: Pitman; 1984; p. 13.

IAA in cytoplasm may occur by carrier-mediated, energy-dependent mechanisms.

The mechanism of action whereby auxin produces growth seems to involve second messengers and the plant cell wall. It is described by Bandurski and Nonhebel:

> When IAA-induced growth occurs, the solution bathing the cell wall becomes more acid and the wall becomes more easily deformed. This change in the plasticity of the wall seems to be due . . . . to enzyme-induced changes in the wall. Whether this enhanced enzymatic activity is attributable to more enzyme secreted into the wall or to enhanced activity of enzymes already in the wall is not known.[4]

Auxin, IAA, is in the chemical family of indoles that includes serotonin and melatonin. Serotonin and melatonin have been shown to function in the regulation of daily rhythms in vertebrates. Perhaps auxin also plays some role in the daily cycles, such as leaf movement rhythms, of plants.

GIBBERELLINS IN PLANTS

The gibberellins (GAs) are over 60 different diterpene acids that have been isolated from a fungus, *Giberella fujikuroi*. They are widely distributed in higher plants as well as in the fungi. Gibberellins are variously synthesized from 3R-mevalonic acid. The effects of gibberellins include shoot elongation, increased stem diameter, and flowering in conifers; growth and development of ferns, algae, and fungi; and a multitude of responses in higher plants. For example, GAs promote growth in higher plants by stimulating cell division and/or by stimulating cell expansion. Jones and MacMillan suggested a mechanism of action for gibberellins that is similar to the actions of auxin:

> The action of GA_3 in all target tissues may therefore be via its effect on the transcriptional process. This could be a quantitative effect, where GA_3 could accelerate the synthesis of all

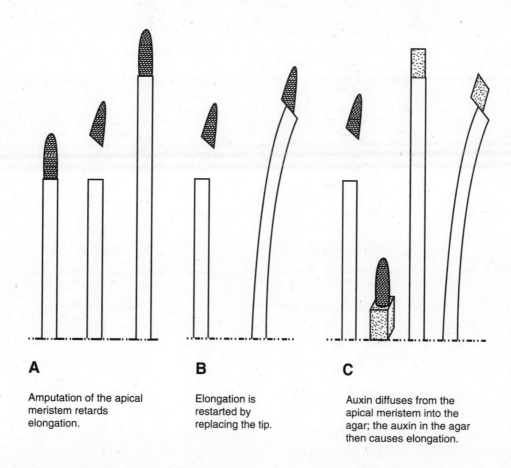

A

Amputation of the apical
meristem retards
elongation.

B

Elongation is
restarted by
replacing the tip.

C

Auxin diffuses from the
apical meristem into the
agar; the auxin in the agar
then causes elongation.

Figure 21.1 The diagrams show three experiments that demonstrate auxin function in higher plants. Each vertical bar represents a shoot of an individual plant such as an oat coleoptile. The height of the bar represents the amount of growth or elongation. The hatched region is the apical meristem which is the growing tip of the plant and which is a source of auxin. The block represents agar. Bending also occurs depending on the placement of the tip or agar block; elongation on the side that receives the most auxin is responsible for the bending. Modified, with permission. J.W. Mavor. General Biology, Fifth Edition. New York: Macmillan; 1959.

classes of RNA, as has been reported for castor bean, or its effect could be qualitative by the induction of specific enzymes, as in the cereal aleurone.[5]

CYTOKININS IN PLANTS

A cytokinin is "a compound which, in the presence of optimal auxin, induces cell division in the tobacco pith or similar assay (e.g., carrot phloem or soybean callus) grown on an optimally defined medium."[6]

Chemically, the natural cytokinins are substituted purines. Names of some specific cytokinins are N6 (benzyl) adenine, dihydrozeatin, and ß-D-ribofuranosyl adenosine. Bioassays for the cytokinins are based on promotion of cell division or expansion, senescence retardation, or pigment synthesis induction. Cytokinins are found in some tRNA species so tRNA turnover is a potential source of the substances. But they may also be

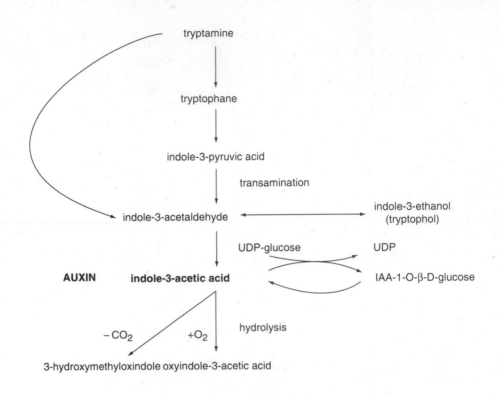

Figure 21.2 The figure illustrates the biosynthesis and some metabolites of auxin (IAA). The structure of IAA (indole-3-acetic acid) is shown. For storage or transport, auxin also combines (e.g., with glucose) to form high and low molecular weight ester conjugates. After Bandurski, R.S.; Nonhebel, H.M. Chapter 1: Auxins. In Wilkins, M.B. Advanced Plant Physiology. Marshfield, MA: Pitman; 1984; p. 1–20.

synthesized de novo from adenine in plant tissue.

The ratio of cytokinin/auxin affects the type of plant organ that is formed in culture; for example, in tobacco pith tissue cultures, changing the ratio determined whether the cells formed roots or buds. Cytokinins increase bean and radish leaf size by enlarging the cells. Senescence in leaves is marked by the disappearance of chlorophyll and the breakdown of proteins—the rates of both of these are slowed by cytokinins. There is a role of light in the function of cytokinins in chloroplast development, in pigment synthesis, and in seed germina-

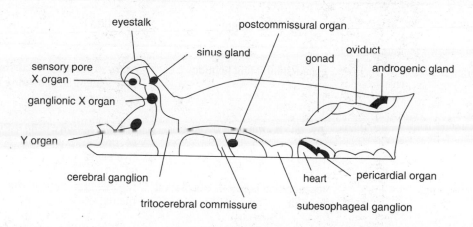

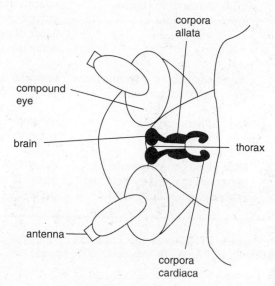

Figure 21.3 The figure shows the anatomy of some aspects of the endocrine systems of invertebrates. (Upper) The diagram shows the upper portion of the body of a generalized crustacean with the head on the left and the approximate location of the endocrine structures. (Lower) Diagrammatic representation of the head of a cockroach showing the location of the endocrine structures. Redrawn, with permission. Turner, C.D.; Bagnara, J.T. General Endocrinology, Sixth Edition. W.B. Saunders; Philadelphia, PA; 1976; pp. 550, 564.

tion. For example, cytokinins can substitute for the light requirement in the germination of light-sensitive lettuce seeds. Cytokinins affect the opening of the stomata of some plant species to increase the rate of transpiration.

INHIBITORS IN PLANTS

Milborrow describes the **inhibitors** as substances that block plant growth and are involved in plant self-defense:

Table 21.2 Invertebrate Chemical Messengers

Invertebrate	Chemical messenger	Function
starfish radial nerves	gonad-stimulating peptide	ovary to secrete 1-methyladene-nine leading to spawning and oocyte maturation
polychaete worms	juvenile hormone of cerebral ganglia	inhibits epitoky (transformation of immature worm to reproductive adult)
polychaete worms	regeneration hormone of cerebral ganglia	regeneration of posterior segments
earthworms	sex hormone from supraesophageal ganglia	inhibits gonad maturation, involved in egg laying, maintenance of clitellum, gamete differentiation
leeches	gonad-stimulating hormone from brain neurosecretory cells	testicular development
slugs	gonadal hormone	development and function of accessory genital complex.
octopus	optic gland gonad-stimulating hormone regulated by light and brain subpedunculate lobe	ovary follicle cell development and yolk deposition, spermatogenesis

Based on remarks in Turner, C.D.; Bagnara, J.T. Chapter 17: Endocrine mechanisms in the invertebrates, General Endocrinology, Sixth Edition. Philadelphia, PA: W. B. Saunders; 1976; pp. 545–580.

...most plants contain from a few to many secondary products, polyketide, terpenoid or alkaloidal compounds...[which may function] to comprise a static chemical defence against insect or fungal attack. Others are classified as phytoalexins....which are synthesized rapidly in response to attack by a pathogenic organism or damage to a tissue.[7]

One way that growth might be inhibited is by the action of **diphenolic acids** (e.g., *p*-coumaric acid) that may stimulate the activity of IAA oxidase; however, the issue is clouded by the fact that nonophenolic acids (e.g., caffeic acid) inhibit activity of the oxidase.

Abscisic acid (ABA) is a growth inhibitor that may accelerate abscission (the autumn leaf fall). Bioassays for the abscisic acid include abscission of petiolar cotton stumps, wheat embryo germination inhibition, barley aleurone amylase synthesis, and stomata closure in epidermal strips. Abscisic acid is generally found in all tissues of higher plants but not in most fungi, bacteria, algae, or liverworts. Abscisic acid functions in growth inhibition, root geotropism, dormancy,

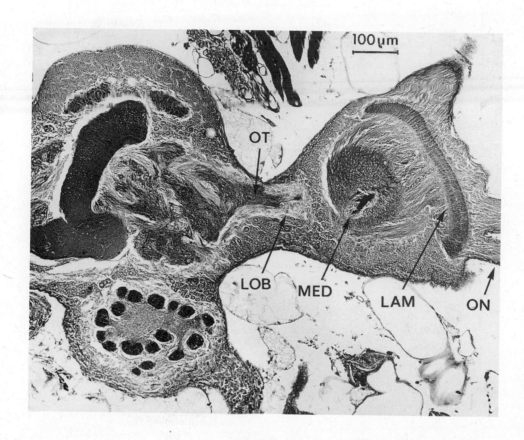

Figure 21.4 The photograph shows a histological section of half of the brain of a cockroach. OT = optic tract; LOB = lobula of optic lobe; MED = medulla of optic lobe; LAM = lamina of optic lobe; ON = optic nerve. The top of the page is anterior; the left of the page is the center of the brain. The photograph was a gift from Shepherd K. Roberts.

fruit ripening and development, parthenocarpy, flowering, turgor, injury resistance, solute movement, and enzyme production have been investigated. Concentrations vary from 3–500 µg/kg. Some other inhibitors are lunularic acid, baratasins, jasmonic acid, seselin, avocado inhibitors, and eucalyptus inhibitors.

ETHYLENE IN PLANTS

Ethylene[8] (C_2H_4) is a gaseous substance whose effects are seen at the times of fruit ripening,

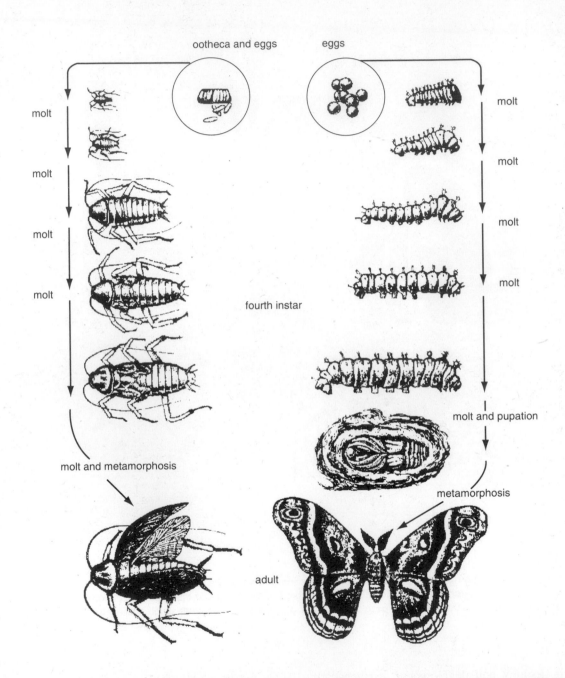

ootheca and eggs   eggs

molt

molt

molt

molt

molt

molt

molt

molt

fourth instar

molt and pupation

molt and metamorphosis

metamorphosis

adult

Figure 21.5 Two routes of insect development are shown. Incomplete (hemimetabolous) metamorphosis is shown for cockroaches on the left; complete (holometabolous) metamorphosis is shown on the right for the giant silkworm moth. Cockroaches develop with the instars as immature insects (left). In the giant silkworm moth (right), the immature insects, or instars, are caterpillars; eclosion is the emergence of the mature insect from its pupa. Modified, with permission. Turner, C.D.; Bagnara, J.T. General Endocrinology, Sixth Edition. Philadelphia, PA: W.B. Saunders; pp. 550–564.

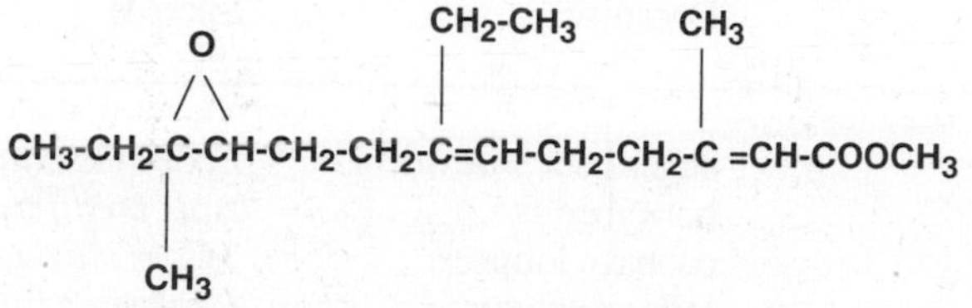

juvenile homone

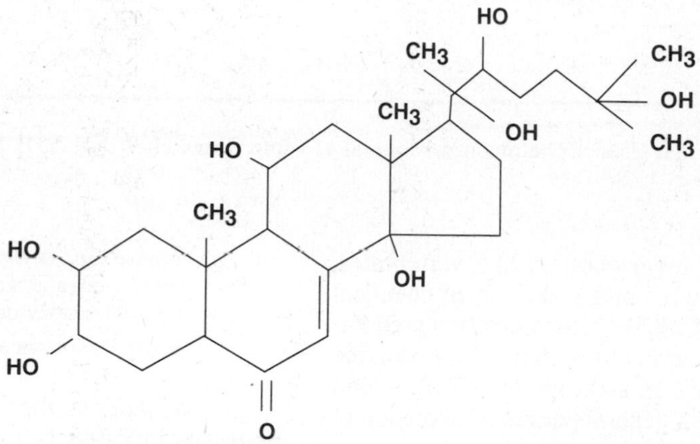

ecdysone

Figure 21.6 The figure illustrates the structures of juvenile hormone (JH, upper) and ecdysone (a steroid, lower).

dormancy termination, abscission, flowering, and modification of reproduction.

The production rate for ethylene varies from 0.02 nl per gram per hour in fruits to 6000 nl per gram per hour in the fungus *Penicillium digitatum*. The pathway for production of ethylene is methionine to S-adenosylmethionine (SAM) to ACC (1-aminocyclopropane-1-carboxylic acid) to ethylene.

Auxin stimulates conversion of SAM to ACC. In most cases, high auxin content corresponds with high ethylene production. Stress stimulates ethylene production so that the compound is an indicator of stress (chemicals, chilling, drought, flood, radiation, insects, diseases, mechanical wounds).

Carbon dioxide and silver are ethylene antagonists. Cut carnations can be treated with silver compounds to extend their vase-life. A compound whose trade name is Ethrel® is used to promote fruit ripening, accelerate abscission, increase rubber and sugar production, synchronize pineapple flowering, and increase tobacco leaf senescence.

INVERTEBRATE CHEMICAL MESSENGERS

Invertebrate chemical messengers also fail the test of the classical hormone in being trans-

Table 21.3 Insect Sex Pheromones

Pheromone	Organism	Species
valeric acid	sugar beet wireworm	*Limonius californicus*
9-keto-2-decenoic acid	honeybee	*Apis mellifera*
cis-7-dodecen-1-ol	cabbage looper	*Trichoplusia ni*
cis-9-tetradecen-1-ol	fall army worm	*Laphygma frugiperda*
trans-3-*cis*-5-tetra-decadienoic acid	black carpet beetle	*Attagenus megatoma*
trans-10-*cis*-12-hexadecadien-1-ol	silk-worm moth	*Bombys mori*
d-10-acetoxy-*cis*-7-hexadecen-1-ol	gypsy moth	*Porthetria dispar*
propylure	pink bollworm	*Pectinophora gossypiella*
2,3-dihydro-7-methyl-1 H-pyrrolizidin-1-one	male butterfly	*Lycorea ceres ceres*
cetyl acetate		
cis-vaccenyl acetate		

Regnier, F.E., Law, J.H. Insect pheromones. Journal of Lipid Research 9: 541-551; 1968.

ported by blood. Invertebrates, like vertebrates, have secretory systems and make use of chemical messengers (Figure 21.3). Neurosecretion predominates in most of the invertebrates with endocrine glands present in the arthropods. Turner and Bagnara describe the general pattern of evolution of endocrine function:

> Neurosecretory cells, producing chemical messengers (neurohormones) for prolonged action at a distance, are the first elements of this kind to appear during the phylogeny of animal organisms. These glandlike neurons function together with purely nervous elements to adjust the organism to environmental changes. Epithelial endocrine glands appear to be absent in coelenterates and annelids, neurosecretory mechanisms operating alone to control such processes as growth and reproduction. The same is probably true of flatworms, nemerteans and nematodes, though these groups have not been explored in sufficient detail. The cephalopod molluscs appear to be the first organisms to achieve a structural organization requiring the presence of endocrine glands. Circumscribed endocrine glands in-

crease in complexity through the arthropod and vertebrate classes, but neurosecretory cells continue to be of great importance.[9]

Chemical messengers found in invertebrates are in Table 21.2. Generally, neurosecretory cells are found in the nervous systems and the neurohormones function to control maturation and reproduction.

CRUSTACEAN HORMONES

The crustaceans are the group in which lobsters and crabs are found. Crustaceans have clusters of neurosecretory cells, neurohemal organs, and endocrine glands.

Two **X organs** located in the eyestalks or head are believed to be neurosecretory along with aggregates of neurosecretory cells in the tritocerebral commissure, the esophageal connective ganglia, the thoracic ganglia, and the brain.

The **sinus glands**, also in the eyestalks, are viewed as "reservoirs for the storage and discharge of neurohormones derived from the axons of neurosecretory neurons. The sinus gland is an example of a neurohemal organ in which circulatory vessels are in close association with the terminals

Table 21.4 Stimulation of Courtship in Male Fruit Flies

Stimulus	Courtship index ± SEM
virgin female	16 ± 2
extract from 1–8 hour males	31 ± 3
extract from 3–6 day old males	3 ± 1

The courtship index is the percentage of courtship observed in a male *Drosophila melanogaster* during ten minutes of observation. It was measured by watching the fruit flies (N = 10 tests). Tompkins, L.; Hall, J.C.; Hall, L.M. Courtship-stimulating volatile compounds from normal and mutant *Drosophila*. J. Insect Physiol. 225: 689–697; 1980; p. 691.

of neurosecretory cells. The X-organs and sinus glands may secrete a molt-inhibiting neurohormone.

The **Y organs**, in the anterior part of the animal, may secrete a molting hormone under control of eyestalk hormones. Eyestalk and Y organ secretions may control metabolism by changing sugar concentration and hypodermis glycogen. An octapeptide, **distal retinal pigment hormone**, was isolated. The hormone from the eyestalk controls adaptation to changes in dark and light which, in crustaceans, involves movement of pigment in the ommatidia that form the compound eyes.

The **pericardial organs** release a neurohormone that controls heartrate and contraction amplitude. These organs have terminals from axons that originate in the esophageal connective ganglia and the brain. The pericardial organ hormones may include peptides and serotonin.

Like vertebrates, crustaceans can change color rapidly with chromatophores. Chromatophores in crustaceans may be under hormonal control by **chromatophorotrophins** from the neurosecretory cells Black, white, red, yellow, brown, and blue pigments can aggregate or disperse in crustacea to achieve background adaptation. The neurohemal posterior commissure organ and the tritocerebral commissure contain high concentrations of chromatophorotrophins. An octapeptide has been purified that acts as a red pigment-concentrating hormone.

Sexuality in crustaceans is a reversible phenomenon dependent upon which gonads and hormones are present. The **androgenic glands** are along the vas deferens, are distinct from the testes, regulate spermatogenesis and secondary sex characteristics, and are likely controlled by X-organ and sinus gland secretions. The **ovaries** may have two hormones which function to produce female secondary sex characteristics. An ovarian inhibiting hormone prevents vitellogenesis and may come from the eyestalks, ganglionic X organs, and/or sinus gland.

INSECT CHEMICAL MESSENGERS

Insects, like crustaceans, have chemical messengers that function in development and reproduction and in other functions.[10] Clusters of neurosecretory cells are found in insect subesophageal ganglion, ganglia of the ventral chain, and in medial and lateral protocerebrum or brain (Figure 21.4). The hormones function in development and metamorphosis (Figure 21.5). Insect physiologists have gone so far as to give the chemical messengers names that include the word "hormone."

The **brain neurosecretory cells** make hormones (Figure 21.6). Brain hormone (prothoracic gland-stimulating factor, prothoracotropin) is probably a polypeptide and is required for pupation. The brain also makes a hormone that stimulates egg maturation in blowflies. Bursicon (tanning hormone) is a 40,000 molecular weight protein hormone that causes darkening of cuticle in blowflies. The brain medial neurosecretory cells make eclosion hormone.

The paired or fused **corpora cardiaca**

Table 21.5 Insect Recruiting Pheromones

Pheromone	Organism	Species
geraniol geranial neral geranoic acid nerolic acid	honeybee	*Apis mellifera*
2-methyl-6-methylene-7-octen-4-ol 2-methyl-6-methylene-2,7-octadien-4-ol cis-verbenol	bark beetle	*Ips confusus*
brevocomin	beetle	*Dendrotonus brevoconus*

Regnier, F.E., Law, J.H. Insect pheromones. Journal of Lipid Research 9: 541–551; 1968.

arise at the posterior edge of the brain by the dorsal aorta and are an aggregate of neurosecretory cells. They are neurohemal organs that are believed to act both in storage-release and in secretion. The corpora cardiaca may release a polypeptide that raises the concentration of trehalose (circulating carbohydrate), a peptide that increases heart rate, and eclosion hormone.

The **corpora allata** originate near mouth parts and are also near the back of the brain. The corpora allata secrete a **juvenile hormone** (JH) that acts with molting hormone to delay metamorphosis. In reproduction, JH functions in yolk deposition, spermatophore formation, and oviduct secretion. Some parasites alter host growth and development by secreting a substance with effects similar to JH.

The **ventral glands or prothoracic glands** (named for their location in a particular species) secrete the steroid **ecdysone** (molting hormone) under control of brain hormone. Some plants make steroids with ecdysone activity and can those plants influence the metamorphosis of the insects that feed upon them.

There are other glands and hormones in insects. **Proctodone** from gland-like cells in the end of the abdomen participates in diapause termination. The testes of some species, such as fireflies, have masculinizing properties and may have an androgenic hormone. The fused thoracic ganglia, corpora allata, or brain may be the source of **antidiuretic neurohormone**, probably a polypeptide, which acts on the Malpighian tubules.

INSECT USES OF CHEMICALS

Stadler summarizes the ubiquitous role of chemicals in the lives of insects: "In insects, the chemistry of the environment is a dominant modality mediating adaptive behavior, including the choice of food and feeding, avoidance of danger, location of a sexual partner and the choice of a habitat for the progeny."[11]   Termites, for example, use chemicals in their foraging strategies, caste regulation mechanisms, and defensive strategies.[12] Insects are equipped with specialized organs to secrete and to detect chemical signals. For instance, contact chemoreceptive sensilla typically have a single pore at the tip of the sensillum and 2–10 unbranched dendrites from 2–10 cells reaching to the tip. The sensilla are variously found on the head, thorax, abdomen, wings, tarsi, and the ovipositor.

Monarch and viceroy butterflies defend themselves from blue jays with a digitalis-like cardiac glycoside toxin that is distasteful. They feed on milkweed to obtain the toxin. Names of some of the glycosides are calotropin, calotoxin, and calactin. Insects in general defend themselves from

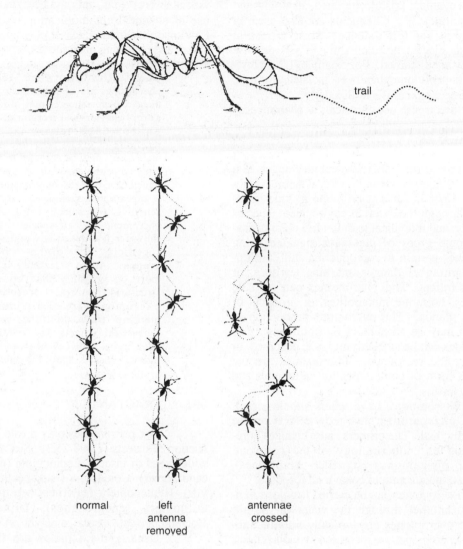

Figure 21.7 The figure illustrates the way that ants lay pheromone, or odor, trails. The upper sketch shows an ant in the process of laying a trail by applying a line of pheromone with the tip of its abdomen (right). The lower illustration shows an idealization of ant trail following. On the left is the normal weaving trail-following method where the worker ant moves from one side of the trail to the other detecting the strength of the odor differential with its antennae. The center represents the behavior of an ant with its left antenna removed; the ant overcorrects to its right side. The right illustration represents the disoriented behavior of an ant with its antennae glued in crossed position. Modified, with permission. After Wilson, E.O. Chemical communication among workers of the fire ant Solenopsis saevissima (Fr. Smith). 1. The organization of mass-foraging. 2. An information analysis of the odor trail. 3. The experimental induction of the social responses. Animal Behavior 10: 134–164; 1962; and Hangartner, W. Spezifitat und inaktivierung des spurpheromons von *Lasius fuliginosus* Latr. und orientierung der arbeiterinnen im duftfeld. Zeitschrift fur Vergleichende Physiologie 57: 103–136; 1967.

predators with chemical deterrents. Identified toxins include cardiac glycosides, histamine, acetylcholine, hydrogen cyanide, aristolochic acid, alkaloids, and benzoquinones.[13]   Chemicals are also used by other insects for self defense. Some terrestrial arthropods eject a noxious fluid in self defense when they are disturbed. For example, 1,2-dialkyl-4(3H)-quinazolinones has been isolated from the defensive secretion of the millipede.[14]

Insects also use chemicals as pheromones.

PHEROMONES

Pheromones are chemical messengers that carry information between individual members of a species. Criteria for a pheromone include transmission through the external environment, species specificity, and individual to individual communication. Some types of messages signaled using pheromones pertain to reproduction and development, warning of danger, marking territory, or marking trails. The pheromones can also be hormones, hormone metabolites, or products of exocrine glands. The pheromone production or secretion may be stimulated by hormones. The pheromones can be smelled, ingested, absorbed, or tasted by the recipients. Pheromones are the dominant form of communication in animals and microorganisms.[15]

Pheromones have been subclassified. **Primer pheromones** have slow effects on the target individual. The primers cause changes in reproduction or endocrinology of the recipient. **Releaser pheromones** (signaller pheromones), in contrast, initiate a rapid behavioral response.

Pheromones can be carried from one individual to another through the water or the air. Airborne pheromones are typically volatile substances. Pheromones are identified by their actions; some of their structures have been determined. Experienced investigators can often easily identify the occupants of an animal colony by the pungent odors emanating from the animal rooms. For example, a colony containing mice smelis differs from that of hamsters and both differ in aroma from a colony of ground squirrels and all differ from the perfume of cockroaches. Early attention was directed toward the chemical identification of the pheromones and delineation of their action; more recent focus has shifted to the receptors and the means by which the pheromones exert their actions.[16]   Some specific examples of pheromones

give a perspective on the variety of substances and responses that may be involved. In particular, the "social insects" (e.g., ants and bees) make extensive use of chemical communication.[17] Regnier and Law subdivide insect releaser pheromones into sex, alarm, and recruiting pheromones:

> Chemically identified releaser pheromones are of three basic types: those which cause sexual attraction, alarm behavior, and recruitment. **Sex pheromones** release the entire repertoire of sexual behavior. Thus a male insect may be attracted to and attempt to copulate with an inanimate object that has sex pheromone on it. It appears that most insects are rather sensitive and selective for the sex pheromone of their species. Insects show far less sensitivity and chemospecificity for **alarm pheromones**. Alarm selectivity is based more on volatility than on unique structural features. **Recruiting pheromones** are used primarily in marking trails to food sources. Terrestrial insects lay continuous odor trails, whereas bees and other airborne insects apply the substances at discrete intervals.[18]

SEX ATTRACTANTS IN INSECTS

Sex pheromones play a role in the reproduction of insects (Table 21.3). Sex attractants are widespread in insects: Lepidoptera (moths, sugarcane borers), Coleoptera (bark beetles, boll weevils), Hymenoptera (sawflies, bee queens, ants), Orthoptera (cockroaches), Diptera (flies), Homoptera (scale insects, mealybugs).

Usually the females are the emitters. Typically, they release volatiles from a gland located at the end of their abdomen. However there are also males with attractants—oriental fruit flies and salt marsh caterpillars. Sometimes both sexes emit pheromones which play roles in the attraction and courtship repertoire. For the female American cockroach, the pheromone emitted elicits "increased rates of location, upwind movement, and wing-raising by males." Wing raising is attractive to females when they are only a few centimeters away. The sex attractants are notorious for their long distance potency. A female Dipteran sciarid, *Bradysia impatiens*, releases a pheromone that at

Table 21.6 Insect Alarm Pheromones

Pheromone	Species
heptan-2-one	*Iridomyrmex pruinosis,*
	Apis mellifera,
	Conomyrma pyramica,
	Atta texana
tridecan-2-one	*Acanthomyops cliviger,*
	Lasius umbratus
undecane	*Acanthomyops cliviger,*
	Lasius umbratus
tridecane	*Acanthomyops claviger*
2-*trans*-hexan-1-al	*Crematogaster africana*
2-methyl-2-hepten-6-one	*Tapinoma nigerrimum,*
	Iridomyrmex dectu,
	I. conifer, I. nitidiceps
	Tapinoma nigerrimum
2-methylheptan-4-one	*Pogomyrmex barbatus,*
4-methylheptan-3-one	*P. badius, P. californicus,*
	P. occidentalis,
	Atta texana
2,6-dimethyl-5-hepten-1-al	*Acanthomyops cliviger*
2,6-dimethyl-5-hepten-1-ol	*Acanthomyops claviger*
citronellal	*Acanthomyops claviger*
citral	*Acanthomyops claviger,*
	Atta sexdens
isoamyl acetate	*Apis mellifera*
α-pinene	*Nasuititermes exitiosus*

Regnier, F.E., Law, J.H. Insect pheromones. Journal of Lipid Research 9: 541–551; 1968.

tracts males from at least a mile downwind.

Not all pheromones are volatile. For example, female *Drosophila melanogaster* make pheromones that coat the cuticle.[19] They are waxy long-chain hydrocarbons that protect the cuticle from desiccation. They stimulate taste receptors on males' legs. The courtship-stimulating pheromone synthesized by mature virgin females is 7,11-heptacosadiene. Immature flies of both genders synthesize two courtship-stimulating pheromones, 11- and 13-tritriacontene.[20] Mature males synthesize at least one inhibitory pheromone.[21]

There are a variety of insect parts that secrete pheromones—organs on the thorax and legs, mandibular glands, labial glands on the proboscis, abdominal glands, etc.[22]

Bark beetles make use of pheromones to aggregate in trees for breeding, a so-called "mass attack" (from the viewpoint of the tree). Male *Ips paraconfusus* releases an aggregating pheromone along with the feces from its hindgut. The three component pheromone (ipsenol, ipsdienol, and cis-verbenol) have been isolated from the boring dust and faeces (frass) produced by males boring into ponderosa pines.[23]

Virgin female cockroaches and pink bollworm moths secrete a male attractant.[24,25] **Disparlure** is the pheromone sex attractant of the female gypsy moth, *Lymantria dispar*. Mark Jerome Walters extolls the powers of disparlure:

The gypsy moth releases disparlure from a specialized gland on her abdomen, then fans it on its way through the air by flapping her wings. Since the females don't fly, they send out these chemical messages and wait in a tree. . . . The male's elaborate antennae, each covered by some 15,000 pheromone-sensitive hairs, will fire in the presence of a single molecule of the attractant, and can detect a female from great distances—perhaps up to seven miles away. One 250-trillionth of an ounce of the aphrodisiac will cause neurons in its antenna to fire at a rate of 200 pulses a second, sending its brain the message for the individual to fly upwind.[26]

Walters continues describing how the USDA was able to use a form of the sex attractant isolated from female gypsy moths to attract males to traps. The role of sex pheromones in the reproduction of a butterfly is described by Meinwald, Meinwald, and Mazzocchi:

Males of the queen butterfly, *Danaus gilippus berenice*, deprived of the two extrusible brushlike 'hairpencils' at the rear of their abdomen, are capable of courting females but incapable of seducing them. In normal courtship, an aphrodisiac secretion associated with the hairpencils is transferred by way of tiny cuticular 'dust' particles to the antennae of the females. Of the two substances identified from the secretion, one (the ketone) acts as the chemical messenger that induces the females to mate. The only known function of the other compound (the diol) is to serve as a glue that sticks the dust to the female.[27]

There are also daily cycles in the attraction of male butterflies to female pheromone extract.[28]

In another example, the courtship-stimulating volatile compounds of fruit flies (*Drosophila melanogaster*) were examined with gas chromatography and behavioral assays (Table 21.4). Extracts from virgin females stimulate the most courtship (courtship index, 68 units) while that from mature males did not elicit the courtship behavior (courtship index, 2 units). The gas chromatograms of fly extracts from the females differed from the males. Interestingly, the courtship behavior in male flies was also elicited by young males.[29]

Parenthetically, it is interesting to note that sex determination in *Drosophila* is by the ratio of X chromosomes to autosomes (not the presence or absence of the Y chromosome). Signal genes relay information about the X:autosome ratio in each cell to the sex-lethal gene whose transcript is spliced in a gender specific manner. The presence of female-specific sex-lethal gene products initiates a cascade of gene activities that results in the cell's developing and functioning as a female cell; if the female-specific sex-lethal gene products are not synthesized in a cell, it develops and functions as a male cell.[30]

ANT TRAILS

Ant trail laying is an example of the use of recruiting pheromones (Table 21.5). Some years ago, during a student project in a graduate course, the author had a chance to observe the effects of ant trail pheromone (Figure 21.7). The trailblazers were tiny red ants that inhabited the university Biology Building. The ants could find a food source in fifteen minutes; when they departed, they left invisible trails that could be traced by following the scout ant with a pencil line. More ants quickly appeared heading toward the food on the lines marking the trails. In considering pheromones, recall that many species have much more sensitive senses of smell than do humans. Moreover some of them function in the dark. Odors add a dimension of silent and nonvisual communication in species that lack telephones, writing, radios, and television sets.

MALE-TO-MALE INHIBITION IN INSECTS

Sex attractants are not the only way pheromones are used in reproduction. Hirai and coworkers describe a male-to-male inhibitory pheromone:

The behavioral function of a pheromone released by males of the army-worm moth *Pseudaletia unipuncta* was investigated both in laboratory wind-tunnel experiments and in experiments with moth-baited traps in the field . . . . the only obvi-

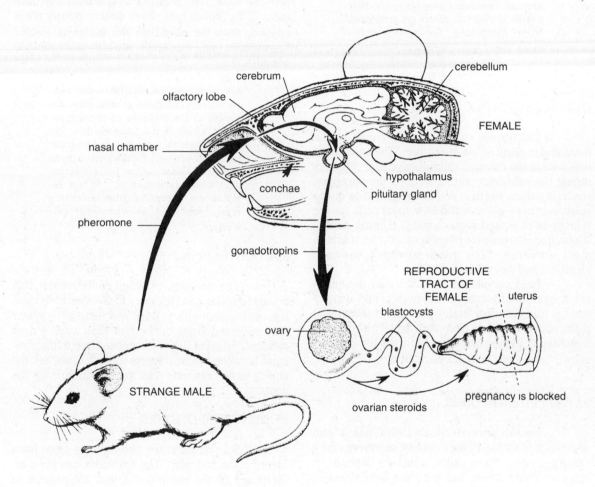

Figure 21.8 Pregnancy can be blocked by exposing a female mouse to a mouse of a different strain, the Bruce effect. The female mouse perceives pheromones of the male mouse with her olfactory epithelium. A chain of neuroendocrine events results in a decrease in gonadotropins. The ovary does not produce the hormones necessary to develop and maintain a uterine environment appropriate for pregnancy. Modified, with permission. Paxton, M.J.W. Endocrinology: Biological and Medical Perspectives. Dubuque, IA: Wm. C. Brown Publishers; 1986.

ous effect of the *P. unipuncta* male pheromone was upon other males, decreasing their tendency to approach sexually receptive pheromone-releasing females and to exhibit copulatory behavior when near those females. The adaptive significance of the male pheromone may be related to the increased reproductive efficiency that results if multiple males are prevented from competing for a single female."[31]

QUEEN SUBSTANCE IN BEES

The **queen substance** is secreted by the mandibular gland of the queen bee. The hormone is involved in the colony's reproductive life. Workers ingest the substance and it inhibits their ovaries, rendering them sterile. Workers exposed to queen substance also fail to build new royal cells for the rearing of new, and rival, queens. During nuptial flight, queen substance plays another role; it acts as a sex attractant. The queen substance has been identified as 9-ketodecanoic acid.

Bees use chemicals other than the queen substance. Bumble bees lick objects and thereby mark a trail for other males that guides their flight paths with a secretion from their labial glands. The mandibular gland secretions are used for defense, alarm, fungistasis, and sex attraction.[32]

ALARM PHEROMONES

Social animals sometimes use alarm pheromones to alert other colony members that a danger exists. Alarm pheromones are common in insects (Table 21.6), but they are also found in other creatures. Earthworms have an alarm pheromone. When earthworms are disturbed (by handling, pinching, severing, electric shock—or presumably when baited on a hook) they secrete extra mucus. The mucus was avoided by other members of the species as was determined by measuring escape speed latency in naive (undisturbed) worms. The hypothetical pheromone was most effective when on dry surfaces, it was insoluble in cold water, and it was still potent after three months.

CRAB-MOLTING PHEROMONE

A pheromone is involved in crab molting and reproduction. Premolt female crabs elicit display and search behavior in male crabs (they walk high, they extend their red chelae, they try to copulate). The water from premolt female crabs will provoke the female behavior in less than five minutes. If the female crabs have their excretory pores capped, then the effect on the males is lost.[33] Crustaceans (e.g., true crabs) are also susceptible to sex attractants:

Males of the species *Portunus sanguinolentus* display a behavioral response to the presence of premolt females which is the same as their behavior when they are exposed to water in which premolt females have been kept. Release of a sex-attractant pheromone is indicated. When females are prevented from releasing urine, there is no evidence of the attractant."[34]

RECOGNITION IN FISH

The question of whether individual fish could recognize specific water from other individual fish was tested with **yellow bullheads**.[35] Water was collected from donor fish that were fed or shocked. Blinded fish were able to learn to discriminate between the two waters in 26.2 trials, but the ability to discriminate was lost by cauterizing the nares.

RODENT PHEROMONES

Several roles for pheromones have been identified in rodents. The emphasis has been on discovery of the pheromones that are present in male urine, particularly those that participate in reproduction.[36]

The **Lee-Boot effect** has to do with the suppression of reproduction in female mice. The effect is postulated to depend on a female pheromone(s). When female mice are housed in groups of four or more, the corpora lutea are maintained, even in the absence of copulation and pregnancy.[37] Sixty-one percent of female mice housed together show evidence of pseudopregnancy (prolonged diestrus) whereas isolated females have an incidence of only 0.2%.

The **Whitten effect** is shortening estrous cycle length by males.[38,39,40] Evidence was presented that the Whitten effect depends on a pheromone in male mouse urine. A male mouse, his cage bedding, or his urine shortens the estrous cycle of female mice. Experiments to demonstrate that the effect was airborne involved placing cages of 48–56 female mice upstream, next to, and downstream from male mice in a wind tunnel with an airflow 6 m/min. The mice were checked for estrus after 48, 72, and 96 hours in the wind tunnel. In the upstream cage, 35% female mice were in estrus. In the cage adjacent to the male, 84% of the females were in estrus. In the downstream cage, 70% of the females were in estrus. The increased incidence of estrus in the female mice in proximity to the males or bathed in male mouse effluent air was taken as evidence that the effect was airborne. The production of the pheromone is dependent on androgens.

The **Vandenbergh effect** has to do with precocious puberty. The effect is thought due to a pheromone in male mouse urine. The urine of a male mouse or the mouse himself can cause early puberty to occur in female mice. The puberty effect is dramatic, being advanced by several weeks. Likewise, mature female mouse perfumes advance puberty in young male mice.

The **Bruce effect** involves pregnancy termination (Figure 21.8).[41] The effect is believed to be caused by a pheromone that is probably secreted into the urine by the preputial glands of male mice. The pregnancies of newly pregnant female mice can be terminated by exposing the female mice to a strange male, his urine, or his cage bedding. Within a week the female goes into estrus. The female response to the urine can be abolished by removing her olfactory bulbs, thereby rendering her anosmic (unable to smell).[42] The Bruce effect may be accomplished by inhibition of prolactin by hypothalamic dopamine.

SEX ATTRACTANTS IN MAMMALS

Dogs make use of pheromones in their reproduction. In the dog, the sex attractant (methyl p-hydroxybenzoate) in the vaginal secretions of estrous females attracts male dogs.[43] Female rodents are believed to use olfaction in courtship and copulatory activities, and the males have scent glands which enlarge in the breeding season.[44]

Walters discusses the possibility of a mammalian sex attractant in pigs. Pigs were discovered to secrete musky smelling androgen, which the pigs also find in truffles. The substance, transferred from the pig's testes to his saliva, causes female pigs to assume a mating stance. The same chemical, also found in human armpits, has prompted speculations about the possibility of human pheromones.[45]

The possibility of a human male sex pheromone with aphrodisiac or attractant effects on human females has been a topic of popular science articles. It is rumored that the androgen-dependent substance smells like sandalwood and is present in high quantities in horses. Kloek found that the various steroids have distinct smells and that one that smells like sandalwood is testosterone.[46] It may be a mistake to attribute women's interest in perfumes to an effort to attract males; rather, the women's interest in perfumes may derive from their own attractions to odors.

Changes in the odors emitted by women over the menstrual cycle have been studied.[47] In particular, the sex-hormones and their metabolites have been candidates for interactions between the sexes.[48] It has been suggested that odors play a role in psychosexual development (e.g. Oedipus complex and establishment of sexual identity).[49]

ALLOMONES AND KAIROMONES

There are words that describe chemical messengers that act between members of different species. Allomones are the chemical messengers whose effects favor the species that secretes the substance. Kairomones favor the recipients. Presumably, essence of skunk is an example of an allomone. A charming description of interspecies chemical communication appears in Farley Mowat's entertaining book, *Never Cry Wolf*. Mowat describes an incident in which he was able to successfully mark and defend his own "territory" by urinating at its perimeter in the manner of canines:

> The territory owned by my wolf family comprised more than a hundred square miles, bounded on one side by a river but otherwise not delimited by geographical features. Nevertheless there *were* boundaries, clearly indi-

cated in wolfish fashion.

Anyone who has observed a dog doing his neighborhood rounds and leaving his personal mark on each convenient post will have already guessed how the wolves marked out *their* property. Once a week more or less, the clan made the rounds of the family lands and freshened up the boundary markers -- a sort of lupine beating of the bounds.

. . . . One evening, after they had gone off for their regular nightly hunt, I staked out a property claim of my own, embracing perhaps three acres, with the tent in the middle, and *including a hundred-yard long section of the wolves' path.*

Staking the land turned out to be rather more difficult than I had anticipated. In order to ensure that my claim would not be overlooked, I felt obliged to make a property mark on stones, clumps of moss, and patches of vegetation at intervals of not more than fifteen feet around the circumference of my claim. This took most of the night and required frequent returns to the tent to consume copious quantities of tea; but before dawn brought the hunters home the task was done, and I retired, somewhat exhausted, to observe results.

I had not long to wait. At 0814 hours . . . the leading male of the clan appeared over the ridge behind me, padding homeward with his usual air of preoccupation. As usual he did not deign to glance at the tent; but when he reached the point where my property line intersected the [wolf] trail, he stopped as abruptly as if he had run into an invisible wall. He was only fifty yards from me and with my binoculars I could see his expression very clearly.

His attitude of fatigue vanished and was replaced by a look of bewilderment. Cautiously he extended his nose and sniffed at one of my marked bushes. . . . Briskly, and with an air of decision, he . . . began a systematic tour of the area I had staked out as my own. As he came to each boundary marker he sniffed it once or twice, then carefully placed *his* mark on the outside of each clump

of grass or stone."[50]

REFERENCES

1. Riddiford, L.M.; Williams, C.M. Volatile principle from oak leaves: Role in sex life of the polyphemus moth. Science 155: 589–590; 1967.
2. Bandurski, R.S., Nonhebel, H.M. Chapter 1: Auxins. In Wilkins, M.B. Advanced Plant Physiology. Marshfield, MA: Pitman; 1984; pp. 1–20.
3. Dennison, D.S. Chapter 7: Phototropism. In Wilkins, M.B. Advanced Plant Physiology. Marshfield, MA: Pitman; 1984; p. 149.
4. Bandurski, R.S.; Nonhebel, H.M.; Op. cit.; p. 16.
5. Jones, R.L.; MacMillan, J. Chapter 2: Gibberellins. In Wilkins, M.B. Advanced Plant Physiology. Marshfield, MA: Pitman; 1984, pp. 21–52.
6. Horgan, R. Chapter 3: Cytokinins, in Wilkins, M.B. Advanced Plant Physiology. Pitman, Marshfield, MA: Pitman; 1984; pp. 53–75.
7. Milborrow, B.V. Chapter 4: Inhibitors. In Wilkins, M.B. Advanced Plant Physiology, Marshfield, MA: Pitman; 1984; pp. 76–110.
8. Beyer, E.M.; Morgan, P.W.; Yang, S.F. Chapter 5: Ethylene. In Wilkins, M:B. Advanced Plant Physiology. Marshfield, MA: Pitman; 1984; pp. 111–126.
9. Turner, C.D.; Bagnara, J.T. General Endocrinology, Sixth Edition. Philadelphia, PA: W.B. Saunders; 1976; p. 545.
10. Regnier, F.E.; Law, J.H. Insect pheromones. Journal of Lipid Research 9: 541–551; 1968.
11. Stadler, E.S. Contact chemoreception. In Bell, W.J.; Carde, R.T., editors. Chemical Ecology of Insects. Sunderland, MA: Sinauer Associates, Inc., Publishers. 1984; p.3.
12 . House, P.E. Sociochemicals of termites. In Bell, W.J.; Carde, R.T., editors. Chemical Ecology of Insects. Sunderland, MA: Sinauer Associates, Inc., Publishers. 1984; pp. 474–519.
13. Huheey, J.E. Warning, coloration, and mimicry. In Bell, W.J.; Carde, R.T., editors. Chemical Ecology of Insects. Sunderland, MA: Sinauer Associates, Inc., Publishers. 1984; pp. 257–297.
14. Meinwald, Y.C.; Meinwald, J.; Eisner, T.

1,2-dialkyl-4(3H)-quinazolinones in the defensive secretion of a millipede (*Glomeris marginata*). Science 154: 390–391; 1966.

15. Shorey, H.H. Animal Communication by Pheromones. New York: Academic Press; 1976; pp. 1–168.

16. Prestwich, G.D. Chemistry of pheromone and hormone metabolism in insects. Science 237: 999–1006; 1987.

17. Wilson, E.O. Chemical communication in the social insects. Science 149, 1064–1071, 1965

18. Regnier, F.E.; Law, J.H. Insect pheromones, Journal of Lipid Research 9: 541–551; 1968; p. 541.

19. Antony, C.; Jallon, J. The chemical basis for sex recognition in Drosophila melanogaster. J. Insect Physiol. 28: 873–880; 1982.

20. Shaner, A.M.; Dixon, P.D.; Graham, K.J.; Jackson, L.L. Components of the courtship-stimulating pheromone blend of young male Drosophila melanogaster: (Z)-13-tritriacontene and (Z)-11-tritriacontene. J. Insect Physiol. 35: 341–345; 1989.

21. Tompkins, L.; Hall, J.C. Drosophila males produce a pheromone which inhibits courtship. Z. Naturforsch. 36C: 694–696; 1981.

22. Carde, R.T.; Baker, T.C. Sexual communication with pheromones. In Bell, W.J.; Carde, R.T., editors. Chemical Ecology of Insects. Sunderland, MA: Sinauer Associates, Inc., Publishers. 1984; pp. 355-383.

23. Birch, M.C. Aggregation in bark beetles. In Bell, W.J.; Carde, R.T., editors. Chemical Ecology of Insects. Sunderland, MA: Sinauer Associates, Inc., Publishers.; 1984; pp. 331–353

24. Barth, R.H. Insect mating behavior: Endocrine control of a chemical communication system. Science 149: 882–883; 1965.

25. Jones, W.A.; Jacobson, M.; Martin, D.F. Sex attractant of the pink bollworm moth: Isolation, identification, and synthesis. Science 152: 1516–1517; 1966.

26. Walters, M.J. The Dance of Life. New York: Argor House, William Morrow; 1988; pp. 90-91.

27. Meinwald, J.; Meinwald, Y.C.; Mazzocchi, P.H. Sex pheromone of the queen butterfly: Biology. Science 164: 1170–1175; 1969.

28. Comeau, A.; Carde, R.T.; Roelofs, W.L. Relationship of ambient temperatures to diel periodicities of sex attraction in six species of Lepidoptera. Can. Ent. 108: 415–418; 1976.

29. Tompkins, L.; Hall, J.C.; Hall, L.M. Courtship-stimulating volatile compounds from normal and mutant Drosophila. J. Insect Physiol. 26: 689–697; 1980.

30. Hodgkin, J. Drosophila sex determination: A cascade of regulated splicing. Cell 56: 905–906; 1989.

31. Hirai, K.; Shorey, H.H.; Gaston, L.K. Competition among courting male moths: Male-to-male inhibitory pheromone. Science 202: 644–645; 1978.

32. Duffield, R.M.; Wheeler, J.W.; Elckwort, G.C. Sociochemicals of bees. In Bell, W.J.; Carde, R.T., editors. Chemical Ecology of Insects. Sunderland, MA: Sinauer Associates, Inc., Publishers. 1984; pp. 387–428.

33. Ryan, E.P. Pheromone: Evidence in a decapod crustacean. Science 151: 340–341; 1966.

34. Ryan, E.P.; Ibid.

35. Todd, J.H.; Alema, J.; Bardach, J.E. Discrimination of donor fish by smell not eyes or mucous. Science 158: 672–673; 1967.

36. Doty, R.L. A cry for the liberation of the female rodent: Courtship and copulation in Rodentia. Psychological Bulletin 81: 159–172; 1974.

37. Stoddart, D.M. Mammalian Odors and Pheromones. London: Edward Arnold Publishers Ltd.; 1976.

38. Bronson, F.H.; Marsden, H.M. Male-induced synchrony of estrus in deermice. Gen. Comp. Endocrinol. 4: 634–637; 1964.

39. Bronson, F.; Whitten, W.K. Oestrus-accelerating pheromone in mice: Assay, androgen-dependency, and presence in bladder urine. J. Reprod. Fert. 15: 131; 1968.

40. Bronson, F. H.; Eleftheriou, B.E.; Dezell, H.E. Strange male pregnancy block in deermice: Prolactin and adrenocortical hormones. Biol. Reprod. 1: 302; 1969.

41. Bruce, H.M. Pheromones. Brit. Med. Bull. 26: 10; 1970.

42. Parkes, A.S.; Bruce, H.M. Olfactory stimuli in mammalian reproduction. Science 134; 1049–1054; 1961.

43. Goodwin, M.; Gooding, K.M.; Regnier, F. Sex pheromone in the dog. Science 203: 559–561; 1979.

44. Doty, R.L. A cry for the liberation of the female rodent: Courtship and copulation in Rodentia. Psychological Bulletin 81: 159–172; 1974.

45. Walters, M.J. The Dance of Life. NewYork: Argor House, William Morrow; 1988; pp. 90–91.

46. Kloek, J. The smell of some steroid sex-hormones and their metabolites. Reflections and experiments concerning the significance of smell for the mutual relation of the sexes. Psychiat. Neurol. Neurochir. 64: 309–344; 1961; p. 322.

47. Doty, R.L.; Ford, M.; Preti, G. Changes in the intensity and pleasantness of human vaginal odors during the menstrual cycle. Science 190: 1316–1317; 1975.

48. Kloek, J.; Op.cit.

49. Kalogerakis, M.G. The role of olfaction in sexual development, Psychosomatic Medicine XXX: 420–432; 1963.

50. Mowat, F. Never Cry Wolf. Bantam Books: New York; 1983; pp. 54–57.

CHAPTER 22

EPILOGUE

This chapter collects an assortment of endocrine ideas. It begins with some unifying concepts (rheostasis, APUD cells, development, time courses, neuroendocrine transducers). It discusses some hormones that have behavior aspects to their function (endorphins, cholecystokinin, steroids, homosexuality). Areas of promise for the future in hormones are touched upon (weight control, fertility regulation, light therapy, molecular biology).

BIOLOGICAL VARIATION

One concept that can get lost in discussions of the general properties of a system, such as an endocrine system, is the concept of biological variation. The menstrual cycle is not 28 days long, 28 days is just the mode of the human menstrual cycle. Even human body temperature, a very common measurement, is rarely reported other than by a single number, 98.6°F. But body temperature has wide individual variations (Figure 22.1).[1] So also, all the hormones fluctuate because of many variables: species, individual variation, age, time of day, day of the reproductive cycle, time of year, feast or famine, wet or dry, hot or cold, etc.

HOMEOSTASIS AND RHEOSTASIS

There are some unifying concepts in endocrinology. Homeostasis, Claude Bernard's concept of a constant internal environment, was defined in 1926 by Walter B. Cannon. It is still a useful concept. Jane C. Kaltenbach describes homeostasis as the "maintenance of a relatively stable environment with in the body [which] enables cells to function under optimal conditions, thereby enabling organisms to be independent of the sometimes widely fluctuating factors outside the body."[2] The idea of homeostasis is that an organism needed to keep its physiology processes within narrow ranges in a relatively constant balance, or "steady state." In homeostasis, physiological processes are automatically coordinated to maintain steady state. After an environmental challenge that disturbs the steady state, the organism returns to its steady state. Hormones, with their stimulations and inhibitions, are ideally suited for maintenance of a steady state and restoration of an organism after a perturbation.

The finding that an organism's physiology varies with time of day and season of the year modifies our concept of homeostasis. The steady state that is maintained in the morning is different than that maintained at night; the steady state in summer is different than that in winter. Recently, Myrsovsky reexamined the concept of homeostasis. He points out its limitations, that sometimes physiological mechanisms promote change in the internal environment. In other words, there are changes in regulated levels. He offers an alternative term, rheostasis, which he proposes to "describe regulation around shifting set-points."[3] The adjustable

phenomena have sometimes been attributed to physiological equivalents of thermostats. So, according to Myrsovsky, physiologically, in organisms, there are thermostats that respond to temperature changes, there are baroreceptors to respond to pressure changes, there are osmostats to respond to changing salt concentrations, and there other mechanisms that act like they have set points (chemostats, alphastats, gonadostats, mechanostats, and lipostats).

EVERYTHING AFFECTS EVERYTHING

Endocrinologists attempting to make models for hormone interactions often find that "everything affects everything." An endocrine system can be extraordinarily complex when all the hormones and their impinging controlling factors are taken into account (Figures 22.2 and 22.3). The models with multiple interactions are often very useful because they show relationships and they provide a shorthand list of the various factors that impinge on a system. It is possible to make useful predictions of physiological consequences from these models (many of which have appeared in the chapters of this book), but the only way to determine what will actually transpire is to measure the various parameters in an experiment.

APUD CELLS

Another unifying concept ties together many of the endocrine glands and parts of the nervous system by proposing a common ancestry, embryological origin from neural crest cells.

"On account of our findings it now becomes necessary to postulate that some 300 million years ago, in our earliest vertebrate ancestors, a distinct system of nerve cells arose from the neural crest. Their power of locomotion spread them effectively throughout the organism, where they came to rest particularly, but not exclusively, in entodermal tissues of the foregut. The cells came to respond to stimuli not by relay to a more central cell in the nervous system but by local discharge of one or more of their products. In a few of the cells belonging to the APUD cell system the secretion product can be considered to have remained fixed as

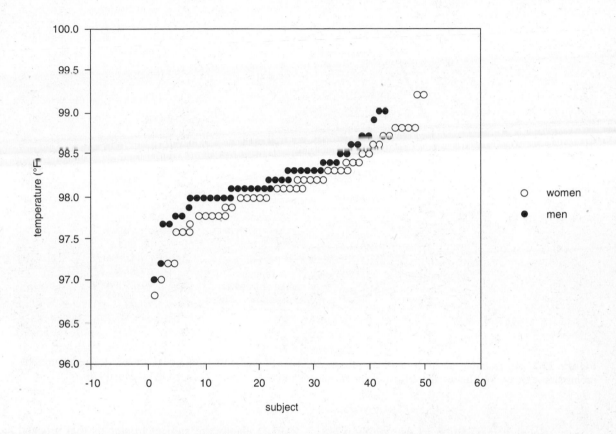

Figure 22.1 Body temperatures in a class of 50 female and 43 male endocrinology students attending college at Temple University in 1992 averaged 98.149°F. Temperatures were measured during class with mercury fever thermometers at 10:52 a.m. and ranged from 96.8–99.2°F. There was no difference between genders. Data collected by S. Binkley and R. Opiekun.

the ancestral biogenic amine but in the majority, presumably through environmental influences, modifications of their amine-storing proteins have given rise to polypeptides which, in the case of 9 of the members of the APUD series, are now recognized as hormones. The APUD cell system thus constitutes a peripheral neuroendocrine system, analogous to the central neuroendocrine systems of the hypothalamus.[4]

This is the Pearse APUD (Amine Precursor Uptake and Decarboxylation) hypothesis of a diffuse neuroendocrine system. It probably has to be modified because some of the cells develop from endoderm. The APUD cells (Table 22.1) have common properties which include the following:

First, the cells possess the biochemical ability to take up amine precursors (e.g., 5-hydroxytryptophan) and to decarboxylate these precursors. The cells then secrete peptide and amine products (epinephrine, norepinephrine, dopamine, serotonin) as hormones and neurotransmitters. The gut and nerve cells are so similar that the gut cells have been called the "diffuse endocrine system."

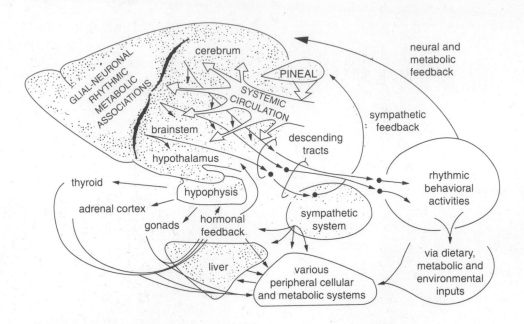

Figure 22.2 An example of an "everything affects everything" model of hormone function. Reproduced, with permission. Quay, W. Endocrine effects of the mammalian pineal. Amer. Zool. 10: 237–246; 1970.

Second, in addition to the common biochemistry, and probably explaining that common ability, was the suggestion that the APUD cells all originated from neural crest cells or neuroectocytes during development (Figure 22.4).

Third, the concept explains disorders where multiple endocrine glands are involved (MENs). The MENs usually involve the adrenal, pancreas, thyroid, pituitary, and parathyroid. The explanation is that the cause is somehow related to the glands' common APUD properties.

Fourth, the cells have common staining properties (enterochromaffin, argentaffin, argyrophil clear cells, and fluorogenic amine content).

The main organs suggested for pacemaking vertebrate daily rhythms are the eyes, the suprachiasmatic nuclei of the hypothalamus, the pineal gland, and the eyes. These organs also are at the top of the endocrine hierarchies. The latter two of these organs, pineal and hypothalamus, are already identified as APUD and most of the other

APUD glands are subject to signals that proceed through hierarchies under these organs. Virtually all of the hormones of the APUD tissues have daily rhythms. Physiology involving oscillations and cycles may be another feature shared by APUD cells.

There is some controversy over what cells actually come from neural crest:

Studies using quail and chick embryos have disputed the claim that the APUD cells of the gastrointestinal tract and pancreas originate from neural ectoderm. However, the endocrine cells of the gastrointestinal tract and pancreas contain an enzyme specific to neural cells (neuronal-specific enolase, NSE), which supports the postulate of a common neural origin. Regardless or their origin, it is clear that the endocrine cells of the gut are remarkably similar to other cells of

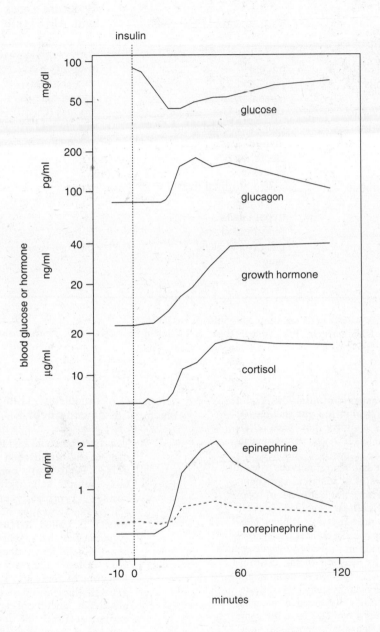

Figure 22.3 The graphs show that injected insulin alters glucose and certain hormones that regulate glucose. The data were obtained from six men given intravenous injections of insulin (0.15 U/kg). Redrawn, with permission. Gerber, A.J.; Cryer, P.E. et al. The role of adrenergic mechanisms in the substrate and hormonal response to insulin-induced hypoglycemia in man. J. Clin. Invest. 58: 7; 1976.

Table 22.1 APUD and the Endocrine System

APUD cell types	Tissues with APUD cells	Endocrine glands with APUD cells
MSH-secreting cells	pituitary	pituitary axis
ACTH-secreting cells	pituitary	pineal gland
chromaffin cells	adrenal medulla	hypothalamus
melanophores	skin	thyroid (C cell)
ultimobranchial cells	ultimobranchial gland	parathyroid
C-cells	thyroid gland	placenta
carotid body cells	carotid body	
islet cells	pancreas	
gastrointestinal hormone secreting cells	gastrointestinal tract	
	hypothalamus	
	pineal gland	
	parathyroid gland	
	lung	
	placenta	

Endocrine glands with APUD cells are from Mulvihill, S.J.; Deveney, C.W.; Way, L.W.; Tebas, H.T. Regulatory peptides of the gut. In Greenspan, F.S., editor. Basic and Clinical Endocrinology, Third Edition. Norwalk, CT: Appleton & Lange; 1991; p. 573.

the hypothalamic-pituitary axis and to neurons within the gut wall....even though its validity has been challenged, the [APUD] concept is appealing because it posits a common origin for gut and central nervous system cells with almost identical cytochemical characteristics (storage of peptides) and cellular functions (release of peptide messengers). It helps clarify why identical peptides are synthesized, stored, and released by gut epithelial cells, neurons of the gastrointestinal tract, and nerve cells in the central nervous system. Peptide-releasing neurons and peptide-releasing epithelial cells actually have the same function–release of a chemical messenger.[5]

HORMONES IN DEVELOPMENT

The same hormones that have been the characters in this book are key players in the development of organisms. Gilbert summarizes the functions of **development**:

> The first function involves the production and organization of all the diverse types of cells in the body...muscle cells, skin cells, neurons, lymphocytes, blood cells....The generation of cellular diversity is called **differentiation**; the processes that organize the differentiated cells into tissues and organs are called **morphogenesis** (creation of form and structure) and **growth** (increase in size). The second major function of development is **reproduction**: the continued generation of new individuals of the species.[6]

The roles that hormones play in reproduction have already been discussed in this book in the chapters that deal with testosterone, estrogens, and

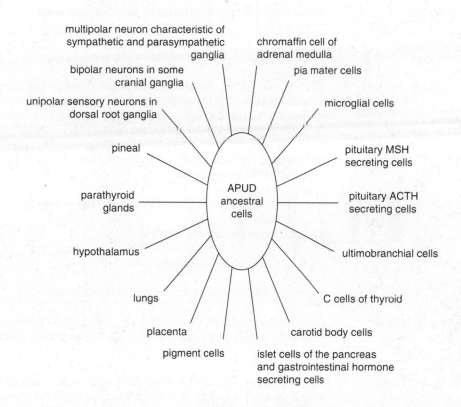

Figure 22.4 The figure is intended to illustrate the plethora of cells and tissues suggested to have a neural crest (neuroectoderm or neuroendocrine ectoblast) origin. The model should be modified because some of the cells develop from endoderm. Most of the cells come to rest in the brain or in the endocrine glands. The APUD hypothesis is a unifying concept in which the cells have common biochemical abilities to take up amines and to decarboxylate them. The APUD endocrine cells all produce peptide and amine hormones.

progesterone. Hormone influence on growth was discussed in the chapter that covered growth hormone. Metamorphosis provides more examples. Triiodothyronine causes metamorphosis of amphibians. Prolactin, on the other hand, inhibits metamorphosis. Dopamine, which increases at the time of metamorphosis, inhibits prolactin, and thereby acts to promote the onset of metamorphosis. Metamorphosis in insects likewise involves hormones. A prothoracic hormone from brain neurosecretory cells stimulates the prothoracic gland to produce the steroid hormone ecdysone, which, when

secreted in pairs of pulses, promotes molting. Juvenile hormone from the corpora allata blocks metamorphosis. Another area where examples can be found is in reproduction. The production of testosterone during fetal life is necessary for the development of male reproductive organs. But there are other roles for chemical messengers in development.

In development of higher organisms, there is a sequence of anatomical events. The main body of work of embryologists comprises the description of these events in various species. Central ques-

Table 22.2 Chemical Messengers in Development

Chemical messenger	Process(es) that may be affected by chemical messenger
fibroblast growth factor (FGF)	induction of mesoderm by vegetal cells; binds to heparin
transforming growth factors (TGf-ß-factors)	TGF-ß2 may induce dorsal mesoderm (notochord and axial muscles); stimulates growth of fibroblast cells and embryonic endothelial cells; TGF-ß inhibits division of kidney cells in culture, lung carcinoma, mammary carcinoma, and melanoma cells
mesenchymal factor	induction of the differentiation of pancreatic epithelial cells by a glycoprotein from mesenchyme
retinoids (compounds related to vitamin A)	possible morphogens involved in limb bud development
cyclic AMP	aggregation of slime mold amoebae
thyroid hormones	promotes amphibian metamorphosis
dopamine	inhibition of prolactin in amphibian metamorphosis
growth hormone and somatomedins	coordinated regulation of mammalian growth, IGF-I permits cells to pass from the G_1 (gap) phase to the S (DNA synthesis) phase of the cell cycle
nerve growth factor (NGF)	130,000 dalton glycoprotein which may prevent neuronal death and which act as chemotactic agent to help axons reach their targets
platelet derived growth factor (PDGF)	stimulates division of smooth muscle cells, fibroblasts, and glial cells; cells pass from G_0 (quiescent) phase to G_1 (gap) phase of the cell cycle

tions of embryology surround the mechanisms by which the anatomical changes take place.[7] **Induction** is the word used by embryologists for "the process by which one embryonic region interacts with a second region to cause the latter tissue to differentiate in a direction it otherwise would not [differentiate]."[8] Chemical messengers between cells obviously have potential for participating in the means by which induction occurs. There are three possibilities for induction: (i) diffusion of inducers between cells, (ii) induction of change in one cell by the matrix of another cell, and (iii) contacts between the inducing cell and the responding cell.

The "inducers" are variously referred to by embryologists as "substances" or "factors." Some of these inducers, many of which are believed to be similar to mammalian growth factors, are listed in Table 22.2. The possibility of diffusible inducers has been proved with experiments involving transfer of induction medium "conditioned" by pretreating it with development embryonic cells. Diffusible inducers were also investigated with experiments where inducing and responding tissue were placed on two sides of membranes with pores so small they prevented cells from touching but

Table 22.2 Chemical Messengers in Development (continued)

Chemical messenger	Process(es) that may be affected by chemical messenger
epidermal growth factor (EGF)	stimulates cell division and development in epidermis, mammary epithelium, esophagus, mouth, cornea, accelerates mouse eyelid opening and tooth eruption, cells progress from G_1 (gap) to S (DNA synthesis) phase
G_1 epidermal growth inhibitor	blocks cells from beginning S (DNA synthesis) phase
G_1 epidermal growth inhibitor	stops cell division after DNA replication
ß-interferon (ß-IFN)	cell growth inhibitor; blocks cell cycle between G_0 (quiescent) and G_1 (gap) phases and blocks cell cycle between G_1 (gap) and S (DNA synthesis)
testosterone	causes development of epididymus, vas deferens, and seminal vesicles from Wolffian duct; causes development of scrotum and penis from urogenital swellings and sinus
anti-müllerian duct factor(AMDF)	müllerian duct atrophy
maturation-promoting factor (MPF)	progesterone-induced factor in cytoplasm permitting oocyte nuclei to resume divisions
cytostatic factor (CSF)	protein that stops oocyte in second meiotic metaphase
calcium ions	from endoplasmic reticulum; destroy CFS permitting meiosis to proceed and the fusion of pronuclei to occur; with CSF and MPF, regulates biphasic cell cycle of early blastomeres

The cast of characters in development is similar to that in endocrinology. Some as yet unidentified chemical messengers in development may yet turn out to be hormones. Gilbert, S.F. Developmental Biology, Second Edition. Sunderland, MA: Sinauer Associates, Inc.; 1988; 843 pages.

with pores large enough for molecules to pass through (i.e., pore size 0.5μm).

The concept of diffusible chemical messengers appeared again in the hypothesis of morphogens. A **morphogen** is hypothesized as a morphogenetic substance that is produced at a "source," moves by diffusion, and ends at a "sink." Morphogens are used to explain pattern formation. Pattern formation is the process(es) whereby location of a cell can determine whether it becomes muscle or cartilage and determine the direction of growth of nerve axons.

Another concept in embryology is the idea that factors may be distributed unevenly, as in gradients. The original gradient idea was proposed to explain polarization within oocytes. Experimental observations based on development of sea urchin embryos required the hypothesis of **double or dual gradients** that are at different angles, or even opposed to, each other to explain development in three dimensions. The ideas of gradients have also been applied to cellular migration,

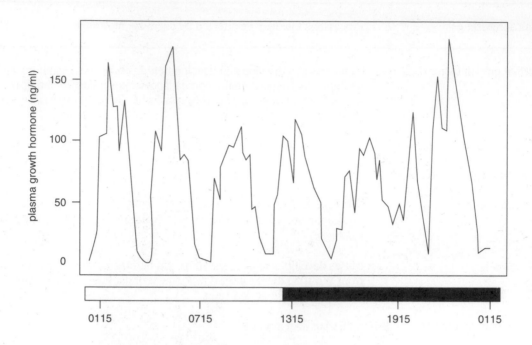

Figure 22.5 The graph shows the ultradian cycles (peaks more than once a day) in rat plasma growth hormone. The rats were kept in a light-dark cycle (LD12:12; time is indicated by the bar below the record). Redrawn after data of Tannenbaum, G.S.; Martin, J.B. Evidence for an endogenous ultradian rhythm governing growth hormone secretion in the rat. Endocrinology 98; 1976; p. 565.

morphogens, marking on butterfly wings, polarity in hydra, neuronal migration, chick retina cells, and zebra stripes.

Chemotaxis is another area where chemical messengers have been suggested to play a part in development. For example, nerve axons must traverse long distances to connect nerve cell bodies with the cells on which the axons terminate. The idea that the target might secrete soluble molecules has been proposed as a **chemotactic hypothesis**. The soluble molecules from the target would form a gradient that could be followed by the growing axon. Nerve growth factor has been considered one possible chemotactic molecule. Serotonin, another chemotactic factor, can inhibit the growth of some axons while sparing the growth of others.

The way that many of the developmental chemical messengers affect growth is believed to be by modifying the cell cycle. The cell cycle has stages, or phases, which are in a sequence: mitosis (M), prereplication gap (G_1), DNA synthesis (S), premitotic gap (G_2), mitosis (M), etc. A cell cycle clock, or cytochron, was proposed by Edmunds,[9] who correlated cell cycles and circadian rhythms. The mitosis rhythm is often 24 hours long, with the beginning of the cycle (G_1) starting at lights-on and cell division (M phase) commencing at lights-off. Ehret and Trucco[10] developed a molecular model, the chronon model, which explains the timing of circadian rhythms based on the sequence of transcription and translational events of molecular biology. If the developmental messengers act on the cell cycle, and the cell cycle is controlled by a daily clock, then the developmental messengers share the pervasive nature of daily rhythmicity

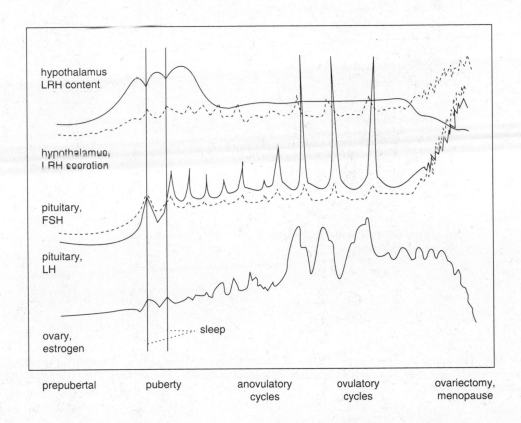

hypothalamus
LRH content

hypothalamus,
LRH secretion

pituitary,
FSH

pituitary,
LH

sleep

ovary,
estrogen

prepubertal   puberty   anovulatory   ovulatory   ovariectomy,
                                    cycles   cycles   menopause

Figure 22.6 A simplified diagrammatic representation of the cycles in female reproductive hormones: life cycle (menarche to menopause), daily sleep cycle, and menstrual cycle. The time scale (horizontal axis) and
hormone scales are not linear and have been modified to attempt to accomodate all the cycles. The hormones have
similar responses to ovariectomy or menopause. Redrawn, with permission. Rebar, R.W.; Yen, S.S.C.
Endocrine rhythms in gonadotropins and ovarian steroids with reference to reproductive processes. Krieger, D.,
editor. Endocrine Rhythms. New York: Raven Press; 1979; p. 260.

that is apparent in the daily changes in hormone
concentrations. The mechanism for these daily
signals is thus likely to be important to understanding development as well as endocrine systems.

    Strictly considered, chemical messengers
during development may lack the blood borne quali-
fication of classical hormones. However, the
chemical inducers certainly fit the idea of chemical
messengers and are considered by some as true
hormones.

TIME COURSES AND RHYTHMS

    Temporal organization, the occurrence of
events at certain times and in timed sequences is a
unifying feature common to the endocrine system.
As shown throughout this book, this organization
is apparent in the daily oscillations (e.g., in pineal
enzymes and melatonin production) and seasonal
rhythms (e.g., in reproduction) of hormones and
functions controlled by the endocrine glands. The
timing can be astonishingly precise. Knowledge of

try-gly-gly-phe-met   methionine enkephalin

tyr-gly-gly-phe-leu   leucine enkephalin

tyr-gly-gly-phe-met-thr-ser-glu-lys-ser-   β-endorphin
glu-thr-pro-leu-val-thr-leu-phe-lys-asn-
ala-ile-val-lys-asn-aln-his-lys-lys-gly-
gln

tyr-gly-gly-phe-leu-arg-ile-arg-pro-lys-   dynorphin
leu-lys-trp-asp-asn-gln

Figure 22.7 The amino acid sequences of some of the opioid peptides are shown. ß-endorphin is named for the "morphine within" and may be an internally produced natural analgesic. The peptides share the same four amino acids (tyr-gly-gly-phe).

the 24-hour production is now essential for many kinds of endocrine diagnoses, but especially for those hormones that are secreted at night or in cyclic fashion (Figure 22.5). The interactions of episodic release, daily cycles, and life cycles produce a complex pattern of normal hormone values (Figure 22.6).

Some of the fascinating puzzles remaining for endocrinologists to solve are the exact means by which major events of reproduction—puberty, ovulation, climacteric, parturition—are timed.

NEUROENDOCRINE TRANSDUCERS

The interactions of the nervous and endocrine systems provide more unifying ideas. As mentioned in the preface, the timing of events can be subdivided into very quick, short duration responses (less than a second) and slower, longer duration responses (hours and more). Nerve cells and the nervous system usually bear the responsibility for the quick events; typically the endocrine system is appropriate for the slower responses. But the two systems are not totally distinct; they function in concert so that environmental events can be translated into endocrine changes. The phrase "neuroendocrine transducer" was used to describe the interactions of photoreceptors and three endocrine glands by Wurtman, Axelrod, and Kelly:

The primary and perhaps only photoreceptor in the adult mammal is the retina. Light, impinging on its rod and cone cells, generates nervous impulses. This information, along with impulses produced by other exogenous and endogenous stimuli, is carried by specific tracts in the brain to the neuroendocrine transducers, which respond by secreting appropriate amounts of their characteristic hor-

Table 22.3 Hormones and Fat

A. Hormones and lipolysis

RAPID STIMULATION	SLOW STIMULATION	SUPPRESSION
catecholamines	growth hormone	insulin
β_1 agonists	glucocorticoids	PGE1
glucagon		GIP
secretin		
α-MSH		
β-MSH		
VIP		

B. Causes of obesity

EXCESS LIPID DEPOSITION	REDUCED LIPID METABOLISM	LESSENED LIPID UTILIZATION
food intake increase	lipolytic hormone decrease	aging
lesions of the hypothalamus	adipose cell lipolysis defect	lipid oxidation defect
adipose cell hyperplasia	abnormal autonomic innervation	thermogenesis defect
hyperlipogenesis		inactivity
lipoprotein lipase activity increase		

Bierman, E.L.; Glomset, J.A. Disorders of lipid metabolism, pages 876–906, and Bierman, E.L., Hirsch, J. Obesity, pages 907–921. In Williams, R. H., editor. Textbook of Endocrinology, Sixth Edition. Philadelphia, PA: W. B. Saunders; 1981.

mones into the blood. [1] One neuroendocrine transducer, the hypothalamic median eminence, secretes its hormones into a portal circulation; they are then delivered selectively to the anterior pituitary gland where they influence the release of its tropic hormones (e.g., ACTH and the gonadotropins) into the general circulation. [2] The adrenal medulla responds to stimulation of its sympathetic nerves by releasing adrenaline directly into the venous blood. [3] The [mammalian] pineal gland's . . . activity is controlled by nervous signals generated by environmental lighting and transmitted to the pineal by its sympathetic nerves. In response to absence of a light input, the mammalian pineal synthesizes its characteristic hormone, melatonin, and releases this compound into the bloodstream."[11]

THE OPIATE WITHIN

Upon first encountering the body of endocrine knowledge, the student is sometimes surprised to find that the physical appearance of an individual is dependent on, and can even be changed by, hormones. Equally disturbing is the information that comes from research in the area of hormones and behavior. The disturbing aspect of this research is that it implies that some of our behavior is a function of our hormonal milieu and casts the concept of "free will" in new light.

Endorphins are peptide hormones named for actions that are similar to opiate drugs (e.g., morphine). The name, "endorphin," was coined from "the morphine within." It is believed that the brain naturally contained **opiate receptors** to which the opioid peptides bind. Opiate receptors of five subtypes (designated with Greek letters) that bind 18 peptides have been identified in the brain.

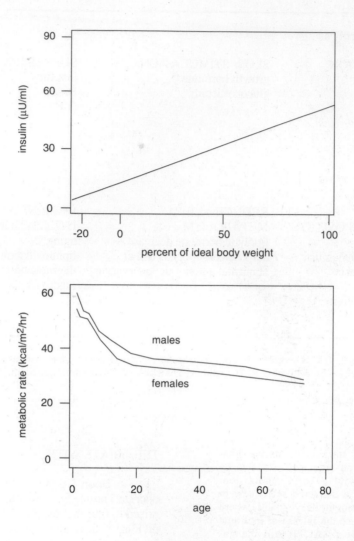

Figure 22.8 The graphs show relationships of insulin and body weight, and of metabolic rate and age. Redrawn, with permission. Bagdale, J.D.; Bierman, E.L.; Porte, D. The significance of basal insulin levels in evaluation of the insulin response to glucose in diabetic and nondiabetic subjects. J. Clin. Invest. 46: 1549; 1967; p. 1551; Spector, W.S., editor. Handbook of Biological Data. National Academy of Sciences, National Research Council. Philadelphia, PA: W. B. Saunders; 1961.

There are drugs that are opiate antagonists (e.g., **naloxone**) that also bind to the receptors. Hadley explains why the endorphins are considered the "morphine within":

Because it is reasonable to conclude that such highly specific [opiate] receptors have not evolved to interact with exogenous opiate alkaloids, it was suggested that endogenous opiatelike substance might exist as natural ligands for the identified opiate receptors.[12]

Included in the endorphins are a group of molecules whose synthesis, like that of the melanotropins, derives from pro-opiomelanocortin (for synthesis of the opioid peptide: ß-endorphin and met-enkephalin). The peptides are metabolized by enzymes (enkephalinase A, enkephalinase B, aminopeptidase). The opiate peptides (Figure 22.7) are distributed in brain (substantia nigra) and gastrointestinal nerve endings. The endorphins and the related enkephalin molecules are referred to collectively as the **opiate peptides**.

What are some examples of the actions of endorphins? Opiate peptides have short-term (five minutes) **analgesia**, or pain killing, effects when they are injected into the brainstem. In contrast, the analgesia produced by morphine lasts four hours. A typical test for analgesia uses the mouse hot plate test. A mouse is placed on a hot plate (52°C or 126°F). The investigator measures the time from placing the mouse on the plate to the time the mouse first licks a hind paw or the time before the mouse makes an escape jump. The times, or latencies, are a test for analgesia. Normal mice exhibit 80–100 second latencies, mice injected with naloxone reduce latencies to 60 seconds, and mice given morphine increase latencies to 160 seconds (indicating analgesia). There is probably also a daily rhythm in the opiate receptors because there is a rhythm in analgesia with the maximum latency in the afternoon at 1500 and the minimum latency at 0800. It has also been noticed that the endorphin concentrations rise during stress and that the pain threshold changes accordingly. It has even been suggested that the endorphins play a role in acupuncture:

> . . . the firing rate of cells in the spinal cord is greatly increased in response to painful stimuli. Acupuncture suppressed this increased electrical activity, but this effect of acupuncture was completely blocked by the specific opiate antagonist, naloxone . . . . It has also been shown that acupuncture analgesia in mice is blocked by naloxone and abolished by hypophysectomy.[13]

The opiate peptides cause euphoria and, like abused opiates, can produce dependency, toler-

ance, and addiction. ß-endorphin can produce a state similar to catatonic schizophrenia: muscular rigidity, loss of righting reaction, lack of spontaneous movement, failure to blink the eyelids, 2°C body temperature drop, and brain EEGs like epileptic seizures. The state produced by endorphins is reversible by naloxone. Morphine and the enkephalins act on the central nervous system and cause euphoria, sedation, analgesia, vomiting, muscular rigidity, and respiratory depression. Discovery of the opiate peptides heralded a new age in the field of mental health since they offered the possibility of a chemical basis for mental health disorders. Schizophrenics had higher spinal fluid endorphins and the symptoms of schizophrenia could be treated with naloxone.

The opiate peptides have endocrine effects. They decrease intestinal motility. The effects of enkephalins, which are gastrointestinal peptides, on the gut are constipation, initial contractions of gastrointestinal parts (stomach, duodenum, jejunum), later distension and lack of motion in gastrointestinal parts (stomach, duodenum, jejunum), colon contraction without peristalsis, and anal sphincter contraction. ß-Endorphin releases pituitary hormones (prolactin, growth hormone, arginine vasopressin, MSH, LH, and FSH). For example, 200 μg/kg injected into a rat causes an increase in plasma arginine vasopressin in 25 minutes.

The endorphins play roles in neurotransmission. It has been suggested that the peptides may act as neurotransmitters and ß-endorphin blocks acetylcholine release. When considering the opiate peptides and their effect on behavior, it is appropriate to mention the effects of MSH and ACTH and related molecules on behavior. These effects include alteration of learning behavior, and as Hadley notes: "There is evidence that MSH- and ACTH-like peptides may function in a role opposite that of opioid peptides in controlling pain sensitivity."[14] They are even supposed to cause stretching and yawning in mice.[15]

THIN AND FAT

A major area of medical concern has to do with weight and lipid disorders—anorexia nervosa, bulimia, malnutrition in the elderly, obesity, hyperlipidemia, atherosclerosis, and cholelithiasis—which all involve hormones and diet.

In particular, consider the many roles that hormones play in fat and cholesterol metabolism.

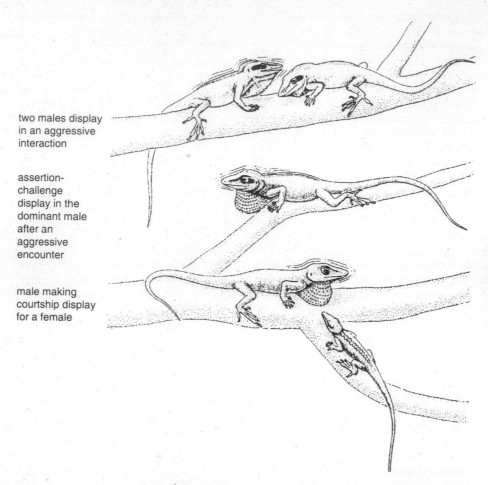

two males display
in an aggressive
interaction

assertion-
challenge
display in the
dominant male
after an
aggressive
encounter

male making
courtship display
for a female

Figure 22.9 The displays of a lizard, *Anolis carolinensis*, depend on androgen. The displays involve disten-
tion of the dewlap, a bright red region of the throat, and head bobbing, or push-ups. Modified, with permission.
Crews, D. Integration of internal and external stimuli in the regulation of lizard reproduction. In Greenberg, N.;
MacLean, P.D., editors. The Behavior and Neurology of Lizards. Rockville, MD: NIMH; 1978; pp. 149–171.

Hormones stimulate fat synthesis and breakdown
(Table 22.3). Hormones stimulate fat deposition
(prolactin, insulin) and fat breakdown (ß-lipotropin,
glucocorticoids, catecholamines, thyroid hormones,
glucagon, and GH). Fat provides a reservoir for
some hormones (estrogen and melatonin) and
stimulate the secretion of others (cholecystokinin).
Hormones of the gastrointestinal tract promote food
absorption. Cholesterol is a precursor of steroids
(e.g., estrogen).

Parts of the nervous system are implicated
in the control of feeding behavior. The brain, in
particular the hypothalamus, controls feeding behavior. Recall that the glucostatic cells that can detect blood glucose levels reside in the ventral medial hypothalamus (VMH) and lateral hypothalamus. **Hyperphagia** (increased feeding) results
from VMH lesions. The VMH reduces electrical
activity during hunger. Electrical stimulation of
the VMH blocks feeding behavior. So the VMH
may be the brain region that prevents feeding.
Aphagia (reduced food intake) and anorexia can result from lesions of the lateral hypothalamus.
Electrical activity of the lateral hypothalamus increases during hunger and feeding onset. Electrical
stimulation of the lateral hypothalamus causes feed-

ing behavior. The lateral hypothalamus may be a brain region that enhances feeding.

Transfused blood from fed rats will reduce the food intake of other rats deprived of food. This is evidence for a humoral factor controlling satiety. It is possible that **cholecystokinin** (CCK), and structurally related molecules such as caerulein, are the chemical messengers that are responsible. In experiments, CCK injected into the VMH reduced food intake, prolonged intermeal interval, and limited feeding. Cholecystokinin (CCK) induces satiety in humans. We can envision a scenario whereby food that is eaten enters the duodenum causing the secretion of CCK. CCK in turn acts to promote activities that aid in digestion of the food, and, at the same time, signals the brain that food has been eaten.

Insulin is a main character in discussions about the etiology and consequences of fat and obesity. Metabolically, insulin promotes triglyceride storage and fatty acid esterification via glycerol phosphate; at the same time insulin suppresses lipolysis. Taken together, these effects mean that insulin promotes fattening. Insulin correlates with percent of ideal body weight (Figure 22.8; r = 0.72).[16] Factors that antagonize insulin (obesity, uremia, corticosteroids, growth hormone, estrogen, etc.) cause the pancreas to secrete more insulin (compensatory hyperinsulinism). The increased insulin stimulates the liver endogenous triglyceride synthesis which leads to excess triglycerides. Insulin receptors on muscle, liver, monocyte, and fat cells decrease in obesity. When insulin is deficient, as in diabetes mellitus, one symptom is accelerated fat catabolism which causes ketoacidosis, anorexia, nausea, vomiting, air hunger, coma, and even death. Insulin varies with normal physiology; for example, insulin increases during pregnancy, insulin peaks about 7 p.m. at night in humans, and insulin decreases during fasting.

Bierman and Glomset discount the idea that hormones cause obesity:

> . . . . the metabolic consequences [of obesity] are predictable. They appear to relate only to fat cell size, and virtually all metabolic disturbances tested are inducible with weight gain and reversible with weight reduction. . . .although numerous hormonal imbalances have been described in obesity, they are likely to be consequences of the obese state, not causes

> of it. . . . the metabolic alteration with the most profound influence on metabolism is the acquired resistance to the action of insulin on glucose utilization by fat and muscle cells.[17]

However, there is good reason to suspect hormones for roles in regulation of body weight, and this area deserves more attention. CCK affects satiety and feeding behavior. There are drugs that inhibit fat-promoting hormones (e.g., bromocriptine inhibition of prolactin, or catecholamines which inhibit insulin release). ß-Lipotropin and thyroid hormones stimulate fat breakdown. It would seem that thyroid hormone (or TSH or TRH) might be ideal for use in weight loss programs. However, overdoses of thyroid preparations may cause tachycardia, angina pectoris, diarrhea, nervousness, sweating, headache, and increased pulse action. Thyroid hormone self-administration, usually among medical and paramedical personnel (to counteract fatigue or to promote weight loss), is the cause of a syndrome of hyperthyroidism (thyrotoxicosis factitia).[18]

STRONG AND WEAK

Anabolic steroids have captured world wide attention because of their use by athletes to enhance athletic performance. The anabolic steroids that have been used are derivatives of testosterone. Testosterone androgenizes males at puberty—the penis elongates and increases diameter, the prostate and scrotum develop, and the hair (pubic, axillary, facial) appears. In addition, testosterone has anabolic effects—accelerated linear growth, enlargement of the larynx and thickening of the vocal cords, development of libido and sexual potential, increase in muscle bulk and strength, decrease in body fat, and increase in aggressive and sexual behavior.

Anabolic steroids and other drugs are prohibited by sports-governing bodies. Nevertheless, many athletes take anabolic steroids (usually testosterone, alkylated testosterone analogs, or testosterone esters). The anabolic steroids have variations in their properties—the alkylated testosterones have a longer half-life than testosterone; the testosterone esters are more lipid soluble which means they are absorbed more slowly from an intramuscular oil injection. The usual technique is

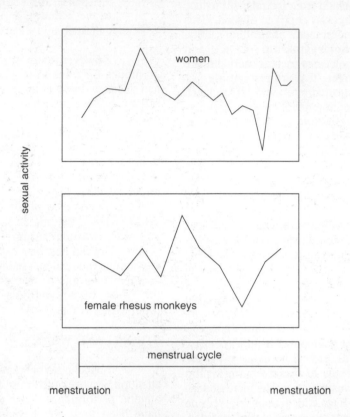

Figure 22.10 The graphs show the changes in sexual activity during the menstrual cycle in primates. Herbert, J. Behavioral patterns. In Austin, C.R.; Short, R.V., editors. Reproduction in Mammals, Book 4: Reproductive Patterns. New York: Cambridge University Press: 1972; p. 48.

administration in 6–12 week "cycles." Enanthate (hepanoate) and cipionate (cyclopentylproprionate esters) can be taken every two or three weeks. Taking more than one steroid at a time for synergistic effects is referred to as "stacking." Anabolic steroid users may use an overlapping pattern to avoid tolerance (plateauing). A "pyramid" pattern is an incremental increase from low daily doses at the beginning of a cycle to higher doses and then tapering the doses toward the end of the cycle. They may also use stimulants, diuretics, antiestrogens, HCG, HGH, anti-acneiform medications, and anti-inflammatories. This polypharmacy is called an "array." Sprinters and endurance athletes take

doses closer to those used clinically for replacement therapy in males with hypogonadism. Athletes in strength sports (weight lifters, throwers) may use 10 to 100 times the replacement dose.

The numbers of steroid users vary depending on the exact study, but in one example developed for high school students, 5–12% of the boys and 0.5–2.5% of the girls self-reported anabolic-androgenic steroid use. More than a third of users in some studies were nonathletes who used the drugs "to look good" or to get "big."[19]

Do the anabolic steroids work for athletes who want to win? The answer is controversial but generally supports the finding that anabolic steroids slightly enhance muscle strength in previously trained athletes. The effects on other aspects related to competition—attitude, diligence in training, agility, competitive spirit—are more difficult to document. A placebo effect has been suggested.

Side effects are dose dependent and have been learned from studies of clinically approved treatments for deficiencies. Individuals who use anabolic steroids near replacement levels, those with hypogonadism, have relatively minimal untoward effects. Puberty is normal and they are able to maintain adult male strength, libido, and sexual function. Medically indicated use of anabolic steroids is for boys with delayed puberty, for infant boys with microphallus, or to promote growth in girls with Turner's syndrome.

More serious side effects in males are associated with large doses. There is paradoxical impotence and lack of sperm production despite heightened sexual drive. This may be explained by negative feedback on the hypothalamus and anterior pituitary gland which abolishes circulating LH and FSH. Circulating FSH is an absolute requirement for sperm to mature. Some feel that abnormal lipid profiles, liver function tests, and concentrations of hormone-binding proteins in the blood of anabolic steroid users may mean there is a propensity toward atherosclerotic arterial lesions. Liver toxicity is attributed particularly to the 17-akyl-substituted androgens taken orally.

It is suspected that anabolic steroids may promote aggressive behavior, but the idea is controversial. Rogal and Yesalis mention the experiments of Brown-Sequard "who attempted (he was his own experimental subject) to show that aqueous extracts of dog and guinea pig testes contained substances that in addition to their androgenic effects, affected vitality, energy, and youthfulness."[20] Investigators who have done psychological/behavioral studies in athletes have reported mood swings, arousal, increased self-confidence, increased pain threshold, increased motivation, reduction in fatigue after exercise, and increased aggression. A serious association of excess anabolic steroids with violent behavior has repeatedly been suggested, but not fully accepted.

One disturbing side effect is called priapism (sustained penile erection). Acne, gynecomastia, and edema because of sodium and chloride retention are other side effects. When anabolic steroid users with problems were asked to voluntarily attend a steroid clinic they reported problems of changes in libido, acne, hirsutism, psychiatric problems, GI upset, severe headaches, aggression, insulin reaction, and injection reaction. Examination findings included gynecomastia, testicular atrophy, and baldness.[21]

In females, anabolic steroid use can cause clitorimegaly, hirsutism, amenorrhea, and deep "masculine" voice (from effects on the larynx). Some of these effects (amenorrhea) are reversible; others (masculine voice) are irreversible.[22,23]

Dependency and withdrawal symptoms have been suggested for anabolic steroid users. Dependency is indicated by preoccupation with drug use, difficulty stopping, and drug craving. Withdrawal effects include violent behavior, mood swings, rage, and depression. Disturbing as the side effects of anabolic steroid use, dependency, and withdrawal may be, there has been no epidemic of severe side-effects and death to deter users. Dietary supplements (e.g., chromium picolinate, gamma oryzanol from rice bran oil and other plant sterols, L-carnitine) are also used without much evidence for efficacy or much information about potential dangers.[24]

Perhaps ironically, the World Health Organization is evaluating the use of 200 mg/week of testosterone ethanate as a male contraceptive. Moreover, anabolic steroids are not the only hormones involved in athletics. Growth hormone also has potential for changing physique. So the opportunity, or problem, for using hormones to manipulate physique is being enlarged.

REPRODUCTIVE BEHAVIOR

An area of behavioral endocrinology that always attracts interest is consideration of the roles that reproductive hormones play in behavior. Some of these have already been discussed in the chapters dealing with testosterone, estrogen, and progestogens. Androgens likewise have well known influences on male behavior in animals, such as head-bobbing in lizards (Figure 22.9). The popular press likes to propound ideas that hormones cause behavior. For example, it was asserted that "when levels of estrogen were high, the women showed greater verbal fluency and used their hands more skillfully than when levels were low."[25]

Of particular interest has been the possibility of a natural aphrodisiac. In addition to the libido-producing effects of androgens and estrogens,

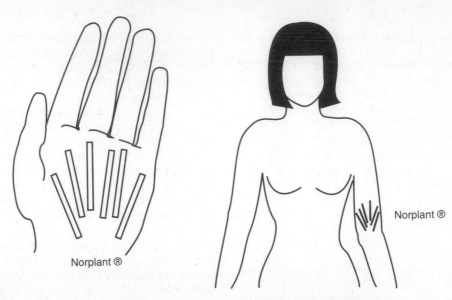

Norplant ®

Norplant ®

Figure 22.11 Norplant® tubes filled with progestin are implanted under the skin of a woman's upper arm to provide contraceptive protection for up to five years. Redrawn. Purvis, A. A pill that gets under the skin. Time; December 24, 1990; p. 66.

a role in stimulating sexual interest has been suggested for luteinizing hormone-releasing hormone (LRH, LH-RH, and GnRH). Jean Marx summarized the central role that LRH plays in reproduction.[26] LRH is thought to increase at puberty and decreased LRH responses may initiate menopause. Variations in sexual activity have been correlated with phases of the menstrual cycle (Figure 22.10)

Not only do reproductive hormones affect behavior, behavior also affects reproduction. LRH disruption has been associated with infertility. In particular, women athletes (ballerinas, runners, gymnasts) may develop anovulation and amenorrhea. The spontaneous restoration of fertility occurs in 70% of the women when they reduce their exercise, but 30% do not resume cycles without medical intervention. One medical intervention that restores cycling is the opiate antagonist naloxone. Thus there is a hypothesis that exercise increases endorphins which in turn cause a decline in LRH which results in amenorrhea and anovulation.

Yet another intriguing hypothesis surrounds LRH. LRH-secreting cells have been found along the terminal nerve leading from the nose to the forebrain which is along the path the cells travel during development. It has been observed that children with Kallmann syndrome fail to de-

velop sexually, can't smell, have clusters of LRH cells in the nose, and do not have clusters of LRH cells in the brain. The coincidence of the LRH cells in the nose and the use of the nose by many species for detecting pheromones was noticed.[27]

Postpartum depression, or "baby blues," is a psychological phenomenon that is observed in 50–80% of women in the weeks just after birth.[28] There may be a physical explanation in the tremendous plunge in estrogen and progesterone that occur at parturition and/or the hormone changes that accompany lactation.

HOMOSEXUALITY

Repeated, mostly unsuccessful, attempts have been made to link homosexuality in humans to hormones. There is circumstantial evidence for a biological basis in the statistics that more men are homosexuals and fewer women are lesbians. The absence of evidence for unusual levels of sex steroids in gay individuals is noteworthy. Investigators have turned to hormonal "programming" of developing brains in search of a hormonal connection with gay behavior. The Merck Manual contains a suggestion concerning the possibility of a hormonal basis for homosexuality:

Table 22.4 Symptoms of SAD and PMS

SAD symptoms	PMS symptoms
sadness	depression
anxiety	anxiety
irritability	irritability
decreased physical activity	energy disturbances
increased appetite	increased appetite
interpersonal difficulties	emotional lability
increased sleep time	sleep disturbances (hypersomnia)
increased weight	weight gain
carbohydrate craving	difficulty concentrating
earlier sleep onset	negative self-perception
later waking	breast swelling
interrupted, not refreshing, sleep	headache
daytime drowsiness	bloating
decreased libido	edema
difficulties around menses	constipation
work difficulties	

Sack, D.; Rosenthal, N.; Parry, B.; Wehr, T. Biological rhythms in psychiatry. In Meltzer, H., editor. Psychopharmacology. New York: Raven Press; 1987; pp. 669–685. SAD and PMS have some common symptoms and there is research showing that light alleviates the symptoms of both.

Constitutional factors involving hormonal programming of the brain during fetal life may be a significant factor [in homosexuality]. Some support for this hypothesis is to be found in the higher-than-expected prevalence of homosexual fantasies and behavior in men and women whose mothers received diethylstilbestrol (DES) during pregnancy.[29]

Animal research offers a few clues. Castrated young male rats subsequently show female characteristics such as lordosis. Newborn female animals given testosterone or estrogens during a critical period develop masculine sexual behavior. A "conversion hypothesis" suggests that the brain is initially bipotential and is feminized early in life by estrogen. In the hypothesis, the feminizing effects of estrogen are prevented by estrogen-binding proteins in serum; but in males, testosterone is converted to estradiol in the brain causing defeminization; in addition, the testosterone has its own virilizing effects.[30]

HUMAN FERTILITY CONTROL

The area of fertility control has long been important to endocrinology. Reproductive control is an important aspect of farm animal husbandry. There has been considerable recent interest in using pineal hormones (e.g., melatonin) to control fertility and time births in seasonally breeding animals such as sheep. In humans, there is interest in contraceptive means to limit fertility on the part of individuals, a larger concern for worldwide population control, and also a focus on means for barren couples to bear children. The wide availability of contraceptive pills in the late 1960's sparked a sexual revolution. However, the "pill," the IUD, and more traditional birth control methods still have failure rates.

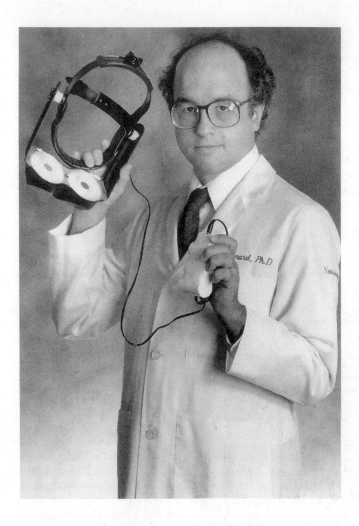

Figure 22.12 The photograph is Dr. George Brainard holding an early version of a visor apparatus to provide portable light therapy. The apparatus is worn on the head; lights in the front of the visor shine into the subject's eyes. Alternatively, a subject can sit in front of a bank of fluorescent lights. Dr. Brainard removed this constraint by affixing a fluorescent light beneath the brim of a safari helmet. Light visors (Bio-Brite) might be used to treat seasonal affective disorder, jet lag syndrome, and shift work maladapation. Photograph courtesy Thomas Jefferson University in Philadelphia.

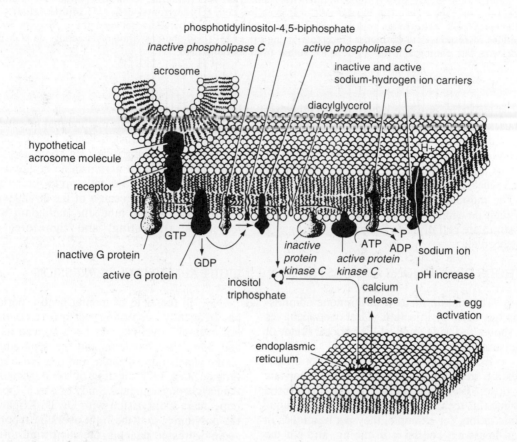

Figure 22.13 The diagram shows Gilbert's model for fertilization based on interaction of proteins in the sperm acrosome membrane with the proteins of the cell membrane of the ovum; the membrane of the endoplasmic reticulum is incorporated into the model. Modified, with permission. Gilbert, S.F. Developmental Biology, Second Edition. Sunderland, MA: Sinauer Associates; 1988; p. 65.

Norplant® is a method of birth control that is expected to come into wide use.[31] Norplant® consists of six progestin-stuffed silicone tubes (Figure 22.11). The tubes are implanted just beneath the skin in a woman's upper arm. The progestin is released continuously for about five years. Fertility resumes 48 hours after the tubes are removed. The method has advantages: daily pills need not be remembered and the total cost may be less than the expense of five years of pills. Irregular menstrual bleeding is a negative side effect that occurs in 75% of women.

In the area of fertility, the possibilities are enormous, and to some, are disturbing. **Fertility drugs** such as Clomid® have been used to stimulate ovulation in infertile women. **Artificial insemination** has been used to provide semen with a higher sperm count and to make use of surrogate mothers. *In vitro* **fertilization** has been accomplished using human eggs and sperm. *In vitro* fertilization did not come as a surprise to biologists. Developmentalists routinely taught embry-

Figure 22.14 (Opposite) The photomicrograph shows the retina. It is a half micron epoxy section of a chick retina two days after hatching (bar = 20 μm. Superimposed are drawings of Golgi stained cell families adapted from Cajal's 1892 study of the chick retina. (A) amacrine cell (amicrine cells are peptidic, dopaminergic, serotonergic, or colinergic), (B) bipolar cell, (G) ganglion cell, (H) horizontal cell, (M) Muller (glial) cell, (P) photoreceptor cell. The retina makes the hormone, melatonin, and parallels between the mediation by cyclic nucleotides of responses to hormones (receptors acting via cAMP) and photons (rhodopsin acting via cGMP) have been drawn. The photograph was a gift to the author from Joel Sheffield.

ology students to provoke ovulation by injecting pituitaries into female frogs, squeeze out the frog eggs, and fertilize the eggs in a Petri dish with sperm released from mashed frog testes. Observed under the microscope, the buff and black frog eggs rotated when fertilized so that the black side was up. The tadpoles were easily raised in order to study their development. The careful student could even stimulate cell division by pricking a frog egg with a needle.

METHODS OF HORMONE ADMINISTRATION

The classic method of hormone administration has been by injection. Oral contraceptives have shown the wide applicability of oral routes of administration.

However, both the injection and oral techniques are treatments that supply a bolus, or one time, dose. Endocrinologists for years have used experimental techniques that produce continuous administration; for example, they put hormones in melted beeswax, cooled it in tubing, and cut the tubing up to make pellets which they implanted.

Norplant® is a widely known application of continuous hormone administration technology that has been in use for years. The technology is not limited to reproductive hormones. For example, researchers implanted Silastic® tubes filled with steroids or melatonin into animals. Lipid soluble hormones pass through the tubing at a low constant rate and the dose of the hormone can be controlled with the length of the tubing.[32,33]

There are also implantable devices, such as Alzet® minipumps, that deliver hormones continuously. The minipumps have a balloon reservoir for the fluid to be injected. A semipermeable membrane surrounds the tube. Fluid from the animal passes through the membrane and presses on the balloon ejecting its contents slowly over one to two weeks. The pumps have the advantage that they can be used for hormones that are water soluble.

In an ingenious method that he called programmable microinfusion, Harry Lynch combined the pump with a long tube. He alternated a melatonin solution and a nonmiscible solution in the tube. Then he used a minipump to force the contents out the tube. Because of the arrangement of the solutions in the tube, the melatonin was released in alternating, and therefore, cyclic pulses.[34,35]

LIGHT ALLEVIATES DEPRESSION

In the field of mental health, periodicity has frequently been observed to be a component. For example, cyclicity has been noticed in mania and depression, catatonia and schizophrenia, psychotic attacks, dipsomania, and premenstrual syndrome. At a 1972 meeting of the Association for the Psychophysiological Study of Sleep, the author remembers a discussion with Dr. D. Kripke about the possibility that the light aversion reported by some depressed patients, the southward migration of northerners on winter vacations, and the role of light in controlling the production of hormones that lower body temperature, such as melatonin, might hint at a role for light in depression which would mean that depression could be treated by altering the illumination of a patient's environment. One of these illnesses that involves wintertime blues has recently been named Seasonal Affective Disorder abbreviated SAD (Table 22.4).[36] Some people who suffered from depression experienced the illness only during certain seasons, mainly winter when the daylengths were short. A considerable advance was the discovery that the illness could be successfully treated with supplemental artificial light exposure. Remission of depression is usually achieved in SAD subjects within a few days of commencing two-hour daily light treatments (phototherapy). The initial methods have been cumbersome with the patients forced to sit in front

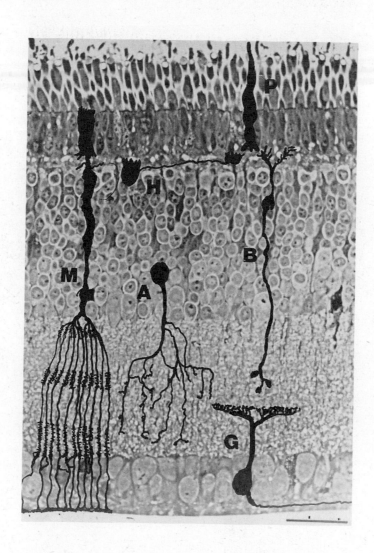

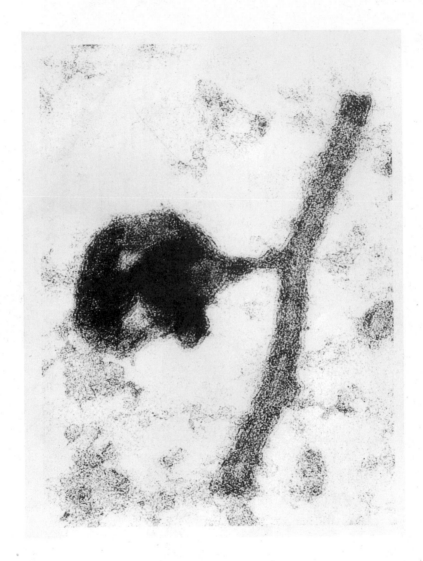

Figure 22.15 The photomicrograph shows a microtubule and an attached vesicle. The microtubules, about 250 angstroms in diameter, were obtained from mouse brain. Microtubules may participate in the movement of particles in cells; they are directly of interest for their role in the movement of microsomes in physiological color change and its control by hormones. The photograph was a gift to the author from Richard Weisenberg.

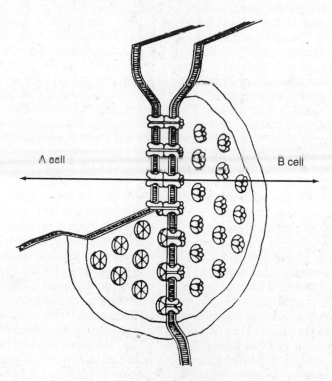

A cell   B cell

Figure 22.16 An example of nonendocrine communication between cells is shown. Chemicals can pass directly between two adjacent cells through special channels. The figure shows a pancreatic A cell and a pancreatic B cell with gap junctions. Each junction has six subunits that contain a channel that penetrates each cell. The arrow shows bidirectional passage of small molecules (<1000 molecular weight—ions, sugars, amino acids). With permission, Orci, L. Macro- and microdomains in the endocrine pancreas. Diabetes 31: 538–565; 1982.

of a wall or box of fluorescent light for several hours. Recent methods using visors promise to free the individual from this restraint (Figure 22.12). A hormonal explanation of SAD based on melatonin (excess melatonin in winter causes depression) has been considered but has so far not been proved.

LARGE QUANTITIES OF HORMONES FROM MOLECULAR BIOLOGY

Molecular biology has been a breakthrough for endocrinology because it allows the synthesis of many enzymes and hormones in large quantities. Prior to this breakthrough, polypeptide hormones were priceless because of their scarcity. To obtain a peptide hormone for research or clinical treatment usually requires its isolation from dis-

sected glands, often glands only obtained from humans during autopsies. But we can now make hormones using the same biochemical machinery as living cells.

To find the specific gene or to make its peptide product, the structure of the peptide hormone must first be worked out. The gene is the DNA containing the blueprint needed for the synthesis of a peptide hormone. Fortunately for endocrinologists, the sequencing of the amino acids of most peptide hormones has already been accomplished. The nucleotide sequence of the DNA for the hormone can be deduced from the amino acid sequence of the protein. For molecular work, the DNA can be produced by chemical synthesis, or it can come from chromosomal DNA, or it can be DNA which is produced by reverse transcription. To make a segment of DNA by reverse transcription, scientists begin with cells that produce the desired peptide hormone, that is, the cells of a hormone-synthesizing gland. Messenger ribonucleic acid (mRNA) that is responsible for synthesizing the peptide hormone is isolated from cells. The DNA is produced as the complement of the mRNA using the enzyme **reverse transcriptase**. The reverse transcriptase is found in retroviruses. The sneaky retroviruses place their genetic information into other cells using reverse transcriptase. Reverse transcriptase synthesizes DNA by making the complement of a single strand of RNA. The DNA that is made by copying RNA is **complementary DNA** (cDNA). The cDNA has the code, or sequence of nucleotides, that can program the sequence of amino acids in the peptide hormone.

Plasmids are used to transfer genes. Plasmids are small circles of double stranded DNA (dsDNA) which usually range in size from 1 to 20 kilobases (a kilobase is a thousand bases or "rungs" of the ladder). Plasmids were discovered to be naturally occurring molecules in many species of bacteria and a few species of plants. They function in bacteria to move segments of DNA from cell to cell. We can use them in molecular biology for the same purpose—i.e., as vectors to move segments of DNA from cell to cell. A gene for human protein made by reverse transcriptase can be inserted into a plasmid.

Genes are inserted into plasmids using enzymes called "restriction endonucleases" (also called "restriction enzymes") which cut DNA sites that consist of a specific sequence of nucleic acids. For example, the restriction endonuclease, EcoRI, will cut DNA at the double stranded sequence of bases GAATTC. The enzyme cuts the DNA asymmetrically so as to leave ends of unpaired DNA termed "sticky ends." The DNA that is cloned from an amino acid sequence using reverse transcriptase can be made so that it has a set of sticky ends at either end of the cDNA (complementary DNA made by copying RNA) which corresponds to the recognition site of a restriction endonuclease. A plasmid is cut using a restriction enzyme that has the same recognition site as the ends of the cDNA that is to be inserted. The cDNA is then combined with the cut plasmid and ligated, or inserted, into the plasmid using an enzyme called "DNA ligase." The result is a plasmid containing a cCNA for a given protein. This plasmid is then inserted into bacteria where it is replicated and transcribed by the DNA-replicating and transcribing machinery of the bacterial cell.

The insertion process by which plasmid-cDNA is introduced into bacteria is termed **transformation** (not to be confused with the use of the word "transformation" in the steroid mechanism of action). Transformation involves chemically treating bacteria so that they become "competent," or permeable, to DNA and they take up the plasmids. The bacteria that is usually used is *Escherichia coli* (*E. coli*) which normally lives in intestines. *E. coli* can be cultured in the laboratory and has been the servant of molecular biologists and geneticists.

In the process of cell transformation, not all of the bacterial cells incorporate plasmids. **Antibiotics** can be used to select the cells of *E. coli* which contain the inserted plasmid carrying the cDNA. The bacterial cell resists an antibiotic when it contains a plasmid with a gene for an enzyme that breaks down the antibiotic. Adding the antibiotic to the bacterial culture medium kills the *E. coli* that do not have the plasmid with the antibiotic resistance. The bacteria with the desired plasmid possessing the desired cDNA remain.

A **clone** is a line of cells that has a single parent cell and a unique piece of cDNA (e.g., for a peptide hormone). Clones containing single plasmids can be grown. Thus it is possible to produce a huge number of bacteria containing the plasmid cDNA. The cDNA can be isolated from the bacteria. The restriction enzyme used to get the initial cDNA can cleave the new cDNA from the plasmid. The plasmid DNA and the cDNA can be separated with electrophoresis.

A piece of single-stranded DNA or RNA (one upright and half of each of the rungs of the chemical ladder) can combine with, or anneal, by base pairing to a complementary strand of DNA or RNA. This is called **hybridization**. A **probe** is a piece of radiolabeled DNA. A probe can be used to find a complementary piece of DNA or RNA (e.g., on an electrophoresis gel). A probe will also radioactively label the colony of bacteria that contains a plasmid with complementary cDNA. A probe can be used to measure how much of a particular sequence of mRNA is present. Monoclonal antibodies provide another kind of probe. Homogeneous antibodies are "raised" or "grown" in large quantities. They come from one parent cell type and they recognize only one antigen. For hormones, the monoclonal antibodies can be used to detect and measure hormones or receptors.

Recombinant methods promise mass production of polypeptide hormones, "raising" peptide hormones, that were previously only available in miniscule quantities obtained from living organisms, their dead carcasses, their blood, or their urine. This means that hormones will now be clinically available. The first hormone that was made was somatostatin.[37] Gertz and Baxter discuss how protein hormones can be produced with direct expression:

> ...sequences that encode the desired proteins must be inserted in the regions of plasmids downstream from bacterial regulatory sequences. The region would include a promoter; the sequences encoding a ribosomal binding site; and an AUG codon, which codes for methionine and is necessary in mRNA to initiate translation. The bacterial regulatory sequences are responsible for directing the synthesis of the desired proteins [hormones]. By this method of direct expression, the synthesized proteins [hormones] can frequently be obtained in yields that represent several percent of the total bacterial proteins.[38]

They also discuss an alternative approach, used for human insulin and ß-endorphin, which involves cleavage of the protein hormone from a fusion (hybrid) protein.

MOLECULAR DETECTION AND REPAIR OF GENETIC DISORDERS

Genetic disorders involving hormones can be detected and repaired. Some endocrine disorders are believed to have a genetic, or inherited, cause because they tend to run in families. In some cases, the etiology is clearcut; for example, congenital adrenal hyperplasia is due to inability to synthesize specific adrenal enzymes that can be inherited. Abnormal DNA coding (due to mutations, deletions, insertions, or a missing gene) for the sequence of a particular hormone is the culprit. In other cases, the genetic cause is not so clearcut; it appears that what is inherited is a susceptibility to developing a disease. Some examples of endocrine diseases with a genetic component are:

Type II diabetes mellitus

Dwarfism
Testicular feminization
Pseudohypoparathyroidism
Congenital adrenal hyperplasia
Type I diabetes mellitus (susceptibility)
Multiple endocrine neoplasia syndromes (susceptibility)

An individual person's DNA can be used for diagnosis of genetic disorders. The diagnosis is possible even before the symptoms of the disorder appear. The DNA can come from cells obtained from biopsy, blood, or, in the case of embryos, from amniotic fluid. Such tests are already available for detections of sickle cell anemia and phenylketonuria. **Polymorphism analysis** is one way of detecting a genetic disease without determining the detailed DNA sequence:

> Somewhere in or around the affected gene [of the diseased individual are] additional differences in comparison to other people. Occasionally, these differences result in the generation of loss of a restriction endonuclease cleavage site. In this case, cleavage of the affected individual's DNA with the restriction enzyme will result in DNA fragments that differ in size from those of other people. Subjecting the fragments to size fractionation on a gel, transferring them to nitrocellulose filters, and performing hybridization to a radiolabeled probe from the gene will allow identification of the aberrant fragment. Since the restriction site polymorphism will be inherited along with the mutation that results in disease susceptibility, this polymorphism can be used as a genetic marker for the disease."[39]

New genes can't be administered in pills. Real hope of repairing genetic disorders is the stuff of genetic engineering. The idea would be to insert genes for normal hormone production. For example, an insulin gene would be placed in a diabetic to repair the insulin deficiency. Sound impossible? Methods exist to place DNA into cells: the DNA can be injected into the cell nucleus or plasmid cDNA can be sent by electroporation. Cells will eat DNA calcium phosphate precipitates. Viruses and bacteria can deliver cDNA to target cells.

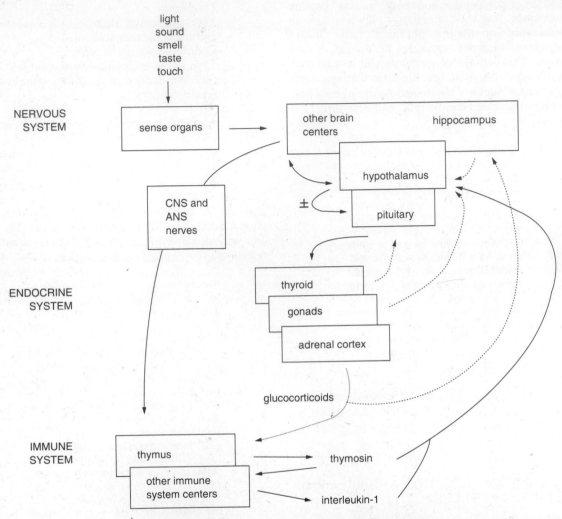

Figure 22.17 The scheme shows the interactions of the neuroendocrine system with the immune system. After Arking, R. Biology of Aging. Englewood Cliffs, NJ: Prentice-Hall; 1991; p. 180.

SHARED IDEAS IN ENDOCRINOLOGY

Ideas about natural organization have common elements. For example, Gilbert shows a model for fertilization that bears similarities with hormone mechanisms of action (Figure 22.13). The use of chemical factors for the induction of development and growth draws on ideas from the way that hormones act, and indeed, some of the chemical messengers are the classical hormones. Relatively few kinds of atoms are used to make up hormones and, indeed, the other molecules of living things, and enzymes do double duty to synthesize more than one product. The activities of slime molds bear similarities to the activities of leucocytes. In short, there appear to be simple principles that underlie the physiology of living things.

IMAGING

Imaging studies are useful in clinical applications of endocrinology.[40] They are used to find the location of abnormalities and to describe details about that location such as its size and its relationship to the surrounding tissues. Imaging is also used to place needles in glands for various treatments (e.g., fine-needle aspiration to confirm a parathyroid tumor). Sonography (ultrasound) is used to visualize the thyroid, parathyroid, pancreas, scrotum, and adrenal glands. Radioisotopes (e.g. ^{131}I and ^{125}I) are used to make scintillation scans which image the thyroid gland and thallium and technetium are used in making whole body and parathyroid scans related to diseases of the thyroid and parathyroid. Magnetic resonance imaging is used to visualize the thyroid and parathyroids. Computed tomography (CT), magnetic resonance imaging (MR, MRI). and scintigraphy are used to scan the adrenal glands, ovaries and the pancreas. Arteriography and venous sampling have been replaced by noninvasive imaging in localization of endocrine tumors, but are still used for some localizations and differential diagnoses (Cushing's syndrome, hyperparathyroidism, insulinoma, gastrinoma, hyperaldosteronism, virilizing tumors) because they provide direct information about endocrine function. Several kinds of imaging techniques (photon densitometry, absorptiometry, quantitative CT, ultrasound) are used to measure bone mineralization which is important in the evaluation of osteoporosis. Magnetic resonance imaging can be used to examine the pituitary and pineal regions.

MYSTERIES

Students confronted with fat textbooks and interminable lectures might get the impression that everything that can be done has been done in endocrinology. Yet many mysteries remain in the science of the endocrine glands themselves and in the overall way they act together to regulate a complex function. For example, the function of the third eye—is it a radiation dosimeter? is it a photoreceptor for rhythms? is it a predator detector?—is still a matter of debate. In another example, we now know that the retina can make melatonin, a hormone (Figure 22.14). What is retina function in hormone production? Should it be considered an "endocrine" tissue?

Chemical communication might be viewed in the larger sense as a continuum—within the cytoplasm (Figure 22.15), between two cells (Figure 22.16), between two tissues by way of the blood (hormones), and between two individuals (pheromones). New opportunities arrive with new technology such as those brought by molecular bi-

ology and recent advances in imaging technology. New chemical messengers remain to be discovered.

The reader of endocrine textbooks or research papers might go away with a view of circumspect glands sedately producing their secretions in an orderly fashion. But the disciplined writings of scientists probably belies the violence and excitement of the actual events at the microscopic and molecular levels. Lights flash on. Retina pigment bleaches. Jolting electrical signals race along nerves. Neurohumors are belched into synapses. Receptors are wrenched into new shapes. Molecules sluice a cascade of enzymes. Cell factories churn out hormones, spit them through tubes, and expel them in wrapped packages. The hormones ride tsunamis of flowing blood. Receptor magnets grab the hormones from the surging fluid. Target cells gobble receptor-hormone complexes. Endocrine reality, therefore, is indeed exciting and dynamic.

PUTTING IT ALL TOGETHER

The genes we are born with determine what hormones are made; the genes are the blueprint, the instructions. The instructions are converted to proteins which act as hormones or which act as enzymes catalyzing the production of the hormones. The hormones convey the instructions. The receptors and mechanisms of action in the target organs amplify the hormone signals.

In this book, we have looked at the endocrine system in bits and pieces. One attempt at an overview, which also shows the interaction with the immune system is presented in Figure 22.17.

REFERENCES

1. Mackowiak, P.A.; Wasserman, S.S.; Levine, M.M. A critical appraisal of 98.6°F, the upper limit of the normal body temperature, and other legacies of Carl Reinhold August Wunderlich. JAMA 268: 1578–1580; 1992.

2. Kaltenbach, J.C. Endocrine aspects of homeostasis. Amer. Zool. 28: 661–773; 1988.

3. Myrsovsky, N. Rheostasis: The Physiology of Change. New York: Oxford University Press; 1990; p. 528.

4. Pearse, A.G.E. Cytochemical evidence for the neural crest origin of mammalian ultimobranchial

C cells. Histochemie 27: 96–102: 1971; p. 101.

5. Mulvihill, S.J.; Deveney, C.W.; Way, L.W.; Tebas, H.T. Regulatory peptides of the gut. In Greenspan, F.S., editor. Basic and Clinical Endocrinology, Third Edition. Norwalk, CT: Appleton & Lange; 1991; p. 573.

6. Gilbert, S.F. Developmental Biology, Second Edition. Sunderland, MA: Sinauer Associates, Inc.; 1988; p. 4.

7. Spemann, H.; Mangold, H. Induction of embryonic primordia by implantation of organizers from a different species. In Willier, B.H.; Oppenheimer, J.M., editors. Foundations of Experimental Embryology. New York: Hafner; 1924; pp. 144–184.

8. Gilbert, S.F. Developmental Biology, Second Edition. Sunderland, MA: Sinauer Associates, Inc.; 1988; p. 299.

9. Edmunds, L.N. Cellular and Molecular Bases of Biological Clocks: Models and Mechanisms for Circadian Timekeeping. New York: Springer-Verlag, New York, Inc.; 1988; 497 pages.

10. Ehret, C.F.; Trucco, E. Molecular models for the circadian clock. I. The chronon concept. J. Theoret. Biol. 15: 240–262; 1967.

11. Wurtman, R., Axelrod, J., Kelly, D. The Pineal. New York: Academic Press; 1968; p. 108.

12. Hadley, M.E. Endocrinology, Second Edition. Englewood Cliffs, NJ: Prentice Hall; 1988; p. 497.

13. Hadley, M.E.; Ibid.; p. 501.

14. Hadley, M.E.; Ibid.; p. 514.

15. Novales, R.R. Actions of melanocyte-stimulating hormone. In Greep, R.O.; Astwood, E.B., editors. Handbook of Physiology Section 7; Endocrinology Volume IV Part 2. Baltimore: Williams & Wilkins Co.; 1974; p. 347.

16. Bagdade, J.D.; Bierman, E.L.; et al. The significance of basal insulin levels in the evaluation of the insulin response to glucose in diabetic and nondiabetic subjects. J. Clin. Invest. 46; 1549; 1967.

17. Bierman, E.L.; Glomset, J.A. Obesity. In Williams, R.H., editor. Textbook of Endocrinology, Sixth Edition. Philadelphia, PA: W. B. Saunders; 1981; pp. 912–913.

18. Berkow, R. The Merck Manual of Diagnosis and Therapy. Rahway, NJ.: Merck Sharp & Dohme Research Laboratories; 1987; p.1040.

19. Rogol, A.D.; Yesalis, C.E. Anabolic-androgenic steroids and athletes: What are the issues? J. Clin. Endo. Metab. 74: 465–469; 1992.

20. Rogol, A.D.; Yesalis, C.E.; Ibid.

21. Frankle, M.; Leffers, D. Athletes on anabolic-androgenic steroids: New approach diminishes health problems. The Physician and Sports Medicine 20: 75–87; 1992.

22. Cowart, V.S. Dietary supplements: Alternatives to anabolic steroids? The Physician and Sports Medicine 20: 189–198; 1992.

23. Rogol, A.D.; Yesalis, C.E. Anabolic-androgenic steroids and the adolescent. Pediatric Annals 21: 175–188; 1992.

24. Cowart, V.S.; Op. cit.

25. Are your hormones up? Time. November 28, 1988; p. 87.

26. Marx, J.L. Sexual responses are—almost—all in the brain. Science 241: 903–904: 1988.

27. Clark, M. Nose for sex. Discover; September, 1990; p. 28.

28. Toufexis, A. Why mothers kill their babies. Time; June 20, 1988; p. 82–83.

29. Berkow, R. The Merck Manual, Fifteenth Edition. Rahway, NJ: Merck Sharp & Dohme Research Laboratories; 1987; p. 1501.

30. Gilbert, S.F. Developmental Biology, Second Edition. Sunderland, MA: Sinauer Associates, Inc., Publishers; p. 759.

31. Purvis, A. A pill that gets under the skin. Time; December 24, 1990; p. 66.

32. Binkley, S.; Mosher, K. Oral melatonin produces arrhythmia in sparrows. Experientia 41: 1615–1617; 1985.

33. Turek, F.; McMillan, J.; Menaker, M. Science 194: 1441; 1976.

34. Lynch, H. J.; Rivest, R.; Wurtman, R. Artificial induction of melatonin rhythms by programmed microinfusion. Neuroendocrinology 31: 106–111; 1980.

35. Binkley, S. The Pineal. Englewood Cliffs, NJ: Prentice Hall; 1988.

36. Wehr, T.; Jacobsen, F.; Sack, D.; Arendt, J.; Tamarkin, L.; Rosenthal, N. Phototherapy of seasonal affective disorder. Arch. Gen. Psychiatry 43: 870–875; 1986.

37. Itakura, K.; Hirose,R.; Crea, R.; Riggs, A.; Heyneter, H.; Bolivar, F.; Boyer, H. Expression in Escherichia coli of a chemically synthesized gene for the hormone somatostatin. Science 198: 1056–1062; 1977.

38. Gertz, B.J.; Baxter, J.D. Gene expression and recombinant DNA in endocrinology and metabolism. In Greenspan, F.S.; Forsham, P.H.,

editors. Basic and Clinical Endocrinology. East Norwalk, CT: Lange Medical Publications; 1986; p. 670.

39. Gertz, B.J.; Baxter, J.D. Gene expression and recombinant DNA in endocrinology and metabolism. In Greenspan, F.S.; Forsham, P.H., editors. Basic and Clinical Endocrinology. East Norwalk, CT: Lange Medical Publications; 1986; p. 672.

40. Gooding, M.D.; Higgins, C.B.; editors. The Radiologic Clinics of North America 31: 967 1188; 1993.

APPENDIXES

GLOSSARY OF TERMINOLOGY AND ABBREVIATIONS

Scientific names of species are usually italicized.
> means greater than; < means less than.

ABP androgen-binding protein

Ac acetyl, acetyl group

acetyl coenzyme A AcCoA; acetyl CoA; an acetyl group donor in melatonin biosynthesis

ACH acetylcholine (Ach)

acrophase peak time of a cosine wave matched to a daily cycle using cosinor analysis

ACTH adrenocorticotropic hormone, corticotropin

actinomycin D RNA synthesis inhibitor

adenohypophysis part of the pituitary gland

ADH antidiuretic hormone, vasopressin

ADP adenosine diphosphate

adrenalin epinephrine

adrenarche increased secretion of adrenal androgens at puberty

afferent incoming, carrying to, carrying toward

affinity attraction, for example between a hormone and a receptor

agonist a substance with similar actions

AI angiotensin one, (AII = angiotensin two, AIII = angiotensin three)

ala alanine, a neutral amino acid, (A)

alloxan causes experimental diabetes by destroying beta cells of the islets of Langerhans in the pancreas which secrete insulin

amenorrhea absence of menstruation

amine derivative of an amino acid, for example, hormones derived from tyrosine or tryptophane

AMP adenosine monophosphate

anabolism synthesis of large molecules from small molecules

analogue a substance that is similar to another or produces the same response, usually a synthetic substance is the analogue

ANF atrial natriuretic factor, ANP

anorexia nervosa starvation syndrome which is accompanied by amenorrhea

ANP atrial natriuretic peptide, ANF

antagonism opposite action

antagonist substance (e.g., a hormone) with the opposite action

aphrodisiac drug or food that stimulates sexual desire

APUD amine precursor uptake and decarboxylation cells or hypothesis

arg arginine, a basic amino acid (R)

ase -ase, a suffix indicating an enzyme

asn asparagine, an acidic amino acid (N)

asp aspartic acid, acidic amino acid (D)

atherosclerosis a condition where the blood vessels have fatty degeneration and there is infiltration of the arterial walls by lipids; the term is generic and includes a number of diseases wherein arterial wall elasticity is lost due to thickening; the condition is characteristic of aging vessels and is a cause of cardiovascular disease and stroke

ATP adenosine triphosphate

atresia disappearance of follicle from the ovary by a natural degenerative process

autoimmune diseases diseases where the body uses the immune system to attack itself as if it were foreign

autoradiography photographic detection of the localization of radioactive compounds, used to localize hormones to locations within cells of targets for example

avidin a protein produced by the chick oviduct in response to progesterone

AVP arginine vasopressin

AVT arginine vasotocin

axoplasmic transport the mechanism by which hormone precursor packages are moved from the cell body of a neurosecretory cell to the terminal of a neurosecretory cell

baroreceptor cells that respond to changes in pressure (e.g., neurons of heart and blood vessels)

BDI 3-BDI, 3-ß-hydroxysteroid dehydrogenase

BH brain hormone

BHL 11-BHL, 11-ß-hydroxylase or 21-BHL, 21-ß-hydroxylase

BRAC basic rest activity cycle; approximately a 90-minute cycle of which the sleep cycle is the night-time manifestation

C the element carbon, or the amino acid cysteine

CA catecholamine

CaBP calcium-binding protein

cAMP cyclic adenosine 3'5'-monophosphate

carbohydrate class of organic compounds that includes sugars, starches, cellulose, dextrin, saccharides

catabolism large molecules breaking down into smaller molecules

catalytic subunit part of an enzyme responsible for the enzyme's ability to speed a reaction

CBG corticosteroid-binding globulin

CCK cholecystokinin

CDR calmodulin

cGMP cyclic guanosine monophosphate

chlorpromazine antagonist for dopamine receptors

cholelithiasis the presence of gallstones, or calculi, in the gall bladder or its duct

chromatography means for separating mixtures of substances based on their chemical properties; chromatography may be paper chromatography, thin layer chromatography (TLC), gas chromatography (GC), or liquid chromatography

circadian rhythm repeating cycles with a period near 24 hours which persist in the absence of external 24-hour time cues

climacteric the end of the reproductive years, menopause is the female climacteric

CNS central nervous system

cobalt chloride destroys pancreatic islet alpha cells which secrete glucagon

coitus sexual intercourse, the act of mating

colchicine microtubule disruptor

collagen protein found in connective tissue synthesized by bone osteoblasts

colloid a milky or cloudy dispersion of particles of a substance in a liquid, found in thyroid follicles

COMT catechol-O-methyltransferase

conjugation reaction in which a hormone combines with a glucuronide or sulfate, usually for the purpose of inactivation and excretion

CRF corticotropin-releasing factor (CRH)

CRH corticotropin (ACTH)-releasing hormone

CS chorionic somatomammotropin

CSF cerebrospinal fluid

CT calcitonin (TCT)

cycloheximide a poison that is a protein synthesis inhibitor

cyproterone acetate antiandrogen that acts as a testosterone receptor antagonist

cys cysteine, an amino acid that contains sulfur, forms disulfide bonds (C)

cytochalasin B microfilament disruptor

Δ delta, means change in the parameter that follows the symbol

DBcAMP dibutyryl cyclic AMP, a cyclic AMP analogue

DBH dopamine ß-hydroxylase, an enzyme in the pathway for synthesis of catecholamine hormones

de novo anew

deoxyglucose 2-deoxyglucose, a substance that inhibits glucose uptake and utilization and thereby acts as a metabolic inhibitor; used experimentally to detect cell and tissue glucose use

DES diethylstilbestrol, or diffuse endocrine system

dexamethasone a steroid that is a synthetic agonist of glucocorticoids; 37.5 times the anti-inflammatory activity of cortisone

DG 2-DG, 2-deoxyglucose

DHCC 1,25 DHCC, 1,25 dihydroxycholecalciferol, active form of vitamin D

DHEA dehydroepiandrosterone, a steroid precursor of testosterone

DHT dihydrotestosterone, an active androgen produced from testosterone by 5-α-reductase in target tissues

diabetes diseases of the pituitary (diabetes insipidus) or the pancreas (diabetes mellitus) where excess water is excreted

DIT diiodotyrosine, a precursor of thyroid hormones

DM diabetes mellitus

DNA deoxyribonucleic acid

DOPA dihydroxyphenylalanine, a precursor of epinephrine

drug medicine, a substance used for treating diseases

E epinephrine, adrenalin

E. coli a bacterium, *Escherichia coli*, used commonly in research, normal inhabitant of vertebrate intestine

e.r. endoplasmic reticulum, a cellular organelle

ECF extracellular fluid

effector a cell or cell group (e.g., muscle or a gland) that responds to a hormonal signal or to a nerve impulse

efferent outgoing, carry away from

EGF epidermal growth factor

electrolyte molecule that can ionize, responsible for plasma osmolarity, can carry electric currents

ELISA enzyme-linked immuno-absorption assay

endo. endocrinology

endocrinol. endocrinology

endocytosis ingestion of substances by cells into their cytoplasm

endogenous inside the organism

enzyme protein that can catalyze, or speed up, a chemical reaction

episodic periodic release of a hormone, bursts of

hormone released several times an hour, pulsatile secretion

ergot alkaloids chemicals that are dopamine receptor agonists; LSD is derived from ergot

estrus heat or sexual receptivity

exocrine glands glands that use ducts to secrete their products

exocytosis extrusion of substances from their cytoplasm by cells

exogenous from outside the organism

fat a class of neural organic compounds which make up adipose tissue and which are a component of food; glyceryl esters of oleic, palmitic, and stearic acid; they produce and store energy (9.3 Calories/g)

FGF fibroblast growth factor

follicle a spherical group of cells in the ovary or the thyroid gland that forms a space, or hollow, that is filled with fluid or colloid

freerun a rhythm in the absence of time cues (e.g., for the perching rhythm of a sparrow, its circadian freerun period is 24.5 hours in constant dark).

FSH ovarian follicle-stimulating hormone

GDP guanosine diphosphate

GH growth hormone

GHRH growth hormone-releasing hormone

GIP gastrointestinal peptide

gla γ-carboxyglutamic acid, an acidic amino acid

gln glutamine, an acidic amino acid (Q)

glu glutamic acid, an acidic amino acid (E)

gluconeogenesis the production of glucose from noncarbohydrates (e.g., proteins or fat)

gly glycine, a neutral amino acid (G)

glycogen the storage form of glucose, a large carbohydrate molecule

glycogenoloysis glycogen breakdown to produce glucose

glycolysis the sequence of reactions that break down glucose to form lactic acid or pyruvic acid

glycoprotein compound of amino acids and carbohydrate units

GMP guanosine monophosphate

GnRH gonadotropin-releasing hormone (LRH)

goiter enlargement of the thyroid that produces (often visible) swelling of the neck

GR glucocorticoid receptor

GRE glucocorticoid response element

GRH growth hormone-releasing hormone

GTP guanosine triphosphate, a nucleotide

H the element hydrogen, also the amino acid histidine; H$^+$ hydrogen ion

HCC 25HCC, 25-hydroxycholecalciferol, an intermediate in vitamin D production

HCG human chorionic gonadotropin (hCG)

HCS human chorionic somatomammotropin (human CS)

HIOMT hydroxyindole-O-methyltransferase, an enzyme characteristic of the pineal gland

hirsutism hairiness

his histidine, a basic amino acid (H)

HPA hypothalamo-pituitary adrenal axis

HPL human placental lactogen

HT 5-HT, 5-hydroxytryptamine, serotonin

hydroxylation a reaction whereby a hydroxyl (-OH) group is added to a molecule, can be catalyzed by a hydroxylating enzyme

hyl hydroxylserine, a basic amino acid

hyp 4-hydroxyproline, an imino acid

hyperlipidemia excessive blood fat

hypertension high blood pressure

IGF-I insulin-like growth factor I

IGF-II insulin-like growth factor II

immunoassay assay that depends on the use of an antigen-antibody reaction; if radioisotopes are also used, then it is called a radioimmunoassay (RIA)

impotence inability of the male to attain erection and accomplish coition

in vitro experimentation in "artificial" culture conditions—organ culture, cell culture, perfusion, superfusion

in vivo in the living organism; in endocrinology the phrase usually denotes experimentation with living animals

infertility inability to successfully reproduce on the part of either sex for any of a variety of reasons

iso isoleucine, a neutral amino acid; alternatively, isoproterenol, a catecholamine agonist (ISO)

JGA juxtaglomerular apparatus

K potassium, K$^+$ potassium ion

L liter, also abbreviated lower case (l)

LATS long-acting thyroid stimulator

leu leucine, a neutral amino acid (I)

LH luteinizing hormone, or, unfortunately, lateral hypothalamus

LH-RH gonadotropin-releasing hormone (LRH)

lordosis arching of the back in response to a male's advances, female rats assume a swayback posture

LPH ß-LPH, lipotropin, a hormone

LRH gonadotropin-releasing hormone

LVP the hormone, lysine vasopressin

lys lysine, a basic amino acid (K)

M melatonin, a pineal hormone; also abbreviated MT or MEL

MAO monoamine oxidase, monamine oxidase

MCH melanophore-concentrating hormone

melanin a brown or black pigment synthesized from tyrosine in melanophores and melanocytes; it is also found outside cells (cytocrine melanin); the pigment contributes to hair and feather color

menarche the onset of menstrual cycling at puberty

menopause the end of menstrual cycling, the female climacteric

menstruation bleeding from the vagina that recurs periodically in primate females when the uterine lining sloughs

metabolism anabolism and catabolism, the chemical processes that take place in cells

metamorphosis developmental change in shape to attain an "adult" form

methylation reactions in which a methyl group (-CH3) are transfered to another molecule; some enzymes that catalyze methylations are PNMT, HIOMT, and COMT; the methyl donor is often acetyl coenzyme A

methylxanthines drugs that inhibit phosphodiesterase; include caffeine and theophylline; raise intracellular cAMP

μg micrograms

mg% milligrams per 100 milliliters

MIF MSH release-inhibiting factor, melanostatin

MIT monoiodotyrosine, a precursor of thyroid hormones

mittelschmerz abdominal pain associated with the time of ovulation in women

ml milliliter; also mL

MOD maturity onset diabetes

MRF MSH-releasing factor

MRF müllerian regression factor

mRNA messenger ribonucleic acid

MSH melanophore-stimulating hormone, melanotropin

MSH-RH MSH-releasing hormone

MT melatonin

N the element nitrogen

NA noradrenalin, norepinephrine

Na the element sodium, Na^+ sodium ion

nadir the minimum, as of a daily cycle

NE noradrenalin, norepinephrine, one of the catecholamine hormones

neural crest cells that separate from neural ectoderm during formation of the nervous system in embryos; endocrine glands that produce peptide and amine hormones may develop from the cells, see APUD

nucleus a central structure in a cell where the genetic material (DNA) resides; or, alternatively, a group of cells in the brain

O the element oxygen

OCS oral contraceptive steroids

optic chiasm where the optic nerves cross, near the hypothalamus and the pituitary gland

osmolarity solute concentration in a solution (osm, Osm)

osmoreceptor cell that responds to changes in blood osmolarity

osteoblasts bone cells that secrete the organic bone matrix of proteins and polysaccharides

osteoclasts bone cells that release calcium by reabsorption of bone; multinucleate

osteocyte living cells of mature bone

osteogenic cells cells that develop into bone cells

osteomalacia a disease that is also called Rickets

osteopenia decreased mass of bone

osteoporosis a kind of osteopenia where there is a loss both of the matrix and minerals of the bone

P probability

Paget's disease a disease with abnormal bone resorption

parturition the process of giving birth, childbirth

PBI protein-bound iodine

PDGF platelet derived growth factor

peptide a molecule consisting of amino acids connected by peptide bonds, usually less than 10 amino acids

PG prostaglandin; abbreviations for prostaglandins usually have three letters starting with PG

PGE2 prostaglandin E_2

PGF2α prostaglandin $F_{2\alpha}$

PGI2 prostaglandin I_2

PGSI prostaglandin synthesis inhibitor

pH negative logarithm of the hydrogen ion concentration

phagolysosome a cell organelle that is a lysosome. Examples are the lysosomes that consume colloid droplets containing thyroglobulin in the thyroid

phe phenylalanine, an aromatic amino acid

photoperiodism a response that is dependent on day (or night) length

PIF prolactin-inhibiting factor

PIH prolactin-inhibiting hormone

PKC protein kinase C, an enzyme

plasma the fluid portion of lymph or blood

PLC phospholipase C

plexus network, can be nerves or vessels

PMS premenstrual syndrome or pregnant mare serum

PNMT phenylethanolamine-N-methyltransferase, an enzyme in the synthesis of catecholamine hormones

polydipsia excess drinking

polypeptide a molecule consisting of amino acids connected by peptide bonds, usually less than 100 amino acids

polyuria excess urination

POMC pro-opiomelanocortin

PP pancreatic polypeptide

PRA plasma renin activity

precursor a substrate, a molecule out of which another molecule is made by a chemical reaction

PRF prolactin-releasing factor, dopamine

PRL prolactin

pro proline, an imino acid (P); alternatively, the element, phosphorus

product in an enzyme reaction, the substance(s) produced by the reaction

progestagens synthetic progesterones (norethynodrel, norethindrone); progestens, progestins

progestins progestens

prohormone precursor molecule, e.g., proopiomelanocortin or proinsulin

protein a molecule consisting of amino acids connected by peptide bonds, usually more than 100 amino acids; all enzymes and many hormones are proteins

PTH parathyroid hormone, parathormone

puromycin protein synthesis inhibitor

R- part of a molecule whose detailed structure is not shown

radioactive isotopes forms of elements that are radioactive

range a statistic, the maximum value minus the minimum value

receptor protein on cell membrane or within the cell that specifically binds with (recognizes) a hormone or other molecule

regulatory subunit portion of protein kinase that binds to cAMP and then dissociates from protein kinase to release the catalytic subunit

rer rough endoplasmic reticulum

RIA radioimmunoassay; assay that uses radioisotopes and antibodies to measure a substance such as a hormone

RNA a macromolecule, ribonucleic acid; mRNA is the messenger form, tRNA is the transfer form

RRA radioreceptor assay, assay that uses radioisotopes and receptors to measure a substance such as a hormone

rT_3 reverse T_3; reverse triiodothyronine

S sulfur; also, the amino acid serine.

SAD seasonal affective disorder

Saralasin a chemical that is an angiotensin II receptor antagonist

SCG superior cervical ganglion, part of the pathway by which pineal glands are regulated

SCN suprachiasmatic nuclei; portions of the hypothalamus that appear to be the site of origin, or pacemaker, of the mammalian circadian rhythm

SD standard deviation, a measure of statistical variability

second messenger a substance that carries the hormone's (first messenger) message from the cell membrane to control events in the cytoplasm, e.g., cAMP

SEM standard error [of the mean], a measure of statistical variability

ser serine, a hydroxyl substituted amino acid (S), or alternatively, smooth endoplasmic reticulum of a cell

Sertoli factor inhibin

serum fluid remaining after blood has been allowed to clot; fluid containing antibodies

SON supraoptic nucleus of the hypothalamus

specificity a word used in endocrinology in several ways. One way is the concept that there is a fixed relationship between two molecules which permits them to recognize each other and to exclude other molecules; such biochemical specificity occurs in antibody-antigen and in hormone-receptor interactions. Another way is to describe the fact that some peptide hormones function best in the species from which they come—called species specificity

spinnbarkeit a measure of the "stretchability" of the cervical mucus

SRIF somatostatin

SRP signal recognition particle

STH somatotropin, GH

substrate in an enzyme reaction, the compound(s) on which the enzyme acts, a reactant

suckling nursing

synergism acting together

T$_3$ triiodothyroine

T$_4$ thyroxine

TBG thyroxine-binding globulin

TBPA thyroxine-binding prealbumin

TCT thyrocalcitonin, CT

tetany muscle cramps

TGF transforming growth factor, there are alpha and beta TGFs

thr threonine, a hydroxyl substituted amino acid

thyrotoxicosis the effects of excess thyroid hormone

titer (titre) a term previously used to denote amounts of solute in a solution, or of a hormone in blood (e.g., grams/milliliter)

transcription synthesis of RNA using the nucleotide sequence of DNA

transformation change in shape of a hormone-receptor complex

translation synthesis of proteins from the message contained in RNA

translocation movement of a hormone-receptor complex within a cell to the cell nucleus

TRH TSH-releasing hormone

trophic pertaining to feeding, nutrition, digestion

tropic -tropic, turning

try tryptophan (tryptophane), an aromatic amino acid (W)

TSH thyroid-stimulating hormone

TXA$_2$ thromboxane A$_2$

tyr tyrosine, an aromatic amino acid (Y)

tys sulfated tyrosine

val valine, a neutral amino acid (V)

VIP vasoactive intestinal peptide

VMA vanillylmandelic acid, a catecholamine metabolite

VMH ventromedial hypothalamus

VP vasopressin, ADH; AVP is arginine vasopressin; LVP is lysine vasopressin

witch's milk lay term for drops of secretions, or milk, from the nipples of newborn infants

zf zona fasiculata of the adrenal cortex

zg zona glomerulosa of the adrenal cortex

zr zone reticularis of the adrenal cortex

ANNOTATED BIBLIOGRAPHY OF BOOKS IN ENDOCRINOLOGY

Abrams, W. B.; Berkow, R.; editors. The Merck Manual of Geriatrics. Rahway, NJ: Merck Sharp & Dohme Research Laboratories; 1990; 1267 pages. Many clinicians contributed sections to this geriatric medical manual. It was first published in 1990 and intended for physicians to use as a manual in caring for the elderly.

Aschoff, J.; Ceresa, F.; Halberg, F.; editors. Chronobiological Aspects of Endocrinology. Stuttgart-New York: F. K. Schattauer Verlag; 1974; 463 pages. The collection of research papers is from a meeting (April 8–10, 1974) in a Symposium Capri volume .

Ashcroft, F.M.; Ashcroft, S.J.H.; editors. Insulin: Molecular Biology to Pathology. New York: Oxford University Press; 1992; 421 pages. Sections by 31 contributors discuss the pancreatic ß-cell, insulin (biosynthesis, secretion, action, receptor, deficiency) and diabetes (immunology, genetics, aetiology). The book is intended to provide an "up-to-date account of what is known about insulin" and it has a useful glossary.

Austin, C. R.; Short, R. V.; editors. Reproduction in Mammals I: Germ Cells and Fertilization. London: Cambridge University Press; 1972, 133 pages. Articles by individual authors cover primordial germ cells, oogenesis and ovulation, spermatogenesis and the spermatozoa, cycles and seasons, and fertilization. The five volumes in this series have simple diagrams, are concise, and are individually indexed. A second edition was published in 1984.

Austin, C. R.; Short, R. V.; editors. Reproduction in Mammals II: Embryonic and Fetal Development. London: Cambridge University Press; 1972; 153 pages. Articles by individual authors cover the embryo, sex determination and differentiation, the fetus and birth, manipulation of development, and pregnancy losses and birth defects.

Austin, C. R.; Short, R. V.; editors. Reproduction in Mammals III: Hormones in Reproduction. London: Cambridge University Press; 1972; 143 pages. Articles by individual authors cover reproductive hormones, the hypothalamus, role of hormones in sex cycles, role of hormones in pregnancy, and hormonal control of lactation.

Austin, C. R.; Short, R. V.; editors. Reproduction in Mammals IV: Reproductive Patterns. London: Cambridge University Press; 1972; 156 pages. Articles by individual authors cover species differences, behavioral patterns, environmental effects, immunological influences, and aging.

Austin, C. R.; Short, R. V.; editors. Reproduction in Mammals V: Artificial Control of Reproduction. London: Cambridge University Press, London; 1972; 152 pages. Articles by individual authors cover increasing reproductive potential in farm animals, limiting human reproductive potential, chemical methods of male contraception, control of human development, reproduction and human society, and the ethics of manipulating reproduction in man.

Austin, C. R.; Short, R. V.; editors. Reproduction in Mammals VII: Mechanisms of Hormone Action. London: Cambridge University Press; 1979; 239 pages. Articles by individual authors cover the releasing hormones, pituitary and placental hormones, prostaglandins, androgens, estrogens, and progesterone.

Austin, C. R.; Short, R. V.; editors. Reproduction in Mammals VIII: Human Sexuality. London: Cambridge University Press; 1980; 176 pages. The articles cover the origins of human sexuality, human sexual behavior, variant forms of human sexual behavior, contemporary patterns of behavior, constraints on behavior, and perennial morality.

Austin, C. R.; Short, R. V.; editors/ Reproduction in Mammals VI: The Evolution of Reproduction. London: Cambridge University Press; 1976; 189 pages. Articles by individual authors cover the development of sexual reproduction, the evolution of viviparity in mammals, selection for reproductive success, origin of species, and specialization of gametes.

Bagnara, J.T.; Hadley, M., Chromatophores and Color Change. Englewood Cliffs, NJ: Prentice Hall; 1973; 202 pages. The book is an enthusiastic and readable monograph reviewing skin color changes in lower vertebrates with interesting illustrations.

Bell, W.J.; Carde, R.T.; editors. Chemical Ecology of Insects. Sunderland, MA: Sinauer Associates, Inc., Publishers; 1984; 524 pages. The book includes chapters written by experts on the subjects of insect pheromones and hormones. Topics covered include contact chemoreception, olfaction, odor dispersion, chemo-orientation in walking and flying insects, plant-herbivore relationships, parasite-host relationships, alarm pheromones, warning coloration and mimicry, aggregation, sexual communication with pheromones, and socio-chemicals of bees and ants and termites.

Bentley, P. Comparative Vertebrate Endocrinology. London: Cambridge University Press; 1976; 415 pages. This book is organized by function, rather than by gland, which provides a useful perspective. Chapters describe hormone involvement in nutrition, calcium metabolism, skin, water balance, and reproduction.

Berkow, R.; editor. The Merck Manual, Fifteenth Edition. Rahway, NJ: Merck Sharp & Dohme Research Laboratories of Merck & Co., Inc.; 1987; 2695 pages. The Merck's Manual of the Materia Medica was originally a 262-page volume in 1899 intended to provide a "reminder" for general practitioners to use in selecting medicine. The modern edition is a medical "Bible" in wide use by medical students and physicians.

Binkley, S. The Clockwork Sparrow. Englewood Cliffs, NJ: Prentice Hall; 1990; 262 pages. The volume is an introductory textbook aimed at senior biology and beginning graduate students on the subject of circadian rhythms in vertebrates.

Binkley, S. The Pineal: Endocrine and Nonendocrine Function. Englewood Cliffs, NJ: Prentice Hall; 1988; 304 pages. The book is a textbook to introduce graduate students to the subject of the pineal gland. The first of a series of endocrine subspecialty books; the series editor is Mac Hadley.

Bolander, F.F. Molecular Endocrinology. San Diego, CA: Academic Press; 1989; 318 pages. The book was written as a textbook for a course in molecular endocrinology. Includes chapters on receptors, calmodulin, gene regulation, histone and nonhistone proteins, and molecular evolution.

Brown, J.; Barker, S. Basic Endocrinology, Second Edition. Philadelphia, PA: F.A. Davis; 1966; 219 pages.

Crapo, L. Hormones, The Messengers of Life. New York, NY: W. H. Freeman; 1985; 194 pages. Written for the lay science audience, the book presents historical aspects, pictures of some of the fathers of endocrinology, and basic endocrinology in an entertaining manner.

Epple, A.; Brinn, J.E. Comparative Physiology of the Pancreatic Islets. Springer-Verlag: New York; 1987; 223 pages. The monograph covers evolution of the islet, ontogeny of gnathostone pancreas, comparative islet cytology, exocrine pancreas, insulo-acinar interactions, neural and hormonal regulation, function of the islet, insulin, glucagon, pancreatic polypeptide and somatostatin.

Epple, A.; Scanes, C.; Stetson, M.H. Progress in Comparative Endocrinology. Wiley-Liss: New York; 1990.

Epple, A.; Stetson, M.; editors. Avian Endocrinology. New York: Academic Press; 1980; 577 pages. The book is a collection of papers presented at the Second International Symposium on Avian Endocrinology, held in Benalmadena, Spain, May 4–9, 1980.

Euler, U.S. von; Heller, H.; editors. Comparative Endocrinology, Volume II. New York: Academic Press; 1963; 282 pages. The book includes articles intended to provide a critical and up-to-date picture of the comparative aspects of endocrinology to the medical scientist and zoologist and research worker. Volume two contains articles on invertebrate hormones of reproduction and molting, invertebrate neurosecretory systems, and tissue hormones. Volume one covers the glandular hormones.

Ezrin, C.; Godden, J.; Volpe, R.; Wilson, R. Systematic Endocrinology. New York: Harper & Row; 1973; 509 pages. The introductory medical textbook consists of 17 chapters for a system-based curriculum written by 12 "young authorities" in the Toronto area. The editors set forth to produce a book which met the standard of Peter Mere Lathan: "A good book, though it be not necessarily a hard one, contains important facts, duly arranged and reasoned with care."

Fraser, C.M.; editor. The Merck Veterinary Manual, Sixth Edition, Rahway, NJ: Merck & Co. Inc.; 1966; 1677 pages. As subtitled, a handbook of diagnosis, therapy, and disease prevention and control for the veterinarian. The section on the endocrine system describes the animal correlates of human endocrine disorders.

Fregly, M.; Luttge, W. Human Endocrinology: An Interactive Text. New York: Elsevier Biomedical; 1982; 365 pages. Textbook concerning a portion of topics in endocrinology. The work is aimed at preprofessional and graduate students in the health sciences. Written in the "Socratic" fashion, the chapters in this book are followed by sections of questions and answers. The book covers pituitary, thyroid, adrenal, reproduction, glucose regulation, and calcium regulation.

Frieden, E. H. Chemical Endocrinology. New York: Academic Press; 237 pages. The textbook "begins with a brief description of the biological functions of the products of the endocrine glands. The main body of the work is organized around detailed descriptions of the chemistry of the several hormones . . . [The] principles of hormone bioassay, and bioassay procedures for most of the hormones are described in considerable detail."

Frieden, E.; Lipner, H. Biochemical Endocrinology of the Vertebrates. Englewood Cliffs, NJ: Prentice Hall; 1971; 164 pages. A small book which succeeded nicely in providing a concise overview of basic endocrinology.

Fuchs, F.; Klopper, A. Endocrinology of Pregnancy, Third edition. New York: Harper & Row; 1983; 306 pages. The book is 15 chapters by 17 authors intended for an audience of obstetrical trainees. The book is a "review within a single volume of the diverse aspects of the endocrinology of pregnancy, parturition, and lactation."

Ganong, W. Review of Medical Physiology, Fourteenth Edition. Norwalk, CT: Appleton & Lange; 1989; 673 pages. A concise summary of physiology for medical students. The sections on endocrinology are particularly strong and include information in the introduction, 165 pages of chapters on endocrine glands, and useful sections in other chapters (e.g., gastrointestinal hormones in the chapter on gut).

Gilbert, S.F. Developmental Biology, Second Edition. Sunderland, MA: Sinauer Associates, Inc., Pubs.; 1988; 843 pages. A textbook of embryology and development with a 36-page chapter on hormones and other sections in which growth factors are important.

Gooding, G.A.; Higgins, C.B. The Radiolologic Clinics of North America: Endocrine Radiology. Philadelphia, PA: W. B. Saunders Co.; 1993; pages 967-1188. Endocrinopathies are usually diagnosed by clinical symptoms and with chemical studies of hormones and their metabolites. Imaging techniques, the subject of this volume, are used to locate the source of a functional abnormality and to describe the details of its size, relationship to surrounding tissue, and other characteristics. Techniques which are covered include thyroid and parathyroid sonography and radioisotope evaluation, magnetic resonance imaging in hyperparathyroidism and of the pancreas and ovary, scintigraphic evaluation of adrenal cortex and medulla in hypertension, Conn's and Cushing's syndrome, endocrine angiography, ultrasound of the adrenal and pancreas and scrotum, radiologic diagnosis of osteoporosis and its use for hypothalamus and pituitary pathology.

Goodman, M. H. Basic Medical Endocrinology. New York: Raven Press; 1988; 346 pages. The book on human endocrinology is based on the author's teaching of first year medical students.

Gorbman, A.; Bern, H. A Textbook of Comparative Endocrinology. New York: John Wiley and Sons; 1962; 468 pages. The first textbook of the field of comparative endocrinology covers the endocrine aspects of comparative physiology, embryology, and evolution.

Gorbman, A.; Dickhoff, W.; Vigna, S.; Clark, N.; Ralph, C. Comparative Endocrinology. New York: John Wiley & Sons; 1983; 572 pages. The textbook is oriented to "consider endocrine mechanisms [as] adaptive systems that play a basic role in making each species fit into its environmental niche."

Greenspan, F.; editor. Basic and Clinical Endocrinology, Third Edition. Norwalk, CT: Appleton & Lange; 1989; 786 pages. The editor hoped to "provide a compact yet comprehensive and authoritative review of the rapidly expanding field of endocrinology, in which new concepts, new diagnostic techniques, and new therapeutic methods are continually being developed." The book has 29 chapters written by dozens of endocrinologists and a useful table of normal hormone test results in humans.

Greer, Monte A.; editor. The Thyroid Gland. New York: Raven Press; 1990; 594 pages. The volume is in the Comprehensive Endocrinology series, Luciano Martini, Editor-in-Chief. Sixteen contributed articles cover thyroid gland ontogeny, phylogeny, anatomy, biochemistry, control of thyroid function, extrathyroidal hormone metabolism and thyroid hormone action, and diseases of the thyroid gland.

Griffen, J.E.; Ojeda, S.R. Textbook of Endocrine Physiology, Second Edition. New York: Oxford University Press; 1992; 351 pages. The book for beginning medical students was written by 13 contributors from the University of Texas Southwestern Medical School. Subjects covered in chapters are genes, mechanisms of action, pituitary, hypothalamus, water metabolism, sexual differentiation, reproductive function, growth, development, thyroid, adrenal glands, calcium homeostasis, glucose metabolism, lipid metabolism, and protein metabolism.

Hadley, M. Endocrinology, Third Edition. Englewood Cliffs, NJ: Prentice Hall; 1992; 608 pages. The book is an undergraduate biology textbook. The book includes insightful speculations and thoughtful analyses in comparative endocrinology by the author. There are chapters on all the classical endocrine glands and on the pineal gland and on the melanotropins. The melanotropins are Dr. Hadley's special area of expertise.

Hawker, R. Notebook of Medical Physiology: Endocrinology. New York: Churchill Livingstone; 1978; 189 pages. The book is a review text for medical students preparing for examinations in medicine and surgery such as the FRCS, FRACS, FFA, MRCP, and FRACP examinations. It contains sample questions.

Hazelwood, Robert L. The Endocrine Pancreas. Englewood Cliffs, NJ: Prentice-Hall; 258 pages. The book is intended to "update what is known about the endocrine pancreas [and to] give the student . . . a reference source." Chapters are devoted to histology, embryology and anatomy, biochemistry, mechanisms of action, hormone circulation and clearance, islet hormone message:receptor-signal transduction, physiology, hyper- and hyposecretion of islet hormones, and comparative aspects.

Kashgarian, M.; Burrow, G. The Endocrine Glands. Baltimore, MD: Williams and Wilkins; 1974; 147 pages. The authors combine their expertise as pathologist and clinical endocrinologist to explain and illustrate endocrinopathies.

Katchadourian, H.A.; Lunde, D.T. Fundamentals of Human Sexuality, Second Edition. New York: Holt Rinehart and Winston; 1975; 595 pages. The informative book is a well illustrated basic college introductory textbook.

Krieger, D.T., editor. Endocrine Rhythms. New York: Raven Press; 1979; 332 pages. Contains research contributions by many authors which "consider the basic classification, causation, and properties of endocrine rhythms."

Lardy, H.; Stratman, F. Hormones, Thermogenesis, and Obesity. New York: Elsevier; 1989; 528 pages. The book is a symposium volume with articles on metabolism and thermogenesis, brown adipose tissue, humoral factors, the role of the thyroid in thermogenesis, dehydroepiandrosterone, and phenethanolamine/ß agonists effects on fat and lean mass disposition.

Le Baron, R. Hormones: A Delicate Balance. New York: Bobbs-Merrill Co., Inc.; 1972; 178 pages. An introductory book for nonbiologists.

Martin, C. Endocrine Physiology. Oxford University Press; 1985; 1009 pages. The comprehensive endocrinology textbook groups hormones by functions in sections including carbohydrate and protein and lipid metabolism, water balance, calcium and phosphate, reproduction, and body size. It ends with a section that covers hypothalamus, pituitary, pineal, and thymus glands. The book is for students who have completed college level animal physiology and biochemistry.

McCann, S.M. Endocrinology: People and Ideas. Bethesda, MD: American Physiological Society; 1988; 471 pages. Fifteen chapters by 18 contributors discuss "the main pathways of development and highlights the prominent investigators [to provide a] picture of the evolution of this exciting area of physiology and the people involved in its growth." The book is one of the few places that photographs of endocrinologists are available.

Mishell, D.R.; Davajan, V. Infertility, Contraception, and Reproductive Endocrinology. Oradell, NJ: Medical Economic Books; 1986; 688 pages. The authors achieve their goal of a simple and comprehensive description of diagnostic and therapeutic methods in gynecology. Sections cover the normal and abnormal reproductive endocrinology, infertility, and contraception.

Mundy, G.R. Calcium Homeostasis: Hypercalcemia and Hypocalcemia, Second Edition. United Kingdom: Martin Dunitz Ltd.; 1990; 272 pages. The book's purpose is "to provide a simple and straightforward account of the physiological mechanisms which regulate the concentration of calcium in the extracellular fluid, and the diseases which upset the homeostasis of calcium."

Norman, A.; Litwack, G. Hormones. Orlando, FL: Academic Press; 1987; 806 pages. The textbook was written for first year medical students, graduate students, and advanced undergraduate students in the biological sciences.

Norris, D.O. Vertebrate Endocrinology. Philadelphia, PA: Lea and Febiger; 1980; 524 pages. The textbook is for advanced undergraduate zoology majors. It includes chapters on chordate evolution, migratory behavior in animals, and water balance in fishes. The book is enlivened with endocrine cartoons.

Pang, K.T.; Schreibman, M.P.; editors. Vertebrate Endocrinology, Volume 3. Regulation of calcium and phosphate. San Diego, CA: Academic Press, Harcourt Brace Janovich, San Diego; 1989. The book is the third in a series of collections of reviews in comparative endocrinology. The first volume is on morphological considerations; the second volume is on regulation of water and electrolytes.

Paxton, M.J. Endocrinology: Biological and Medical Perspectives. Dubuque, IA: Wm. C. Brown; 1986, 368 pages. An introductory endocrinology textbook for upper division undergraduate students and beginning graduate students. The book contains a useful chapter on measurement of hormones and an extensive glossary.

Peter, R.E.; Gorbman, A. A Student's Guide to Laboratory Experiments in General and Comparative Endocrinology. Englewood Cliffs, NJ: Prentice-Hall, Inc.; 1970; 209 pages. The book describes experiments with animals for a college laboratory course. The experiments are conducted with frogs, mice and insects.

Postlethwait, S.N. Human Sexuality. Philadelphia, PA: W. B. Saunders; 1976. The book is in workbook format and is an introductory book for a "minicourse." Clear diagrams and glossaries illustrate the human reproductive system, sexual maturation, pregnancy, birth control, and venereal diseases.

Ralph, C.L., editor. Comparative Endocrinology: Developments and Directions.. New York: Alan R. Liss; 1985; 190 pages. The book is a collection of papers by comparative endocrinologists deriving from a symposium. Contributions cover neuropeptides, vitellogenesis in *Drosophila*, prolactin, gonadotropin-releasing hormone, comparative reproductive endocrinology, avian growth hormone, and embryonic diapause in a marsupial.

Schneeberg, N. Essentials of Clinical Endocrinology. St. Louis, MO: C. V. Mosby; 1970; 449 pages.

Schreibman, M.P.; Scanes, C.; Pang, P.K.T.; editors. Endocrinology of Growth, Development, and Metabolism in Vertebrates. San Diego: Academic Press; 1993.

Schultz, S.G.; Makhlouf, G.M.; Raunder, B.B.; editors. Handbook of Physiology: Section 6: Volume II, Neural and Endocrine Biology. The Gastrointestinal System. Bethesda, MD: American Physiological Society; 1989; 722 pages. Twenty-eight chapters were contributed by experts to mark the "coming of age of neural and endocrine biology of the gut." The book was formerly Section 6: Alimentary Canal in the Handbook of Physiology.

Shorey, H.H. Animal Communication by Pheromones. New York: Academic Press; 1976; 168 pages. In his review of the introductory textbook, E.O. Wilson (Science 195, 570–571, 1977) wrote that "Shorey has written a useful account of our present knowledge of chemical communication, shorter but better organized and more easily read than the multiauthored Pheromones (1974) edited by M.C. Birch. [Shorey's book] is a primer of the subject, quickly covering the main principles with well-chosen examples and figures but backed up by a thorough bibliography of 726 titles."

Slaunwhite, W. Fundamentals of Endocrinology. New York: Marcel Dekker; 1988; 422 pages. An introductory textbook for medical and dental students that is organized by function rather than by gland or hormone.

Tortora, G.J.; Anagnostakos, N.P. Principles of Anatomy and Physiology, Sixth Edition. New York: Harper & Row; 1990; 956 pages. The book is a textbook for an introductory course in anatomy and physiology for health professional courses (nurses, technicians, paramedics, etc.). The book is replete with colorful illustrations. There is a 46-page chapter on the endocrine systems and there are other chapters on reproduction and subjects with endocrine information.

Turner, C.D.; Bagnara, J. Endocrinology, Sixth Edition. Philadelphia, PA: W. B. Saunders; 1976; 596 pages. A comparative endocrinology textbook written for undergraduate biology students. Contains a list of books published in the area of comparative endocrinology on page 26.

Welty, J.C. The Life of Birds, Second Edition. Philadelphia, PA: Saunders College Publishing; 1982; 754 pages. The college textbook is on the subject of avian physiology. The author says it addresses the question posed by Aristophanes: "My question, answer in the fewest words, What sort of life is it among the birds?"

Wendt, H. The Sex Life of the Animals. New York: Simon and Schuster; 1962; 383 pages. An entertaining and informative volume described by its author as an "evolutionary history of reproduction."

Wilkins, M.B.; editor. Advanced Plant Physiology. Marshfield, MA: Pitman Publishing; 1984; 514 pages. The advanced textbook is about the physiology of plants with multiple contributors many of whose chapters deal with plant hormones, their chemistry, their function, and their transport.

Williams, R.; editor. Textbook of Endocrinology: Philadelphia, PA: W.B. Saunders; 1987; 1270 pages. The clinical textbook has chapters by a multiplicity of endocrine experts. The tome includes chapters on psychoendocrinology, obesity, autoimmunity, aging, and cancer.

Wilson, E. O. The Insect Societies. Cambridge, MA: The Belknap Press of Harvard University Press; 1971; 548 pages. The fascinating book on insect sociology includes the role of chemical messengers in their social interactions.

Wilson, E. O. Sociobiology, The New Synthesis. Cambridge, MA: The Belknap Press of Harvard University Press; 1975; 697 pages. The influential book includes information on pheromones.

ENDOCRINE-RELATED PERIODICALS

Acta Endocrinologica (Acta Endocrinol.)
Advances in Cyclic Nucleotide Research (Advan. Cyclic Nucl. Res.)
American Journal of Physiology (Am. J. Physiol.)
American Zoologist (Amer. Zool.)
Annales d'Endocrinologie (Ann. d'Endocrinol.)
Annual Reviews of Medicine, Physiology, and Biochemistry
Biology of Reproduction (Biol. Reprod.)
Chronobiologia
Chronobiology International (Chronobiol. Int.)
Clinical Endocrinology (Clin. Endocrinol.)
Diabetes
Endocrine Journal (Endocr. J.)
Endocrine Research (Endocrine Res.)
Endocrine Research Communications (Endo. Res. Commun.)
Endocrine Reviews (Endocr. Rev.)
Endocrinologica Japonica (Endocrinol. Jap.)
Endocrinology
Endokrinologie
Experimental and Clinical Endocrinology
Experimental and Clinical Endocrinology (Exp. Clin. Endocrinol.)
General and Comparative Endocrinology (Gen. Comp. Endocrinol.)
Hormone and Metabolic Research (Horm. Met. Res.)
Hormone Research (Horm. Res.)
Hormones and Behavior (Hormone Behav.)
Journal of Biological Rhythms (J. Biol. Rhythms)
Journal of Clinical Endocrinology and Metabolism (J. Clin. Endocrinol. Metab.)
Journal of Clinical Investigations
Journal of Comparative Physiology B (J. Comp. Physiology))
Journal of Endocrinology (J. Endocrinol.)
Journal of Endocrinology (J. Endocrinol.)
Journal of Interdisciplinary Cycle Research
Journal of Physiology
Journal of Pineal Research (J. Pineal Res.)
Molecular and Cellular Endocrinology (Mol. Cell. Endocrinol.)
Neuroendocrinology
Physiology & Behavior
Proceedings of the National Academy of Sciences, USA (Proc. Natl. Acad. Sci. USA)
Prostaglandins
Psychoneuroendocrinology
Recent Progress in Hormone Research (Rec. Prog. Horm. Res.)
Thyroid
Vitamins and Hormones (Vit. Horm.)